HUTCHISON'S CLINICAL METHODS

25th Edition

HUTCHISON'S
CLINICAL
METHODS

An integrated approach to clinical practice

Edited by

Michael Glynn MA MD FRCP FHEA

Consultant Gastroenterologist
Royal London Hospital
London, United Kingdom
Former National Clinical Director
GI and Liver Diseases, NHS England

William M. Drake DM FRCP

Professor of Clinical Endocrinology, Consultant Endocrinologist
Queen Mary University of London
St Bartholomew's Hospital
London, United Kingdom

ELSEVIER

ISBN: 978-0-7020-8265-8
      978-0-7020-8266-5

Content Strategist: Jeremy Bowes
Content Project Manager: Shravan Kumar
Design: Ryan Cook
Illustration Manager: Nijantha Priyadharshini P
Marketing Manager: Deborah Watkins

Printed in India

Last digit is the print number: 9 8 7 6 5 4 3 2 1

Working together to grow libraries in developing countries

www.elsevier.com • www.bookaid.org

Preface to the Twenty-fifth Edition

Hutchison's Clinical Methods is a book for students of all ages and all degrees of experience. Although the scope, complexity and technology of clinical medicine continues to evolve with great speed, the aim of this text is exactly as it was when Robert Hutchison published the very first edition 125 years ago in 1897: to provide a detailed guide to the acquisition of the traditional clinical skills of history taking and physical examination leading to the formulation of a differential diagnosis and management plan. This approach remains as essential as ever to providing good patient care; indeed, as the array of potential investigations expands (and the overall cost continues to rise), it is imperative that traditional methods are not ignored, because diagnosis based solely on investigation generates as many problems as it solves. Even though many patients now have easy access, via the Internet, to information about disease and diagnosis, it is the editors' experience that patients need time spent listening to their symptoms, careful physical examination and simple human compassion. Although the circumstances of clinical practice of the readers will vary hugely across the world (with different structures and levels of funding of healthcare), a sound clinical method is indispensable. The layout of this edition adheres to Hutchison's original approach, with sections on the overall patient assessment, assessment in particular situations, the core body systems and key clinical specialties. Overall, this forms a logical sequence if read straight through but also allows study of each section separately.

As in previous editions, new contributors have joined the book. Some have written entirely new chapters and others have modified the work of their predecessors. All the contributors are accustomed to working closely together and the book reflects how a team of specialists working closely together can best serve patients. It has been the editors' responsibility to integrate the chapters into a single text with a logical narrative, but the expertise lies with the contributing authors, whose time and dedication is gratefully acknowledged, as are the extensive contributions of previous experts.

Some of the changes to the previous edition have been made as a result of formally gathered feedback from the International Advisory Board. In addition, a reader survey elicited a range of positive suggestions for improvements to the book. Constructive readers' comments direct to the editors are always welcome.

Michael Glynn and Will Drake
Barts Health NHS Trust

Sir Robert Hutchison MD FRCP
(1871–1960)

CLINICAL METHODS

A GUIDE TO THE PRACTICAL STUDY
OF MEDICINE

BY

ROBERT HUTCHISON, M.D., M.R.C.P.
DEMONSTRATOR IN PHYSIOLOGY, LONDON HOSPITAL MEDICAL COLLEGE

AND

HARRY RAINY, M.A., F.R.C.P.Ed., F.R.S.E.
UNIVERSITY TUTOR IN CLINICAL MEDICINE, ROYAL INFIRMARY, EDINBURGH

WITH 137 ILLUSTRATIONS AND 8 COLOURED PLATES

CASSELL AND COMPANY, LIMITED
LONDON, PARIS & MELBOURNE
1897
ALL RIGHTS RESERVED

Clinical Methods began in 1897, three years after Robert Hutchison was appointed Assistant Physician to The London Hospital (named the Royal London Hospital since its 250th anniversary in 1990). He was appointed full physician to The London and to the Hospital for Sick Children, Great Ormond Street in 1900. He steered *Clinical Methods* through no less than 13 editions, at first with the assistance of Dr H. Rainy and then, from the 9th edition, published in 1929, with the help of Dr Donald Hunter. Although Hutchison retired from hospital practice in 1934, he continued to direct new editions of the book with Donald Hunter, and from 1949 with the assistance also of Dr Richard Bomford. The 13th edition, the first produced without Hutchison's guiding hand, was published in 1956 under the direction of Donald Hunter and Richard Bomford. Dr A. Stuart Mason and Dr Michael Swash joined Richard Bomford on Donald Hunter's retirement to produce the 16th edition, published in 1975, and following Richard Bomford's retirement prepared the 17th, 18th and 19th editions. Dr Swash edited the 20th and 21st editions himself and was joined by Dr Michael Glynn for the 22nd edition. On Dr Swash's retirement Prof William Drake joined Dr Glynn as a co-editor from the 23rd edition. In keeping with the tradition that lies behind the book, each of these editions has been revised with the help of colleagues at The Royal London Hospital, and the other hospitals which now form Barts Health NHS Trust, namely St Bartholomew's Hospital, Whipps Cross University Hospital and Newham University Hospital.

Sir Robert Hutchison died in 1960 in his 90th year. It is evident from the memoirs of his contemporaries that he had a remarkable personality. Many of his clinical sayings became, in their day, aphorisms to be remembered and passed on to future generations of students. Of these, the best known is his petition, written in 1953, his 82nd year:

'From inability to let well alone;
from too much zeal for the new
and contempt for what is old;
from putting knowledge before wisdom, science
before art, and cleverness before common sense;
from treating patients as cases;
and from making the cure of the disease more
grievous than the endurance of the same, Good
Lord, deliver us.'

Michael Glynn and Will Drake
Royal London Hospital

Contributors

Nicola Byrne MBChB MSc MRCPsych
Consultant Psychiatrist
South London and Maudsley NHS Foundation
Trust
London, United Kingdom

Peter Byrne MA MD MRCPsych
Consultant Liaison Psychiatrist
Royal London Hospital
London, United Kingdom

Rino Cerio BSc MBBS FRCP (Lond.) FRCPath
Professor of Dermatopathology, Consultant
Dermatologist
Queen Mary University of London
Royal London Hospital
London, United Kingdom

Tahseen Chowdhury MBChB MD FRCP
Consultant in Diabetes and Honorary Professor
Royal London Hospital
London, United Kingdom

Andrew Coombes BSc MBBS FRCOphth
Consultant Ophthalmologist
Royal London Hospital
London, United Kingdom

**Teresa Cutino-Moguel DipLSHTM MSc PhD
FRCPath**
Honorary Clinical Senior Lecturer,
Consultant Virologist
Queen Mary University of London
Royal London Hospital
London, United Kingdom

Ceri Davies MD FRCP
Consultant Cardiologist
St Bartholomew's Hospital
London, United Kingdom

William M. Drake DM FRCP
Professor of Clinical Endocrinology,
Consultant Endocrinologist
Queen Mary University of London
St Bartholomew's Hospital
London, United Kingdom

Laurence Dufaur MBBS BSc MRCP DipGUM
Specialist Training Registrar, Sexual Health & HIV
Royal London Hospital
London, United Kingdom

Sophie Edwards MBBS FRCP
Consultant Physician, Older Peoples Services
Royal London Hospital
London, United Kingdom

David Gallagher MA MRCP PhD
Consultant Neurologist
Royal London Hospital
London, United Kingdom

Michael Glynn MA MD FRCP FHEA
Consultant Gastroenterologist
Royal London Hospital
London, United Kingdom
Former National Clinical Director
GI and Liver Diseases, NHS England

Ali Jawad OBE MBChB MSc FRCP DCH
Consultant Rheumatologist
Royal London Hospital
London, United Kingdom

Stephen Kelly MBChB MSc MRCP PhD
Consultant Rheumatologist
Department of Rheumatology
Royal London Hospital
London, United Kingdom

Rehan Khan MRCOG DipIPM
Consultant in Obstetrics and Gynaecology
Royal London Hospital
London, United Kingdom

Geraint Morris BMedSC MBBS FRCP FRCEM
Consultant in Emergency Medicine
Homerton University Hospital
London, United Kingdom

Shankar Ramaswamy MBBS MD FRCA FFPMRCA
Consultant in Pain Management and Anaesthesia
Royal London Hospital
London, United Kingdom

Anna Riddell MBBS BSc MRCPCH
Consultant Paediatrician
Royal London Hospital
London, United Kingdom

Caryn Rosmarin MBBCh DTM&H FCPath(SA) FRCPath(UK)
Consultant Microbiologist
Royal London Hospital
London, United Kingdom

Liat Sarner MBBS FRCP DipGUM DFSRH
Consultant Physician, Sexual Health & HIV
Royal London Hospital
London, United Kingdom

Saksena Sushma MBBS MD DM FRCP
Consultant Hepatologist and Associate Dean (Education)
Queen Mary University of London
Royal London Hospital
London, United Kingdom

Michael J. Wareing MBBS BSc FRCS(ORL-HNS)
Consultant ENT Surgeon
Royal London Hospital
London, United Kingdom

Elinor Warner MA MBBS MRCS DOHNS
Specialist Training Registrar in ENT
Royal London Hospital
London, United Kingdom

Veronica White MBBS MSc MD FRCP
Consultant Respiratory Physician
Royal London Hospital
London, United Kingdom

Sajeda Youssouf MBChB MRCP MD
Consultant Nephrologist
Royal London Hospital
London, United Kingdom

International Advisory Board

Acknowledgements

The Editors would like to acknowledge the contribution of all past authors to this textbook. Each new edition builds on the expertise of the many writers whose work has shaped this book over more than a century. In particular we would like to acknowledge the following who stepped down after the last edition to allow new authors to take their place: Adam Feather, James Green, Lina Hijazi, Richard Langford, John Peters, Andrew Rochford, Trevor Turner and Rodney Walker.

The Editors and Publishers would like to thank all the students and doctors who have provided valuable feedback on this textbook and whose comments have helped shape this new edition. We hope we have listed all those who have contributed and apologise if any names have been accidentally omitted.

Contents

SECTION 1

General patient assessment

Doctor and patient: 1
General principles of history taking

Michael Glynn

Introduction

If asked why they entered medicine, most doctors would say that they wish to relieve human suffering and disease. To achieve this aim for every patient, it is essential to understand what has gone wrong with normal human physiology in that individual and how the patient's personality, beliefs and environment are interacting with the disease process. History taking and clinical examination are initial, but crucial, steps to achieving this understanding, even in an era in which the availability of sophisticated investigations might suggest to a lay person that a blood test or scan will give all the answers. In addition, even though many diseases are now curable, the relief of symptoms is usually what the patient expects from the medical process.

The phrase 'Clinical Methods' is used less than it used to be. It can be defined as the set of skills doctors use to diagnose and treat disease and the manner in which doctors approach clinical problems and relate to patients. The skills that make up Clinical Methods are acquired during a lifetime of medical work, and they evolve and change as new techniques and new concepts arise and as the experience and maturity of the doctor develop. Clinical Methods are acquired by a combination of study and experience, and there is always something new to learn.

The aims of any first consultation are to understand patients' own perceptions of their problems and to start or complete the process of diagnosis. This double aim requires knowledge of disease and its patterns of presentation, together with an ability to interpret a patient's symptoms (what the patient reports or complains of, e.g. cough or headache) and the findings on observation or physical examination (called physical signs or, often, simply 'signs'). Appropriate skills are needed to elicit the symptoms from the patient's description and conversation and the signs by observation and by physical examination. This requires not only experience and considerable knowledge of people in general, but also the skill to strike up a relationship, in a short space of time, with a range of very different individuals.

The two main steps to making a diagnosis:
1. Establishing the clinical features by history and examination, which represents the clinical database.

2. Interpreting the clinical database in terms of disordered function and potential causative pathologies, whether physical, mental, social or a combination of these.

This book is about this process. This first chapter introduces the basic principles of history taking and examination; more detail about the history and examination of each system (cardiovascular, respiratory, etc.) is set out in individual succeeding chapters. Without prejudice, and except in specific scenarios involving female patients, the patient is referred to as 'he' throughout the book, the editors preferring this to 'he/she' or 'they'.

Setting the scene

Most medical encounters or consultations do not occur in hospital wards or Emergency Departments, but in primary care or outpatient settings. Whatever the setting, a certain familiarity to the context of the consultation, including the consulting room itself, the waiting area and all the associated staff, makes the process of clinical diagnosis easier. Patients are less often assessed in their own home than previously, and many doctors now find this a strange concept.

Meeting the patient in the waiting room allows the doctor to make an early assessment of his demeanour, hearing, walking and any accompanying persons. It is good to offer a greeting and careful introduction and to observe the response unobtrusively but with care. It is important to remember that patients are easily confused by medical titles and hierarchies. All the following questions should be quickly assessed:
- Does the patient appear relaxed and smiling or furtive and anxious?
- Does the patient make good eye contact?
- Is he frightened or depressed?
- Are posture and stance normal?
- Is he short of breath or wheezing?

In some conditions (e.g. congestive heart failure, acute asthma, Parkinson's disease, stroke, jaundice), the general nature of the problem is immediately obvious. It is very important to identify the patient correctly, particularly if he has a name that is very common in the local community. Carefully check the full name, date of birth, address and any numerical identifier used by the local health system (in the United Kingdom all patients will have an NHS number or hospital registration number).

Pleasant surroundings are very important. It is essential that both patient and doctor feel at ease and, especially, that neither feels threatened by the encounter. Avoid looking at the patient full-face across a desk. Note-taking is important during consultations while being able to see the patient and establish eye contact and to show sympathy and awareness of his needs during the discussion of symptoms, some of which may be distressing or even embarrassing. If the doctor is right-handed and the patient sits on the doctor's left, at an angle to the desk, the situation is less formal, and clues, such as agitated foot and hand movements, are more evident. If other people are present, arrange the seating to make it clear that it is the patient who is the centre of attention rather than any others present. Increasingly doctors are entering information directly into a computer, rather than writing, and this affects positioning. It can be helpful for the patient to be able to see the screen to confirm what the doctor is noting there.

Emergency presentations

If the patient is being seen as an emergency, the whole process of history taking is altered according to the surroundings and the degree of illness. No history may be obtainable from a severely ill or unconscious patient, but collateral history from bystanders, relatives or emergency medical personnel is important to gather. In retrospect this information can be hard to get later on in the patient's illness and can be crucial to the diagnosis (e.g. was the patient seen to have a grand mal seizure, or did he complain of sudden pain, before a collapse?).

History taking

Having overcome the strangeness of meeting and talking with a wide variety of people that he might not ordinarily meet, the new medical student usually feels that history taking ought to be fairly simple, but that physical examination is full of pitfalls such as unrecognized heart murmurs and confusing parts of the neurological examination. However, the experienced doctor comes to realize that history taking is immensely skilled, and that the extent to which this skill goes on increasing with experience is probably greater than for clinical examination.

Beginning the history

The process of gathering information about a patient often begins by reading any referral documentation and with the immediate introduction of doctor and patient.

Box 1.1	Areas of questioning that can be covered at the beginning of history taking

- Confirm date of birth and age
- Occupation and occupational history
- Past medical history
- Smoking
- Alcohol consumption
- Drug and treatment history
- Family history

Blood Rev. 2003;17(3):131–142.

However, once the social introductions are achieved, the doctor usually will begin with a single opening question. Broadly, there are two ways to do this.

A single open-ended question along the lines of 'Tell me about what has led up to you coming here today' gives the opportunity for the patient to begin with what he feels to be most important to him and avoids any prejudgement of issues or exclusion of what at first hearing may seem less important. However, at this stage the patient may be very anxious and nervous and still making his own assessment of how he will react to the doctor as a person. A beginning that focuses on issues which may be more factual and less emotive can be more rewarding and lead to a more satisfactory consultation. Box 1.1 lists some of the areas of questioning that can be usefully included at the beginning of the history. It is important to inform the patient that this is going to be the order of things so that he does not feel that his pressing problems are being ignored. A statement along the lines of 'Before we discuss why you have come today, I want to ask you some background questions' should be sufficient to inform the patient satisfactorily.

A particular logic exists in taking the past medical history at this stage. For many conditions, the distinction as to what is a current problem and what is past history is unclear and arbitrary in the patient's mind. A patient presenting with an acute exacerbation of chronic obstructive pulmonary disease may have a history of respiratory problems going back many years. Therefore, taking the history along a 'timeline' will often build up a much better picture of all of the patient's problems, how they have developed and how they now interact with life and work.

Once these preliminaries have been completed, the doctor should use a simple and open-ended question to encourage the patient to give a full and free account of the current issues. This could be something along the lines of 'Tell me what has led up to you coming here today'. This wording leaves as open as possible any question about the cause of the patient's problems and why he is seeing a doctor, and could give rise to an initial answer beginning with such varied phrases as 'I have this pain …', 'I feel depressed …', 'I am extremely worried about

Box 1.2	Particular gestures useful in analysing specific pain symptoms

- A squeezing gesture to describe cardiac pain
- Hand position to describe renal colic
- Rubbing the sternum to describe heartburn
- Rubbing the buttock and thigh to describe sciatica
- Arms clenched around the abdomen to describe mid-gut colic

Box 1.3	Words and phrases that need clarification

Ordinary English words

- Diarrhoea
- Constipation
- Wind
- Indigestion
- Being sick
- Dizziness
- Headache
- Double vision
- Pins and needles
- Rash
- Blister

Medical terms that may be used imprecisely by patients

- Arthritis
- Sciatica
- Migraine
- Fits
- Stroke
- Palpitation
- Angina
- Heart attack
- Diarrhoea
- Constipation
- Nausea
- Piles/haemorrhoids
- Anaemia
- Pleurisy
- Eczema
- Urticaria
- Warts
- Cystitis

…', 'I don't know but my family doctor thought …', 'My wife insisted …' or even 'I thought you would already know from the letter my family doctor wrote to you'. All of these answers are perfectly valid, but each gives a different clue as to what are the real issues for the patient, and how to develop the history-taking process further for that individual. This part of history taking is probably the most important and the most dependent on the skill of the doctor. It is always tempting to interrupt too early and, once interrupted, the patient rarely completes what he was intending to say. Even when he appears to have finished giving his reasons for the consultation, always ask if there are any more broad areas that need discussion before beginning to discuss each in more detail.

Developing themes

This stage of the history is likely to see the patient talking much more than the doctor, but it remains vital for the doctor to steer and mould the process so that the information gathered is complete, coherent and, if possible, logical. Some patients will present a clear, concise and chronologically perfect history with little prompting, although they are in the minority. For most patients, the doctor needs to do a substantial amount of clarifying and summarizing with statements such as 'You mean that …', 'Can I go back to when …', 'Can I check I have understood …', 'So up to that point you …', 'I am afraid I am not at all clear about …' and 'I really do not understand, can we go over that again?' If a patient clearly indicates that he does not wish to discuss particular aspects of the history, then this wish must be respected and the diagnosis based on what information is available, although it is also important to explain to the patient the limitations that may be imposed by this lack of information.

Non-verbal communication

Within any consultation, non-verbal communication is as important as what the patient says. There may be contradictions, such as a patient who does not admit to any worries or anxieties but who clearly looks as if he has many. Particular gestures during the description of pain symptoms can give vital clinical clues (Box 1.2). While concentrating on the conversation with the patient, the doctor should keep a wide awareness of all other clues that can be gleaned from the consultation. These include the patient's demeanour, dress and appearance, any walking aids, the interaction between the patient and any accompanying people and the way that the patient reacts to the developing consultation.

Vocabulary

It is very important to use vocabulary that the patient will understand and use appropriately. This understanding needs to be on two levels: he must understand the basic words used, and his interpretation of those words must be understood and clarified by the doctor. Box 1.3 lists words and phrases that may be used in the consultation that the doctor needs to be very careful to clarify with the patient. If the patient uses one of the ordinary English words listed, its meaning must be clarified. A patient who says he is dizzy could be describing actual vertigo, but could just mean light-headedness or a feeling that he is going to faint. A patient who says that he has diarrhoea could mean liquid stools passed hourly throughout the day and night or could mean a couple of urgent soft stools passed first thing in the morning only. Therefore, the doctor needs to use words that are almost certainly going to be clearly understood by the patient, and the doctor must clarify any word or phrase that the patient uses to avoid any possibility of ambiguity.

Indirect and direct questions

Broadly, questions asked by the doctor can be divided into indirect or open-ended and direct or closed. Indirect or open-ended questions can be regarded as an invitation for the patient to talk about the general area that the doctor indicates to be of interest. These questions will often start with phrases such as 'Tell me more about …', 'What do you think about …', 'How does that make you feel …', 'What happened next …' or 'Is there anything else you would like to tell me?' These questions inform the patient that the agenda is very much with him, that he can talk about whatever is important and that the doctor has not prejudged any issues. If skilfully used, and if the doctor is sensitive to the clues presented in the answers, a series of such questions should allow the doctor to understand the issues that are most important from the patient's point of view. The patient will also be allowed to describe things in his own words.

Many patients are in awe of doctors and have some conscious or subconscious need to please them and go along with what they say. If the doctor prejudges the patient's problems and tends to 'railroad' the conversation to fit his assumed diagnosis too early in the process, then the patient can easily go along with this and give simple answers that do not fully describe his situation. Box 1.4 illustrates this extremely simple, common and important pitfall of history taking.

Disease-centred versus patient-centred

An interview that uses lots of direct questions is often 'disease-centred,' whereas a 'patient-centred' interview will contain enough open-ended questions for patients to talk about all of their problems and be given enough time to do so. This will also help to avoid the situation in which the doctor and the patient have different agendas. Often there can appear to be a conflict if the patient complains of symptoms that are probably not medically serious, such as tension headache, while the doctor is focusing on some potentially serious but relatively asymptomatic condition, such as anaemia or hypertension. In this situation, a patient-centred approach will allow the patient to air all of his problems and will allow a skilled doctor to educate the patient as to why the other issues are also important and must not be ignored. A general practitioner (GP) may rightly refuse a demand for antibiotics for a sore throat that is likely to be viral but should use the opportunity to educate and inform the patient about the true place of antibiotic

Box 1.4	Example of a history that leads to a poor conclusion

A GP is seeing a 58-year-old man who is known to be hypertensive and a smoker. The receptionist has already documented that he is coming in with a problem of chest pain. The GP makes an automatic assumption that the pain is most likely to be angina pectoris, because that is probably the most serious cause and the one that the patient is likely to be most worried about, and therefore starts taking the history with the specific purpose of confirming or refuting that diagnosis.

GP: I gather you've had some chest pain?

Patient: Yes, it's been quite bad.

GP: Is it in the middle of your chest?

Patient: Yes.

GP: And does it travel to your left arm?

Patient: Yes—and to my shoulder.

GP: Does it come on when you walk?

Patient: Yes.

GP: And is it relieved by rest?

Patient: Yes—usually.

GP: I'm afraid I think this is angina and I will need to refer you to a heart specialist.

The GP has asked only very direct and closed questions. Each answer has begun with 'Yes'. The patient has already been quite firmly tagged with a 'label' of angina, and anxiety has been raised by the specialist referral.

Alternatively, the GP keeps an open mind and starts as follows:

GP: Tell me why you have come to see me today.

Patient: Well, I have been having some chest pain.

GP: Tell me more about what it's like.

Patient: It's in the centre of my chest and tends to go to my left arm. Sometimes it comes on when I've been walking.

GP: Tell me more about that.

Patient: Sometimes it comes when I am walking and sometimes when I'm sitting down at home after a long walk.

GP: If the pain comes on when you are walking, what do you do?

Patient: I usually slow down, but if I'm in a hurry I can walk on with the pain.

GP: I am a little worried that this might be angina, but some things suggest it might not be, so I am going to refer you to a heart specialist to make sure it isn't angina, or plan treatment if it is.

The GP has asked questions which are either completely open-ended or leave the patient free to describe exactly what happens within a directed area of interest. Clarifying questions have been used. While being reassuring, the GP expresses some concern about angina and is clear about the exact reason for the specialist referral (for both clarification and treatment).

treatment and the risks of excess and inappropriate use of them. The doctor needs to grasp the difference between the disease framework (what the diagnosis is) and the illness framework (what are the patient's experiences, ideas, expectations and

Box 1.5	Areas of everyday life that can be used as a reference for the severity, importance or clarification of symptoms

Exercise tolerance: 'How far can you walk on the flat going at your own speed?', 'Can you climb one flight of stairs slowly without stopping?', 'Can you still do simple housework such as vacuum cleaning or making a bed?'

Work: 'Has this problem kept you off work?', 'Why exactly have you not been able to work?'

Sport: 'Do you play regular sport and has this been affected?'

Eating: 'Has this affected your eating?', 'Do any particular foods cause trouble?'

Social life: 'What do you do in your spare time and has this been restricted in any way?', 'Has your sex life been affected?'

Box 1.6	Suggested headings for basic history taking

- Name, age, occupation, country of birth, other clarification of identity
- Main presenting problem
- Past medical history: 'Before we talk about why you have come, I need to ask you to tell me about any serious medical problems that you have had in the whole of your life'
- Specific past medical history: e.g. diabetes, jaundice, tuberculosis, heart disease, high blood pressure, rheumatic fever, epilepsy
- History of main presenting complaint
- Family history
- Occupational history
- Smoking, alcohol, allergies
- Drug and other treatment history
- Direct questions about bodily systems not covered by the presenting complaint

feelings) and to be able to apply both frameworks to a clinical situation, varying the degree of each, according to the differing demands.

Judging the severity of symptoms

Many symptoms are subjective and the degree of severity expressed by the patient will depend on his own personal reaction and also on how the symptoms interact with his life. A tiny alteration in the neurological function of the hands and fingers will make a huge impression on a professional musician, whereas most others might hardly notice the same dysfunction. A mild skin complaint might be devastating for a professional model but cause little worry in others.

Assessing how the symptoms interact with the patient's life is an important skill of history taking. A simple question such as 'How much does this bother you?' might suffice. It may be helpful to ask specific questions about how the patient's daily life is affected, with comparison to events that many patients will experience. Box 1.5 illustrates some of the relevant areas. Patients do not want exaggerated or 'fake' sympathy, but occasional interjections such as 'That must be difficult, given your work' will provide reassurance that you are assessing their symptoms against the backdrop of their lives.

Medical symptomatology often involves pain, which is more subjective than almost any other symptom. Many patients are stoical and bear severe pain uncomplainingly, whereas others seem to complain much more about apparently less severe pain. A simple pain scale can be very helpful in assessing pain severity. The patient is asked to rate his pain on a scale from 1 to 10, with 1 being a pain that is barely noticeable and 10 the worst pain he can imagine or the worst pain he has ever experienced. It is also useful to clarify what the reference point is for '10,' which for many women will be the pain of labour. The pain scale assessment is useful in

diagnosis and in monitoring disease, treatment and analgesia. Assessing a patient with pain is discussed in more detail in Chapter 11.

Which issues are important?

A problem for those doctors wishing to take the history in chronological order—'Start at the beginning and tell me all about it'—is that people usually start with the part of the problem that they regard as the most important. This is, of course, entirely valid from the patient's viewpoint, and it is also important to the doctor, because the issue that most bothers the patient is then brought to attention. Curing disease may not always be possible, so it is important to be aware of the important symptoms because, for example, pain may be relieved even though the underlying cause of the pain is still present. It is very common for the doctor to be pleased that one condition has been solved, but the patient still complains of the main symptom that he originally came with.

A schematic history

A suggested schematic history is detailed in Box 1.6. In many clinical situations it will be clear that a different scheme should be followed. An important part of learning about history taking is that each doctor develops his own personal scheme that works for him in the situations that he generally comes across. Nevertheless, it is useful to start with a basic outline in mind.

Direct questions about bodily systems

Within the variety of disease processes that may present to doctors, many have features that occur in many of the bodily systems which at first may not seem to be related to the patient's main complaint. A patient presenting with back pain may have had some haematuria from a renal cell carcinoma that has

Box 1.7	Bodily systems and questions relevant to taking a full history from most patients

If the specific questions have been covered by the history of the presenting complaint, they do not need to be included again. If the answers are positive, the characteristics of each must be clarified

Cardiorespiratory

- Chest pain
- Intermittent claudication
- Palpitation
- Ankle swelling
- Orthopnoea
- Nocturnal dyspnoea
- Shortness of breath
- Cough with or without sputum
- Haemoptysis

Gastrointestinal

- Abdominal pain
- Dyspepsia
- Dysphagia
- Nausea and/or vomiting
- Degree of appetite loss
- Weight loss or gain
- Bowel pattern and any change
- Rectal bleeding
- Jaundice

Genitourinary

- Haematuria
- Nocturia
- Frequency
- Dysuria
- Menstrual irregularity: women
- Urethral discharge: men

Locomotor

- Joint pain and/or swelling
- Change in mobility

Neurological

- Seizures
- Collapses
- Dizziness
- Eyesight
- Hearing
- Transient loss of function (vision, speech, sight)
- Paraesthesia

Box 1.8	List of clarifications for a complaint of pain

- Site
- Radiation
- Character
- Severity
- Time course
- Aggravating factors
- Relieving factors
- Associated symptoms

alert to all aspects of the patient's health and not just the area or problem that he has presented with. For example, a GP would not ignore a high blood pressure reading in a patient presenting with a rash, even though the two are probably not connected. This function of any consultation can be regarded as 'screening' the patient. In health economic terms, a true screening programme for a particular disease across a whole population (such as for cervical cancer) has to be evaluated as being useful, economic and with no negative effects. However, once the patient with a complaint has attended a doctor, a simple ('opportunistic') screening process can be incorporated into the consultation with little extra time or effort. The direct questions (and full routine examination) encompass this screening function as well as contributing to solving the patient's presenting problems.

Clarifying detail

One of the basic principles of history taking is not to take what the patient says at face value but to clarify it as much as possible. Almost all of the history will involve clarification, but there are specific areas where this is particularly important.

Pain

Whenever a patient complains of pain, a series of clarifying questions as listed in Box 1.8 should follow. A simple pain scale has been described above. The other characteristics are vital in analysing what might be causing the pain. Some painful conditions have classic sites and radiation patterns (myocardial ischaemia is classically felt in the centre of the chest radiating to the left arm). Pain from a hollow organ is classically colicky (such as biliary or renal colic). The pain of a subarachnoid haemorrhage is classically very sudden, 'like a hammer blow to the head'. Some pains have clear aggravating or relieving factors (peptic ulcer pain is classically worse when hungry and better after food). Colicky right upper quadrant abdominal pain accompanied by jaundice suggests a gallstone obstructing the bile duct; a headache accompanied by preceding flashing lights suggests migraine. It is always worth making sure that any symptom of pain has been clarified in this way, and although some of the points will come out

spread and is the cause of the presenting symptom. For this reason, any thorough assessment of a patient must include questions about all the bodily systems and not just areas that the patient perceives as problematic. This area of questioning should be introduced with a statement such as 'I am now going to ask you about other possible symptoms that could be important and relevant to your problem'. A list of such question areas is given in Box 1.7.

In addition, during any medical consultation, however brief, it is the duty of the doctor to be

---

Box 1.9   Clarifying questions in the drug history

- Can you tell me all the drugs or medicines that you take?
- Have any been prescribed from another clinic, doctor or dentist?
- Do you buy any yourself from a pharmacy?
- Are you sure you have told me about all tablets, capsules and liquid medicines?
- What about inhalers, skin creams or patches, suppositories or tablets to suck?
- Were you taking any medicines a little while ago but stopped recently?
- Do you ever take any medicines prescribed for other people, such as your spouse?
- Do you use herbal or other complementary medicines?

Box 1.10   Details of the family history

Are there any illnesses that run in your family?

Occasionally this will reveal major genetic trends, such as haemophilia. More often there will be an answer such as 'They all have heart trouble'.

Basic family tree of first-degree relatives

This should be plotted on a diagram for most patients, including major illnesses and cause and age of any deaths.

Specific questions about occurrence of problems similar to the patient's

Ask the patient about items in the developing differential diagnosis, for example 'Does anyone in your family have gallstones/epilepsy/high blood pressure?' if these seem a likely diagnosis for the patient under consideration.

---

in the open-ended part of the history taking, others will need specific questions.

Drug history

At first glance, asking a patient what drugs he is taking would seem to be one of the simplest and most reliable parts of taking a history. In practice, this could not be further from the truth, and there are many pitfalls for the inexperienced. This is partly because many patients are not very knowledgeable about their own medications and also because patients often misinterpret the question, giving a very narrow answer when the doctor wants to know about medications in the widest sense. The need for clarification in the drug history is given in Box 1.9. The drug history, almost more than any other, benefits from being repeated at another time and in a slightly different way. For example, in trying to define a possible drug reaction as a cause of liver dysfunction, it is not unusual to find that the patient has taken a few relevant tablets (such as over-the-counter nonsteroidal anti-inflammatory drug) just before the onset of the problem and only remembered or realized it was important to say so when asked repeatedly and in great detail.

Family history

Like the drug history, the family history would seem at first glance to be simple and reliably quoted. In general this is true, but it can be dissected into sections that will uncover more information. These are set out in Box 1.10.

Occupational history

It is always useful to know the patient's occupation, if he has one, because it is such an important part of life and one with which any illness is bound to interact. In some situations, a patient's occupation will be directly relevant to the diagnostic process. The classic industrial illnesses, such as lead poisoning and other toxic exposures, are now extremely rare in developed industrial countries, but accidental exposure continues to occur. Other problems, such

---

Box 1.11   Probing the alcohol history

Doctor: Do you drink any alcoholic drinks?
Patient: Oh yes, but not much—just socially.
Doctor: Do you drink some every day?
Patient: Yes.
Doctor: Tell me what you drink.
Patient: I usually have two pints of beer at lunchtime and two or three on my way home from work.
Doctor: And at the weekend?
Patient: I usually go out Saturday nights and have four or five pints.
Doctor: Do you drink anything other than beer?
Patient: On Saturdays I have a double whisky with each pint.

The first answer does not suggest a problem, but based on the figures in Box 1.12, the actual amount adds up to 70 units per week, which clearly confers considerable health risks to this patient.

---

as asbestosis or silicosis, produce effects many years after exposure, and a careful chronological occupational history may be required to elucidate the exposure. For patients with nonorganic problems, the work environment can often be the trigger for the development of the problem.

Alcohol history

The detrimental effects of alcohol on health cause a variety of problems, and the frequency of excess alcohol use means that up to 10% of adult hospital inpatients have a problem related to alcohol. To make an accurate estimate of alcohol consumption and any possible dependency, it is essential to enquire carefully and not to take what the patient says at face value, but to probe the history in different ways (Box 1.11). For documentation, the reported amount should then be converted into units of alcohol per week (Box 1.12). If the reported amount seems at all excessive then an assessment should be made of possible dependency for which the CAGE questions are very useful (Box 1.13). AUDIT-C.

Box 1.12 Units of alcohol (1 unit contains 10 g of pure alcohol)

The units of alcohol can be determined by multiplying the volume of the drink (in ml) by its % alcohol by volume (abv) and dividing this by 1000. For example, 1 pint (568 ml) of beer at 3.5% abv contains: (568 × 3.5) / 1000 = 1.988 units.

It is important to bear in mind that alcohol strength varies widely within each category of drink, but here is a guide to the most common alcoholic drinks:

- Standard-strength beer (3.5% abv): 1 pint = 2 units
- Very strong lagers (6% abv): 1 pint = 3.5 units
- Spirits (whisky, gin, etc., 40% abv): 1 UK pub measure (about 25 ml) = 1 unit
- Wine (12%): 1 standard glass (175 ml) = 2 units

The UK government now recommends that to minimize alcohol-related health effects, both men and women should keep to less than 14 units of alcohol per week.

Box 1.13 The CAGE assessment for alcohol dependency

- C – Have you ever felt the need to Cut down your alcohol consumption?
- A – Have you ever felt Angry at others criticizing your drinking?
- G – Do you ever feel Guilty about excess drinking?
- E – Do you ever drink in the mornings (Eye-opener)?

Two or more positive answers could indicate a problem of dependency.

Retrospective history

The concept of retrospective history taking is a refinement of taking the past medical history and develops the theme of never taking what the patient says at face value. Many patients will clearly say that they have had certain illnesses or previous symptoms using medical terminology. This information may not be accurate, either because the patient has misinterpreted it or because he was given the wrong information or diagnosis in the first place. This area becomes particularly important if any new diagnosis is going to rely on this type of information. For instance, in assessing a patient presenting with chest pain at rest, a history of angina of effort will be considered a risk factor for acute myocardial infarction and will increase the likelihood of that as the current diagnosis. However, on closer questioning, it might become clear that what the patient was told was angina (perhaps by a relative and not even a doctor) was in fact a vague chest ache coming on after a period of heavy work and not a clear central chest pain coming on during exertion.

Clearly the possibility of retaking the history for everything the patient says about his medical past may not be practical in the time available, but the possibility and value of doing this should always be borne in mind and can completely alter the developing differential diagnosis.

Box 1.14 A typical 'garrulous' history

Doctor: Tell me about what has led to you coming here today.

Patient: Well doctor, you see, it was like this. I woke up one day last week; I am not quite sure which day it was; it might have been Tuesday; or, no, I remember it was Monday because my son came round later to visit; he always comes on a Monday because that's his day off college; he's studying law; I'm so pleased that he's settled down to that; he was so wild when he was younger; do you know what he did once …?

Doctor (interrupting): Can you tell me what did happen when you woke up last Monday?

Patient: Oh yes; it was like this; I am not sure what woke me up; it may have been the pain; no, more likely it was the dustmen collecting the rubbish; they do come so early and make such a noise; that day it was even worse because their usual dustcart must have been broken and they came with this really old noisy one …

Doctor (interrupting): So you had some pain when you woke up then?

Patient: Yes. I think it must have been there when I woke up because I lay in bed wondering where on earth there might be some indigestion remedy. I knew I had some but I am one of those people who can never remember where things are; do you know what I managed to lose last year …?

Doctor (interrupting): Was the pain burning or crushing?

Patient: Well, that depends on what you mean by …

Doctor (interrupting): Yes, but did you have any crushing pain?

The doctor gradually changes from very open-ended to very closed questions in order to try to get some information that is useful to building up the diagnostic picture—eventually a question is asked that just has a yes/no answer.

Particular situations

It is true to say that, although many themes, patterns and common areas to history taking and some areas of history taking might seem routine, the process of history taking for different patients will never be identical. Some particular and often challenging situations deserve some further description.

Garrulous patients

A new medical student will soon meet a patient who says a huge amount without really conveying any of the information that goes towards a useful medical history. This will be in marked contrast to some other patients who, from the first introductory question (e.g. 'Tell me about what has led up to you coming here today'), will reveal a perfect history with virtually no prompting. A fictitious but typical history from the former type of patient is given in Box 1.14. When faced with such a patient, the doctor needs to alter significantly the balance of open-ended and direct questions. Open-ended questions will tend to lead to such a patient giving a long recitation but with little useful content. The doctor will have to use many more clear and direct questions which may just have yes/no answers. The overall history will inevitably be less satisfactory, but it is not possible to get the 'perfect' history in every patient.

Angry patients

Only a few patients are overtly angry when they see a doctor, but anger expressed during a clinical consultation may be an important diagnostic clue but, at the same time, get in the way of a smooth diagnostic process. Some patients will be angry with the immediate circumstances, such as a late-running outpatient clinic. Others will have longer-term anger against the surgery, department or institution that will be more difficult to address. It is always important to acknowledge anger and to try to tease out what underlies it. Even if it is not the doctor's immediate fault that the clinic is running late or there have been other problems, it is always worth apologizing on behalf of the unit or institution.

For some patients, anger may be part of the symptomatology or expressed as a reaction to the diagnosis or treatment. This will be particularly true in patients with a nonorganic diagnosis who insist that there is 'something wrong' and that the doctor must do something. Many types of presentation will fall into this group, including tension headache, irritable bowel and back pain. There may be obvious secondary gain for the patient (such as staying off work and claiming benefits) and challenging this pattern of behaviour may provoke anger.

It is the duty of a doctor to attempt to work with and help a wide variety of patients, and those who are angry are no exception. However, occasionally it may be best to acknowledge that the doctor–patient relationship has broken down and that facilitating a change to another doctor may be in the best interests of the patient.

The well-informed patient

In the last century, doctors often looked after patients for a long time without really explaining their illness to them, and patients were reasonably happy taking the attitude that 'the doctor knows best'. This approach is no longer acceptable and it is the duty of a doctor to give the patient as much information about his illness as possible, particularly so that he is able to make informed choices about treatments. This change of approach has led to many patients seeking out information about their problems from many other sources, particularly the Internet. It is not unusual for a patient to come into the first consultation with a new doctor, armed with printouts from various websites that he feels are relevant, or to show information on his smartphone.

Doctors must take all this in their stride, go through the information with the patient and help him by showing what is relevant and what is not. Many websites with medical content are created by individuals or groups without proper information for a sound basis of knowledge, but it can be difficult for the patient to make a judgement about this. Being able to inform patients of a few relevant and reliable websites can be very helpful. In general, it is easy and more rewarding to look after well-informed patients, provided they do not fall into the very small group that have such fixed and erroneous ideas about their problems that the diagnostic and treatment process is impeded.

Accompanying persons

Some people come to consultations alone and others with one or more friends or family members. Always spend time during the initial exchange of greetings identifying who is present and getting some idea of the group dynamics. If the patient appears to be alone, ask whether there is someone waiting outside. There is always a reason people come accompanied, but if there appear to be too many people present or if the presence of others might threaten the relationship with the patient at any time in the consultation, it is appropriate to consider asking the others to leave, even if only briefly. It is reasonable, if in doubt, to ascertain why others wish to be present, and certainly whether this is also the patient's wish. It is very important to know if the patient does want to object to the presence of others, but feels unable to do so. This is particularly difficult if the doctor does not speak the patient's language and can only speak to those accompanying. Consider whether specific questions about the history should be asked of those accompanying, either with the patient or separately, with specific consent.

Be aware of a situation in which the accompanying people answer all the questions, even if there is not a language difficulty. Many clues to diagnosis may be masked if direct communication with the patient is not possible (using an interpreter/advocate for patients who do not speak the same language as the doctor is discussed below). There may be many reasons that the patient does not speak for himself. These may include embarrassment in front of those accompanying (such as a teenager with his parents). In such circumstances, it may be necessary to leave parts of the history until those accompanying can reasonably be asked to leave, such as during the examination. Occasionally it is clear that the patient will not talk for himself, in which case the history from those accompanying will have to be the working information.

Using interpreters/advocates

Particularly in the cities of Western countries, there will often be found a large immigrant population who do not speak the first language of the country, even if they have been resident for some years, and it is impractical for each patient to be looked after by health professionals who speak their language. In these circumstances, the medical consultation has to be undertaken with an interpreter. The most immediate solution may be to use a family member; however, if the issues are private or embarrassing, this often does not work well. It is also unethical to use an underage family member as an interpreter (under 16 years of age).

The best solution is to have available an independent interpreter/advocate for the consultation, although in areas where many patients are not native speakers, many interpreters may be needed for a range of languages. Another solution for infrequently encountered languages is a telephone-based interpreting service.

When taking a history via an interpreter/advocate, the overall style usually has to change. The breadth of history and the clinical clues that can be obtained from a good initial open-ended question may well be lost in the double translation, and the doctor often changes to a much more direct style of questioning for which the answers will be unambiguous even when going through the double translation. It is also not unusual for the interpreter/advocate and the patient to have a few minutes of conversation following an apparently simple question from the doctor, but then a very short answer is returned to the doctor. This leaves the doctor bemused as to what is really going on with the patient. Finally, history taking via an interpreter/advocate usually takes considerably longer than when the doctor and the patient speak the same language.

Analysing symptoms

The objective of the history and examination is to begin identifying the disturbance of structure and function responsible for the patient's symptoms. This is done by analysis of the symptoms and signs leading to a differential diagnosis (a list of possible diagnoses that will account for the symptoms and signs, usually set out in descending order of likelihood). This list of possibilities is then often refined by the use of special investigations, but in up to 80% of patients the likely diagnosis is reasonably clear after the initial history. The process of analysis can be likened to detective work, in which the symptoms and signs are the evidence. When a medical student is first faced with the myriad data gleaned on taking a history, he is often baffled as to how to start the analysis, but the student can be reassured that the process becomes easier as more medical knowledge is acquired. An analysis of symptoms from a medical student is more based on facts learned from textbooks, whereas an experienced doctor will tend to base the analysis more on patterns of disease presentation that he has encountered many times. Whereas the analytical process is largely acquired through this type of experience, some principles can be described. This topic is discussed further in Chapter 3.

Box 1.15	'Hard' and 'soft' symptoms

'Hard' symptoms

- Pneumaturia: almost always caused by a colovesical fistula
- Fortification spectra: if associated with unilateral headache, strongly suggests classic migraine
- Rigors: strongly suggests bacteraemia, viraemia or malaria
- A bitten tongue: if associated with a seizure, strongly suggests a grand mal fit
- A sudden severe headache 'like a hammer blow': strongly suggests a subarachnoid haemorrhage
- Pleuritic chest pain: strongly suggests pleural irritation caused by an infection or by a pulmonary embolus
- Itching: if associated with jaundice, indicates intra- or extrahepatic cholestasis

'Soft' symptoms

- Dizziness
- Light-headedness
- Tiredness
- Back pain
- Headache
- Wind

'Hard and soft' symptoms

A detective analysing evidence of a crime will put a lot of weight on fingerprint or DNA evidence and less weight on identification evidence. The same principles apply to analysing symptoms. A 'hard' symptom can be thought of as one that, if clearly present, adds a lot of weight to a particular diagnosis. A 'soft' symptom may be thought of as one which is either reported by patients so variably that its true presence is often in doubt, or one which is present in such a variety of conditions as not to be useful in confirming or refuting a diagnosis. Examples of these two groupings are given in Box 1.15.

Time course

A simple algorithm would be that the character of the symptom suggests the 'anatomy' of the problem and the time course the 'pathology' of it. For instance, a vascular event, such as a myocardial infarct, stroke or subarachnoid haemorrhage, usually has a sudden onset, whereas something that gradually progresses or for which the onset cannot be exactly dated by the patient, such as weight loss or dysphagia, may be a malignant process. Some pitfalls in this type of analysis must be borne in mind to avoid confusion.

Disease processes that gradually progress may start off by being asymptomatic and the patient may only notice symptoms when they start to interfere with his lifestyle and activities. For example, exertional breathlessness in a largely sedentary patient may develop late in a cardiorespiratory disease process, whereas a patient who actively exercises is likely to notice symptoms much earlier. This phenomenon is also seen where the relevant bodily organ or system has a lot of reserve and the symptom may show itself only when the reserve is used up. This could be true for a relatively chronic liver disease, such as primary biliary cholangitis, apparently presenting acutely. The proverb of the 'straw that broke the camel's back' is a good analogy of this sort of situation (a camel is steadily loaded up with straw until suddenly it appears that a single piece of straw is sufficient to make the camel collapse). In addition, the disease process may have a step-wise worsening rather than a linear decline, such as in a situation of multiple small strokes when the patient may not present until a single small stroke makes a big difference to his functional ability.

Pattern recognition versus logical analysis

It is important to realize that in some clinical situations the diagnosis may be clear based on previous experience; in others the diagnosis has to be built up through a process of logical analysis of symptoms, signs and special investigations. The fact that the process of gaining information from symptoms, signs and special investigations is never completely exact must also be borne in mind so that the patient with an atypical presentation is not assigned the wrong diagnosis. The area of medicine that probably most often uses pattern recognition is dermatology, but recently skin biopsies are used much more to clarify diagnoses that were previously assumed. A patient presenting with chest pain and signs of underperfusion may easily be thought to be having a myocardial infarction, but a brief history of the character of the pain (tearing and going through to the back) may prompt a search for a dissecting aortic aneurysm.

Negative data

An experienced history taker will begin the analysis from the outset of the clinical encounter. This means that during the initial process and without the need for so much later review, questions can be asked for which a negative answer is as important as a positive one. These questions are usually very specific and direct, often with a yes/no answer. A patient whose presenting complaint is exertional chest pain can immediately be asked if the pain is worse on increased exertion and how long a period of rest is needed to relieve it. Pain that is not predictably produced by exertion and is not reliably relieved by rest may well not be angina pectoris. However, it remains very important that interjected questions of this type do not spoil the flow of the patient's story.

What does the patient actually want?

If a patient comes to a doctor with a long history, it is always worth trying to find out why he has come

Box 1.16	General reasons that patients come to see doctors (other than for a severe or acute problem)

- Cannot tolerate ongoing symptoms and wants to be rid of them
- Someone else noticing specific problems (e.g. jaundice)
- Another doctor noticing specific problems (e.g. high blood pressure)
- Worry about underlying diagnosis (often induced by relatives, friends, books, media or Internet)
- Spouse or relative worried about patient
- Cannot work with symptoms
- Colleagues/bosses complaining about patient's work or time off
- Requirement of others (insurance, employment benefit, litigation)

for medical help and what he actually wants from the consultation. There may be various scenarios, as listed in Box 1.16. It is always worth trying to find out which might apply to the individual patient, because it sets the scene for giving advice and treatment, particularly if an exact diagnosis or a complete treatment cannot be provided. It is often much easier to reassure a patient that nothing seriously is wrong rather than giving him an exact diagnosis or fully relieving his symptoms.

Retaking the history

It is clear that history taking is an inexact process, heavily influenced by the doctor and by the patient. The logical conclusion of this is that no two histories taken from the same patient about the same set of symptoms will be identical, even if the same doctor repeats the process. Given two slightly or significantly different histories, it may be hard to know on which one to base the diagnosis, or whether to regard history taking for that patient as so unreliable as to be useless. The main message is that a single attempt at the history may not suffice and repeated histories taken at different times by different people and in different ways may provide just as much extra information on which to base a diagnosis as more and more detailed special investigations. When a patient is seen for a second or alternative opinion, the doctor usually spends more time on retaking the history than on repeating the examination.

Note-taking

When making notes, it is important to keep eye contact with the patient. Notes should not be made only at times that might suggest to the patient what items of information are regarded as important. It is better to listen carefully and just record enough to help remember the important points later. A fuller account can be written up or dictated afterwards for typing, or by voice recognition. In the fuller record,

Box 1.17	Duties of doctors registered with the UK General Medical Council (2013)

Knowledge, skills and performance

- Make the care of your patient your first concern
- Keep your professional knowledge and skills up to date
- Recognize and work within the limits of your competence

Safety and quality

- Take prompt action if you think that patient safety, dignity or comfort is being compromised

Communication, partnership and teamwork

- Protect and promote the health of patients and the public
- Treat patients politely and considerately
- Respect patients' right to confidentiality
- Listen to, and respond to, patients' concerns and preferences
- Give patients the information they want or need in a way they can understand
- Respect patients' right to reach decisions with you about their treatment and care
- Support patients in caring for themselves to improve and maintain their health

Maintaining trust

- Be honest and open and act with integrity
- Never discriminate unfairly against patients or colleagues
- Never abuse your patients' trust in you or the public's trust in the medical profession
- You are personally accountable for your professional practice and must always be prepared to justify your decisions and actions

the exact history, the weight placed on various items and, most importantly, what the patient actually said can be recorded. What patients say, word for word, is often as important as any later reconstruction of the history. Increasingly doctors are entering information directly into computers, rather than writing, during a consultation. If an experienced doctor starts this for the first time, it can feel intrusive, but can soon be mastered so as to become second nature. Patients will generally accept the presence of the computer as being part of the fabric of modern life.

Conclusion

History taking is the cornerstone of medical practice. It combines considerable interpersonal skill and diversity, with the need for logical thought based on a wealth of medical knowledge and represents the beginning of treating and caring for patients in the widest sense. Almost all the attributes of good medical practice as set out by the UK General Medical Council (Box 1.17) are encompassed in good history taking. Taking a detailed history while getting to know a patient and arriving at a likely diagnosis is as rewarding in itself as performing a technical procedure for a patient or seeing him get better in the end.

General patient examination and differential diagnosis | 2

William M. Drake and Tahseen A. Chowdhury

Introduction

The separation of the history from the examination is artificial because the latter starts with the first greeting and ends when the patient departs. Some physical findings may prompt further questioning; do not be concerned that your history taking was inadequate, but revisit these areas at the conclusion of the examination or during it. From the outset, the clinician is assimilating potentially relevant information from the patient's posture, appearance, speech, demeanour and response to questions. Who is this patient? What kind of person is he? What are his anxieties? What is the reason for consulting a doctor at this time? In the outpatient setting, note the patient's grooming and appropriateness of dress. If the patient is in hospital, are there outward signs of social support, such as get-well cards or indicators of a religious faith?

General examination of a patient

Many patients are apprehensive about being examined; the environment is unfamiliar, they may feel exposed and are likely to have anxieties about the findings. Be open about your status as a medical student or junior doctor. Reassure the patient that the extra length of time you take to complete your examination compared with someone more senior is because you are less experienced but that does not necessarily imply the findings are worrying. Many students, early in their training, are anxious about touching and examining patients. Persevere; with practice and experience, confidence will come quickly.

The examination should be conducted in a warm, private, quiet area. Daylight is preferable to artificial light, which may make the recognition of subtle changes in skin colour (e.g. mild jaundice) difficult. A cold room increases anxiety levels and shivering muscle generates strange noises on auscultation of the chest. In hospital, you may need to ask neighbouring patients to turn down the volume on their television or radio. Prior to conducting a clinical examination, ensure that your hands are thoroughly washed and dried.

A thorough examination requires adequate exposure of the patient. Patients should be asked to undress completely or at least to their underclothes and then to cover themselves with a sheet or an examination gown. If the patient keeps his underclothes on, do not forget to examine the covered areas (buttocks, breasts, genitalia, perineum). Ideally a chaperone should be present when a male doctor examines a female patient and is essential for intimate examinations, such as of the rectal, vaginal and breast areas. This is to reassure the patient and to protect the doctor from subsequent accusations of impropriety. Although the patient's attendance at a consultation suggests he is happy to be examined, this may not be the case and it is always courteous to ask permission. Check to be sure he is able to prepare for the examination by disrobing and mounting the couch unaided. Do not embarrass him by waiting for him to fail and ask for help.

For most patients, start the examination on the right side of the bed/couch with the patient semi-recumbent (approximately 45°). Do not dent the confidence of an already anxious patient with heart failure or peritonitis by moving him unnecessarily from the position he finds most comfortable. From the right-hand side of the patient, it is easier to examine the jugular veins, apex beat and abdominal viscera, although left-handed students will take longer to master this approach. Try to expose only the area you are examining at the time. With practice, you will become adept at using the gown or drape to cover the body part just examined as you proceed to the next. Regular attention to the patient's comfort, such as adjustment/replacement of pillows, helps strengthen the professional bond and reassures him that you are concerned about his welfare.

Quickly make a global assessment of the severity of the patient's illness. Ask yourself: 'Does this person look well, mildly ill or severely ill?' If the patient is severely ill then it is appropriate to postpone a detailed examination until the acute situation has been resolved. Do not put severely ill patients to inconvenience or distress that is not essential at that moment.

Posture and gait

In the outpatient or primary care setting, observe your patient from the moment you meet him in the waiting area. Does he rise easily from a chair? Does he walk freely, stiffly or with a limp; confidently or apparently fearful of falling; aided or unaided? In the hospital setting, note the patient's posture in bed. Healthy people adjust their position at will, without difficulty. In disease, this ability is lost to variable degrees, and severely ill patients may be sufficiently helpless that they adopt positions that are very uncomfortable. Patients with left-sided heart failure typically find that lying horizontally worsens their sense of breathlessness (orthopnoea). The pain of peritonitis typically compels patients to lie supine, sometimes with the legs drawn up, still and quiet, with shallow breathing movements in order to minimize the pain that movement induces. This contrasts with the restlessness of renal colic, in which the patient often rolls around in a futile attempt to find a position free from pain. With acute inflammatory or infective joint disease, the affected limbs often lie motionless. In severe cases of meningitis, the neck may bend backwards and appear to burrow into the pillow.

Speech and interaction

Much information comes from the first interaction. The face, particularly the eyes, indicate real feelings better than words. Did your patient smile when you introduced yourself? Was it symmetrical or was there obvious facial weakness? Did he make eye contact? Was the face animated or expressionless, as in Parkinson's disease? Was the voice hoarse because of laryngeal disease, recurrent laryngeal nerve palsy or myxoedema? Was the speech pressured, as in thyrotoxicosis or mania or monotonous, and expressionless, as in severe depression? Was it slurred from cerebellar disease or a previous stroke?

Physique and nutrition

The nutritional state of a patient may provide an important indicator of disease, and prompt correction of a deficient nutritional state may improve recovery. The more detailed methodologies available for nutritional assessment and management in the context of complex gastrointestinal disease are covered in Chapter 14. In the general survey, note if the patient is cachectic, slim, overweight or obese (Box 2.1). If obese, is it generalized or centrally distributed? Wasting of the temporalis muscle leads to a gaunt appearance, and recent weight loss may result in prominence of the ribs (Fig. 2.1). Other clues to poor nutrition include cracked skin, loss of scalp and body hair and poor wound healing. Malnutrition, together with acute or chronic illness, often leads to hypoalbuminaemia with associated oedema, making overall body weight an unreliable marker of malnutrition. A smooth, often sore tongue without papillae (atrophic glossitis, Fig. 2.2) suggests important vitamin B deficiencies. Angular stomatitis (cheilosis, a softening of the skin at the angles of

Box 2.1	Body mass index

$$BMI = weight\ (kg)/height\ (m)^2$$

In Europeans:
- Normal BMI: 20–25
- Overweight: 25.1–30
- Obese: 30.1–35
- Grossly obese: >35.1

In Asians:
- Normal BMI: 18–23
- Overweight: 23.1–28
- Obese: 28.1–33
- Grossly obese: >33.1

Figure 2.1 A patient with marked cachexia, showing widespread muscle and soft tissue wasting. (From Forbes CD, Jackson WF. Color Atlas and Text of Clinical Medicine, ed 3. 2002. Mosby, Edinburgh.)

Figure 2.2 Atrophic glossitis in a patient with severe vitamin B12 deficiency. Also seen is angular stomatitis from severe iron deficiency. (From Forbes and Jackson. Color Atlas and Text of Clinical Medicine, ed 3. 2002. Mosby, Edinburgh. Reproduced by kind permission.)

Figure 2.3 Pellagra as a result of niacin deficiency. (From Forbes CD, Jackson WF. Color Atlas and Text of Clinical Medicine, ed 3. 2002, Mosby, Edinburgh. Reproduced by kind permission.)

Figure 2.4 Dupuytren's contracture. (From Forbes CD, Jackson WF. Color Atlas and Text of Clinical Medicine, ed 3. 2002, Mosby, Edinburgh. Reproduced by kind permission.)

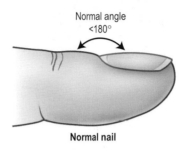

Normal angle
<180°

Normal nail

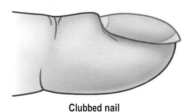

Clubbed nail

Figure 2.5 Lovibond's angle refers to the angulation between the nail plate and the skin below the nail, when viewed laterally. Normally it is less than 180°. When clubbing is present, the angle is at least 180°, or more.

the mouth followed by cracking) may occur with a severe deficiency of iron or B vitamins. Niacin deficiency, if profound, may cause the typical skin changes of pellagra (Fig. 2.3).

Temperature

Body temperature may be recorded in the mouth, axilla, ear or rectum. A 'normal' mouth temperature is 35.8° to 37°C. Those in the ear and rectum are 0.5°C higher and in the axilla 0.5°C lower. There is a diurnal variation in temperature; the lowest values are recorded in the early morning with a maximum between 6 and 10 pm. In women, ovulation is associated with a 0.5°C rise in temperature. In hospitalized patients, regular temperature measurements may identify certain characteristic patterns of disturbance. A persistent fever is one that does not fluctuate by more than 1°C during 24 hours; a remittent fever oscillates by 2°C during the course of a day; and an intermittent or spiking fever is present for only several hours at a time before returning to normal. None has great sensitivity or specificity for any particular diagnosis, but changes over time may provide useful information about the course of a disease.

Hands

Examine the hands carefully because diagnostic information from a variety of pathologies may be evident. The strength of the patient's handshake may be informative with regard to underlying neurological or musculoskeletal disorders. Characteristic patterns of muscular wasting may accompany various neuropathies and radiculopathies (see Chapter 16). Make note of any tremor, taking care to distinguish the fine tremor of thyrotoxicosis or recent beta-adrenergic therapy from the rhythmical 'pill rolling' tremor of Parkinsonism (see Chapter 16) and from the coarse jerky tremor of hepatic or uraemic failure

(sufficiently slow to be referred to as a metabolic 'flap') or the intention tremor of cerebellar disease.

Feel for Dupuytren's contracture in both hands, the first sign of which is usually a thickening of tissue over the flexor tendon of the ring finger at the level of the distal palmar crease. With time, skin puckering in this area develops, together with a thick fibrous cord, leading to flexion contracture of the metacarpophalangeal and proximal interphalangeal joints. Flexion contracture of the other fingers may follow (Fig. 2.4).

Check for clubbing of the fingers. Normally, the angle of the fingernail and the nail base (Lovibond's angle) is approximately 180° and the base feels firm to palpation (Fig. 2.5). As clubbing develops, the tissues at the base of the nail are thickened and Lovibond's angle is lost. Subsequently, the nail becomes more convex, both transversely and longitudinally, and seems to 'float' in a softened nail bed. In normal nails, when both thumbnails are apposed, a diamond-

Figure 2.6 Clubbing of the fingers. This case is very marked. (From Forbes CD, Jackson WF. Color Atlas and Text of Clinical Medicine, ed 3. 2002, Mosby, Edinburgh. Reproduced by kind permission.)

Figure 2.7 Small dermal infarcts in infective endocarditis. (From Forbes CD, Jackson WF. Color Atlas and Text of Clinical Medicine, ed 3. 2002, Mosby, Edinburgh. Reproduced by kind permission.)

Figure 2.8 Splinter haemorrhages. (From Forbes CD, Jackson WF. Color Atlas and Text of Clinical Medicine, ed 3. 2002, Mosby, Edinburgh. Reproduced by kind permission.)

shaped gap is created, called Schamroth's window. With clubbing, a combination of the thickened nail bed and the loss of Lovibond's angle indicates that this window is reduced or even obliterated. In gross cases (usually owing to severe cyanotic heart disease, bronchiectasis or empyema), the volume of the finger pulp increases (Fig. 2.6) and becomes bulbous like the end of a drumstick. The toes may also be affected. Lesser degrees of clubbing may be seen in bronchial carcinoma, fibrosing alveolitis, inflammatory bowel disease and infective endocarditis. The last of these may also be associated with Osler's nodes—transient, tender swellings caused by dermal infarcts from septic cardiac vegetations (Fig. 2.7). Splinter haemorrhages (Fig. 2.8) and nail-fold infarctions (Fig. 2.9) may be signs of a vasculitic process, but may also be the result of trauma in normal individuals and are therefore rather non-specific.

Trophic changes may be evident in the skin in certain neurological diseases and in peripheral circulatory disorders, such as Raynaud's syndrome, in which vasospasm of the digital arterioles causes the fingers to become white and numb, followed by blue/purple cyanosis and then redness owing to arteriolar dilatation and reactive hyperaemia (Fig. 2.10).

In koilonychia the nails are soft, thin and brittle and the normal convexity replaced by a spoon-shaped concavity (Fig. 2.11). It is a rare feature

Figure 2.9 Nail-fold infarction. (From Forbes CD, Jackson WF. Color Atlas and Text of Clinical Medicine, ed 3. 2002, Mosby, Edinburgh. Reproduced by kind permission.)

Figure 2.10 Raynaud's syndrome in the acute phase with severe blanching of the tip of one finger. (From Forbes CD, Jackson WF. Color Atlas and Text of Clinical Medicine, ed 3. 2002, Mosby, Edinburgh. Reproduced by kind permission.)

Figure 2.12 Leuconychia in a patient with chronic liver disease. (From Forbes CD, Jackson WF. Color Atlas and Text of Clinical Medicine, ed 3. 2002, Mosby, Edinburgh. Reproduced by kind permission.)

Figure 2.11 Koilonychia. (From Forbes CD, Jackson WF. Color Atlas and Text of Clinical Medicine, ed 3. 2002, Mosby, Edinburgh. Reproduced by kind permission.)

of longstanding iron deficiency and is owing to defective collagen formation, which can also cause blue sclerae. Leuconychia (opaque white nails) may occur in chronic liver disease and other conditions associated with hypoalbuminaemia (Fig. 2.12), but are not particularly useful for making a clinical diagnosis of chronic liver disease.

Beau's lines are horizontal (transverse) depressions in the nail that may result from any disease process, illness, chemotherapy or malnutrition that constitutes a sufficient insult to affect the growth plate of the nail. Fingernails grow at a rate of 0.1 mm per day, so the timing of the disease onset can be estimated by measuring the distance from the Beau's line to the nail bed. They disappear over several months as the nail grows out.

Odours

Certain odours may provide diagnostic clues. The odour of alcohol on the patient's breath is easily recognizable, but do not assume that an alcoholic foetor implies alcoholism or that all the patient's current symptoms

and signs are related to alcohol intoxication. Patients with alcohol dependence may have reversible problems, such as hypoglycaemia or a subdural haematoma. The odour of diabetic ketoacidosis resembles acetone ('pear drops' or nail varnish remover) and those of hepatic failure and uraemia have been described as 'ammonia-like' or 'mousy,' respectively, but such terms are rather subjective and their use is limited. Halitosis (bad breath) is common in patients with suppurative lung diseases and in those with gingivitis owing to poor dental hygiene. As with all smells, they are difficult to describe but can be characteristic when previously experienced and learned.

Face and neck

In addition to the important expressions and features of mood and attitude noted above, important diagnostic clues may easily be apparent on inspection of the face. Examination of the cranial nerves is covered in Chapter 16, but palsies of the III (Fig. 16.5) and VII (Fig. 2.13) nerves may be obvious simply on inspection. Parotid swellings are usually easily apparent; the tender bilateral parotid swelling of mumps or the unilateral swelling with reddening of the skin from acute parotitis contrasts with the non-tender bilateral enlargement that sometimes accompanies chronic alcohol use (and possibly accompanying liver disease). Some patients with mitral stenosis have a bright, circumscribed flush over the malar bones, and in some patients with systemic lupus erythematosus there is a red raised eruption on the bridge of the nose extending onto the cheeks in a 'butterfly' distribution (Fig. 2.14). Telangiectasias, minute capillary tortuosities, may be seen on the face of patients with liver disease and, rarely, as a hereditary disorder (Fig. 2.15). In systemic sclerosis, radial puckering (furrows) may be seen around the mouth (Fig. 2.16) that, as the skin becomes tighter, limits the extent to which the mouth may be opened (Fig. 2.17).

Figure 2.13   A, B. Lower motor neuron palsy of the right facial nerve (Bell's palsy).

Figure 2.14   Classic butterfly wing rash in a young patient with systemic lupus erythematosus.

Figure 2.15   Hereditary telangiectasia. The telangiectasia can be seen at the margin of the lips and on the lower lip.

Neck swellings are usually best felt from behind the patient. The general principles of lymph node palpation are described below, and the details of examination of the thyroid are covered in Chapter 19.

Lymph glands and lymphadenopathy

Details pertaining to the examination of specific lymph node groups may be found in the relevant chapters (e.g. Chapter 22 for cervical lymphadenopathy). Here, the general principles of palpating for lymphadenopathy will be covered. Lymph nodes are interposed along the course of lymphatic channels, and their enlargement should always be noted. Lymph from the arm drains into the axillary nodes. These should be examined routinely, but particularly in conjunction with examination of the breast

The neck should be inspected and palpated. Examination of the jugular venous pulse is described in detail in Chapter 13, but it is an important part of the examination in all patients, not just those with suspected cardiovascular disease. It may contribute useful information regarding the severity of lung disease, and its careful assessment is particularly important in patients suspected of having a disturbance of fluid and electrolyte balance.

Figure 2.16   Radial puckering (furrows) around the mouth in systemic sclerosis.

Figure 2.17   Limited mouth opening in systemic sclerosis.

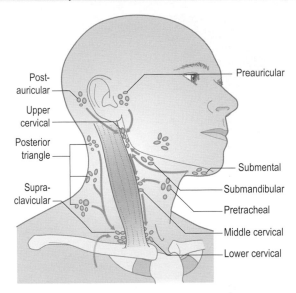

Figure 2.18   The cervical lymph node groups.

Examination of lymph nodes involves inspection and palpation. Inflammation of the overlying skin and any associated pain usually implies an infective aetiology, whereas malignant lymphadenopathy is usually not tender. To palpate for lymphadenopathy, use the pulps of your fingers (usually the index and middle but, for large nodes, the ring finger as well) to move the skin overlying the potentially enlarged node(s). Determine the size, position, shape, consistency, mobility, tenderness of the node and whether it is an isolated lymph node or whether several coalesce. For the head and neck nodes, it is often helpful to tilt the head slightly towards the side of examination in order to relax the overlying muscles. Feel for each of the groups shown in Figure 2.18 in whatever order you find most efficient and reliable. Muscles and arteries in the neck and groin may be mistaken for lymph nodes. If in doubt, try to move the structure in question in two directions (laterally and superior to inferior). It should be possible to move a lymph node in two directions, but not an artery or muscle.

Determining whether a lymph node is pathological can be difficult and requires practice and experience. In general, small, mobile, discrete lymph nodes are frequently found in normal individuals, particularly those who are slim and have little overlying adipose tissue. The finding of an enlarged lymph node should prompt the question 'Is this consequent upon local pathology, for example infection or malignancy, or is it part of a more generalized abnormality of the reticuloendothelial system (including other lymph node groups, liver and spleen)?' (Fig. 2.19).

Axillae

Most information from examination of the axillae comes from palpation for possible lymphadenopathy (Fig. 2.20), but inspection may reveal an absence/

(see below). Lymph from the lower limbs drains via deep and superficial inguinal nodes, although only the latter can be palpated and, in turn, comprise a vertical and horizontal group. The vertical inguinal nodes lie close to the upper part of the long saphenous vein and drain the leg. The horizontal group lies above the inguinal ligament and drains the lower abdominal skin, anal canal, external genitalia (excluding the testes), buttocks and lower vagina.

Figure 2.19 Gross enlargement of supraclavicular and cervical lymph nodes. (From Forbes CD, Jackson WF. Color Atlas and Text of Clinical Medicine, ed 3. 2002, Mosby, Edinburgh. Reproduced by kind permission.)

Figure 2.20 Gross (in this case, painless) axillary lymph node enlargement. (From Forbes CD, Jackson WF. Color Atlas and Text of Clinical Medicine, ed 3. 2002, Mosby, Edinburgh. Reproduced by kind permission.)

Figure 2.21 Acanthosis nigricans (sometimes seen in insulin resistance and gastric cancer) visible in the axilla.

Figure 2.22 Freckling and neurofibromas in von Recklinghausen's disease.

of insulin resistance and occasionally gastric cancer, Fig. 2.21), or (very rarely and almost always in the presence of café au lait spots elsewhere) the characteristic freckling of von Recklinghausen's disease (Fig. 2.22).

Support the weight of the patient's arm by holding his arm at the elbow with your non-examining hand so that the patient's pectoral muscles are relaxed. With the fingers of your right hand cupped together, probe the apex of the left axilla, then slide them downwards against the chest wall to feel for lymphadenopathy. Next, 'sweep' your fingers along the inside of the anterior and posterior axillary folds, feeling for enlargement of the pectoral and subscapular lymph nodes, respectively. Use your left hand in the same way to examine the right axilla.

Skin

Examination of the skin with respect to specific dermatological diagnoses is covered in Chapter 20. In the context of the general examination, the most important features relate to temperature, hydration, pallor, colour/pigmentation and cyanosis. Use the back of your fingers to assess the temperature of the skin. This complements rather than replaces the formal measurement with a thermometer. You

paucity of secondary sexual hair in either gender (most commonly in association with chronic liver disease, but also in certain endocrinopathies), abnormal skin colouring, such as the dark velvety appearance of acanthosis nigricans (characteristic

Figure 2.23 Advanced scleroderma. (From Forbes CD, Jackson WF. Color Atlas and Text of Clinical Medicine, ed 3. 2002, Mosby, Edinburgh. Reproduced by kind permission.)

Figure. 2.24 Jaundiced skin. The deep yellow colour is caused by high levels of conjugated bilirubin. This patient also had gynaecomastia owing to chronic liver disease. (From Forbes CD, Jackson WF. Color Atlas and Text of Clinical Medicine, ed 3. 2002, Mosby, Edinburgh. Reproduced by kind permission.)

may note generalized warmth in febrile illness or thyrotoxicosis or localized warmth if there is regional inflammation. Cold skin may be localized, such as when a limb is deprived of its blood supply, or generalized in states of circulatory failure, when the skin feels clammy and sweaty.

Lift a fold of skin and make note of its thickness, mobility and how easily it returns to its original position (turgor). The skin on the back of the hand is often thin and fragile in elderly patients; it may show decreased mobility in scleroderma (Fig. 2.23) or in oedematous states and have reduced turgor in the presence of dehydration. The skin of patients who are acromegalic is typically thick and greasy.

Note the colour of the skin (the following description is less relevant to people with dark skin). Normal skin colour varies considerably; some people have a fresh complexion and others, although completely healthy, a pale one. Pallor may be seen temporarily in the context of haemorrhage, shock and intense emotion. Patients who are anaemic are often pale, but not all pale people are anaemic. The colour of the mucous membrane of the eyelids and mouth is a better indication of anaemia than the colour of the skin.

Yellowness of the skin is usually caused by jaundice (Fig. 2.24). A pale lemon-yellow tinge is characteristic of haemolytic jaundice, whereas in obstructive jaundice there is a dark yellow or orange tint, sometimes accompanied by scratch marks from itching caused by bile salts. Lemon tinge may also be associated with uraemia, which may occasionally also cause a 'frosting' of the lips or forehead, the so-called 'uraemic frost,' which only occurs when the blood urea has been very high for several days.

An important determinant of skin colour is the relative amount of oxyhaemoglobin and deoxyhaemoglobin. Oxyhaemoglobin is a bright red pigment. An increase in its flow beneath thinned facial skin causes the characteristic plethora of Cushing's syndrome (Fig. 2.25), whereas a decrease in flow causes pallor. As blood passes through the capillary bed, oxygen is given up to metabolizing tissues to produce deoxyhaemoglobin. This has a darker, less red, more bluish pigment, and its presence in peripheral blood vessels in increased amounts causes the clinical sign of cyanosis. There are two physiological types of cyanosis:

Figure 2.25 The characteristic plethoric appearance of a patient with Cushing's syndrome. (From Forbes CD, Jackson WF. Color Atlas and Text of Clinical Medicine, ed 3. 2002, Mosby, Edinburgh. Reproduced by kind permission.)

peripheral and central. Peripheral cyanosis is associated with increased extraction of oxygen from capillaries when peripheral blood flow is slowed, often owing to vasospasm caused by cold, heart failure or anxiety. The cyanosed extremity is usually cold and the tongue is unaffected. Any condition causing slowing of the peripheral circulation may lead to peripheral cyanosis because there is more time for oxygen extraction. Central cyanosis is caused by inadequate oxygenation of blood, in turn owing to heart failure, serious respiratory disease or mixing of venous and arterial blood across a right to left cardiac shunt. In the latter situation, a proportion of deoxygenated blood passes directly from the right to the left side of the

Figure 2.26 Central cyanosis in a patient with severe respiratory disease (*left*) compared with the tongue of a (*right*) normal person. (From Forbes CD, Jackson WF. Color Atlas and Text of Clinical Medicine, ed 3. 2002, Mosby, Edinburgh. Reproduced by kind permission.)

heart, without passing through the pulmonary circulation, thereby 'missing out' on the opportunity to become oxygenated. Central cyanosis is generalized and the peripheries are often warm. At least 5 g/dL of reduced haemoglobin is necessary to produce central cyanosis; therefore, it is less marked in patients who are anaemic. The cyanosis of heart failure is often towing to both peripheral and central causes. The presence of central cyanosis is best appreciated at the lips, mucous membranes and conjunctivae, where the keratinized skin is thinnest (Fig. 2.26).

Pulses

Arterial pulses are detected by compressing the relevant vessel against a firm underlying structure, usually a bone. Details of the characteristic pulse abnormalities that help in the diagnosis of various cardiac disorders are described in Chapter 13, but palpation of all the peripheral pulses should form part of the general examination of all patients. Some may be difficult to feel and you may need to vary the degree of pressure in order to pick up the relevant pulsation. On occasion, you may confuse the patient's pulse with your own. Feel your own pulse on the side of your forehead with your other hand and compare it with the patient's, as they will usually differ.

The radial pulse is palpated by gentle pressure of the artery against the distal shaft of the radius, using the tips of the index and middle fingers. It provides information about rate and rhythm, although significant abnormalities in character may also be detected. If the rhythm is regular, it is safe to count the number of beats for 15 seconds and multiply by 4 for the rate. Irregular and very slow pulses require palpation for a full minute. Palpating both radial pulses simultaneously can give useful information in selected patients. Atheromatous narrowing of the axillary artery may cause reduced strength of one radial pulse compared with the other, as may aortic dissection or compression of a subclavian artery by a cervical rib.

To palpate the femoral pulse, press deeply below the inguinal ligament, midway between the anterior superior iliac spine and the symphysis pubis. The pulse is usually easily felt against the underlying femur. In obese patients it may be useful to use two hands, one on top of the other. Occasionally, such as in young patients with hypertension, it may be appropriate to examine for radio-femoral delay. Here, the radial and femoral pulses on one side of the body are palpated at the same time. The pulsation should occur simultaneously; any delay may suggest coarctation of the aorta, in which the aorta is constricted just beyond the subclavian artery. Blood flow to the arms is good, but to the legs is poor such that the pulse is weak and delayed.

The popliteal pulse is the most difficult to palpate. Flex the knee to approximately 120° with the foot on the bed, and, with your thumbs on the patella, place your fingers in the popliteal fossa such that they meet in the midline. Occasionally, it may be necessary to have the patient lie prone with the knee flexed to 90° and the leg resting against the shoulder or upper arm; press the thumbs deep into the popliteal fossa.

The dorsalis pedis pulse is palpated by pressing against the tarsal bones just lateral to the extensor tendon of the great toe, although in some patients it may be necessary to explore the dorsum of the foot more widely. In general, it is most convenient to use the right hand to examine the left dorsalis pedis pulse; the right pulse is often best felt with the right hand from the left side of the patient.

To feel the posterior tibial pulse, with the patient's foot relaxed between plantar- and dorsiflexion, press your curved fingers against the distal part of the tibia, approximately 1 cm behind and below the medial malleolus. The posterior tibial pulse may be difficult to feel and require extra patience and pressure in obese or oedematous patients.

Blood pressure

The physiology of blood pressure measurement (including a description of the Korotkoff sounds) is given in Chapter 13. Many doctors and medical students neglect to measure the blood pressure routinely in the belief that it is somehow a 'nursing' observation. This is a poor habit to adopt, not least because, once the technique has been mastered, it can be combined easily with simultaneous, unobtrusive observations of the patient that may provide useful diagnostic information without him feeling self-conscious. Although not necessary or appropriate to perform routinely, assessment for postural (orthostatic) hypotension is frequently informative in older patients, particularly those with symptoms of unsteadiness, syncope or presyncope, or those taking medication for hypertension. It is

Figure 2.27   Peripheral vascular disease. Seen are pallor, loss of hair and early ulceration on the dorsum of three toes. (From Forbes CD, Jackson WF. Color Atlas and Text of Clinical Medicine, ed 3. 2002, Mosby, Edinburgh. Reproduced by kind permission.)

defined as a drop in blood pressure of greater than 20/10 mmHg within 3 minutes of changing from a supine to an upright position. Various 'protocols' are adopted; the authors favour measurement of blood pressure supine after a period of calm rest and then every minute for 3 minutes after moving to a vertical position. Together with assessment of the jugular venous pulse, it can provide important information about volume status in the evaluation of patients with fluid and electrolyte abnormalities and those with recent gastrointestinal bleeding.

Legs and feet

Examination of the legs requires adequate exposure from the groins and buttocks to the toes. Note the colour and texture of the skin. Peripheral vascular disease often makes the skin shiny and hair does not grow on ischaemic legs or feet (Fig. 2.27). Pressure on the toes of ischaemic feet will cause blanching of the characteristic purple colour, with subsequent slow return. Passive elevation of an ischaemic leg leads to marked pallor of the foot as perfusion against gravity falls (Buerger's test). Painless trophic lesions, often with deep ulceration, may be seen in diabetic peripheral neuropathy. The posterior aspect of the heels is a particularly important area to inspect in elderly, emaciated or neurologically impaired patients, all of whom are vulnerable to pressure ulcers caused by obliteration of arteriolar and capillary blood flow to the skin.

Inspect the legs for easily seen oedema (fluid in the subcutaneous tissue that appears as swelling) and examine for pitting oedema. Press firmly but gently behind the medial malleolus, over the dorsum of the foot and on the shin. If oedema is present, a depression/concavity will form and persist for some time (Fig. 2.28). The skin over oedematous feet and shins has a pallid, glossy appearance and

Figure 2.28   Pitting oedema in a patient with cardiac failure. A depression remains in the oedema for several minutes after firm fingertip pressure is applied. (From Forbes CD, Jackson WF. Color Atlas and Text of Clinical Medicine, ed 3. 2002, Mosby, Edinburgh. Reproduced by kind permission.)

Figure 2.29   Varicose veins. (From Forbes CD, Jackson WF. Color Atlas and Text of Clinical Medicine, ed 3. 2002, Mosby, Edinburgh. Reproduced by kind permission.)

a characteristic doughy feel. The best place to look for mild degrees of oedema in cardiac disease is behind the malleoli in patients who are ambulant and over the sacrum in those who are confined to bed. Usually, 5 to 10 seconds of finger pressure is sufficient to produce the typical shallow pit, but it may be necessary to press for 20 to 30 seconds to avoid overlooking mild degrees of oedema. Some doctors grade oedema on a 4-point scale (slight and short-lived after relief of pressure to very marked and long lasting), although the system is poorly standardized. Oedema owing to cardiac disease or to conditions associated with a low plasma protein level is bilateral. In local venous obstruction the oedema is confined to the parts from which the return of blood is impeded. Thus, oedema of an arm occurs when malignant lymph nodes constrict the axillary vein, and unilateral leg oedema will develop if the ileofemoral vein is occluded. The oedema of lymphatic obstruction does not pit on pressure.

Varicose veins should be sought with the patient standing (Fig. 2.29). Superficial varicosities are generally obvious in this position, whereas the efficiency of the valves of the long saphenous vein should be assessed by Trendelenburg's test. With the patient lying, the saphenous vein is emptied by elevating the leg. Occlude the upper end of the vein by finger pressure on the saphenous vein opening (alternatively use a tourniquet) and ask the patient to stand while maintaining this pressure. If the valves are incompetent, the veins will rapidly fill from above when the pressure is released.

Venous thrombosis is rare in healthy mobile persons but frequently complicates enforced bed rest, particularly after surgery. The affected limb will be swollen. The circumference of the calf should be measured and compared with the unaffected leg at the same distance below the tibial tuberosity. A discrepancy of more than 1 cm is significant. The affected leg is also tender and warmer than normal, with dilated superficial veins, which do not collapse when the leg is elevated. Forceful dorsiflexion of the foot may cause pain in the calf (Homan's sign). Sometimes a deep vein thrombosis may extend up the thigh leading to a tender, hard, palpable femoral vein.

Breasts

Breast examination should form part of the routine clinical assessment, usually at the time of chest examination. It requires tact and sensitivity and should be conducted with a chaperone. With the patient disrobed to the waist, the arms should be in a relaxed position by the sides, usually starting with the patient sitting or standing. By inspection, note the size, symmetry, contour (e.g. any dimpling) and colour of the breasts. Inflammatory breast cancer with oedema of the overlying skin may produce a characteristic look and texture termed peau d'orange (orange peel skin). Note any asymmetry or nipple inversion. Simple, longstanding inversion is often a normal phenomenon, but associated retraction of the areola and recent nipple inversion are both more sinister. Ask the patient to raise her arms above her head. This manoeuvre allows inspection of the inframammary fold and may expose subtle contour abnormalities. Now, with the patient supine, ask the patient to rest one arm above her head. This helps spread the breast tissue more evenly across the chest and makes palpation of any nodules easier. For ease of annotation, the breast is usually divided into four quadrants, with the upper outer quadrant extending into an axillary tail. Use the pads of your middle three fingers to palpate the breast, using rotatory movements gently to compress the tissue against the chest wall. Proceed systematically to examine all quadrants, the tail and areola. Sometimes it is useful to support the breast with the other hand in order to aid examination, especially when the breasts are large.

Breast tissue varies among patients, ranging from smooth to granular, and may change in a given individual with the menstrual cycle. For any nodule, note its size, shape, consistency, tenderness, mobility and the presence of any tethering or skin ulceration. Ask the patient to press her hands against her hips. If the lump becomes less mobile, it is likely to be attached to the pectoral muscles. Fixation to skin may be assessed by moving the skin overlying the lump independently. If this is not possible then skin involvement is likely.

Swelling of male breast tissue is usually easily apparent (Fig. 2.30). Distinguishing true glandular enlargement from pectoral fat may be facilitated

Figure 2.30 Gynaecomastia in a male patient. (From Forbes CD, Jackson WF. Color Atlas and Text of Clinical Medicine, ed 3. 2002, Mosby, Edinburgh. Reproduced by kind permission.)

with the patient's arms above his head. At some stage of puberty, most boys will have a palpable disc of breast tissue.

Putting it all together

The information given in this and subsequent chapters describes techniques of physical examination that *may* be helpful in elucidating the cause of a patient's symptoms. It is not implicit that *all* of these examinations should be performed for *all* patients. For example, it is not appropriate to make a detailed assessment of the neurological system in someone in severe respiratory distress owing to pulmonary oedema or in abdominal pain from peritonitis. Initially, both alone and during teaching, you will probably practise examining individual systems (e.g. the cardiovascular system). Soon, however, you will be ready to conduct a complete examination. The following is a suggested order for the student to practise, and doctor to perform, in all hospitalized patients who are not acutely ill, in order to exclude any major abnormality in the various bodily systems.

General

- Overall appearance (well, unwell, severely ill; neglected or well-cared for).
- Posture and gait.
- Nutrition, obesity, oedema.
- Skin colour, cyanosis, jaundice, anaemia.

- Skin lesions (spider naevi, vitiligo, purpura, petechiae).
- Body hair (distribution, quantity).
- Vital signs (temperature, pulse, respiration rate).
- Obvious features of endocrine disease (e.g. Cushing's, acromegaly, hyperlipidaemia).

Mouth and pharynx

- Odours, lips, tongue (ask to protrude), teeth, gums, buccal mucous membrane, tonsils.

Hands

- Clubbing, tremor, wasting, arthropathy, metabolic flap, Dupuytren's contracture, splinter haemorrhages, nailfold infarcts, koilonychia, leuconychia, nicotine stains.

Cardiovascular and respiratory (anterior, patient semi-recumbent)

- Radial pulse: rate, rhythm, character.
- Blood pressure, lying and standing.
- Jugular venous pulse.
- Carotid pulses, separately, both sides.
- Inspection for symmetry, scars, dilated vessels, breasts, nipples.
- Praecordial palpation: apex beat, thrills, heaves.
- Auscultate the heart sounds.
- Palpate tracheal position.
- Chest expansion.
- Tactile vocal fremitus.
- Percuss the lungs.
- Auscultate the breath sounds.
- Vocal resonance.

Cardiovascular and respiratory (posterior, sitting forward)

- Inspect for symmetry of movement, scars.
- Chest expansion.
- Tactile vocal fremitus.
- Percuss the lungs.
- Auscultate the breath sounds.
- Vocal resonance.
- Inspect for sacral oedema.

Neck (while sitting forward)

- Thyroid palpation.
- Cervical, submandibular lymphadenopathy.

Abdomen

- Inspection: size, distension, asymmetry, scars, abdominal wall movements, dilated vessels, visible peristalsis, pulsations, pubic hair, spider naevi.

- Palpation: tenderness, rigidity, hyperaesthesia, masses, organomegaly, hernial orifices, inguinal lymphadenopathy, genitalia, digital rectal (where relevant).
- Percussion: organomegaly, masses.
- Auscultation: bowel sounds, bruits.

Upper limbs

- Inspection: fasciculations, wasting, trophic changes.
- Test for tone, power, reflexes, coordination and cutaneous sensation.
- Test joints for swelling, pain and movement, if relevant.

Lower limbs

- Inspection: fasciculations, wasting, trophic changes, ulceration, varicose veins, oedema.
- Test for tone, power, reflexes, coordination and cutaneous sensation.
- Test joints for swelling, pain and movement, if relevant.
- Peripheral pulses.

Cranial nerves

- Visual acuity, pupillary responses, visual fields, extraocular movements, nystagmus fundoscopy.
- Facial movements and sensation.
- Rinne and Weber test.
- Palatal elevation, tongue appearance and protrusion.

Documentation and communication

An accurate, concise record of a clinical episode is crucial for effective care. It serves as a tool for ordering the doctor's thoughts as he reviews the findings before constructing a provisional differential diagnosis. It may identify errors or missing data (did I examine the reflexes?). It serves as a reminder of those thought processes at future consultations as the results of investigations become available and/or the condition evolves, and it allows colleagues to pick up the 'thread' of a case if the initial assessing doctor is unavailable. Furthermore, as rising expectations and increasing availability of medical information via the Internet embolden more patients to question the quality of their care, accurate documentation is vital in order to provide the evidence for the quality of the decision-making and assessment in the event of a disagreement between patient and doctor. All medical note entries should be dated, timed and signed and each page should have the patient's name and hospital record number clearly written. In many countries, this is now automatic on account of the increasing use of electronic (paperless) medical records. Although, in many ways, a major

advance, the increasing use of electronic records carries new possibilities for error, particularly for patients with chronic illness or those whose hospital stay is prolonged. 'Cutting and pasting' the original assessment and problem list into the clinical record at subsequent inpatient or outpatient encounters has the potential to perseverate (well-intentioned) error that may have arisen from incomplete information and/or lack of availability of initial results. It is the authors' view that, in the era of electronic notes, maintaining diagnostic rigour and 'open-mindedness' requires extra discipline; something it is never too early to practice.

The style and extent of note-taking will vary according to circumstance. For example, a postoperative visit to a surgical outpatient clinic after a routine hernia repair is likely to focus exclusively on issues relating to pain and scar healing, with brief documentation. In contrast, the initial consultation at a falls clinic will involve the expert in elderly medicine gathering potentially relevant information about past medical history, current medication, social support and the history of the current problem, and will certainly require a comprehensive physical examination. A General Practitioner likely already knows the details of the patient's family, social, past medical and drug histories, so in the limited time available will focus on the current problem. In all of these situations, however, the clinician should avoid being constantly engaged in writing notes or, increasingly, looking at a computer screen. Maintain eye contact as the patient talks about his problems. The following suggestions refer to a new patient consultation in the outpatient clinic or a non-acutely ill hospitalized patient. The goal is to write a complete yet concise record of the patient's problem that can be followed easily as a logical narrative by the next doctor to see that patient.

Start with the routine social data: name, address, marital status, occupation, dependent family members and children. The order in which the family, past medical and presenting complaint histories are documented is not rigidly set. For those patients who have enjoyed good health to the point of the current illness, the presenting complaint and history of the current problem fall naturally out of the context of the above background information. Medical notes for such a patient with (for example) a spontaneous pneumothorax might read as follows:

Mr JW, aged 32, manual labourer, married, 2 children. Generally in excellent health and symptom free.
  Keen sportsman.
No relevant past medical history.
Presenting complaint (PC): Breathlessness.
History of presenting complaint (HPC):

- Sudden-onset right-sided chest pain.
- Worse on inspiration.
- Associated severe breathlessness; unable to get comfortable.

- No cough or sputum or haemoptysis.
- No injury or trauma to chest.
- No previous similar episodes.
- No recent periods of immobility.
- No leg swelling or pain.

Past medical history (PMH):
- Appendectomy age 6.
- Varicocoele found and surgically corrected age 25 following assessment for primary infertility.

An important differential diagnosis in a patient with pneumothorax is pulmonary embolism, sometimes with prior deep venous thrombosis. The 'negative' features of the history (no leg symptoms, no recent immobility) 'steer' the narrative and any subsequent reader of the history away from this diagnosis, but they serve as a focus for its consideration. If a rigid system were recommended of documenting all *potentially* relevant past medical and family history prior to the presenting problem, the same history might read:

Mr JW, age 32, manual labourer, married, 2 children. Generally in excellent health and symptom free. Keen sportsman.

No family history of deep vein thrombosis or pulmonary embolism. No family history of tall stature, lens dislocation, valvular heart disease (all features of Marfan's syndrome, an important association with pneumothorax in young patients). Varicocoele surgery age 25 with no history of postoperative deep vein thrombosis or pulmonary embolism.

PC: Breathlessness.

HPC:
- Sudden-onset right-sided chest pain.
- Worse on inspiration.
- Associated severe breathlessness; unable to get comfortable.
- No cough or sputum or haemoptysis.
- No injury or trauma to chest.
- No previous similar episodes.
- No recent periods of immobility.
- No leg swelling or pain.

Although used as an extreme example, such a style of documentation could 'obstruct access' to the presenting complaint. For many patients, however, it *is* appropriate to detail a pertinent family history and/or past medical history prior to the current problem or as an 'introduction/context' to it. Good examples of this would include a middle-aged man with rectal bleeding and a strong family history of carcinoma of the colon, or a young person, breathless on exertion, who underwent corrective surgery for congenital heart disease as a child. For other patients, the current problem is the latest development of a long-standing illness, such as cough and breathlessness in a patient with chronic obstructive pulmonary disease. This skill of interweaving the past/family history with the current problem will develop with experience, so do not be disheartened if your notes initially seem disjointed.

Box 2.2	Example of a cardiovascular system statement

- Pulse 76 regular, peripheral pulses normal
- Neck veins not distended. No peripheral oedema
- BP 130/80
- Apex beat not displaced
- Heart sounds I and II heard in all areas
- No murmurs, lungs clear

Many patients have had medical and surgical episodes in their history that are essentially 'closed events'; for example cataract removal, hernia repair or tonsillectomy as a child. Although they may seem irrelevant to the current problem, they may subsequently provide important useful information and it is important to document them meticulously. For example, knowing that a bilateral oophorectomy was performed at the time of a hysterectomy is helpful information in the assessment of a woman with ascites. The past medical history (if accurate) makes a diagnosis of carcinoma of the ovary highly improbable. Documentation of any surgical procedures, however minor, can provide reassuring or helpful anticipatory information in patients likely to undergo general anaesthesia. Recording of the history concludes with the full list of drugs, dosages and dosing intervals, any adverse reactions to previously prescribed medicines and documentation of the review of systems (see Chapter 1).

Details of the physical examination should be documented in a clear, structured framework. Start with a general, non-judgemental comment about the patient's overall appearance, such as 'well man with moderate generalized adiposity' or 'drawn, anxious woman, breathless on undressing'. Record important positive and negative features on general examination, for example jaundice, clubbing, rash, fever, lymphadenopathy. The remainder of the examination should be documented under bodily systems: cardiovascular, respiratory, gastrointestinal (often referred to as abdominal), nervous system, skin, limbs and joints. Negative findings are often as pertinent as positive ones. Simple line drawings are often particularly effective. A concise summary of the findings in the cardiovascular system might read as in Box 2.2.

The case notes should conclude with a brief summary of the history and the major abnormalities found on examination, which leads to the differential diagnosis and management plan (Boxes 2.3 and 2.4).

Presenting a case

It is very valuable to your learning to practice making short summaries of your findings, emphasizing both important positive findings and relevant negative ones. The summary should begin with the name, age, sex and occupation of the patient and end with a

| Box 2.3 | Framework of pathological processes informing a differential diagnosis |

- Congenital
- Degenerative
- Infective/inflammatory
- Metabolic
- Neoplastic
- Nutritional
- Toxic
- Traumatic
- Vascular

| Box 2.4 | Order of tasks to follow when constructing a provisional management plan |

1. List the monitoring/nursing recommendations that are imperative to the patient's immediate comfort, wellbeing and safety.
2. List the investigations that need to be done immediately (e.g. blood cultures and malaria film in a patient returning from overseas with a fever of unknown origin).
3. Document the medications you propose to prescribe, including the dosages and frequency of administration (this includes intravenous fluid therapy).
4. List the investigations that may need to be done at some stage in order to provide further diagnostic information.

brief statement of the problem. Another important skill to acquire is that of oral presentations of the cases you see to colleagues; the ultimate test is the ability to communicate a difficult problem to a senior colleague on the telephone. The history and findings on examination should be communicated in temporal, coherent order, making an interesting and easily grasped narrative.

Summary

Ultimately, the goal is for the clinician to use a combination of experience, knowledge and appreciation of the accuracy and limitations of history taking and examination to try to come to a correct diagnosis, or diagnoses, and facilitate the best treatment with the least discomfort and anxiety for the patient. As with everything described in this chapter, no substitute exists for practice and an open-ended willingness to learn from both success and error.

The next steps: 3
Differential diagnosis and initial management

Michael Glynn

Introduction

The term 'Differential Diagnosis' used to be very widely used by doctors, but it now seems to be used less, and is less well understood. It might be better termed as 'Differential Diagnoses', because the process of preparing it is to formulate a list of possible diagnoses that cover the presenting clinical situation, usually written in the descending order of likelihood. It is a very important part of the overall treatment of a patient from initial presentation, particularly in the emergency situation. Hopefully, the doctor clerking a patient will write a thorough history and complete a detailed examination. He may write a good plan of treatment, but the intermediate step of preparing the differential diagnoses is often missed or replaced by something which is entitled 'Impression', which often only considers one possibility. Box 3.1 gives three illustrations of situations in which the 'Impression' is too restrictive, whereas a full differential diagnosis would allow the treating doctors to consider the full range of possibilities, including those that are quite rare, but nevertheless vitally important if present.

One of the most common reasons for attendance at an Emergency Department with chest pain is because the patient himself or a referring doctor is worried that the chest pain is of cardiac origin. This is the reason a receiving doctor might write 'chest pain, rule out cardiac cause' as the overall 'impression'. However, there are other causes of acute chest pain, both common and rare. There is often a feeling that suggesting rare diagnoses opens avenues of investigations that are time consuming and expensive, but this is far from the truth. For instance, it may take only brief consideration that the patient may have a dissecting thoracic aortic aneurysm to return to the patient and clarify the character of the chest pain (dissecting aneurysms produce pain that is tearing in nature and clearly going through from front to back) and to check the blood pressure in both arms. Together with a simple chest X-ray, this may be sufficient evidence to exclude a dissecting thoracic aortic aneurysm without the need to resort to an emergency computed tomography (CT) scan.

The most common cause of an acute headache is probably a tension headache. There is no useful test for this and the diagnosis will largely be made

on history. Particularly in the emergency situation, some very serious causes of acute headache must not be missed, such as a subarachnoid haemorrhage or a sagittal sinus thrombosis. Careful and accurate differentiation between these two is clearly imperative because anticoagulation for a suspected sagittal sinus thrombosis would be completely the wrong treatment for a subarachnoid haemorrhage.

The process of differential diagnosis does not mean that every single possible cause needs to be specifically excluded in every clinical situation. However, having the full list of differential diagnoses written down helps the doctor weigh the likelihood of each one and then clarify the situation as is appropriate to the particular clinical situation. This clarification will not necessarily mean arranging complex investigations. It might mean just a mental

Box 3.1	Samples of common emergency medical problems and the contrast between a simple 'impression' and a full list of 'differential diagnoses'

Presenting problem	Impression	Differential diagnoses
Chest pain	Rule out cardiac cause	Acute coronary syndrome Pulmonary embolus Gastro-oesophageal reflux Musculoskeletal pain Dissecting thoracic aneurysm
Severe headache	Likely migraine	Tension headache Migraine Subarachnoid haemorrhage Temporal arteritis Sagittal sinus thrombosis
Apparent stroke	Cerebral infarction	Cerebral infarction (thrombus or embolus) Cerebral haemorrhage Carotid or vertebral dissection Hemiplegic migraine Brain tumour with haemorrhage Cerebral abscess Cerebral vasculitis

Box 3.2	Examples of key questions that help to confirm or refute specific diagnoses

Diagnosis	Key questions
Subarachnoid haemorrhage	▪ Was it the worst headache you have ever had? ▪ Did it start extremely suddenly like a blow on the head?
Diarrhoea caused by irritable bowel	▪ Does the need to open your bowels ever wake you from your sleep (rare in irritable bowel)?
Cardiac chest pain	▪ Does the pain feel like a weight pressing on your chest?
Intermittent claudication or angina pectoris	▪ Does the pain come on with a predictable amount of exercise?

check that the right specific questions have been asked or making sure that particular physical signs have been checked.

This reviewing, checking and clarification process that is mentally undertaken by the doctor clerking the patient is not something that needs to be delayed until the history and examination are completed. As the student and doctor become more experienced in the process of history and examination and the preparation of the differential diagnoses, they will begin to think through the patient's problems as soon as the consultation begins. The consultation will often be punctuated by key questions aimed at confirming or refuting a particular diagnosis that has occurred to the doctor during the course of the clerking process. Box 3.2 is a list of some key questions and the diagnoses to which they refer.

Management plan

Having obtained the history and examination details and formulated a list of differential diagnoses, the student or doctor needs to decide on what should happen next. As with everything clinical, what the patient actually wants is of paramount importance. Box 1.16 in Chapter 1 gives a list of the general scenarios that may lie behind a consultation between patient and doctor. Of particular relevance to the process of differential diagnosis and planning management is the degree to which patients want answers to queries or relief of symptoms. Quite a useful question can be 'Are you worried about your symptoms because of the trouble they give you and you want to be rid of them, because of what might be wrong, or both?' This can be quite a confusing question for the patient, but if explained carefully and answered specifically, it can avoid a lot of unnecessary investigation. In addition, starting out on the right track can make subsequent management much simpler, and it is often much easier to reassure

patients that nothing is seriously wrong than to give them an exact diagnosis or full relief of symptoms. This process particularly applies to a patient who has a fear of cancer. In a relatively young patient with quite harmless symptoms, even if a serious diagnosis is not really suspected, it may be necessary to perform some sort of investigation (such as an endoscopy or a CT/magnetic resonance image scan) to provide the necessary reassurance, even if it is not absolutely necessary for the process of resolving the differential diagnosis.

The priority of different investigations, the order in which they are done and the question of when treatment is given, all have to be considered and planned carefully. There is often quite a strong temptation for the doctor making the initial plan to start off with quite a large series of investigations. This is often done because the doctor assumes the patient needs the reassurance of normal tests and, to some extent, doctors need that reassurance themselves. There may even be a temptation to practice defensive medicine to avoid being accused in the future of under-investigating and missing diagnoses. However, this level of investigation is often not a productive way forward; it can overuse resources, sometimes prevent other patients having their tests in a timely manner, and, according to circumstance, can be financially detrimental to the individual patient. However, there may also be drawbacks to a logical series investigation and planning the next test only when the results of the first one are known. On occasions, this can seem a slow and tedious process for the patient, particularly if the health system allows only relatively infrequent patient review. Box 3.3 illustrates some clinical scenarios and the contrast in investigation style.

What to write in the case notes

Recording the possible differential diagnoses and the thinking behind them at the time of an initial consultation is a very important process, and can be crucial in getting to the correct diagnosis and avoiding the very real risk of neglecting a diagnosis that seemed very possible at the outset, but seems less likely as clinical events change. This is particularly true if the relevant symptoms are likely to become less severe after the initial presentation. An example might be a patient who presents with chest pain and who is hypoxic. When reassessed later, the hypoxia may have resolved and, if the original differential diagnosis is not reviewed, the diagnosis of pulmonary embolus might be overlooked. It is particularly good practice to write down the differential diagnostic list annotated either with confirmatory features for each possible diagnosis or any areas that lack confirmation. Such a list is given in Box 3.4.

Some items on a list of possible differential diagnoses may be more a result of a hunch on the part of the doctor rather than logical derivation

Box 3.3	Examples of clinical scenarios and contrasting investigation styles	
Clinical scenario	**Logical investigation**	**Immediate investigation**
Iron deficiency anaemia with dyspepsia in a man	Gastroscopy—if no ulcer, then colonoscopy—if no colonic source of blood loss, then do coeliac check and exclude or treat for parasites/worms	Gastroscopy and colonoscopy combined and a check for coeliac disease: exclude or treat for parasites/worms
Transient ischaemic attack	Carotid ultrasound—if no clear embolic source, then cardiac ECHO for possible cardiac source of emboli—if normal, then blood tests for hypercoagulability	Carotid ultrasound, cardiac ECHO and blood tests for hypercoagulability all arranged at the same time
Abnormal liver function tests without alcohol excess or medication side-effect	Blood tests for viral hepatitis and ultrasound if no cause found, then blood tests for rarer liver diseases	Do a full 'liver screen' in all patients, including tests for viral hepatitis, fatty liver disease and rarer liver diseases

Box 3.4	A 'model' write-up of a differential diagnostic list in a patient presenting as an emergency with chest pain (see Box 3.1), with relevant positive and negative pointers written down for each possible diagnosis

Differential diagnostic list	Key features
Acute coronary syndrome	Many risk factors, mildly raised initial troponin
Pulmonary embolus	Sudden onset, but pain not pleuritic, not hypoxic and no electrocardiographic change
Gastro-oesophageal reflux	Burning pain but no previous dyspeptic history
Musculoskeletal pain	Tender right lower anterior ribs
Dissecting thoracic aneurysm	Blood pressure same in both arms, no mediastinal widening on chest X-ray

What to say to the patient

Every doctor has a duty to be truthful with patients. However, this does not mean there is duty to tell a patient 'the whole of the medical textbook'. This means that there is a duty to say what is likely and also what is serious, the two not always coinciding. For example, in a patient aged 46 attending a gastro-enterology out-patient clinic with a change in bowel habit of 3 months' duration associated with some cramping abdominal pain and bloating and a few episodes of bright red rectal bleeding, the most likely diagnosis is not serious. A full differential list would include as relatively likely diagnoses, irritable bowel syndrome accompanied by some haemorrhoidal bleeding and also inflammatory bowel disease. A less likely but certainly a serious diagnosis would be the presence of colorectal cancer, which would be unusual at age 46, but certainly not unknown. Rare diagnoses might include gut vasculitis and ischaemic colitis. Good practice would be to say to the patient, 'I think you have irritable bowel syndrome accompanied by some haemorrhoidal bleeding, but to exclude inflammatory bowel disease and the unlikely possibility of bowel cancer, I recommend that you have a colonoscopy' (the rarer diagnoses do not need to be mentioned at this stage).

What to do when the diagnosis is unclear

At the outset, the diagnosis relevant to any clinical situation is almost always unclear. Occasionally the doctor may make a 'spot diagnosis', such as when a patient walks into the consulting room with obvious and previously undiagnosed Parkinson's disease, although the patient may have come with problems and issues that have a different underlying cause. After history and examination, the student or doctor will prepare a list of differential diagnoses

from the available information. This might particularly apply to conditions that have relatively vague presentations rather than with a classical symptom complex. An example might be putting Addison's disease on the differential diagnostic list of a patient who presents with a specific condition but has also been non-specifically unwell, has a relatively low systolic blood pressure and a sodium concentration below the lower limit of normal. The initial focus would be on treating the specific presentation. However, having Addison's disease on the differential list will allow this to be reviewed later and investigations planned, such as basal paired measurements of cortisol and corticotropin. Addison's disease would be a good example of a good style of clinical practice which states 'once you have thought of it, you need to exclude it'. This is particularly true in many areas of medicine which now rely on teamwork and doctors changing their duties from day to day. If the first doctor had considered Addison's disease as a possible diagnosis, it would often be unwise for a second doctor to come along and discard that possible diagnosis without arranging the specific test or at least considering it very carefully. This clinical approach applies in many situations, although each consultation is a clinical episode in its own right, and the doctor must make the best judgement of the clinical circumstance relevant at the time.

and will start a process of confirming or refuting those diagnoses, often with key investigations, or sometimes starting treatment and watching the effect of that treatment.

Doctors must be prepared for the not uncommon situation in which the diagnostic list appears to be exhausted and the patient's condition has not improved. It is at this point that the initial diagnostic list is particularly useful, to double check that it is complete and to rethink what level of testing is needed to confirm or refute any diagnoses. The list may well be reviewed in the light of how the clinical situation has evolved.

One particular issue will often arise that can be posed as the question, 'Which is more likely—a rare condition that has not yet been thought of, or a common condition that has been missed on the first round of testing?' This way of looking at a problem will often lead to the repeat of an examination (e.g. an upper gastrointestinal endoscopy) or an alternative look at the same problem (e.g. an abdominal CT scan following a normal ultrasound scan). It is certainly important to realise that every medical test has an error rate, even with the best quality control in laboratories and the highest standards in departments such as radiology and endoscopy.

Multiple causation

A common challenge facing the doctor is whether to accept the clinical findings on the basis of a single pathological process, or whether to invoke more than one bodily system or pathological process. This skill can be acquired only with time and experience but, in general, younger patients, shorter histories and examination findings confined to a single organ system tend to favour a single cause, whereas multiple causation is more likely among older patients with symptoms and signs in more than one bodily system.

Selecting appropriate investigations

As with history taking and physical examination, judicious selection of appropriate investigations to clarify a patient's diagnosis is a skill that develops through teaching, practice and a willingness to learn from mistakes. This is increasingly true as access to high-definition radiological imaging becomes more widespread and the vast majority of haematological and biochemical investigations are automated and provided as a 'package' rather than individually selected. Although it might instinctively be thought by the student that the easy availability of such data could only be beneficial to a patient (i.e. lead to the fortuitous diagnosis of unsuspected disease), in many cases it can lead to unnecessary expense and patient anxiety. This is because asymptomatic benign lesions identified on imaging or minor disturbances of haematological/biochemical parameters often necessitate further investigation and surveillance.

Ask yourself the following questions when considering which investigations to request:

- Will this test confirm/complement the information derived from the history and examination?
- Will this test provide new information (such as a chest X-ray in a patient with a productive cough and weight loss but no physical findings on examination)?
- Could this test provide useful information over a period of time as a marker of disease progression (e.g. the inflammatory markers erythrocyte sedimentation rate (ESR) and C-reactive protein (CRP) in a patient with infective endocarditis. Neither test is specific for the diagnosis, but changes in both values may be useful markers of disease progression)?
- What are the possibilities of this test yielding clinically irrelevant/distracting information compared with a diagnostically informative result? A good example of this would be the indiscriminate use of cranial computed tomography (CT) scans in patients with ill-defined neurological symptoms (such as dizziness) before a detailed neurological examination has been performed. Meningiomas (benign tumours arising from the meninges) are not-infrequent findings in patients undergoing cranial imaging. In a patient with dizziness without other neurological symptoms or signs, such a finding is likely to be irrelevant and, because the meningioma will need routine surveillance, is likely to cause unnecessary anxiety. In contrast, the finding of a meningioma in a patient with a carefully taken history of focal seizures is likely to be highly relevant (and, in fact, a reassuring finding for many patients because the differential diagnosis includes many other, more aggressive, brain tumours with a bleak outlook).
- What are the potential risks and discomfort to the patient of the proposed test (including the risk of unnecessary anxiety generated by an irrelevant finding demanding further evaluation)? In the case of routine haematological and biochemical tests requiring straightforward venipuncture, the immediate risk (aside from minor discomfort) is extremely low. In the case of coronary angiography, the risk of death is around 0.1% and of serious complication (myocardial infarction, stroke, arrhythmia, cardiac perforation) approximately 1.7%. Following a kidney biopsy, the risk of a haemorrhage sufficiently severe to require an emergency nephrectomy is around 0.0003% (1 in 3000). In these and other situations, the clinician must balance benefit and risk. The benefit can be diagnostic information leading to targeted treatment of a serious illness, or excluding problems for which the treatment has significant risk. The risk is that of the investigation itself or of the anxiety or distress that it may provoke.

■ What information does the laboratory and/or radiology department require to make this test maximally useful? A biopsy or surgical specimen sent to the pathology laboratory is likely to yield much more diagnostic information when accompanied by clinical details and a specific question than if delivered, speculatively, without either.

Conclusion

The process of formulating a set of differential diagnoses is simple, quick, rewarding, and without cost. Clinicians must keep it in the forefront of their mind when attending to patients, after the initial assessment, and then revise and refine as the clinical journey progresses.

Ethical considerations | 4

William M. Drake

Introduction

The cornerstone of a good relationship between doctor and patient is trust. In primary care, this relationship (often in the context of caring for the whole family) may be built up over several years, but in hospital practice or in an emergency, the patient and the doctor may be meeting for the first time. Patients expect a high standard of behaviour and care when they seek medical help. This includes the following expectations:

- They will be consulted about decisions bearing on their treatment.
- They will be informed about their illness.
- They will be informed about the likely outcome of any treatment offered.
- Their right to confidentiality will be respected.

Always assume that a patient is able fully to understand the nature of the medical problem and its implications, regardless of your impression of educational level. Some patients like to discuss what they would like to know early in a consultation and many will say clearly what information they would like to be given to the family. Occasionally, family members may feel that the patient would not be able to comprehend medical information or ask that he be 'protected' from the full details of a serious illness. Patients may insist that they do not wish the family to know about their medical problems or, sometimes, that they themselves do not wish to know the diagnosis. In all such instances, the needs and rights of each individual patient should be considered paramount, over and above those of the family, in the event of conflict.

Autonomy

The fundamental principle underlying medical ethics is autonomy: patients have the right to decide their own medical destiny. This gives rise to the concept of seeking the patient's consent for medical interventions, for research and for teaching. Only in the case of a minor or a mentally disturbed person may consent be sought from the patient's lawful parents or guardians. Assent, but not consent, may be sought from relatives, such as in the case of an unconscious patient in an intensive care unit. The doctor therefore has a duty not only to advise but also to explain. This principle crosses all religious and cultural boundaries.

Consent

The patient's consent should be sought for any treatment, however minor, even when that consent might appear implicit as, for example, by attendance at an emergency unit with injury. Sometimes assessment of a minor symptom discloses a separate, more serious issue. In such circumstances, consent to investigate the new problem is required.

To give consent, a patient must have sufficient, accurate information about the illness in order to make an informed judgement about whether its investigation and treatment are justified. There are four requirements of the doctor discussing an intervention with a patient:

1. The procedure itself must be described, including the technique, its implications and the intended benefit of doing it.
2. Information about the risks and complications must be given, which usually means all the risks, as well as some information about the consequences of any complication.
3. Associated risks (e.g. from anaesthesia or from other drugs that may be necessary) should be described.
4. Alternative medical or surgical investigations or treatments should be discussed, so that the reasons for the specific advice given are clear. In addition, the implications of the 'do nothing' option should be discussed.

Obtaining consent

The amount of information divulged will vary according to the context of the discussion and according to the needs of the patient as they emerge in the consultation. The objective is not to place the patient in the situation of having to decide between conflicting medical data, but to explain why a particular investigation or treatment is being recommended. The patient must not feel under duress.

Setting the scene

Discussions regarding consent for investigation and treatment should be conducted in a suitable environment that is quiet, free of interruptions and away from unnecessary observers, such as other patients or unfamiliar nurses or students. Make time for the discussion and turn off pagers or mobile phones, which, if they interrupt a discussion, can give the impression that you are rushed and fitting the patient into a busier, more important schedule. Use simple language that the patient can understand. Be patient. If necessary, and with the patient's permission, involve relatives. If there is likely to be a language problem, make sure that an interpreter (not a relative) is available. At the end of the discussion, check that the patient has actually understood and document this. A written summary of the information supplied should be given to the patient for later consideration.

Implications of consent or refusal

Some patients, after detailed discussion, decline the recommended investigation or treatment. This should not result in the doctor being any less committed to the patient's welfare. Discussions regarding alternative strategies should commence within the framework of what has been agreed and what is acceptable to the patient.

If explicit consent is given, the patient and doctor should both sign an appropriate consent form. This procedure should be followed for all serious interventions. In hospital, this will be a standardized form; a similar form should be used in family or private practice to verify that the discussion took place. The act of both parties signing the form does not constitute proof that consent has been lawfully given, but merely documents that a discussion took place. It is good practice to make a separate, contemporaneous note describing what was discussed.

Legal requirements for consent

Three aspects of consent are required in law:
1. The patient must be mentally and legally competent to give consent.
2. The patient must have been sufficiently well informed to be able to give consent.
3. Consent must have been given voluntarily, and not under duress.

Competence and capacity for consent

The definition of mental capacity is given in Box 4.1. If the patient does not have capacity to make a decision, the doctor must involve the relatives, although the doctor is still making the final decision. If the patient does not have capacity and has no relatives, in the UK the doctor must involve an

Box 4.1	Criteria for having mental capacity

- The patient can understand what has been explained
- The patient can recall and repeat what has been explained
- The patient can discuss what has been explained and weigh information
- The patient can communicate the decision that he has made

Independent Mental Capacity Advocate (IMCA) to help with decision-making, particularly if consenting for surgery or for making decisions about change of living circumstances.

Special difficulties with consent arise when the patient is unconscious. If treatment is necessary in order to save life, it can and must be given without waiting for consent. If relatives are available, they should be consulted, but their wishes are not necessarily paramount in the decision to initiate life-saving therapy. The relatives may thus assent to treatment, but they cannot legally consent to it (in the UK). This limitation also means that relatives cannot legally refuse treatment that is medically in the best interests of the patient, although a conflict of this kind should be reason to consider, carefully and in detail with the relatives, the reasons for disagreement.

Consent for the treatment of children requires particular consideration. In general, a minor (i.e. a person under the age of 16 years) can be treated without parental consent, provided that care has been taken to ensure the child understands the nature of the treatment proposed and its possible risks, adverse effects and consequences. However, this should be a most exceptional decision. In practice, the parents' agreement should almost always be sought. An obvious exception would be in an emergency, such as after a life-threatening head injury or when non-accidental injury is suspected. Difficult decisions sometimes arise, such as when the prescription of contraceptive drugs to a young girl is requested in circumstances she does not wish her parents to know or parents refusing to allow a bleeding child to have a blood transfusion for religious reasons.

Appropriately informed

The point at which a patient may be considered to be appropriately informed is a matter of judgement. Some patients make it clear that they do not wish for long and involved discussions, whereas others are comfortable only when very full explanations have been given. It is often necessary to strike a balance. It is easy to frighten a patient by reciting unwelcome, but rare, complications of a procedure to such an extent that the patient refuses treatment. This should not be the objective of discussing treatment and is rarely in the patient's best interest.

If a procedure is so risky that the doctor feels it is not justified and is therefore futile, the patient should be advised accordingly rather than being asked to decide for himself.

Consent law in the UK has recently been revised following a particular judgement in the case of Montgomery. The revision centres around the level of risk that needs to be explained to the patient. Previously it was assumed that risks that were rare did not need to be included in the explanation given prior to consent. Now doctors have a duty to take reasonable care to ensure that patients are aware of all 'material risks'. When seeking consent to treatment, the question of what is a 'material risk' is judged from the perspective of what a reasonable person would consider material in the patient's position. This makes understanding how patients would perceive the consequence of any risk particularly important (such as a tiny risk of blood transfusion being needed after a percutaneous biopsy procedure, or the tiny risk that laparotomy and colostomy may be needed after a colonoscopy perforation, which itself has a low risk of occurring).

Confidentiality

The fact that all aspects of the encounter are confidential forms the foundation for the consultation, because it allows the patient freedom of expression in the knowledge that disclosures made within the confines of the consulting room will not be made available to others.

The principle of confidentiality applies also to the medical records. These are held by the doctor or the group practice or, in the case of hospital records, by the hospital itself. Medical records are not available to anyone other than the medical and nursing staff treating the patient and are immune from police powers of search. They are made available, however, with the permission of the patient and, once disclosed, may be used as evidence in court in both civil and criminal cases. Patients have the right to inspect their own medical records after making a written application. In the UK, the principle of confidentiality is rigorously supported by the General Medical Council and its breach is regarded as a serious matter.

The main situations in which confidentiality can be relaxed include the following:

- When the patient or the patient's legal adviser allows it.
- When it is in the patient's interests.
- If there is an overriding duty to society as a whole.
- In cases of statutory disclosure.
- Sometimes after death.

With permission

A common example of relaxation of confidentiality with the patient's permission occurs when a consultation is witnessed (e.g. by medical students or a nurse). The patient should be given the opportunity to ask that others leave.

In the patient's interests

When it is necessary that another family member be informed about the nature of a patient's illness, for example in order to obtain information essential for effective treatment, it may be judged in the patient's best interests to break confidentiality. Another example might arise if a patient was judged mentally incompetent and it became necessary to involve a legal adviser to handle the patient's financial and legal affairs during a severe illness. This generally requires permission from a court.

An overriding duty to society

Occasionally confidentiality may be relaxed in the context of a known or possibly pending violent crime. In the case of an illness such as epilepsy or coronary heart disease that might impair the ability to control a vehicle, the responsibility to inform the authorities rests with the patient. Voluntary disclosure is encouraged, maintaining the principle of confidentiality between doctor and patient, but if the patient clearly does not make the disclosure, the clinician does have discretion to break this principle in circumstances that entail serious public risk (e.g. a patient having regular seizures who clearly has not informed the driving licensing authority).

Statutory disclosure

Confidentiality is breached in the case of certain infectious diseases, such as tuberculosis, that are statutorily notifiable to the public health authorities. There is also a statutory duty for a doctor to help in the identification of a driver involved in a road traffic accident who, for example, might have attended a surgery or accident and emergency department after the accident. The doctor in the witness box is in a state of privilege and is protected against any action for breach of confidentiality when instructed by a court to disclose potentially confidential information. Similarly, a court can ask that medical documents be released to it if they are regarded as necessary for the completion of a fair trial of an accused person.

Inspection of medical records

Patients have a lawful right to inspect their own medical records and can see any reports concerning their own medical condition that have been prepared before they are released to another party. Such reports can only be prepared with the permission of the patient or at the request of a statutory body, as in the context of an order under the Mental Health Act, or in the jurisdiction of a recognized court.

Generally, persons other than the patient have no right to inspect the medical records of an individual in the absence of written permission or when the records are subject to a subpoena from a recognized court.

After death

Generally, the principle of confidentiality should extend to patients who have died. In the cases of a number of deceased public figures of recent years (e.g. Winston Churchill and John F. Kennedy), this principle was not adhered to on the grounds (not universally accepted) that there were matters of public interest involved.

Organ donation

When a tissue that can be replaced by the donor's own tissues, such as blood or bone marrow, is given to another patient, no special ethical problem arises. When a living donor gives an irreplaceable organ, such as a kidney, difficulties arise. The donor must be of sound mind, not under duress and must not be placed in a position to gain financially by the gift. The sale of organs for transplantation is forbidden in all developed countries and is rapidly becoming illegal in all countries. Similar considerations apply to the acquisition of donor organs from a minor, a practice about which it is particularly difficult to issue sound guidelines.

Resuscitation

Resuscitation is generally available in hospitals in the event that cardiopulmonary arrest occurs unexpectedly. However, this is not always successful, and many patients, recognizing the terminal nature of their illness, may request that resuscitation not be attempted. This is an entirely valid request which should be respected once it is certain that the options are clearly understood by the patient.

Not for resuscitation

Sometimes a patient is so seriously ill that resuscitation is deemed inappropriate by medical and nursing staff. Clearly, this implies a value judgement by those concerned that, in some way, the patient's life is not worth saving. The situation most frequently arises when a patient has terminal cancer; resuscitation followed by a few hours or days of further pain and discomfort might be regarded as an unnecessary prolongation of the illness.

The decision to withhold resuscitation is a matter for which it is proper always to seek the patient's full, informed consent. The patient's views are paramount and should be respected whatever the views of the clinicians and nurses or even the relatives. Relatives have no legal rights in a decision about the possible resuscitation of another individual. Although they may be consulted and their views noted, they should not be allowed to influence a decision once it has been made by the individual, unless it is decided that the patient is not competent by reason of dementia or some other impairment of judgement to reach a decision. Overt depression, for example, might be a reason for not accepting a patient's expressed wish not to be resuscitated.

Although it might be thought not helpful to a patient to discuss this issue openly, in fact the reverse is usually the case. Most patients near death are aware of their situation and welcome the opportunity for a full discussion of the issues. The agreement of the patient and medical staff should be signed in the case record; most hospitals now use a formal protocol to document this procedure. Patients should always be resuscitated when cardiopulmonary collapse is unexpected and their wishes are unknown.

Consent for autopsy

Explicit consent is required for autopsy, because tissue samples will be taken and examined and some may be retained for future use. If this is intended or is likely to occur, permission to retain the samples must be obtained as part of the consent for autopsy. This process of consent implies that the family will be given some idea of what studies might be undertaken on the retained samples in the future. It may be appropriate to consider whether any circumstances might develop in which the family might reasonably expect to be informed of the results of any such studies. For example, if information of a predictive or genetic nature were to be obtained in relation to the risk of vascular disease or of specific cancers, then the family might wish to know of this.

Other ethical problems

Several other problems arise in medical practice, many of which are likely to become more important in the coming years.

Medical negligence

Inadvertent adverse events are common in clinical practice, but few of these result in any legal action. Accusations of negligence often imply that a doctor–patient relationship has broken down. For the doctor, such an action is distressing and sometimes professionally damaging, even when shown not justified.

In considering whether there has been negligence, it is necessary to establish breach of professional duty (whether the standard of care afforded the patient fell below what was expected). The standard expected is that of the ordinary skilled practitioner in the field in question, practising in the circumstances pertaining. It is not that of the greatest expert in the land. Thus, in assessing possible negligence, a court will need to establish:

- what the ordinary practice is
- that the doctor did not follow this practice
- that the doctor undertook a course of clinical management that no ordinarily skilled doctor in that specialty would have undertaken if acting with ordinary care.

A mistake in diagnosis is not necessarily negligent, and the test of the standard of care applicable to the ordinary practitioner in the specialty will be applied by the court in considering this.

Doctors are expected to keep up to date in their expertise by continuing medical education, and this is an aspect that is relevant to this judgement. Doctors in training are expected, by and large, to exercise an appropriate standard of care, and no patients should expect a lower standard of care simply because they are cared for by a junior doctor with less experience. This would clearly be wrong. It is imperative, therefore, that in treating a patient, advice and help should be sought from senior colleagues whenever relevant.

If negligence has occurred, the legal process will go on to attempt to establish what harm resulted from the negligence and that the harm would not have occurred if the negligent act had not been committed.

HIV

Testing for HIV requires the consent of the patient or an individual. It is usual to counsel the individual about the consequences of a positive result before testing, as there are implications for lifestyle, future health and even employment hinging on the result of the test.

Genetics

The rapidly evolving availability of relatively accurate genetic testing for susceptibility to inherited diseases, based on the modern understanding of DNA and the genetic code, has raised a number of ethical problems for which most societies are not well prepared. For example:

- Who should have genetic tests done?
- What should be done with the results?
- Who, if anyone, should have access to the information, other than the patient?
- How should expensive treatments that may be possible for genetically determined disorders be made available?
- Is it socially and economically appropriate to prevent such disorders?

The application of genetic information to medical practice is a current major area of change. It can be expected to have profound implications for the management of most aspects of disease and for the ways in which all societies view the acquisition and availability of medical information.

Genetic counselling

Genetic counselling is relatively long established. The clinical geneticist will usually be asked to assess the risks of genetically determined disease in the context of statistical data or a known familial occurrence of a disease, for example Down's syndrome, Duchenne muscular dystrophy or cystic fibrosis. There is knowledge about the genetic causation of each of these conditions, and certain tests with various probabilities of accuracy are available to assess the risk for individuals in a family and for the risk that a planned pregnancy might result in an affected offspring. Major difficulties arise in deciding whether to inform someone who has been shown by genetic testing to be certain to develop a disease in later life, for example Huntington's disease. Ideally, such decisions should be made before testing is undertaken at all. Even when offering counselling about the risks for planned pregnancies, similar difficulties arise. The social costs in terms of unresolved problems to individuals and their families of offering treatment or prevention for genetic disorders are largely undetermined at present. Practice in this context will change as knowledge and experience accumulate.

Decisions regarding the protection of vulnerable patients

Sometimes, in clinical practice, a doctor may have concerns that the environment from which the patient has come for medical care (and to which he may be scheduled to return) is not safe and that the patient is vulnerable to one or more forms of abuse (physical, emotional, financial). Ethical difficulties arise, for example, between the stated desire of a patient, whose judgement may be impaired by dementia or delirium, to return to his home (his liberty) and the concern on the part of the doctor that he may be at risk in doing so. In the UK, Deprivation of Liberty Safeguards (DoLS) were introduced to ensure that vulnerable adults, either in hospital or in community care, are cared for in a way that does not restrict their freedom unfairly or illegally. A patient's liberty or freedom **may** be restricted if:

1. It is in the patient's best interest.
2. There is no other available way to care for this patient.
3. This is safe and follows correct and defensible processes (see below).

DoLS may **only** be applied to adults (over 18 years old) who:

1. Do not retain capacity.
2. Are deemed to have a mental health condition, including delirium and dementia.
3. Are not being detained under the Mental Health Act (1983).

Any doctor contemplating trying to keep a patient in hospital for the patient's own safety should consider the safeguards around depriving patients of their liberty. These include:

- Deprivation of liberty (DoL) is undertaken as a last resort.
- The doctor should be able to demonstrate that he/she has considered all available appropriate

and safe other options prior to depriving patients of their liberty.

- All care should be provided in the least restrictive manner possible.
- The doctor must be able to demonstrate that the DoL is safe, lawful and protects the patient.

To ensure that the DoL follows these criteria, the caring organization (most commonly the hospital trust in the UK) must be able to demonstrate the following:

- An advocate or patient representative has been provided for persons having their liberty deprived.
- The DoL may be legally challenged in the court of protection by patients or their legal representation.
- Mechanisms are in place for review and monitoring of the DoL.

Most UK hospital trusts now have DoLS officers who will ensure all of these criteria are in place. It is crucial that the doctor pre-emptively ensures the issue of DoLS is raised and documented as early as possible when considering keeping a patient in the hospital against his/her will.

In an emergency situation the hospital trust can grant itself urgent/emergency authorization of a DoL. This is valid for 7 days, but a standard authorization made through the local authority or health board must be applied for in this period. A further 7-day emergency DoL may be granted by this authority. The patient's carers, relatives or legal representatives should be kept informed of all developments. These details apply to the UK only; other countries have their own processes and protocols.

Principles of medical ethics

Several modern attempts have been made to encapsulate the principles of ethical medical behaviour in a series of simple statements. The Declaration of Geneva (Box 4.2) represents a modern attempt to restate the Hippocratic Oath in contemporary language. The International Code of Medical Ethics (Box 4.3) was derived from these principles and restates them in more direct terms. The Declaration of Helsinki (1975) sets out recommendations for the guidance of doctors wishing to undertake biomedical research involving human subjects. The recommendations of the Declaration of Helsinki are generally recognized as relevant to the design of research protocols. The UK General Medical Council's duties of doctors are listed at the end of Chapter 1.

Box 4.2 Declaration of Geneva propounded by the World Medical Association in Sydney (1968)

On admittance to the medical profession:

- I will solemnly pledge myself to consecrate my life to the service of humanity
- I will give my teachers the respect and gratitude which is their due
- I will practise my profession with conscience and dignity
- The health of my patients will be my first consideration
- I will respect secrets that have been confided in me, even after the patient has died
- I will maintain by all the means in my power the honour and noble traditions of the medical profession
- My colleagues will be my brothers
- I will not permit considerations of religion, nationality, race, party politics or social standing to intervene between my duty and my patient
- I will maintain the utmost respect for human life from the time of conception. Even under threat I will not use my medical knowledge contrary to the laws of humanity
- I make these promises solemnly, freely and upon my honour

Box 4.3 International Code of Medical Ethics

Duties of doctors in general

- To maintain the highest standards of professional conduct
- To practise uninfluenced by motives of profit
- To use caution in divulging discoveries or new techniques of treatment
- To certify or testify only those matters with which the doctor has personal experience
- To ensure that any act or advice that could weaken physical or mental resistance of an individual must be used only in the interest of that individual

The following are unethical practices

- Any self-advertisement except as expressly authorized in a national code of ethics
- Collaboration in any form of medical service in which the doctor does not have professional independence
- Receipt of any money in connection with services rendered to a patient other than a proper professional fee, even if the patient is aware of it

Duties of doctors to the sick

- There is an obligation to preserve life
- The patient is owed complete loyalty and all the resources of medical science. Whenever a treatment or examination is beyond the capacity of the doctor, the advice of another doctor should be sought
- A doctor must always preserve absolute secrecy concerning all he knows about a patient because of the confidence trusted in him
- Emergency care is a humanitarian duty that must be given, unless it is clear that there are others better able to give it

Duties of doctors to each other

- A doctor must behave to his colleagues as he would have them behave toward him
- A doctor must not entice patients from his colleagues
- A doctor must observe the principles of the Declaration of Geneva

SECTION 2

Assessment in particular groups

Women | 5

Rehan Khan

Introduction

All medical history taking, examination, investigation and management plans are intensely personal matters for patients. In obstetric and gynaecological practice, intimate details must be elicited; this requires tact, discretion, consideration and the maintenance of proper confidentiality. Women may have particular expectations of their doctors and complying with these may not be easy. A gentle manner and a genuine interest in the patient help to develop a good professional relationship. Allow adequate time, but it is essential to keep a sense of direction and purpose so that what is important is quickly separated from the trivial. You must be aware that there may be an expectation on the patient's part that she would be seeing a senior person throughout, so always be very clear about your status as a medical student or doctor in training. As with breast disease, gynaecological and obstetric cases are usually multidimensional in nature; the reported symptoms are experienced and reported against a backdrop of core aspects of the patient's lay beliefs. Developing the necessary skills to gather and interpret the relevant information requires considerable care, insight and reflection.

Gynaecological history

The usual preparations for history taking should be followed: courteous introduction; a statement as to your status as a student or trainee; and a careful check that you have the correct patient, that she understands the language and seemingly has competence. It may be that the patient is younger than the age of competence (16, or 18 if she is in care, in the UK), and awareness of this and its effect on management may be an issue. If a relative, such as a parent, insists on being present during the history, potentially sensitive questions may be reserved for a time when the other person has been asked to leave the room, such as during the examination. Sometimes, it is appropriate to revisit sensitive issues at a future appointment, which the patient may feel more confident to attend alone.

In all consultations, you should describe the process that is about to take place and get an agreement or verbal consent. This will include history taking, an examination, an explanation of the findings and a discussion of a plan of action, which, of course, will include an opportunity for the patient to ask questions.

There are different systems for eliciting a history: the one outlined below is comprehensive and is the author's preferred one. It should, of course, be adapted to the individual patient. For example, in a postmenopausal patient with a urogynaecological problem, detailed menstrual and obstetric histories contribute little. In a younger patient, the history may be more related to menstruation, pregnancy and its complications and sexual activity in general. As a general rule, the introductory part of the history should be taken using open questions to allow a broader response.

Presenting complaint

The presenting complaint is a statement of what the patient perceives to be the problem. As the consultation progresses and the relationship between doctor and patient develops, it may become apparent that the real presenting problem is something separate. Even so, it is important to start with the patient's chief concern as a way of building trust and rapport with someone who is likely to be anxious.

History of presenting complaint

Take a detailed description of the presenting complaint, with an emphasis on the timeline (when the problem started and how it developed over time) and the degree of symptomatology (how much the problem is affecting the patient).

In order to assess a woman's gynaecological wellbeing, certain areas of focused questioning are needed. Many students feel awkward taking a gynaecological history, but this is often unnecessary, because women with gynaecological problems will be expecting such questions. It may be helpful, at least initially, to use pre-prepared direct questions in order to overcome this initial self-consciousness.

Pain history

It can be very difficult to know from the history if lower abdominal pain has its origins in the gynaecological, gastrointestinal or urinary system. The principles of eliciting a pain history outlined throughout this book apply in gynaecological practice. In addition, cyclical pain associated with periods is typically caused by endometriosis, whereas pain that was originally cyclical but later becomes continuous is often caused by adhesions. In all cases it is necessary to take an accurate history of bowel and bladder symptoms, because a substantial number of patients attending the gynaecology clinic with pain symptoms subsequently turn out to have bowel pathology (e.g. irritable bowel syndrome) or bladder pathology (e.g. interstitial cystitis). The two major gynaecological causes of chronic pain are endometriosis and pelvic inflammatory disease; in both cases the symptoms may be caused by the formation of pelvic adhesions.

Menstrual history

For premenopausal women, a menstrual history is mandatory. This can be done quite quickly with practice but is usually dependent on direct questioning. Menstruation (the cyclical loss of sanguineous fluid from the uterus) is recorded as the days of menstrual loss and the duration of the interval from the first day of one period to the first day of the next, for example 5/28. Medical and 'lay' terminologies sometimes overlap confusingly in medicine, although, in this context, the words 'period', 'menstrual period' and 'menstrual cycle' can be used interchangeably by doctor and patient alike. The aim of this section of the history is to establish if the patient's menstrual periods are problematic and, if so, in what way. Box 5.1 shows some examples of direct questions around the menstrual history, together with some points requiring clarification. In addition, Box 5.2 lists several other questions that are required in order to check for bleeding problems not connected to periods.

If the patient is post- or perimenopausal, the history taking should reflect this. Some examples of direct, focused questions that could be asked are the following:

- Are you still having periods? or
- When did you have your last period?
- Has there been any bleeding since your last period? (This relates to a definition of postmenopausal bleeding—generally defined as bleeding 1 year after the last period, unless the patient is taking hormone replacement therapy, in which case it is important to establish which type. Exclusion of organic pathology is mandatory in this situation.)

Occasionally, gynaecological conditions may be associated with cyclical blood loss from the anus or urethra.

Box 5.1	Some examples of direct questions around the menstrual history, together with some points requiring clarification

- How old were you when your periods first started? (Menarche.)
- What was the first day of your last normal menstrual period? (Patients may recall the last day of the period which is not contributory. Whether the period was normal or not is important, as sometimes what the woman thought was a period was in fact bleeding from an abnormal pregnancy that was actually established after the previous period.)
- How often do your periods come?
- How many days are there from the first day of one period to the first day of the next? (It could be that the cycle is irregular; many women keep a diary of their menstrual periods and it is often helpful to see this.)
- For how many days do you bleed?
- How many heavy days are there? (With these two questions you are trying to gauge the level of menstrual loss, so some estimate of the volume of flow is required.)
- Do you use tampons, pads or both? How often do you have to change them? (The use of both tampons and pads together is termed 'double protection' and is strongly indicative of menorrhagia.)
- Do you pass blood clots, and if so how large are they? (The second part of this question is difficult to answer without a frame of reference, and comparison to coins of different denominations can be helpful.)
- Do you ever bleed through your clothes? Is the bleeding like a running tap? (This is called 'flooding'.)
- Does the bleeding interfere with your usual daily activities, e.g. do you have to take time off work? (This is a very important question as it helps to judge the impact of the bleeding problem.)
- Are your periods painful? (Some assessment of the degree of pain is necessary here, e.g. is medication used and, if so, what and how much? Does the pain stop you from carrying out your normal activities?)
- Do you have any other symptoms with your periods? (This is an enquiry about premenstrual syndrome, in which a variety of symptoms can aggregate and then disappear as menstrual flow starts.)

Vaginal discharge

Even if vaginal discharge is not the presenting symptom, routinely enquire about it. If there is a troublesome discharge, enquire about its colour, smell, amount, presence of blood, whether there is an associated vulval itch and, if so, if there are other sites of itching. In women with an abnormal vaginal discharge, questions relating to sexually transmitted disease naturally follow but can be difficult to pose. If the patient is in a sexual relationship, ask about symptoms in her partner(s) and whether either (any) of them is aware of the presence of warts.

- Do you have bleeding between your periods? (If so, how much and when does it occur?)
- Do you have any bleeding after sexual intercourse? (If so, ask for an estimate of how frequently this loss occurs and how heavy it is.)
- What form of contraception are you using? (In the last two questions, it is first necessary to establish whether the patient is in a sexual relationship; this requires additional tact. The pattern of menstruation may be influenced by use of various contraceptive methods, including the combined oestrogen/progestogen pill (combined oral contraception, COC), the progesterone-only pill (POP), injectable progestogens, various intrauterine contraceptive devices and newer progestogen-containing rings placed in the vagina.)

| Box 5.3 | Questions to ask if a prolapse is suspected |

- Do you have a feeling of something coming down?
- Does the feeling go away overnight or when you lie down? (Symptomatic prolapse is gravity dependent except in the most severe cases.)
- Are there occasions when you don't make it to the toilet in time?
- Do you leak urine if you cough or sneeze?
- When you pass urine, do you feel you have completely emptied your bladder?
- When you are passing urine, can you squeeze hard enough to stop the flow? (Arresting flow mid stream is a good test of the strength of the pelvic floor.)
- How often do you get up at night to pass urine?
- Have you ever seen blood in your urine?

| Box 5.4 | Direct questions for patients presenting with pain on sexual penetration |

- How severe is the pain—does sex have to stop?
- Does it happen every time you have sex or only on some occasions? (If intermittent, ask how often this happens.)
- Can you say if the pain is superficial (near the outside) or deep on the inside? (Typical causes of deep dyspareunia include endometriosis and chronic pelvic inflammatory disease.)
- Do you have any other pains in the pelvic region other than the one brought on by sexual activity?
- Is there any bleeding during or after penetrative sex?

Urinary tract and uterovaginal prolapse symptoms

Uterovaginal prolapse refers to a situation in which the uterus 'sinks' or 'slides' down from its normal position in the body. Frequently a woman will notice a bulge ('a lump down below') at the introitus (entrance) of the vagina and may report urinary symptoms consequent upon changes in the pelvic floor muscles that alter the angulation and therefore reliability of the bladder neck. It is very unusual for symptomatic prolapse to occur in women who have not had vaginal deliveries. If this appears to be the presenting complaint, the history can be explored with carefully phrased direct questions (Box 5.3).

It should be clear to the history taker if the reason for any incontinence is in part owing to mobility limitations, but a general enquiry should be made about the layout of the home and symptoms of cough or constipation that may lead to repeated increases in intra-abdominal pressure. Where the history is not clear or needs more objectivity, it is sometimes useful to recommend a simple frequency/volume chart on which the patient can record her symptoms and bring it to a subsequent appointment.

Sexual symptoms

A full sexual history would not be appropriate at the first appointment unless the history taker has specific training in this area. If you know that the patient is in a sexual relationship, it is reasonable routinely to ask her whether she experiences or has experienced pain with sexual intercourse (dyspareunia). Sometimes the patient will present with painful sex on penetration; again, direct but sensitive questions are useful in this context (Box 5.4).

In addition, it is essential to ask whether the patient has had any previous sexually transmitted infections, particularly chlamydia and gonorrhoea, which are associated with pelvic inflammatory disease.

Cervical cytology history

A gynaecological history should always include details of any cervical smears, their dates and whether there have been any abnormalities or treatments. The opportunity also arises to ask if any other screening has taken place, such as mammography and chlamydia, and what the results were.

Past obstetric history

It is inevitable that a gynaecological history will include a truncated obstetric history. This can be a sensitive issue, as medical and lay terminologies regarding lost pregnancies can cause potential confusion and inadvertent distress. Spontaneous abortion is no longer used as the medical term for a miscarriage; what many women refer to as an 'abortion' is a termination of pregnancy in medical language. If the questions are incorrectly constructed, the boundaries of confidentiality can be breached if the history is taken in the presence of a third person.

- How many times have you been pregnant? (Be aware that some patients may not indicate that they have had terminations of pregnancy.)
- What was the weight of the heaviest and the lightest baby?
- How old were you when you had your first pregnancy?
- How old are the children now? or
- How old is the youngest and how old is the oldest?
- How old would he be if he had survived?
- Did you have any difficulty getting pregnant?

No pressure should be placed on a patient during this part of the history, especially in the presence of others. It is important, however, to know the number of pregnancies, their outcome (gestational ages and weights), mode of delivery, age of the children, whether there was any infertility at any time and, if so, the details of any investigations or treatments. Direct questions that may help assimilate this information are listed in Box 5.5.

Past gynaecological history

With the passage of time, many patients forget certain aspects of their past medical history (e.g. tonsillectomy, cataract removal). Women with a gynaecological history do not often forget, so a simple question 'Have you had any gynaecological problems or procedures in the past?' is sufficient to establish any significant gynaecological background, which should then be explored.

Past medical/surgical/anaesthetic history

In order to get a broad view of the patient's medical background, you could ask a simple question such as 'Is there anything in your past medical or surgical history that I should know about?' This is a helpful introductory question that can be followed by more focused enquiry, depending on the case. For example, complicated appendicitis may be related to infertility, or a previous blood transfusion, which has produced blood group antibodies, may be related to a subsequent pregnancy loss. If an anaesthetic is anticipated as part of the patient's management, it is important to assess whether this is likely to be problematic. Ask if she has had an anaesthetic in the recent past and whether there were any problems with it.

Medication or treatment history

Medication and treatment history are standard enquiries and may be contributory. An awareness of medications taken in the past, with their success or failure, is a useful observation. Be aware that patients may take various kinds of supplements which they do not regard as medicines, but which may affect gynaecological health, for example Chinese herbal remedies, agnus castus, black cohosh. Allergic reactions should be recorded and clearly displayed.

Social history

Enquiry as to occupational history, present and past, is appropriate. Even during the course of the relatively short time to take a history, a picture of the patient may emerge indicating how well adjusted she is to her life, her relationships and external influences. These may affect her prospects for recovery from illness or when planning the support of a child. For instance, if the patient is a victim of domestic violence, a request for termination of pregnancy may be considered differently or this may be relevant to antenatal or postnatal care.

Family history

Few purely gynaecological conditions have a familial basis. In the context of infertility, it is important to check whether recurrent familial conditions are present, both on the patient's and her partner's side; recessive and autosomal dominant genetic conditions are often known to patients.

Gynaecological examination

Full awareness of the privacy of the examination is mandatory. A chaperone should be present during any intimate examination (breast or pelvic examination) whether the person performing the examination is male or female. Breast examination is not part of the gynaecological assessment in UK practice unless there is a specific complaint related to the breasts. It is important to ensure that the patient gets undressed in privacy without the doctor or student present, and that she has a suitable covering for the lower half of her body.

For a new consultation, a general examination is necessary and particularly relevant if an anaesthetic is anticipated. Details of the general physical examination are covered in other chapters. In the context of gynaecology, measurements of height and weight (giving the body mass index, BMI) and an assessment of body proportions (e.g. general or central obesity) are important. In 'gynaecological endocrinological' cases, the presence or absence of signs associated with hyperandrogenaemia (hirsutism, male pattern baldness, acne, increased muscle bulk) should be documented.

Abdominal examination

The system of examination described in Chapter 14 is recommended but should focus on inspection

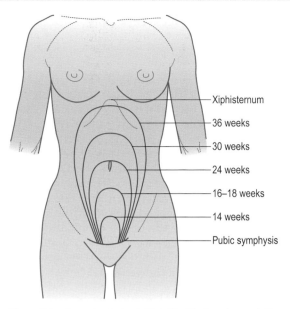

Figure 5.1 Approximate fundal height with changing gestation.

Labels on figure: Xiphisternum, 36 weeks, 30 weeks, 24 weeks, 16–18 weeks, 14 weeks, Pubic symphysis

Figure 5.2 Equipment for the gynaecological examination.

and palpation; percussion and auscultation are less important in gynaecological practice. The presence or absence of scars should be noted. Laparoscopic scars can be subtle, particularly if tucked within the umbilicus. Occasionally (usually to avoid the risk of perforation through adhesions in the lower abdomen) the entry point for laparoscopic surgery may be via Palmer's point in the mid-clavicular line, under the rib cage. Transverse suprapubic (Pfannenstiel's) incisions may also be difficult to see in the suprapubic crease unless specifically looked for.

Suprapubic examination is particularly important because a gynaecological mass arises out of the pelvis and the examining hand cannot get below it. Do this part of the abdominal palpation with the ulnar border of the left hand, starting at or around the umbilicus, and work your way down. When an abdomino-pelvic mass is present, its characteristics and size, either in centimetres measured from the symphysis pubis upwards or estimated as weeks' gestation of an equivalent-size pregnancy, are recorded (see Fig. 5.1). Note its consistency (hard if a fibroid, usually soft if a pregnancy), regularity (subserosal fibroids and ovarian masses are usually irregular) and the presence of any tenderness. It can sometimes be difficult to elicit such signs if there is a scar in the lower abdomen or if the patient is obese. If nothing is palpable arising out of the pelvis, it is reasonable to conclude that any pelvic swelling is less than the size of a 12-week pregnancy. If ascites is suspected, check the supraclavicular and inguinal lymph nodes and look for an associated hydrothorax.

Pelvic examination

In gynaecology, pelvic examination (PE) is usually undertaken vaginally, but it may also be performed

rectally. The instruments used are shown in Figure 5.2. PE should always be preceded by an abdominal examination. To reduce patient anxiety, it is crucial to explain every step sensitively but clearly. Medical students should undertake a PE only in the presence of a supervisor; the same applies to trainees in gynaecology, except where specific permission has been granted by the trainer. In many centres, students begin to learn the technique of PE using artificial manikins and models.

The PE commences with inspection of the perineum in the dorsal (or occasionally left lateral) position and is followed by internal digital examination, using the index and middle fingers (use one finger if the vagina does not accommodate two). Generally, but not always, a speculum examination precedes the digital examination (if it is important to visualize any discharge, take swabs or take a cervical smear, the speculum should always be passed first; Fig. 5.3). If the patient experiences undue discomfort (be it speculum or digital), the examination should cease immediately. Note any inflammation, swelling, soreness, ulceration or neoplasia of the vulva, perineum or anus (Fig. 5.4). Women from certain communities may have been circumcised in childhood: this is known as female genital mutilation (FGM) and can range from scarring of the labia to removal of the external genitalia. Small warts (condylomata acuminata) appearing as papillary growths may occur scattered over the vulva; these are caused by infection with the human papilloma virus. Inspect the clitoris and urethra and ask the patient to strain and then cough to demonstrate any uterovaginal prolapse or stress incontinence. (Fig. 5.5 shows the various types of prolapse.) If the patient has given a history of involuntary incontinence, it is important that the bladder is reasonably full and that more than one

Figure 5.3 Discharge owing to *Chlamydia trachomatis*.

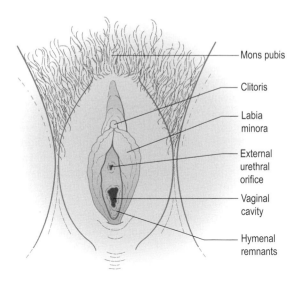

Figure 5.4 The vulva.

Mons pubis

Clitoris

Labia minora

External urethral orifice

Vaginal cavity

Hymenal remnants

substantial cough is taken, because the first cough frequently fails to demonstrate leakage of urine.

For the digital examination, disposable gloves are used and the examining fingers should be lightly lubricated with a water-based jelly. With the patient in the supine position and with her knees drawn up and separated, the labia are gently parted with the index finger and thumb of the left hand while the index finger of the right hand is inserted into the vagina, avoiding the urethral meatus and exerting a sustained pressure on the perineal body until the perineal musculature relaxes. Watch for any sign of discomfort. The full length of the finger is then introduced, assessing the vaginal walls in transit until the cervix is located. At this stage, a second finger can be inserted to improve the quality of the digital examination or, alternatively, a speculum can be used if a cervical smear is required. The examination is continued with the left hand placed on the abdomen above the symphysis pubis and below the umbilicus—the bimanual examination (Fig. 5.6). The hand provides gentle directional pressure to bring the pelvic viscera towards the examiner's fingers in the vagina and serves to assess the size, mobility and regularity of masses. The cervix is then identified; it is approximately 3 cm in diameter, with a variably sized and shaped dimple in the middle, the cervical os. When the uterus is anteflexed and anteverted, the os is normally directed posteriorly. A retroverted uterus means the uterus is tipped backwards so that it aims towards the rectum instead of forward towards the abdomen. The consistency of the cervix is firm and its shape is irregular when scarred. Increased hardness of the cervix may be caused by fibrosis or carcinoma. As a 'soft' cervix indicates the possibility of pregnancy, even greater caution and gentleness are necessary. The mobility of the cervix is usually 1 to 2 cm in all directions and testing this movement should produce only mild discomfort. If the cervix is moved when there is pelvic inflammation, particularly in association with ectopic pregnancy, extreme pain (cervical excitation) results.

It is possible to estimate the size, shape, position, consistency and regularity of the uterus and the relationship of the fundus of the uterus to the cervix (flexion). Uterine size is generally described as normal, bulky or in terms of weeks of gestation (e.g. 6 weeks, 8 weeks, 10 weeks size) even in the absence of pregnancy. Its mobility and shape (symmetrical or non-symmetrical) may be assessed and the ovaries and fallopian tubes (also known as the adnexae) palpated, although these can be difficult to feel in healthy women. Aside from the ovaries in some women, no other swellings should be palpable about the uterus in women of reproductive years. However, adnexal tenderness is an important finding. The pouch of Douglas is then explored through the posterior fornix via the arch formed by the uterosacral ligaments and the cervix.

Pelvic examination in special circumstances

Vaginal bleeding

In most cases, vaginal bleeding dictates that PE should be deferred to another occasion, but if a diagnosis of gynaecological malignancy is suspected, then a PE would be indicated in order to reduce the time taken to reach a diagnosis. As a general rule, consultations should not be cancelled because of vaginal bleeding; the patient can still have a history taken, a general and

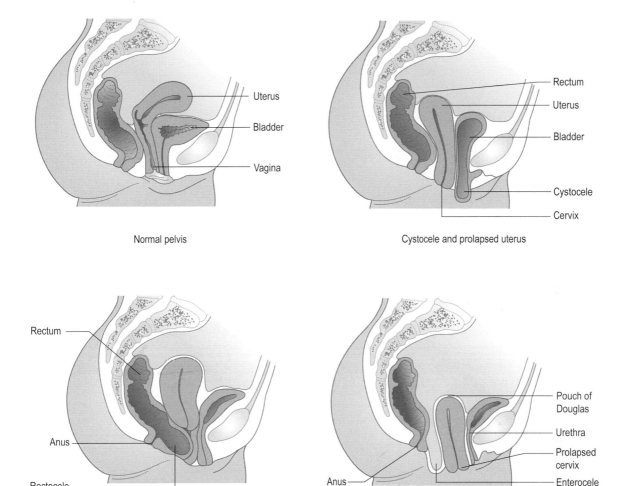

Normal pelvis

Cystocele and prolapsed uterus

Rectocele

Enterocele and prolapsed uterus

Figure 5.5   In cystocele, there is downward prolapse of the anterior part of the pelvic floor, straightening the angulation of the bladder neck and leading to urinary incontinence. In rectocele, the posterior part of the pelvic floor is mostly affected, sometimes with associated faecal incontinence. In some patients, the whole pelvic floor is weak, with double incontinence or prolapse of the uterus. In enterocele, there is a prolapse of viscera from the pouch of Douglas as part of a severe pelvic floor weakness.

abdominal examination, preliminary investigations requested and arrangements made to complete the examination.

Cervical smear

Cervical smears can still be taken in the presence of bleeding and, if the result is inconclusive, it can be repeated. It is essential to involve the patient in the decision-making process. The inconvenience of a repeat visit can be avoided if the smear is taken even if there is bleeding. Patients who have had previous treatment for cervical neoplasia should not have follow-up smears cancelled because of vaginal bleeding.

Examination under general anaesthesia

In some situations, it may be necessary to perform PE under general anaesthesia. The technique for examination under anaesthesia (EUA) is the same as above, but additional care is needed to preserve the

patient's dignity while she is unconscious and unable to take an active part in the proceedings.

Vaginismus

Vaginismus refers to the reflex adduction of the thigh muscles in response to an attempt at vaginal examination. In many cases, the examination has to be abandoned, but mild degrees of vaginismus can sometimes be overcome by asking the patient to clench her fists and place them under her buttocks. This tilts the pelvis in such a way that the examination becomes possible. It is worth attempting this manoeuvre if a cervical smear is required. In any event, a kindly and sympathetic approach by doctor and accompanying chaperone is always necessary.

Intact hymen

The possibility of rupturing or breaking the hymen during PE is an important consideration and it is a particularly sensitive issue for women from many

Bimanual palpation of the uterus

Palpating the uterus

Palpating the lateral fornix

Right-handed clinician

Figure 5.6 Bimanual examination of the pelvis.

communities. In such situations, avoidance of pelvic examination and judicious use of transabdominal ultrasound may often give the appropriate information.

Pregnancy

Vaginal examination in pregnancy is discussed later in this chapter.

Speculum examination

The speculum examination is an essential part of a gynaecological examination. Several types of specula are available for use, including the bivalve type (e.g. Cusco's) used for displaying the cervix (Fig. 5.7) and the single-ended or double-ended Sims' (duckbill) speculum (Fig. 5.8) used to retract the vaginal walls. Occasionally, the Ferguson's speculum is used,

Figure 5.7 Cusco's speculum used to display the cervix.

Figure 5.8   Sims' speculum used to display the anterior vaginal wall.

because it may be required to inspect the cervix when vaginal prolapse is so severe that a bivalve speculum fails to provide a sufficient view. If a cervical smear is to be taken, care should be taken not to get lubricant on the cervix, because this can compromise the quality of the sample, so the taking of the smear before digital examination is good practice without using excessive lubrication. The speculum should be warmed to body temperature and lubricated with water or a water-based jelly. All the necessary equipment, such as spatulas, slides, forceps, culture swabs and so forth, should be prepared before the examination begins (see Fig. 5.2).

Carefully explain to the patient what will happen in the examination. Ask her to lie on her back with her feet together and knees drawn apart, as for the PE. Separate the labia and then the introitus with the thumb and index finger of the left hand and then insert the lightly lubricated bivalve speculum with the handle directly upwards, allowing it to be accommodated by the vagina. When it has been inserted to its full length, the blades of the speculum are opened and manoeuvred so that the cervix is fully visualized (the left hand should now be free to do this; see Fig. 5.7). The screw adjuster or ratchet on the handle is then locked so that the speculum is maintained in place. Any discharge (see Fig. 5.3) and the condition of the cervical epithelium, its colour, any ulceration or scars and retention cysts (nabothian follicles) should be noted.

Taking a cervical (Papanicolaou) smear

Taking a cervical smear involves the technique of liquid-based cytology, in which cells are obtained from the squamocolumnar junction (transformation zone). A spatula placed firmly in the cervical os and rotated through 360° or an endocervical brush may be used. If there is considerable discharge, with or without blood, the cervix can be cleansed using a cotton wool ball and a truer reflection of the cervix will result from the test. Taking a smear through a thick mucoid discharge may result in an unsatisfactory

smear. Samples for *Candida, Trichomonas, Neisseria gonorrhoea, Chlamydia* and herpes may be obtained at the same time (see Chapter 18). The screw of the speculum is then released and the blades freed from the cervix so that the speculum can be gently removed.

Assessment for prolapse

Assessment of the vaginal walls for prolapse or fistula is performed using a Sims' speculum with the patient in the left lateral position. The best exposure is given by the Sims' position, in which the pelvis is rotated by flexing the right thigh more than the left, and by hanging the right arm over the distant edge of the couch. A Sims' speculum is inserted in much the same way as above, using the left hand to elevate the right buttock (Fig. 5.8). The blade then deflects the rectum, exposing the urethral meatus, anterior vaginal wall and bladder base. Ask the patient to strain and note any vaginal wall prolapse. The level of the cervix is recorded as the speculum is withdrawn. The posterior vaginal wall can then be viewed by rotating the speculum through 180°. Uterine prolapse is called first degree if the cervix descends but lies short of the introitus, second degree if it passes to the level of the introitus and third degree (complete procidentia) if the whole of the uterus is prolapsed outside the vulva. Vaginal wall prolapse occurring with, or independent of, uterine prolapse consists of urethrocele, cystocele, rectocele or enterocele (prolapse of the pouch of Douglas). Several of these anatomical variations usually occur together (see Fig. 5.5).

After examination, leave the examination area while the patient dresses, ensuring that she receives any necessary assistance from the nurse chaperone.

History relating to current pregnancy

If a woman tells you she is pregnant, remember that some women may not wish to continue with the pregnancy so it is important to ascertain, as gently as possible, whether the pregnancy is welcome or not. Remember too that whatever the woman's initial reactions, by the time of their birth most babies are genuinely wanted. A review of the current pregnancy can be made. Record the date of the first day of the last menstrual period (LMP), with a note as to its likely accuracy. Ask about the menstrual pattern before conception and whether this was a natural cycle or owing to the use of the contraceptive pill. The expected date of delivery (EDD) of the child can be calculated, assuming there has been a natural 28-day cycle for some months prior to the conception cycle. The EDD is then 9 months and 7 days from the onset of the last menstrual period (i.e. 280 days or 10 lunar months; alternatively, the EDD is 266 days from the date of conception). In some cases, the EDD should be altered at the time of the dating scan.

Later on in the pregnancy, ask about fetal movements. These are usually felt from about 24 weeks' gestation (there is no set number of movements, but it is important to ascertain if the woman suspects that the frequency of movements has reduced). Ask whether there have been any unusual pains or any bleeding. Data are usually assembled chronologically in 3-month episodes (the trimesters); a healthy normal pregnancy has different characteristics and different problems occur at different stages.

If labour is suspected, ask if there has been a 'show' (a brownish or blood-tinged mucus discharge), breaking of the waters or contractions. If the waters have broken, ask about the colour of the water.

Relevant past obstetric history

Here, a reasonably in-depth history is needed. The course and outcome of previous pregnancies must be explored and recorded, because these are an essential guide to the progress of the current pregnancy. Where early loss of pregnancy has occurred, it must be established whether this was by miscarriage, ectopic pregnancy or therapeutic termination of pregnancy ('abortion') and on how many occasions it occurred. The gestation, symptoms leading to miscarriage, complications and any treatment must be noted. If a termination has taken place, ask about the method used (e.g. surgical evacuation or medical management with prostaglandin analogue), any complications and the time taken for the woman to return to a normal menstrual pattern afterwards.

The outcome of each previous pregnancy is recorded as a live birth, a neonatal death or a stillbirth. The birth of a child showing any signs of independent life is recorded as a live birth. This occurs beyond 24 weeks' gestation (or 500 g weight) but, with improved neonatal care, fetal viability may be obtained from an even earlier stage. If such a child dies, that event requires a death certificate in the UK. Also in the UK, a child born after the 24th week of pregnancy who does not, at any time after birth, breathe or show any signs of life is termed 'stillborn' and requires a stillbirth certificate. These are legal requirements. If the child is born dead at an earlier gestation, it is regarded as a miscarriage.

Drug/smoking/alcohol history

As in the gynaecology history, these are all relevant. Prescribed and recreational drugs (including alcohol and tobacco) may harm both mother and fetus. Evidence indicates that some medicinal agents (e.g. methotrexate, both maternal and paternal) have a teratogenic effect when taken prior to the onset of pregnancy. The effect is greater when the relevant agent is taken early in pregnancy (an embryopathy as opposed to a fetopathy; as a general rule, the former has much wider ranging consequences); when in doubt, a full history of exposure time, dosage and gestational age must be taken.

Family history

At some time in the history, taking a genetic history relevant to both partners is required and explored as indicated. Some couples may have had pre-pregnancy counselling if there is a strong family history of a particular disorder. Specific ethnic groups may have particular abnormal genetic predispositions and referral to a clinical geneticist may be indicated. It is especially important to determine whether there is a family history of hypertensive disorders or diabetes, because these can predispose to an increased risk of pre-eclampsia and gestational diabetes, respectively.

Social history

Social history has been discussed under the gynaecology history-taking section and the principles are very similar.

Presentation of obstetric cases

It is common practice in obstetrics to present cases using particular language. Gravidity refers to the condition of pregnancy, regardless of outcome, including the one being presented. It therefore includes any ectopic pregnancies, spontaneous miscarriages and terminations of pregnancy. Para (to bring forth or bear) refers to the number of deliveries over 24 weeks' gestation, or fewer than 24 weeks showing any signs of life. Multiple pregnancies count as one delivery only. Thus, a pregnant woman with one previous healthy child and one previous termination of pregnancy would be described as gravida 3, para 1.

Obstetric examination

General examination

Again, this should follow the approach outlined in Chapter 2. In obstetric practice, height and weight (and calculated BMI) are important. As a general rule, labour is more efficient if the woman is above 152 cm in height; hypertension, gestational diabetes and anaesthetic difficulties are more common if the BMI is above 30 kg/m². Record the blood pressure (it should be 140/90 or lower in a normal pregnancy) and examine carefully for oedema, not only in the ankles but also in the fingers (can she remove her rings easily?) and face. Breast examination is not indicated unless there is a complaint related to the breasts themselves, although it is common for women to ask questions related to breastfeeding.

Abdominal examination in pregnancy

Ask the patient to empty her bladder before the abdominal examination. Make sure the light is good, the room comfortably warm and that there is maximum exposure of the area to be examined (Box 5.6). Look for striae gravidarum ('stretch marks'), linea nigra (a dark coloured midline abdominal stripe), previous caesarean section or other scars and any visible fetal or other movements (unlikely before 30 weeks' gestation, but usually indicative of good health). Ideally the patient is examined semi-recumbent. It is not usually an uncomfortable examination except in certain pathological situations. If part of the examination is likely to be painful, this should be left to the very end.

Ask about any tender areas before palpating the abdomen. Using the flat of the hand as well as the examining fingers can enhance comfort and gentleness; this allows the outline of the pregnant uterus to be delineated more readily. In late pregnancy, palpation may produce uterine contractions, which can obscure details of the uterine contents. Remember that, for women in their first pregnancy, the abdominal musculature (particularly rectus abdominis) has not been previously stretched, such that it is sometimes difficult to be sure about findings on palpation.

The size of the uterus (Fig. 5.9 is a magnetic resonance image (MRI) scan of a normal uterus) is traditionally estimated by the fundal height (see Fig. 5.1), the distance from the symphysis pubis to the fundus (top portion) of the uterus. This is a useful measure, even though it is only one dimension of a globular mass. In a normal pregnancy, the fundal height is just above the symphysis pubis at 12 weeks' gestation, at the umbilicus at 22 weeks and at the xiphisternum at 36 weeks. When the fundus is equidistant from the symphysis pubis and the umbilicus, the gestation is 16 weeks, and when equidistant from the xiphisternum and umbilicus, it is about 30 weeks. From 36 weeks, the fundal height is also dependent on the level of the presenting part, and therefore decreases as the presenting part descends into the pelvis. This is the phenomenon of a 'lightening' sensation experienced by the mother. The height of the fundus above the symphysis is usually recorded in centimetres and, from 20 weeks onwards, the number of centimetres above the symphysis is approximately in accord with the number of weeks of pregnancy, plus or minus 3 cm, up to 38 weeks. This measurement is generally accepted to be objective and, importantly, is reproducible when different healthcare professionals participate in the same woman's care. Common causes of deviation from these measurements include multiple pregnancies, multiple fibroids, maternal obesity, fetal growth restriction and excess or reduced amniotic fluid volume (poly- and oligo-hydramnios, respectively).

Next, determine the lie of the fetus (this is the relationship of the long axis of the fetus to the maternal spine—longitudinal usually, but sometimes oblique or transverse). To confirm the lie, the location of the fetal limbs and back should be identified (Fig. 5.10).

The presentation (the part of the fetus that occupies the lower pole of the uterus) can usually be determined by abdominal palpation if it is cephalic (head), breech (buttocks or feet) or shoulder (Fig. 5.11). Other types of presentation, such as cord and compound, cannot be determined by palpation. At term, over 95% of babies present by the head, but at 30 weeks, because of the greater mobility of the fetus and the relatively larger volume of amniotic fluid, only 70% do so. The breech can usually be distinguished by its size, texture and ability to change shape. However, an ultrasound examination may be needed to confirm this.

The presenting part refers to the part of the fetus that is felt on vaginal examination through the cervix

Box 5.6	Abdominal examination in pregnancy

Inspection

- Striae gravidarum
- Linea nigra
- Scars
- Fetal movements

Palpation

- Fundal height
- Fetal poles and fetal lie
- Presentation: breech, head, etc.
- Attitude
- Level of presenting part
- Fetal movements
- Liquor volume

Auscultation

- Fetal heart rate

Figure 5.9 Magnetic resonance image of the female pelvis. The uterus is arrowed.

Figure 5.10 Method of abdominal palpation to determine fetal lie and location of back.

Figure 5.11 Method of abdominal palpation to determine presenting part.

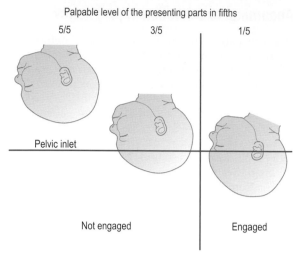

Palpable level of the presenting parts in fifths

5/5   3/5   1/5

Pelvic inlet

Not engaged   Engaged

Figure 5.12 The vertical relationship of the presenting part to the pelvic inlet (the level).

(see Vaginal examination in labour, below). The head may be presenting, but the flexion of the head, or the extension of it, will govern what the presenting part is. In cephalic presentations, the smallest diameters presented to the pelvis occur when the head is well flexed. Thus, in a flexed head, it will be a vertex presentation; in a deflexed head, it will be the brow or even the face. Flexion of the head is termed the attitude. These observations are not usually possible to ascertain on abdominal examination. For a breech presentation, an equivalent assessment is made to determine whether the breech is extended (frank), flexed (complete) or footling (incomplete). Once the presenting part has a relationship to the pelvis, that relationship can be vertical (the level) or rotational (the position). When the flexed head presents, the fetal occiput is termed the denominator. When the face presents, the denominator is the mentum (chin) and when the breech presents, it is the sacrum.

The presenting part is said to be engaged when the largest diameter has passed through the pelvic brim. It is conventional to estimate the number of fifths of the head that can be palpated through the abdominal wall and this indicates its level (Fig. 5.12). Thus, if three or more fifths are palpable, the baby's head will

be unengaged. If less than three-fifths are palpable, then the baby's head is probably engaged in the pelvis, but this does depend on the overall size of the fetal head and of the pelvis. Remember that the pelvic brim has an angle of approximately 45° to the horizontal when the mother is lying flat. If the abdominal wall is reasonably thin, the unengaged head can be palpated by the examiner's fingers passing round its maximum diameter (a manoeuvre known as a 'Pawlik grip'). This means it is above the pelvic brim. When this does not occur, the widest diameter must be below the examining fingers, and fixity of the baby's head in the pelvis is also a guide. This means it is engaged. Engagement will usually occur as the leading edge of the baby's head, on vaginal examination, reaches the level of the ischial spines (zero station).

Fetal movements, both as reported by the mother and observed by the examiner during the examination, are noted. An estimate is made of the fetal size and volume of liquor by a combination of palpation and ballottement. This requires considerable practice. Last, the fetal heart rate (FHR) (normally between 115 and 160 beats/min) is recorded using either a Pinard stethoscope (Fig. 5.13) or now more often with a handheld Doppler device.

Vaginal examination in pregnancy

Vaginal examination (VE) is not usually recommended in early pregnancy. If there is bleeding or retention of urine, it may provide useful information, but the widespread availability of ultrasound scanning has made diagnosis in this situation far less intrusive. In the situation of a threatened miscarriage, it is more appropriate to perform a detailed ultrasound examination, even on the next working day if necessary, than to undertake a VE that may not be particularly helpful. Exceptions to this approach include a suspected ectopic pregnancy with haemodynamic instability

- Is the cervix anterior, mid position or posterior?
- What is the consistency of the cervix—hard, firm or soft?
- Is the cervix dilated?
- Is the cervix effaced (thinned)?
- What is the presenting part? Assuming a head/cephalic presentation, is the presenting part a vertex (posterior fontanelle palpable through the cervical os), a deflexed head (anterior fontanelle palpable) or, unusually, a brow (supraorbital ridges palpable) or face (mentum or chin)?
- What is the station? The station is the relationship in centimetres between the dominator as above and the ischial spine of the pelvis and is measured in centimetres above or below the spines; thus the depth of the presenting part is low when the tip of the presenting part is 2 or 3 cm below the spines.

Figure 5.13 Listening over the fetal back to the fetal heart with a Pinard stethoscope (now largely historical).

or the situation of considerable vaginal blood loss in early pregnancy, in which it is important quickly to diagnose the presence of (and remove) the products of conception at the cervical os. Cervical smears are rarely indicated in pregnancy, unless there is suspicion of a cervical malignancy or one is required for follow-up of known cervical neoplasia.

A case for VE can be made in the situation of possible cervical incompetence. This is a situation in which previous surgery or loop diathermy has led to thinning and dilatation of the cervix such that the weight of the pregnancy sac is too great for the cervix to withstand. The patient, usually somewhere between 16 and 24 weeks into pregnancy, may complain of a small vaginal loss and irregular contractions. If the natural history is allowed to progress, there will be rupture of the membranes followed by a short and painful labour, with subsequent delivery of a fetus (almost always non-viable). Scanning of the cervix in cases at risk has replaced these examinations to some extent, but it remains a difficult problem to diagnose.

Vaginal examination in labour

Assessment of whether a woman is in labour is not always straightforward. A VE may help but is contraindicated if there is painless loss of blood and/or it is known that the patient has a low-lying placenta; potentially dangerous blood loss can occur if a VE disturbs a low-lying placenta.

Vaginal examination in labour should always be preceded by an abdominal examination, as described above, together with observation of any contractions, their intensity, frequency, length of time and whether and how much pain they provoke. The VE aims to answer the questions listed in Box 5.7.

The Bishop score, an amalgam of these findings (excepting the presenting part) at VE, is used to determine whether a woman is in labour. A low

score is indicative of an 'unfavourable cervix' (firm, posterior, long, closed cervix with a high presenting part). In contrast, a 'favourable cervix' is one which is associated with an efficient labour—anterior (easy to reach), soft, open, thinned, with a low presenting part.

By repeating abdominal and vaginal examinations at intervals, the diagnosis and progression of labour can be ascertained. Vaginal examination is a potential introduction of infection and can be unpleasant and uncomfortable, so it is usual not to perform this more frequently than every 4 hours. Once labour is established (i.e. the cervix is fully effaced and dilated at least 4 cm), the cervix should progressively dilate at a rate of at least 0.5 cm per hour.

Investigations in obstetrics and gynaecology

A variety of investigations is available in gynaecological and obstetric practice. The principles of some commonly requested ones are described here.

Pregnancy testing

Most pregnancy tests depend on the detection of human chorionic gonadotrophin (hCG) or its β subunit in urine or blood, respectively. As the chorion produces increasing amounts of hCG from about 10 days post-fertilization, pregnancy diagnosis is possible even before the first missed period. Urine pregnancy test kits may be used at the bedside.

Bacteriological and virus tests

Bacteriological and virus tests used in gynaecology and obstetrics include the following:

- Swabs from the throat, endocervix, vagina, urethra and rectum may be needed to diagnose sexually transmitted diseases (see Chapter 18 for more detail).

Figure 5.14　Ultrasound scan for early dating.

- Cervical scrape brush or liquid cytology samples for human papilloma virus.
- Mid-stream urinalysis (MSU).
- Serum tests for toxoplasma, rubella, cytomegalovirus and herpes simplex (TORCH) detect antibodies from previous infections and may indicate the risk of congenital infection in a future pregnancy.

Imaging

Ultrasound

Transabdominal ultrasound enables a wide field of view, greater depth of penetration and transducer movement. Transvaginal ultrasound, with higher frequency transducers, gives increased resolution and diagnostic power but over a more limited area. More recently, 3-D scanners have been introduced, and these give improved image quality.

In obstetrics, the integrity, location and the number of gestation sacs can be viewed in early pregnancy. By 11 to 13 weeks, mono- or dichorionicity, nuchal translucency, nasal bone development and gross fetal abnormality can be detected (Figs 5.14 and 5.15). Cervical length can be measured, giving an indication of risk of possible late miscarriage or early premature labour. Fetal anatomy surveillance can be carried out using ultrasound from 18 weeks and, if indicated, this can include fetal echocardiography. By 20 weeks, uterine and placental blood flow can be assessed in the form of a uterine artery Doppler test, which can help predict risk of fetal growth restriction and pre-eclampsia. Ultrasound scans in the second and third trimester can be used to measure fetal growth velocity, amniotic fluid volumes, and Doppler examination of blood flow through fetal arteries can be used to ascertain fetal wellbeing.

In gynaecology, ultrasound is useful in the diagnosis of uterine and ovarian pathology and in the assessment of bladder function by measuring residual urine volume and bladder neck activity. It

Figure 5.15　An ultrasound image with shading that gives an impression of three dimensions. Its use scientifically is not yet determined, but patients love it for the view it gives of their babies.

Figure 5.16　An abnormal X-ray hysterosalpingogram: uteri didelphys (double uterus).

is also helpful in the preoperative preparation for repair of anal sphincter damage.

Computed tomography and magnetic resonance imaging

Computed tomography (CT) scanning has proved less useful in gynaecology than was originally anticipated and now is used mainly for staging and follow-up of malignancies. Magnetic resonance imaging, where available, is a better option (see Fig. 5.9). It does not use ionizing radiation and is particularly good at staging gynaecological malignancies.

Hysterosalpingography

Imaging the uterine cavity and Fallopian tubes with X-ray hysterosalpingography (Fig. 5.16) has largely been replaced by the contemporary technique of

Figure 5.17 An endometrial biopsy curette, a pipette cell sampler and fixing medium.

hysterosonography (hysterosalpingo contrast sonography, HyCoSy), in which the flow of saline or galactose microparticles through the tubes and uterus is visualized with a vaginal ultrasound probe, thereby avoiding exposure to radiation.

Endometrial sampling (biopsy)

Sampling of the endometrium is often diagnostically useful. An adequate representative sample of endometrium can be obtained using a Vibra or Pipelle sampling system in the outpatient setting (Fig. 5.17). The definitive assessment of the endometrium is usually by hysteroscopy and directed biopsy. With current miniature fibreoptic systems, this can be done under local analgesia in an outpatient setting.

Colposcopy

Colposcopy permits visualization of the cervix, the vaginal vault (vaginoscopy) or vulva (vulvoscopy) with an illuminated binocular microscope to detect precancerous abnormalities of the epithelium. It can be undertaken on an outpatient basis, by accessing the cervix with a speculum, treating it first with acetic acid then with Lugol's iodine. This aqueous solution of iodine and potassium iodide causes the cervix and the normal mucous membrane, which contain glycogen, to stain dark brown. Those areas of abnormality that fail to take up the stain can then be identified (Schiller's test). The whole cervix is viewed through a colposcope, which gives binocular magnification, to identify the degree, site and extent of the cervical pathology.

Hysteroscopy

In the hysteroscopy technique, the cavity of the uterus is viewed using small-diameter fibreoptic instruments (Fig. 5.18). Diagnostic hysteroscopy using a 4-mm hysteroscope can be performed as both an inpatient and an outpatient procedure for disorders such as abnormal bleeding and subfertility. This technique can also be adapted with larger hysteroscopes to be used operatively for the resection

Figure 5.18 Hysteroscopic view of an intrauterine device in situ.

Figure 5.19 Hysteroscopic view of submucosal fibroids.

of uterine adhesions, polyps, septae, submucous fibroids (Fig. 5.19) and endometrium.

Cystoscopy and cystometry

The pressure/volume relationships of bladder filling, detrusor and sphincter activity and urethral flow rate can be assessed with a cystometrogram. The bladder is catheterized and slowly filled with sterile saline. The volume and pressure at which bladder filling is perceived, and at which a desire to micturate is felt, are noted. The urinary flow rate and postmicturition bladder volume are recorded. Electromyographic (EMG) activity in the external urethral sphincter and/or real-time ultrasound assessment of bladder neck activity and descent may provide further

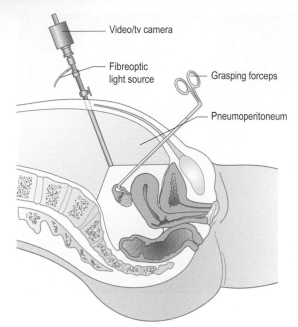

Video/tv camera

Fibreoptic
light source

Grasping forceps

Pneumoperitoneum

Figure 5.20 Diagram of a diagnostic laparoscopy.

information. In stress incontinence, urinary flow commences at low bladder pressures because of sphincter incompetence; in urge incontinence, urinary flow develops at low bladder volumes because of uninhibited detrusor activity. Reflux and overflow also show as urethral leakage. Incontinence can also result from a defect in the anatomical integrity of the urinary tract, such as a congenital abnormality or fistula. Viewing the interior of the bladder by cystoscopy provides information about its condition and allows biopsy of the mucosa or the removal of foreign bodies.

Laparoscopy

Visualization of the pelvic and abdominal viscera is particularly valuable if it can be done without a major injury to the abdominal wall (Fig. 5.20). The abdomen is inflated with carbon dioxide under general or local anaesthesia, so that the anterior abdominal wall is lifted away from the viscera, allowing inspection of the abdominal and pelvic contents using a fibreoptic telescope illuminated by a light source remote from the patient. Laparoscopy may be useful diagnostically (e.g. in the investigation of pelvic pain or infertility) and therapeutically (e.g. sterilization procedures, ectopic pregnancy, division of adhesions, treatment of endometriosis and hysterectomy).

Tests of fetal wellbeing

Besides 'standard' tests of maternal health (haemoglobin, blood glucose, etc.), various investigations may be used to assess fetal wellbeing. In the UK hepatitis B and HIV testing is offered to all pregnant women, and particularly to those in known risk groups, and may also be checked anonymously in order to obtain an estimate of the community prevalence of these infections.

Biochemical tests

Early pregnancy markers

α-Fetoprotein (AFP), unconjugated oestriol, βhCG, inhibin A, PAPP A

These are normal fetal proteins or hormones that pass into the amniotic fluid and maternal serum. The maternal concentration of these substances varies in a predictable way with gestation. For example, at 16 weeks' gestation, increased levels of AFP suggest fetal spina bifida or anencephaly. However, similar levels can be caused by several other conditions, including threatened miscarriage, multiple pregnancy and exomphalos. Decreased levels are associated with Down's syndrome. A computed risk of Down's syndrome can be produced from maternal weight, gestation, parity and race, measured against βhCG and unconjugated oestriol, and the results matched against ultrasound findings. The 'integrated test' for Down's syndrome predicts a risk ratio that depends on such a comparison. Alternatively, the 'combined test' uses the same information plus fetal nuchal translucency at 11 to 13 weeks' gestation.

Late pregnancy

Fetal health in labour can be estimated by checking for the presence of meconium, the responsiveness of the fetal heart rate and by counting fetal movements. In addition to these simple clinical tests, fetal pH measured on a scalp blood sample can be used to detect acidosis and is particularly useful if labour is prolonged, complicated or known to be high risk. Once the membranes are ruptured, the fetal scalp is displayed using an amnioscope and a small sample of capillary blood obtained from a puncture site. If the pH of the sample is below 7.2 then delivery is an urgent priority.

Biological tests

Although biochemical tests provide useful information as the likelihood of a problem with a fetus, biological tests are generally more specific and accurate. It is important before commencing these tests that the woman's attitude to the possible outcomes is explored. Detailed counselling by a trained professional may be required.

Chorion biopsy (chorionic villus sampling, CVS)

Chorion biopsy is a method of obtaining chorionic material at 9 to 13 weeks of pregnancy (usually

Figure 5.21 Multicoloured FISH. The FISH technique is 'fluorescent in situ hybridization'. The picture is not meant for detail but to show the overall multicoloured appearance of the specific nucleic acid sequences on metaphase chromosomes, which allows the antenatal diagnosis of Down's syndrome, X-linked disorders, Turner's syndrome, Klinefelter's syndrome and trisomies 13 and 18.

Figure 5.22 Cardiotocography equipment.

through the abdomen) so that the genetic constitution or biochemical function of fetal cellular material can be determined. It is useful for the diagnosis of Down's syndrome, thalassaemia and a number of other hereditary conditions. Early and rapid diagnosis allows the possibility of therapeutic termination of an abnormal pregnancy, thereby increasing the safety and acceptability of that procedure. There is a small but definite increased risk of spontaneous miscarriage after CVS.

Amniocentesis

Samples of amniotic fluid may be used for the following:
- Chromosome analysis: amniotic fluid is sampled at 13 to 18 weeks' gestation and is currently safer than chorion biopsy. The amount of desquamated fetal cells obtained is much smaller than from chorion biopsy, and cell culture is necessary, so chromosomal analysis is not immediately possible. However, rapid preliminary results can be obtained using the fluorescent in situ hybridization (FISH) technique (Fig. 5.21). This test is mostly used for prenatal diagnosis of Down's syndrome and other chromosomal abnormalities.
- DNA analysis: fetal cells obtained by amniocentesis, CVS or cordocentesis (see below) can be used for DNA analysis of nuclear chromatin in order to test directly for a number of genetically determined diseases in families known to be at risk. DNA testing and chromosomal studies should be carried out only with fully informed parental consent, and with the help of a genetic counselling service.
- Cordocentesis: in this procedure, a needle is inserted through the abdominal wall and into the amniotic sac to obtain fetal blood from the placental insertion of the cord. It is used in special centres when chromosomal abnormality,

haemophilia, haemoglobinopathies, inborn errors of metabolism, fetal viral infections or fetal anaemia are suspected. Although the procedure carries more risk than amniocentesis, it is less traumatic than fetoscopy (which views the amniotic sac contents directly) while still permitting rapid diagnosis.

Non-invasive prenatal testing

Technological advances have meant that it is now possible to detect cell-free fetal DNA in maternal plasma. Because this technique removes the risk of miscarriage associated with invasive testing, it is likely to enter general obstetric practice once cost-effectiveness is established.

Biophysical tests

Fetal movements

In some cases of placental insufficiency, fetal movements decrease or stop 12 to 48 hours before the fetal heart ceases to beat. In a healthy pregnancy, fetal movements generally increase from the 32nd week of pregnancy to term. Subjective reports of reduced movements are likely to be more significant than attempting to use a counting system. A report of reduced fetal movements may indicate that sophisticated and detailed surveillance is required.

Cardiotocography (CTG)

Assessment of the fetal heart rate and its variation with fetal and uterine activity can be recorded antenatally or in labour with ultrasound using the Doppler principle (Figs 5.22 and 5.23). A pressure transducer is attached to the abdominal wall so that variations in uterine activity can be matched with the ultrasound recordings. In labour, once the membranes rupture, a more accurate recording of the fetal heart rate can be achieved by an electrode attached to the

Figure 5.23 An abnormal cardiotocograph showing late variable decelerations during uterine contractions with fetal tachycardia.

Figure 5.24 Fetal scalp electrode.

fetal scalp (Fig. 5.24). The recording is triggered by the fetal electrocardiogram. The information received may be further refined by computerized analysis of the ST segment of the fetal ECG.

Ultrasound visualization

Sequential real-time ultrasonic scanning to detect the presence of symmetrical or asymmetrical growth retardation or changes in fetal activity, breathing, movements, and so forth, can be used to assess placental function. If it becomes clear that fetal growth has halted or the child's survival in utero is in doubt, then urgent assessment of blood flow by Doppler and delivery with neonatal medicine support should be planned.

Doppler blood flow

Studies of changes in the uterine circulation (uterine artery Doppler) may predict the later onset of pregnancy-associated hypertension. Changes in uteroplacental blood flow (absence or reversal of end-diastolic flow in the umbilical arteries) and those in the cerebral fetal circulation (especially the middle cerebral artery) and fetal ductus venosus give further clues to the state of the fetus, or even imminent fetal death, especially in already compromised circumstances.

Children and adolescents | 6

Anna Riddell

Introduction

The skill of clinical examination is the true art of medicine and nowhere more so than in the examination of children. Children are not small adults and, as such, the approach to their examination differs. The examiner needs to be flexible, opportunistic and able to tailor the examination to the individual infant, child or young person. In order to maximize the success of the examination, time must be spent trying to gain the patient's confidence. During most of the examination the child should be contented and any discomfort minimized. Do not give false reassurances as this will result in a loss of trust, which will hinder the examination. It helps if the consulting room has a range of toys suitable for all ages. Younger children may be happier sitting on their parent's lap. If old enough, the child should be allowed to explore the room freely.

As the family enters the room they should be greeted in a friendly manner and introductions made. Adapt the approach according to the age of the child. An adolescent may want to be the focus of the consultation from the start. Younger children usually will want to have time to observe and assess their surroundings before being observed themselves. They will often take a cue from their carer's response. If everyone relaxes and laughs in the first few minutes, the child will relax and the subsequent history and examination will be easier. Ascertain who is with the child. It may not be the mother or father but another family member. Establish at the onset if you will need the help of an advocate to communicate effectively with the family.

For the experienced clinician, much of the information needed to reach a diagnosis for a child is gleaned from careful observation. While talking with the parent, watch and listen to the child. Assess his behaviour and use this information to adapt the approach. Does the child look unwell? Is the child interested in the surroundings and exploring them, or apathetic? Watch the child running around: are there any obvious abnormalities in the gait? Is the face normal, or are there features of abnormal development? Are there any obvious physical abnormalities? Look at the skin, posture, limbs and for any obvious dysmorphic features. Is the breathing unusually noisy? Does the child seem well nourished, or wasted? What is the child's interaction with his/her carer like?

History

The history (Box 6.1) is normally taken from the accompanying carer, but an older child can be invited to give his/her version of events first. It is appropriate to give an adolescent the opportunity for a few minutes of confidential time during the consultation. Use this time to ask questions about alcohol, drugs and sexual activity, which young people may be uncomfortable discussing in front of their parents or carers. Even younger children should be asked simple things in words they can understand. Involve them by asking relevant questions such as the site of the pain, etc. Remember that the carers are giving their versions of the problem, not the child's. Parents may also welcome an opportunity to talk in private away from the child, and it is often during such discussion that the real reason for the consultation emerges. Always take notice of what the carers are saying and listen to their concerns. Any interruptions should be to clarify rather than try and direct the history. Make sure they are given full attention and that they feel their concerns are being taken seriously. All the time they are talking, keep watching everything that the child is doing and his reactions.

Box 6.1	Structure to history taking in children

- Presenting problem(s)
- History of the presenting complaint
- Previous medical history:
  - birth and the newborn period
  - immunizations
  - specific illnesses, accidents, etc.
  - development and behaviour (including milestones)
  - school
  - contacts and travel
- Family history:
  - consanguinity and genetic risk
- Social history
- Drug history (including allergies)

Box 6.2	Pregnancy and infancy

- Did the mother have any particular illnesses or infections, or was she taking any drugs during the pregnancy (including alcohol)?
- Was the baby born at term?
- What were the birth weight and type of delivery?
- Were there any problems in the newborn period: jaundice, breathing problems, fits, feeding difficulties?
- Has the baby had any illnesses?
- How was the baby fed? When were solid foods introduced?
- Were there any intolerances to food?
- Was the weight gain satisfactory?
- What immunizations has the child had?

The structure and focus of the history differ slightly from that of an adult. The core elements of the presenting complaint, a history of the present illness and a history of any previous illness are the same; however, greater emphasis will be placed on aspects such as the developmental history and less on the systems enquiry. Much of the key information will be collected in the history of the presenting complaint. Most children have a single system involved, and enough time needs to be spent evaluating this carefully. Consider the timing of the symptoms; do they tend only to occur at school? Are there any associating or triggering factors? Are the symptoms interrupting daily activities such as sleep, school attendance, participation in sport or play? Is the child's perception of the symptoms different to that of the parent? Ask about symptoms from other systems in relation to the presenting history rather than as abstract questions. For example, a child presenting with cough may be asked about symptoms of gastro-oesophageal reflux, which may be an underlying cause for the cough.

In children, the previous medical history starts from birth and specific attention should be paid to the pregnancy and newborn period (Box 6.2). If the child was born preterm and had a complicated neonatal course ask what impact this has had on his health and activities. Is the child fully immunized? This can be checked in the child's health record, held by the parent, which should have documentation of child health clinic attendances, weights, immunizations, etc. Enquire into the nature and severity of previous illnesses and the age at which they occurred, for example common childhood infections such as chickenpox, admissions to hospital (in particular to intensive care), significant injuries and accidents. Is the child taking any regular medication or allergic to anything? It is important to ask about the child's developmental progress: when did the child first sit up, smile, crawl, walk and talk? Fuller details regarding the 'milestones of development' are given in Table 6.1. Some useful general questions are outlined in Box 6.3.

Family history

Ask about parental age and consanguinity. Find out who are the other children in the family, with age and sex, and who else lives in the family home. Find out if there have been any stillbirths, miscarriages or childhood deaths in the family. Ask if there are any illnesses in the siblings, parents or any near relatives, and if there is any background of inherited disease.

Social history

Approach the social history with diplomacy; sometimes it is more prudent to leave deeper probing to a later occasion in order to develop an initial rapport. The depth of enquiry in a paediatric social history must always be judged on an individual basis. It is useful to know about living conditions and whether either or both parents are employed. Who is the main carer for the child? Is the child in any form of day care? If the child has been separated from the main carer in the past or there is difficulty in the parent's relationship (for example domestic abuse), this may be the basis of a variety of behavioural difficulties. Is there a supportive family structure involving other relatives, for example grandparents? Has the family moved between or within the country frequently and how many languages are spoken in the family? Is the child a looked-after child or is he subject to a child protection plan. For a school-aged child find out which school he attends and whether he requires any additional learning support.

Examination

After forming an impression of the child, the family and their relationship, the examination can now proceed. By now, younger children should have found the occasion so fascinating that they will be prepared to cooperate in most parts of the physical examination, or they may even have fallen asleep. If the child is now crying loudly, things will be difficult and strategies to calm him down to allow examination will be needed.

A key principle in the examination of children is that most of the information needed to make a diagnosis will be obtained during careful observation, including listening to the child and playing with the child. Findings can then be consolidated with the remaining techniques requiring laying on of hands. Try to get down to the level of the child in order to appear less threatening. Undress the child in stages so the examination is complete, but not intimidating. Older children will usually cooperate sufficiently to be examined lying down, and routine physical examination is similar to an adult examination. A younger child should be examined sitting on his carer's lap, as any attempt to get the child to lie down may result in distress. Always talk to children, however young; do not be afraid of looking silly if

Table 6.1 Normal developmental milestones

Age	Movement and posture	Vision and manipulation	Hearing and speech	Social behaviour
6 weeks	When pulled from supine to sitting, head lag is not quite complete When held prone, head is held in line with body When prone on couch, lifts chin off couch Primitive responses persist	Looks at toy, held in midline Follows a moving person	Vocalizes with gurgles	Smiles briefly when talked to by mother
4 months	Holds head up in sitting position, and is steady Pulls to sitting with only minimal head lag When prone, with head and chest off couch, makes swimming movements Rolls from prone to supine	Watches his hands Pulls at his clothes Tries to grasp objects	Turns head to sound Vocalizes appropriately Laughs	Recognizes mother Becomes excited by toys
7 months	Sits unsupported Rolls from supine to prone Can support weight when held, and bounces with pleasure When prone, bears weight on hands	Transfers objects from hand to hand Bangs toys on table Watches small moving objects	Says 'Da', 'Ba', 'Ka' (babbling)	Tries to feed self Puts objects in mouth Plays with paper
10 months	Crawls Gets to sitting position without help Can pull up to standing Lifts one foot when standing	Reaches for objects with index finger Has developed a finger–thumb grasp Object permanence (knows an object exists even when it is removed from view)	Says one word with meaning	Plays 'peep-bo' and 'pat-a-cake' Waves 'bye-bye' Deliberately drops objects so that they can be picked up Puts objects in and out of boxes
13 months	Walks unsupported May shuffle on buttocks and hands	Can hold two cubes in one hand Makes marks with pen	Says two or three words with meaning	Understands simple questions such as 'Show me your shoe?' Tends to be shy
15 months	Can get into standing position without support Climbs upstairs Walks with broad-based gait	Builds a tower of two cubes Takes off shoes	Will say around 12 words, but often understood only by parents	Asks for things by pointing Can use a cup
18 months	Climbs stairs unaided holding rail Runs and jumps Can climb onto a chair and sit down	Builds tower of three cubes Turns pages of a book two or three at a time Scribbles Takes off gloves and socks Can undo a zip	Is beginning to join two words together	Recognizes animals and cars in a book Points to nose, ear, etc. on request Aware of when needs the toilet but not clean and dry Carries out simple orders

the result is a cooperative child. Those parts of the examination that are unpleasant should be left until last; if an attempt is made to examine a child's throat at the outset, the rest of the examination could be jeopardized. Offer the child something to play with—even a stethoscope will be entertaining to a young infant. Children often find it amusing if their toy is examined first. The scheme set out in Box 6.4 can be adapted opportunistically, provided all areas are covered.

Always wash your hands before and after the examination in front of the parent. This will inspire

---

Box 6.3   General questions

- What are the child's present habits with regard to eating, sleeping, bowels and micturition?
- What sort of personality does he have—e.g. extrovert, moody?
- Behaviour: anything unusual that worries the parent?
- How does he get on with other children?
- How does the child compare with siblings or friends of the same age?
- School: which school, does he like it, academic achievement, does he miss much school?

Box 6.4   Scheme for examination of children

- Face
- Head
- Neck
- Feet
- Hands and pulse
- Abdomen
- Chest
- Neurological
- Eyes and fundoscopy
- Genitalia, groins, anus
- Ear, nose and throat
- Routine measurements and simple clinical tests

---

confidence and show that you take infection control seriously. The examination techniques include the usual methods of inspection, palpation, percussion and auscultation; however, no set routine can be followed, and the examination is by regions rather than by systems. The older the child, the more the examination will be akin to that for an adult. Bear in mind the child's age and level of understanding and ability to cooperate when planning the examination. Infants and younger children will need alternative strategies and adapted techniques to elicit clinical signs. The examination may have to be opportunistic, as each child will dictate the order of the examination by his reactions to various procedures.

General examination

If the child appears unwell then the ABCDE approach should be used for assessment (https://www.resus.org.uk/resuscitation-guidelines/abcde-approach/). If not, then proceed as follows.

Note the state of nutrition. Are there any obvious rashes to be seen? Are there any naevi or other skin anomalies? Look at the colour of the child's lips: is there cyanosis or pallor? Listen to the child. Are there any audible noises such as stridor, wheeze or stertor? Is the speech appropriate for the age of the child? Has the child come with any pieces of equipment, such as a feeding pump or portable oxygen? Are there any obvious devices to be seen, such as a central venous line, gastrostomy tube,

Figure 6.1   Plagiocephalic skull.

suprapubic catheter or ventriculoperitoneal shunt? Is the child interacting with the parent and with you as expected for his age? If not, why not? There could be a sensory deficit or a behavioural problem as a reason for this.

The head, face and neck

Look at the child's face and ask the following questions:

- Does it look normal? If not, try to identify which features seem unusual and describe them. Many syndromes are diagnosable by particular facial features.
- If the baby looks dysmorphic, then do not forget to look at the parents to correlate with any family traits. If the appearance is still not clear, ask who the baby looks like.
- Does the child have a large or protruding tongue?
- Are the ears in the normal position, or are they low set and abnormal in any way?
- Are the eyes small (microphthalmus)? Are they set close together or wide apart (hypo- or hypertelorism)?

Next note the shape of the head. This needs to be done by viewing the child's head from the front, sides and from above. It may be small if the baby is microcephalic; globular if the baby is hydrocephalic, sometimes with dilated veins over the skin surface; or brachycephalic (flattened over the occiput), for example in trisomy 21 (Down's syndrome). It is often asymmetrical (plagiocephalic) in normal infants who tend to lie with their heads persistently on one side (Fig. 6.1). This is now much more common because babies are placed on their backs to sleep in order to reduce the risk of sudden death in infancy. It becomes much less noticeable as the child grows older.

Having gained the child's confidence you can now feel his head for fontanelles and sutures. The anterior fontanelle is normally small at birth, enlarges during the first 2 months, and then gradually reduces until final closure at around 18 months. It can close much earlier and has been reported as staying open in a few normal girls until 4 years of age. Delayed closure may be seen, however, in rickets, hypothyroidism and hydrocephalus. An assessment of the tension of the anterior fontanelle is important. In health, it pulsates and is in the same plane as the rest of the surrounding skull. A tense, bulging fontanelle indicates raised intracranial pressure, but it also becomes tense with crying. A sunken fontanelle is a feature of severe dehydration. The posterior fontanelle is located by passing the finger along the sagittal suture to its junction with the lambdoid sutures. It should normally be closed after 2 months of age. Sometimes, when passing the finger along the sagittal suture, a small notch is felt over the vault of the cranium. This is the third fontanelle and, although it can be normal, it is seen in some chromosome abnormalities and in congenital infections such as rubella. While feeling the head, any ridging of the sutures should be noticed, suggesting premature fusion (craniosynostosis). In the neonatal period, the sutures tend to be separated, and there is sometimes a continuous gap from the forehead to the posterior part of the posterior fontanelle. Sutures close rapidly and are normally ossified by 6 months of age. Leave the measurement of the head circumference until near the end of the examination, because some babies find this a little threatening and may start crying.

Having assessed the skull, the neck can be checked, paying particular attention to the presence of lymph nodes. It is common in childhood to feel small lymph nodes in the anterior and posterior triangles of the neck. They can persist for some years and change in size in response to local infections such as tonsillitis (reactive lymphadenopathy). Lymph nodes of greater than 2 cm diameter or rapidly increasing size may indicate significant pathology and should be investigated. Examination of other lymphatic areas can be carried out at a later stage of the examination—the inguinal nodes when the nappy area is checked, and the axillary nodes when the chest is examined. In young babies, the sternomastoid muscles should be checked for the thickened area known as a sternomastoid tumour. This is a benign lesion occurring usually as a result of birth trauma, but it can lead to difficulties with neck movement and an abnormal head and neck posture. Torticollis, a potentially more sinister sign, can be associated with posterior fossa tumours, vertebral osteomyelitis and urinary tract infections.

The limbs

The feet need to be checked for a variety of problems, such as minor varus deformities, overriding toes or flat feet. Genu varum (bow legs) is common in toddlers and usually the legs straighten with age;

Figure 6.2 Baby sitting on mother's lap while the abdomen is examined.

however, it could be a sign of rickets caused by vitamin D deficiency. It is helpful to feel the surface of the legs with your hands to detect muscle wasting or tenderness. Note any bony abnormalities and examine the movements of the knee and ankle. Feel for any swelling or warmth of the joints, which may be suggestive of an arthropathy. At the same time, an assessment of the muscle tone can be made. This part of the examination may be made easier as part of a game. It is easy to notice at the same time whether the skin is dry or lichenified (as in eczema) and to note any skin lesions. All the time the child's reactions should be watched. Is the child still friendly? Be prepared to stop the examination if the child seems to be getting upset, and spend a few minutes trying to re-establish the previous rapport.

The examination can now proceed to the rest of the body. The arms can be examined in the same way as the legs. Do the hands have a single palmar crease, as seen in children with trisomy 21? Is there any clubbing leading to suspicion of underlying cyanotic congenital heart disease or chronic lung disease, such as cystic fibrosis? Are there any limb abnormalities such as syndactyly (fusion of the digits) or polydactyly (extra digits)? Feel the wrists for widening of the epiphyses of the radius and ulna—a sign of rickets. Try to feel the pulse and count it. This is best done at the brachial pulse in a plump, young infant.

The abdomen

The abdomen can be a little difficult to examine if the child is crying, which is why it is important to have gained the child's cooperation by this point in the examination. Most infants and toddlers will need to be examined while sitting on their carer's lap (Fig. 6.2). It is sometimes possible to quieten a crying infant by placing him over his mother's shoulder and examining from behind. Small infants can be given a feed to quieten them. Older children can be asked if they would be happy to lie on an examination couch.

The examination needs to be structured along the three essential components of looking (observation),

Box 6.5	Causes of abdominal distension

- Obesity
- Faeces (constipation, Hirschsprung's disease)
- Ascites (nephrotic syndrome, liver disease)
- Gas (intestinal obstruction, swallowed air)
- Pregnancy in adolescent girls
- Distended bladder (lower abdomen)
- Pyloric stenosis (upper abdomen)
- Abdominal mass caused by a tumour, cyst or collection

Box 6.6	Reasons for a thoracotomy

- Lung surgery
- Persistent ductus arteriosus repair
- Pulmonary artery banding
- Coarctation of the aorta repair
- Blalock–Taussig shunt (also results in unequal radial pulses)

Table 6.2 Causes of hepatomegaly and splenomegaly in children

Hepatomegaly	Splenomegaly	Hepatosplenomegaly
Glycogen storage disorders	Sickle cell disease	Leukaemia
Congenital infections	Spherocytosis	Lymphoma
Heart failure	Malaria	Mucopolysaccharidoses
Haemolytic disease of the newborn		Thalassaemia
		Alpha-1-antitrypsin deficiency

feeling (palpation) and listening (auscultation). Note the presence of any feeding tubes or drains, which may give you valuable information about underlying illness. Look for scars over the abdomen. A laparotomy scar will indicate major abdominal surgery, a 'Mercedes Benz scar' a liver transplant, lower abdominal scars may indicate previous renal surgery. During the first 3 years of life, the abdomen often gives an impression of being protuberant owing to the laxity of the rectus muscles. Causes of true abdominal distension are shown in Box 6.5. Look for any obvious distension or for peristaltic waves (intestinal obstruction or pyloric stenosis). Note the umbilicus and whether or not there is a hernia. Palpation should be gentle initially. Always ask the child if his tummy hurts anywhere and watch his facial expression during palpation. The liver edge can be felt in normal children up to the age of 4 years; it can be anything up to 2 cm below the costal margin. When enlarged, the spleen may be felt below the left costal margin; in infancy it is more anterior and superficial than in the older child or adult. Slight enlargement of the spleen can occur in many childhood infections (EBV, CMV). Causes of hepatosplenomegaly are listed in Table 6.2. Faecal masses can be felt in the left iliac fossa in constipated children. They often feel like a sausage that could be rolled underneath the fingertips. A full or distended bladder presents as a mass arising from the pelvis. Deep palpation of the kidneys can be carried out last. Although it would be logical to examine the groin area at this time, it is often better to do this at a later stage. If the child has cried persistently, it is still possible to examine the abdomen. When the baby breathes in and the abdominal muscles relax, the abdominal viscera and other masses, if present, can be palpated.

The chest

Examining the chest in a child takes in both the respiratory and cardiovascular systems. The basic structure remains the same: first looking, then feeling then listening with the stethoscope. It helps to have let the child play with the stethoscope at an earlier stage of the examination to alleviate any worries about this strange instrument. Observation will give much of the information required for the diagnosis, particularly in younger children and infants. On observation, check for abnormalities that are fixed and those which become obvious on movement. Static deformities in children include pectus excavatum and carinatum, which are a source of great anxiety to many parents but are not usually of any clinical importance. Fixed indentation of the lower ribs at the line of insertion of the diaphragm (Harrison's sulcus) may be seen in obstructive airway disease, owing either to asthma or to a nasopharynx blocked by adenoidal hypertrophy or in conditions leading to increased pulmonary blood flow. Look from the side for an increased anteroposterior diameter of the chest, which could be a sign of a chronic lung disease such as cystic fibrosis. Thickening of the costochondral junction is felt in rickets (rachitic rosary). Note any scars as a result of cardiac surgery. It is important to look for the thoracotomy scar under the arms or even round the back; otherwise you will miss it (Box 6.6). Central sternotomy scars usually indicate the child has had major heart surgery involving valves or closure of septal defects. Asymmetry of the chest becomes more obvious on movement (dynamic deformity) and may indicate an underlying pneumothorax or empyema. Look for any increased work of breathing. This may be indicated by seeing recession (intercostal or subcostal), tracheal tug or flaring of the nares when breathing. The infant may be using accessory muscles, such as the sternomastoids, which results in head bobbing. Count the respiratory rate (Table 6.3) which, in infants, must be done over a minute to be accurate, owing to periodic breathing which is normal in babies. Listen for grunting respiration, which is audible in infants who are attempting to prevent alveolar collapse by creating their own positive airway pressure. The grunting expiration is followed by inspiration and then a pause.

Palpate the anterior chest wall for the cardiac impulse and for thrills. In children under the age of 5 years, the apex is normally in the fourth intercostal space just to the left of the mid-clavicular line. Midline shift can be assessed in this way because palpation for the trachea in the suprasternal notch can be difficult and unpleasant for the child. Vocal fremitus is of less clinical value the smaller the child. This is because of difficulty with cooperation and the small size of the precordium. Expansion is also better assessed by observation for the same reasons. The axillary nodes may now be felt in the same way as in adults.

Chest percussion is useful in older children, but in young children and infants it is rarely of value. Tell the child 'I am going to make you sound like a drum'. Percuss very lightly in babies, directly tapping the chest wall with the percussing finger rather than using another intervening finger. The chest is more resonant in children than in adults.

A stethoscope with a small bell chest piece is suitable for auscultation of the child's chest. Do not use adult-sized chest pieces, because it is impossible to localize added sounds accurately with a chest piece covering such a wide area in a small child. Often it is less threatening to examine the back of the chest first, and much more information about the lungs can be acquired in this way. Listen for the breath sounds and adventitious sounds. Because of the thin chest wall, breath sounds are louder in children than in adults, and their character is more like the bronchial breathing of adults (puerile breathing). Upper respiratory tract infections in children often give rise to loud, coarse rhonchi, which are conducted down the trachea and main bronchi (transmitted upper airway sounds) (Table 6.4). All is not lost if the child is crying, as this is accompanied by deep inspiration giving an opportunity to listen for the character of the breath sounds.

When you are auscultating the front of the chest, the child's immediate instinct is to push the stethoscope away. You can ask the parent to hold the child's hands or try to distract the child with toys held in the hand (Fig. 6.3). It is a good idea to examine a doll or teddy bear first if the child is playing with one. The normal splitting of the first and second sounds is easier to hear in children than in adults. Venous hums and functional systolic flow murmurs are often heard in normal children (Box 6.7). If the murmur does not fit into this classification, remember that most cardiac problems in children occur as a result of congenital heart disease and not acquired as in adults (Table 6.5). Count the heart rate in young children (see Table 6.3). Arrythmias are uncommon in children unless they have had cardiac surgery.

Neurological examination

The neurological examination can usually be carried out in the normal way in older children, but in younger children the extent of the neurological examination will depend on the child's age and willingness to cooperate. Although a great deal should have been learned already from initial observations, still look at the child's static and dynamic posture. Asymmetry may indicate a hemiparesis. A hypotonic child may sit on his back rather than his bottom and an infant may display a 'frog leg' posture when lying down. Children with cerebral palsy may have a characteristic 'windswept' posture (quadriplegic) or have uncoordinated continuous movements (ataxic or dyskinesic). If the child is walking, the gait should have been observed already. Look for toe walking

Table 6.3 Normal observation values at different ages[a]

Age	Respiratory rate (breaths per minute)	Pulse rate (beats per minute)	Blood pressure (systolic mmHg)
Newborn	40–60	90–180	60–90
6 months	25–35	110–180	72–110
1 year	20–30	80–160	72–110
4 years	20–26	80–120	78–112
8 years	18–22	70–110	86–118
12 years	16–20	60–110	90–126

[a](Based on Advanced Paediatric Life Support values.)

Table 6.4 Chest signs of some common respiratory disorders of children

Disorder	Chest movement	Percussion (if carried out)	Auscultation
Bronchiolitis	Restricted, with hyperinflation Often tracheal tug and subcostal recession	Hyper-resonant	Widespread crackles, or wheezing
Pneumonia	Rapid, shallow respirations with audible grunt May be reduced on affected side	Dull or normal	Localized bronchial breathing or crackles May have no abnormal signs
Asthma	Restricted with hyperinflation Use of accessory muscles, and subcostal retraction	Hyper-resonant	Expiratory wheeze
Croup	Inspiratory stridor, with subcostal recession	Normal	Inspiratory coarse crackles with transmitted harsh upper airway sounds

(spastic diplegia), wide-based gait (seen in cerebellar ataxia, but normal in toddlers), limping (antalgic gait) and unilateral sweeping (hemiplegia). Hemiplegia may become more obvious on running as the affected upper limb is brought up closer to the body.

Note any abnormal movements. Tics or habit spasms are repetitive movements, such as shrugging of the shoulders or facial grimacing. Choreiform movements are involuntary, purposeless jerks that follow no particular pattern. Athetoid movements are writhing and more pronounced distally. Fits may be seen as lip smacking or flickering eye movements or as tonic–clonic spasms. Note if they are generalized or focal and if associated with loss of consciousness.

Take the opportunity to check for spinal abnormalities, such as scoliosis or kyphosis, or any evidence of spina bifida, such as a tuft of hair. Be careful to pick up on any signs of a neurocutaneous disorder, such as café-au-lait spots or telangiectasia.

Coordination can best be checked by watching a child at play. It is useful to have toys available that require a degree of coordination. Otherwise, a modification of the finger–nose test using a toy held in the hand can be used. If the child is old enough, watching him dressing or doing up shoelaces is a good way to assess coordination.

Figure 6.3 Attracting the attention of a 10-month-old baby while examining her heart.

| Box 6.7 | The five S's of an innocent murmur |

- Short
- Soft
- Systolic
- Sitting/standing (varies with posture)
- Symptom free

Check muscle tone if this has not already been done. Pick the child up if there is still a friendly relationship. This gives a good idea of the feel of a child and of his muscle tone. A hypotonic (floppy) infant will feel as though he is slipping through your hands. Hypertonia may be regional or generalized, depending on the cause. It will be difficult to move the limbs passively and there may be fixed flexion deformities owing to contractures around the joints. Muscle power is difficult to check in young children, except by watching playing habits and assessing power by ability at a variety of lifting games. Always remember to check for neck stiffness by testing resistance to passive neck flexion rather than by testing for Kernig's sign.

Table 6.5 Categories of key congenital heart disease lesions

Acyanotic (presents with hyperdynamic circulation in heart failure)	Cyanotic (presents with respiratory distress and cyanosis)	Outflow tract obstruction (presents grey and shocked)
Ventricular septal defect (VSD) (pansystolic murmur at left sternal edge)	Pulmonary stenosis (PS) (ejection systolic murmur at the left 2nd intercostal space)	Coarctation of the aorta (ejection systolic murmur over upper left sternal edge radiating to the carotid arteries)
Atrial septal defect (pulmonary flow murmur with fixed splitting of 2nd heart sound)	Tetralogy of Fallot (murmur of PS ± VSD and right ventricular heave)	
Persistent ductus arteriosus (continuous 'machinery' murmur)	Transposition of the great arteries (no murmur)	

Table 6.6 Tanner staging

	Boys (external genitalia)	Girls (breast)	Boys and girls (pubic hair)
Stage 1	Prepubertal	Prepubertal	Prepubertal
Stage 2	Enlargement of scrotum and testes	Breast bud stage	Sparse growth of long, slightly pigmented hair
Stage 3	Enlargement of penis length	Enlargement of breast and areola	Darker, coarser and more curled hair, spreading sparsely over junction of pubes
Stage 4	Increased size of penis with growth in breadth, scrotum skin darker	Areola and papilla form a secondary mound above level of breast	Hair adult in type, but covering smaller area than in adult
Stage 5	Adult genitalia	Mature stage	Adult in type and quantity

Testing of sensation is difficult in young children and less likely to yield useful information. Touch can be tested by observing the reaction when the skin is touched with a cotton wool ball. In older children the approach to assessing sensation is the same as in adults.

Testing the cranial nerves takes a little ingenuity. Eye movements are relatively easy using a toy moved in different directions in front of the baby's face. Young infants will often copy poking out the tongue at them, which will check the 12th cranial nerve. If the child can be made to smile, and even if he is crying, any asymmetry of facial movements can be seen. If a child is able to bite or grimace, the trigeminal nerve is probably intact.

Getting a child's limbs into the correct position to test tendon reflexes may take some time. Often they can be elicited by using a finger rather than a patellar hammer. Tendon reflexes in young infants tend to be brisk, and up to 18 months of age the plantar responses are extensor. The persistence of an extensor response beyond the age of 2 years indicates an upper motor neurone lesion. Note whether primitive reflexes have persisted (Box 6.8), which indicates significant neurodevelopmental dysfunction.

The eyes

The eyes should now be checked. There are signs critical to other systems to look for such as pallor and jaundice. Inspect the eyes for ptosis, conjunctivitis, cataracts or congenital defects, such as colobomata. Watch for spontaneous nystagmus or roaming eye movements which may indicate a visual impairment. It is very important to check for squints, as

ophthalmological referral may be necessary. In infants under 3 months of age there may be a pseudosquint owing to epicanthal folds giving the appearance of a convergent squint. Squints are checked for by shining a light in the eyes from in front of the face and observing the position of the light reflex; it should be at the same position in each cornea. A cover test should then be used (see Chapter 21), using a doll or some other appropriate toy on which the child can focus his gaze. Pupillary accommodation and light reactions can be noted at the same time. Examination of the fundus is particularly difficult in infants and will require dilatation of the pupils. It should be possible to see the red reflex which, if absent, is suggestive of a corneal, lens or vitreous opacity, such as cataract or retinoblastoma. Usually, in an older child, enough of the disc can be seen to detect papilloedema. The testing of vision in young children is included in the section on developmental screening examination.

With the possible exception of the eye examination, nothing so far should have upset a baby unduly. The following examinations should be carried out at the end of the consultation, as they are more likely to upset the child.

The genitalia, groins and anus

The nappy or underpants can now be removed, if necessary, to examine the groin or anus. In boys, notice the penis. The lack of retraction of the foreskin can be a source of worry to parents, but it is normal for it not to retract under the age of 5 years. Forcibly attempting retraction is not only painful but can also result in balanitis. Check the hernial orifices and see whether the testes have descended. To feel the testes, make sure that the examining hand is warm and place a finger in the line of the inguinal canal; advance the finger towards the scrotum. This will stop the cremasteric reflex causing the testes to disappear into the inguinal canal, which tends to happen if the scrotum is approached from below. In young babies, it is not unusual to find a testis in the inguinal canal, but it can usually be pushed into the scrotum without too much difficulty. The testis can be expected to descend into its normal position with increasing maturity.

In girls, check the vulva for redness, soreness or discharge, which are commonly seen in vulvovaginitis. Fusion of the labia is not uncommon, so check that they separate normally. Enlargement of the clitoris may suggest an endocrine disorder. It is important to note that examination for possible sexual abuse should be left to an expert. Check for inguinal lymph nodes and palpate the femoral arteries (simultaneously with the radials) to exclude coarctation of the aorta.

Examination of the anal margin can best be carried out by gently separating the buttocks with one hand on either side; the anal orifice can then easily be seen and inspected for fissures, which are commonly

---

Box 6.8	Primitive reflexes

Rooting reflexes

On touching a baby's cheek, he will turn his head towards the stimulus. Sucking itself is a reflex, and failure of the sucking response beyond the 36th week of gestation suggests significant neurological impairment.

Palmar and plantar grasp

A finger placed across the child's palm or plantar surface of the foot will cause flexion and grasping of the finger. Lost by 2 months of age.

Stepping reflex

When lowered vertically onto a hard surface, the foot presses down and the other leg flexes at the hip and knee in a stepping movement. As this response is alternated from one leg to the other, the baby makes a walking movement. Lost by 2 months of age.

The Moro reflex (see Fig. 6.11)

On dropping the head a few centimetres, the upper limbs abduct and extend symmetrically and then flex. Lost by 6 months of age.

associated with constipation. Rectal examination is rarely necessary in children and, if carried out, should be done with a well-lubricated, gloved little finger, which should be advanced very slowly.

In older children and adolescents puberty is assessed using the Tanner stage (Table 6.6). This will involve examination of the genitalia and looking for breast development and body hair.

The nose, ears, mouth and throat

The most uncomfortable parts of the examination as far as the child is concerned are the nose, ears, mouth and throat.

The nose need only be examined superficially, looking for nasal patency, any deviation of the septum or the presence of polyps or inflamed nasal turbinates. Older children are quite good at sniffing, and this will give some idea of nasal patency.

A cooperative child will allow a look into his ears but, if not, the child should be held by the mother, as shown in Figure 6.4. Held in such a way, the child can be kept still long enough for the eardrums to be inspected. Look carefully for the light reflex, which can be lost if the child has chronic secretory otitis media ('glue ear'). In acute suppurative otitis media, the drum may be bright red and bulging.

The mouth and throat can be examined by encouraging a cooperative child to 'show me your teeth'; an open mouth will then allow a clear view of the mouth and fauces. If uncooperative, the child will need to be held as shown in Figure 6.5. Sometimes it is not too disastrous if the child cries at this point, because this will give a very clear view of the teeth, the tonsils and sometimes even the epiglottis. A spatula is a terrifying instrument to the average child, causing most to clamp their teeth shut. If this happens, the spatula should be advanced to the back of the tongue to induce a gag reflex. Look for the presence of the white patches of candida infection, ulcers seen in inflammatory bowel disease and the Koplik's spots seen in measles.

The general physical examination has now been completed. Hopefully the child is still friendly. Once the child is dressed, the examiner should sit with the parents and explain what has been found. It is always best for the child to have finished dressing before talking to the parents: they are more likely to listen and take in what you have to say if they are not preoccupied with helping their child. Always involve older children in the discussion, as they have every right to know what you have found. Even young children can be given information in terms they will understand. Never, under any circumstances, deceive a child. The eventual truth will result in his losing confidence in you and with later medical attendants.

Signs associated with abuse/child neglect

During the examination of the child you may pick up signs which lead you to be concerned about the possibility of non-accidental injury or other

Figure 6.4   How to hold a baby to allow the ears to be examined. The mother faces the baby to one side and holds him firmly, with one arm around the head and the other around the upper arm and shoulder.

Figure 6.5   How to hold a baby to allow the mouth and throat to be examined. The baby faces the examiner, with the mother holding him firmly with one hand on the forehead and the other holding both arms.

forms of child abuse. These should be noted and considered as part of the differential diagnosis. Any injuries, bruising, scars or burns should be carefully documented on body maps as part of the medical record. Detailed definitions of the four categories of abuse (physical, emotional, sexual and neglect) can be found in Working Together to Safeguard Children: March 2018 (HM Government; http://www.workingtogetheronline.co.uk/). Box 6.9 lists some alerting features of abuse which will help you recognize if abuse is occurring. It is now recognized that safeguarding children is everyone's responsibility, however challenging that may feel. If you do have concerns, make sure you are aware

Box 6.9	Symptoms and signs to help with recognition of abuse/neglect (from NICE guidance 'When to suspect child maltreatment' last updated 2017)	
	Consider maltreatment	**Suspect maltreatment**
Physical abuse	Any serious/unusual injury with absent/unsuitable explanation; oral injuries; burns or scalds; lacerations	Bruising in specific shapes; human bites; lacerations on protected areas of the body; retinal haemorrhage without another medical explanation; bruises on non-bony parts of the body or face, including the eyes, ears and buttocks
Emotional abuse	Fearful/withdrawn; excessive clinginess; overfriendliness; enuresis/encopresis; signs of deliberate self-harm; behavioural or emotional change that has no medical explanation	A combination of several concerning symptoms or signs
Neglect	Severe infestations; dirty clothing/unwashed child; faltering growth/obesity; animal bites; poor school attendance; unimmunized; failure to attend for developmental checks; dental decay	Cold injuries; hypothermia; medical advice not sought; repeated reports of poor living environment, lack of adequate food
Sexual abuse	Gaping anus; anogenital warts; anogenital injury; anal fissure with constipation; vaginal discharge; persistent dysuria	Persistence of anogenital symptoms or signs with no explanation; pregnancy in a child; hymenal injuries; significant anogenital trauma; unusual sexualized behaviours

of your organization's policies and procedures and that you have someone with whom you can discuss them.

Routine measurements

Height and weight

Childhood is a period of growth, the pattern of which may be adversely affected by many disturbances of health as well as social deprivation. Serial measurements of height and weight are therefore essential in the examination of children. In children able to stand, height can be measured against a wall-mounted gauge. Younger children can be measured lying down on special measuring boards. Measurements should be made under standard conditions, and children should be weighed unclothed. If the child keeps on any clothes, this should be noted against the weight so that subsequent weights can be taken with the child wearing the same quantity of clothing. Heights and weights should be compared with those of healthy children of similar sex and age on percentile charts. Figures 6.6 and 6.7 show standard height, weight and head circumference charts drawn from a population of UK boys and girls from birth to 18 years developed by the RCPCH/WHO/Department of Health. Other charts for body mass index (BMI), puberty monitoring and Down's syndrome can be obtained from the RCPCH website.

Comparison should also be made against the parents' height by calculating the mid-parental height. The calculation in centimetres by sex is for boys (Father's **Height** + Mother's **Height** + 13)/2 and girls (Father's **Height** - 13 + Mother's **Height**)/2. Plot the final value in centimetres at the final adult height line (either at 18 years or 20 years of age depending on the chart used) to find the child's expected final centile. A child who fails to grow at an appropriate velocity (growth rate) needs to be investigated further. The term 'failure to thrive' is used to denote children whose weight gain is below that expected (fallen across 2 centiles on the chart). It is the rate of growth rather than a one-off abnormal value which usually gives cause for concern. The child will need a very careful history and examination to be carried out. It is important to pick up any markers of potential chronic disease. There are as yet no satisfactory growth charts for children of Asian origin born in the UK. They tend to be smaller than Caucasian children in the first few years of life; as a rough guide, the mean percentile for an Asian child is the 25th percentile on the standard UK charts. Children of African origin tend to be larger than Caucasian children. There are special growth charts for children with Down's syndrome and Turner's syndrome.

The meaning of the term '10th percentile' is that 10% of all children in the measured population are respectively lighter or shorter at the age concerned. Pre-term infants should be plotted according to their corrected age (chronological age minus the number of weeks born early) up until the age of 2 years.

Head circumference

In infants under the age of 2 years, the head circumference is a good proxy for linear growth and a much more reliable measurement than height or length. The standard measurement is the largest occipitofrontal circumference out of three using a paper tape. Some causes of microcephaly and macrocephaly are listed in Box 6.10. Rather than using a chart showing the head circumference alone,

Figure 6.6 Height, weight and head circumference: boys aged 0–4 years. (© 2009 Department of Health Charts developed by RCPCH/WHO/ Department of Health. Reproduced with permission.)

Figure 6.6, cont'd

Figure 6.7 Height, weight and head circumference: girls aged 0–4 years. (© 2009 Department of Health. Charts developed by RCPCH/WHO/Department of Health. Reproduced with permission.)

Figure 6.7 cont'd

Box 6.10	Causes of microcephaly and macrocephaly

Microcephaly

- Perinatal brain insult—e.g. hypoxic ischaemic encephalopathy
- Fetal alcohol syndrome
- Craniosynostosis syndromes—e.g. Apert and Crouzon syndromes

Macrocephaly

- Hydrocephalus
- Mucopolysaccharidosis
- Excessive brain growth (Canavan and Soto syndromes)

it is more useful to use one that combines head circumference and length and weight percentiles, so that the proportions of each child can be compared to establish if growth is concordant or discordant across the measurements.

Blood pressure

Abnormalities of blood pressure are uncommon in childhood but can be a sign of cardiovascular or renal disease. Measurement can be technically difficult, particularly in small children, and can be significantly affected by pain and distress. An electronic monitor will be used in most paediatric settings as manual methods can be difficult in small children. A variety of cuff sizes should be available and the largest cuff that will fit around the upper arm but not extend to the elbow joint should be used. The use of cuffs which are too small will give erroneously high readings. Doppler techniques more accurately measure blood pressure in children, but these are not always available. The blood pressure should be checked in all four limbs to exclude coarctation of the aorta when congenital heart disease is suspected. Normal values of blood pressure at different ages are listed in Table 6.3.

Temperature

The temperature should be taken if there is a suspicion of an underlying infection or if there is a report from the parent of the child having been hot. Fever is a very common finding in children, which may be caused by exercise and minor infections, as well as severe infections and other serious illnesses. Small infants often respond to infection with low temperatures.

The most common methods used in current practice are axillary measurements using chemical dot strips, or electronic devices giving tympanic membrane readings. These methods are the easiest to use, but readings should be interpreted according to the method used. For example, axillary temperatures are 0.5°C to 1.0°C below core body temperature. Rectal temperature is the best approximation to core temperature but is seldom, if ever, taken. Febrile convulsions may occur in children between 6 months and 6 years of age when the temperature rises rapidly.

Stools

Never be afraid to see a dirty nappy or a stool. This is part of the examination of a baby, and it is important to know the normal appearance of stools in childhood. The stools of a breastfed infant are usually loose and have yellow seeds in them with a characteristic odour. Infants fed on cows' milk formulas pass stools that are a paler yellow colour and more pasty. The character of the stool in older children is more variable than in adults. Some healthy children pass frequent, loose stools containing undigested vegetable matter—'toddler's diarrhoea'. The stools of children with coeliac disease or cystic fibrosis are bulky, particularly smelly and quite characteristic.

Urine

Urine can be tested easily and reliably using modern reagent dipstick methods, but collection of the specimen can be difficult in the younger child. Specially designed collection bags can be attached to the perineum, but these are susceptible to faecal contamination and should never be used to test for a urinary tract infection. This should be done using a 'clean catch' sample specimen into a sterile bowl or other container. Urine samples from children under the age of 2 years should always be double checked for infection in the laboratory. Modern techniques use flow cytometry and results will be available within a few hours. In a septic infant when a specimen is required urgently and an accurate diagnosis needed, the urine may be obtained by catheterization of the bladder using aseptic technique.

Developmental screening examination

The developmental examination assesses the acquisition of learned skills. Development progresses from head to toe (a child needs to be able to hold his head up before being able to sit unsupported). Progress also requires the loss of primitive reflexes (see Box 6.8) at the appropriate age (a child cannot transfer objects between his hands if he still has a grasp reflex). Developmental progress can be affected by emotional difficulties, environment (e.g. lack of stimulation due to neglect) and illnesses.

All infants should have a simple developmental screening examination at regular intervals. Table 6.1 lists the important milestones. Detailed developmental assessment is a specialist subject, but it is important for all those who examine children to be able to carry out a simple developmental screening examination, and to be aware of all the basic milestones.

It is usual to consider development under four main headings:

1. Movement and posture.
2. Vision and manipulation.
3. Hearing and speech.
4. Social behaviour.

Screening for developmental delay involves testing the child's performance of a few skills in each of the four fields of development, and comparing the results with the average for children of the same age. The range of normal developmental progress is wide, and the milestones shown in Table 6.1 are those of an average normal child. Delay in all fields of development is more significant than delay in a single modality, and severe delay is more meaningful than slight delay. Allowance must always be made for those infants who were born prematurely, at least until the age of 2 years, by which time they should have caught up.

By 18 months of age, obvious deviations from normal development should become apparent. Beyond this age, developmental testing is more specialized and is beyond the scope of this chapter. A baby who appears to have delayed development on screening will need further specialized assessment to establish the cause and subsequent management.

Techniques used

The same rules apply to the techniques used in developmental screening as to those of general physical examination. As with all parts of the examination, much more is learned by simply watching a child play and watching his reactions to the surroundings. Time has to be spent gaining the friendship of the child. For example, when offering a 10-month-old baby a small toy, watch to see how he grasps it and reacts to it. Let the baby play with the toys and bricks while sitting on the mother's lap, and if the child remains suspicious, get the mother to offer the various objects.

In the UK, routine developmental screening is usually carried out by a health visitor who is trained in developmental skills and who will refer to a doctor babies about whom there is any suspicion. There is always an assessment at birth, 10–14 days (the newborn review), 6–8 weeks, 9–12 months and 2–2 and a half years of age. If at any point concerns are raised, then the child will be referred to a specialist community team for further assessment. Once at school age, the school nursing team supports their health and development.

Head control

By 4 months, babies can normally keep their head in line with the trunk when pulled from supine to sitting and, when held in the sitting position, will keep their head upright. Before this age, the head lags behind the trunk (Figs 6.8 and 6.9).

Testing vision

Much will be learned about a child's vision by observation. Note whether the child is looking around the room and at particular toys, or staring at nothing in particular, especially if there are nystagmoid or random/roving eye movements, the latter suggesting that the child is unable to see.

Figure 6.8   Head control at 6 weeks of age.

Figure 6.9   Head control at 4 months of age.

When he picks a toy up, is accommodation normal? The routine examination of the eye has been dealt with in the first part of this chapter.

Checks of visual acuity are not easy in young babies. By 6 weeks of age, babies should be following their mother with their eyes, and by 6 months they should be able to follow a rolling ball at 3 metres. This is the basis of one method of visual testing at this age. The ability of the child to follow rolling balls of differing diameters gives an accurate assessment of visual acuity. At the 8-month check, the baby should be able to see and pick up an object the size of a raisin at arm's length. From the age of approximately 2 years, the Sheridan–Gardiner test is used. This is a simple comparison test, with the examiner indicating letters or familiar toys on a board and asking the child to indicate a similar object on a board held by the mother. The acuity is the ability of the child to pick out the smallest objects (see Chapter 21).

Testing hearing

In the past, it was usual to check the hearing for the first time between 6 and 8 months of age using the distraction test (Fig. 6.10). This can still be used as a screening method, but it has a large observer error and has largely been replaced by a national screening programme for all newborn babies, based on otoacoustic emissions. This measures vibration

Figure 6.10 Testing hearing at 8 months: the child is held upright and forward on his parent's lap and distracted by an examiner in front of him. An examiner then presents sounds at 35 dB at different frequencies behind him and observes if the child turns towards the direction of the sound.

reflected from the normally functioning cochlea. Additionally, brainstem auditory evoked potentials are used to assess the more vulnerable babies with the risk factors detailed in Box 6.11. This measures electrical activity in the baby's brain in response to sound. Audiometry and tympanometry are methods used in older children who can cooperate with the tests. They are useful for detecting middle-ear disease or glue ear, which is more common in this group of children (see Chapter 22).

Examination of the newborn

The Apgar score (Box 6.12) is a combined cardio-respiratory and neurological score used immediately after birth and will be the first assessment a baby will have in his life. An Apgar score of 6 or less at 5 minutes after birth is associated with a neurological deficit in about 10% of cases. Assessment of gestational age can be carried out clinically using the Dubowitz score (not detailed here). With more reliable dating scans, this method of assessment is rarely used now.

Every newborn baby is examined within the first 24 hours of life and again before the end of the first week. This is a very important examination designed to assess the general state of health and to detect congenital abnormalities (Box 6.13). It must always be interpreted in the context of the history of the pregnancy and birth and in the knowledge of any known history of inherited disorders in the family.

Weight is measured routinely at birth; the head circumference (occipitofrontal) may not be measured before 48 hours, to allow for moulding to subside. Note whether meconium, the dark green, sticky stool of the newborn baby, has been

---

Box 6.11 Risk factors for hearing impairment

- Family history of deafness
- Congenital malformations (particularly ear, facial and spinal)
- Congenital infections (rubella, cytomegalovirus)
- Perinatal illness (gestation below 32 weeks at birth, low birth weight, jaundice)
- Postnatal illness (meningitis)

Box 6.12 The Apgar score

In each of the five categories, a score of 0, 1 or 2 is awarded, to give a maximum of 10. A score of 7–10 is good, 3–6 is moderate and 0–2 is severe. Scores are carried out 1, 5 and 10 minutes after birth:

- **A**ppearance—skin colour
- **P**ulse
- **G**rimace—reflex irritability
- **A**ctivity—muscle tone
- **R**espiratory effort

Box 6.13 Checklist for examination of the newborn

- Weight, length, head circumference
- Alertness and wakefulness
- Skin colour: cyanosis, jaundice, birth marks
- Face: ears, dysmorphic features
- Head: skull and fontanelles
- Eyes: red reflex
- Mouth and tongue
- Neck: branchial cysts
- Limbs: digits and palmar creases, talipes
- Chest: murmurs
- Abdomen and umbilicus
- Perineum and genitalia
- Spine: sacral development
- Neurological assessment: posture, movements and tone, reflexes, the cry
- Hips

---

passed within the first 24 hours. If not, consider the possibility of Hirschsprung's disease (agangliosis of the rectum).

It provides reassurance to the baby's mother to conduct the examination in front of her. Ask the parent to undress the baby in a warm place and treat the baby gently, leaving the most unpleasant parts of the examination until last. Initially watch the baby, noting the state of awareness. If the baby is awake, seemingly looking around and not crying, take the opportunity to examine the nervous system at this point.

The skin

Note the colour of the skin. Peripheral cyanosis is a common finding in the normal newborn, but central cyanosis may indicate the presence of cardiac or respiratory disease. The head and neck may appear plethoric owing to confluent petechial haemorrhages as a result of prolonged or obstructed labour. Jaundice is common after 48 hours in most preterm and some term babies and is considered physiological. Any baby jaundiced before 48 hours or after 14 days of age needs to be investigated. The most common cause is haemolytic disease of the newborn owing to ABO blood group incompatibility, which normally presents within 48 hours. Late onset jaundice could be caused by liver disease, hypothyroidism, sepsis and haematological factors and so should be investigated.

Look for birthmarks, which are either pigmented lesions or haemangiomata. Many babies have a collection of dilated capillaries on the upper eyelids and nape of the neck (sometimes called 'stork bites'), which fade after a few weeks. Some babies develop a crop of small erythematous papules with a surrounding red flare on the trunk during the first week (erythema toxicum or urticaria neonatorum) which look alarming to the first-time parent but do not have any pathological significance and usually fade after a few days. Superficial peeling of the skin, especially over the periphery, is common and is most apparent in post-term and some small-for-gestational-age babies. Milia are whitish pinhead spots concentrated mainly around the nose. They are sebaceous retention cysts and can be felt with the finger. They usually disappear within a month. Lanugo hair may cover the body, especially in preterm babies and some dark-haired babies. It usually disappears over the first 2 or 3 weeks. Mongolian blue spot is the name given to the normal dark blue areas of pigmentation commonly seen over the sacrum and buttocks or back of the legs in darker skinned babies.

The face

Look at the face for obvious dysmorphic features. Accessory auricles are small, pedunculated skin tags, usually just in front of the ears. Note any lip defect that may indicate an underlying cleft palate.

Once the superficial examination has been completed, more formal examination takes place. As for older babies, this should be regional rather than by systems, starting with the head and working down.

The head

Inspect and palpate the head. The caput succedaneum is an area of oedema of the scalp over the part of the head that presented during labour. It pits on pressure and is not fluctuant. A cephalhaematoma is a subperiosteal haematoma that appears a few days after birth as a large, cystic swelling limited to the area of one of the skull bones. It tends to resolve relatively slowly over a few months and may leave a calcified edge. It should be distinguished from a meningocele, which is usually midline and occipital and associated with an underlying bony defect. The anterior fontanelle varies in size considerably at birth.

The eyes

The eyes are best examined when they are open spontaneously. A bluish tinge to the sclera is usual. Even though newborn infants can see, eye movements tend to be random, often giving the impression of a transient squint. Subconjunctival haemorrhages show as dark red patches covering the sclera, sometimes ringing the cornea, and can occur following normal deliveries. Look for evidence of conjunctivitis, which could be secondary to maternally transmitted infections, and check for other abnormalities as described earlier in this chapter. In particular, check for the red reflex; its absence could indicate a major ophthalmic problem, such as a retinoblastoma or cataract.

The mouth and tongue

Make sure that there is no cleft of the palate and note particularly whether the uvula is normal. A bifid uvula indicates a submucous cleft of the palate, which requires surgery. Epithelial pearls are small white areas, best seen on the hard palate. Occasionally teeth are present at birth. They are usually incisors and can be green in colour. If loose, they are best removed. True macroglossia is seen in babies with congenital hypothyroidism, Beckwith's syndrome and in mucopolysaccharidosis. Children with trisomy 21 appear to have large tongues because their mouths are small, resulting in protrusion.

The neck

The neck of a newborn baby seems rather short and can be difficult to visualize. Rarely, cystic swellings are seen. Cystic hygromas are fluid-filled sacs that occur most commonly on the head or neck of a baby. They occur owing to blockages in the lymphatic system. Dermoid cysts and thyroglossal cysts are seen in the midline or branchial cysts just in front of the upper third of the sternomastoid muscle

The limbs

Examine the limbs for abnormalities. Extra digits on the hand are not uncommon and may be familial, but they are rarer on the feet. Look for a single transverse palmar crease, which is classically seen in babies with trisomy 21, syndactyly (partial fusion of two or more digits) and clinodactyly (in-turning of the tip of the digit). Talipes equinovarus is a serious abnormality of the arrangement of the tarsal bones and requires an orthopaedic referral.

The chest

The general appearance and shape of the chest should be noticed. Breast enlargement with exudation of a milky fluid from the nipples is sometimes seen in newborn infants of either sex. This is caused by transferred maternal hormones and disappears in a few days without causing problems. Listen for stridor, which may be secondary to laryngomalacia or an anatomical obstructive defect. Listen also for grunting. Note the symmetry of the chest wall, the pattern of respiration and whether there is any in-drawing on inspiration. Neonatal breathing is predominantly abdominal and quiet. Palpation, percussion and auscultation are of almost no value in the neonate. Transient systolic murmurs are extremely common in the first few days of life and may reflect the closing ductus arteriosus or non-specific flow murmurs. They should be reviewed when the baby is older.

The abdomen

The abdomen of a newborn baby usually seems a little distended and moves with respiration. Slight divarication of the rectus muscles may occur, and this exaggerates this abdominal bulging. True abdominal wall defects may be present, such as exomphalos. The liver edge is palpable up to 2 cm below the costal margin, and the lower poles of both kidneys can be felt. A very enlarged bladder could suggest a neurological problem such as spina bifida. Check the umbilical stump: it should contain two arteries and one vein. A single umbilical artery is associated with an increased incidence of congenital abnormalities of the renal tract. Sometimes excess granulation tissue accumulates over the stump once the cord has separated to form a small granuloma; this can be simply treated by local application of salt .

The perineum and genitalia

Examine the perineum for hypospadias, hydroceles, inguinal hernias or undescended testicles. Look for patency of the anus: an imperforate anus is easily overlooked unless it is specifically checked for. While looking at the buttocks and anus, inspect for a sacral dimple. If the blind-ending pit can be visualized, it is usually of no significance. However, if the base of the pit cannot be seen an ultrasound will be needed to rule out significant spinal lesions. Make sure that the back is straight and that there are no obvious spinal abnormalities, especially spina bifida. Check female external genitalia for clitoral enlargement, which would suggest a virilizing condition, such as congenital adrenal hyperplasia, and for labial fusion. It is not unusual for girls to have a mucus vaginal discharge and sometimes bleeding. This is the result of transferred maternal hormones and is usually transient. Make sure that the femoral pulses are palpable.

Neurological assessment

Combine a formal neurological examination with observation of the baby's behaviour. Spontaneous movement normally consists of alternating flexion and extension. Any marked difference between the two sides is abnormal.

The normal position of a newborn baby is one of flexion. If the baby is crying, look for any weakness or paralysis in the face, suggesting injury to the facial nerve, or any deficiency of arm movements, suggesting injury to the brachial plexus which may have occurred during delivery (Erb's palsy). Note the limb and truncal tone. Assess power from resistance during undressing. Tendon jerks are difficult to elicit at this age, but can be checked, using a finger rather than a tendon hammer.

Primitive reflexes

Primitive responses are present in the normal newborn infant and disappear at variable times in accordance with developmental progress (see Box 6.8). The absence of one or more of these reflexes in the newborn infant may indicate some abnormality of the brain, a local abnormality in the affected limb or a neuromuscular abnormality. The most well-known startle reflex is the Moro reflex (see Box 6.8 and Fig. 6.11). As it is a startle reflex and may make the baby cry, it should be left until the end of the examination. A clearly unilateral response suggests some local abnormality, such as a fracture or brachial plexus injury in the arm on the side that does not respond. Persistence of primitive reflexes beyond the fourth month of life should alert you to the possibility of developmental delay.

Examination of the hips

Examination of the hips is essential but should be left to the end because it can be uncomfortable for the baby. It is performed by carrying out two provocation manoeuvres to demonstrate that the femoral head can be dislocated and then lifted back into the acetabulum, as illustrated in Figures 6.12 and 6.13. It is usual to differentiate between

Figure 6.11 Eliciting the Moro reflex.

Figure 6.12 Stage 1 (Barlow test) of the examination of the hips: the hips are flexed, rotated medially and pushed posteriorly. This will dislocate dislocatable hips.

Figure 6.13 Stage 2 (Ortolani test) of the examination of the hips: the hips are abducted and a 'click' or a 'clunk' is felt for (see text). Note the position of the examiner's hands, with the thumbs on the medial aspect of the thigh and the fingers over the lateral trochanters.

a tendinous 'click' and the typical 'clunk' of a hip moving in and out of its socket. The latter is more a feeling than an actual noise. Asymmetry of skin creases on the upper posterior thigh and limitation of abduction are signs that do not develop until 6 weeks of age. With any doubt about possible congenital dislocation of the hip, ultrasound examination should be carried out. This is routine for all at-risk newborn babies (breech delivery, a family history of congenital dislocation of the hip, especially if female, and any baby in an unusual intrauterine position).

Having now completed the examination, the baby should be dressed and, as in every examination of children, your findings must be conveyed to the parents.

Summary

Throughout this chapter, emphasis has been placed on getting to know the child and treating him as gently as possible. Time has to be spent gaining the child's confidence. Students and doctors new to working with children have a natural anxiety when approaching young children, and it is only by playing and being with them that confidence in examining them will develop. Developing and practising the skills of the examination of children is a challenge that is immensely rewarding when completed satisfactorily.

Older people | 7

Sophie Edwards

Introduction

'In the end, it's not the years in your life that count. It's the life in your years.'

Abraham Lincoln

At the turn of the twentieth century, there were 65 000 people in the UK aged 85 or older. By 2050, it is projected there will be more than 3 million. Many people still associate old age with frailty, disability and loss of independence. The positive aspects of ageing, such as sagacity, maturity and experience, are too often neglected. Society holds youthfulness in high esteem, but as the burden of morbidity is delayed by improvements in health care and economics it is hoped that these commonly held negative beliefs about growing old will gradually disappear.

Age is traditionally defined in terms of chronological age, but older people are a heterogeneous group and each old person should be respected as an individual, not merely classed according to age. Increasingly the role of 'Frailty' as a syndrome and a more accurate predictor of morbidity and mortality is ensuring that appropriate care and planning is provided to those who need it most, regardless of age.

People age at different rates. It is the complex interplay of environmental, psychosocial, genetic and acquired pathological processes that determines an individual's biological age. The role of Geriatric Medicine is to take a holistic view of this process and to provide care in a way that optimizes a person's function and health.

Presentation of disease in older people

Two major factors influence the recognition of disease processes in older people:

1. Acceptance of ill health, with a delay in seeking help.
2. Atypical presentation of disease processes.

The acceptance of ill health and disease as 'ageing', with its resultant disabilities, means that many older people expect to be frail, rarely complain and often are late seeking help. Coming to terms with some disability or change is necessary at all

ages, and acceptance is part of survival. However, the tacit acceptance of inevitable deterioration, for example in vision, hearing, teeth and memory, may lead to treatable conditions being ignored and result in loss of independence. Table 7.1 illustrates what may be regarded as normal ageing and what is pathological.

As medicine has developed, people now survive illnesses they would previously have died from. Many patients will now present to health care settings with multiple comorbidities, which may be causally linked or not. Managing multiple conditions and pulling out the key problem at any one time is a skill that requires a combination of knowledge, an ability to manage uncertainty and close attention to detail. It is often the 'little things' that count the most.

Proper diagnosis and treatment in older people requires the identification and treatment of amenable clinical problems and recognition of the special needs and the specific clinical presentations of older people. The social aspects of care may be as important as the disease process itself. Understanding this encourages a patient-centred, multi-disciplinary team (MDT) approach. Caring for older people requires clinical acumen and much skill. Geriatricians not only recognize diseases and their presentations in older people but, perhaps equally importantly, act as their patients' advocate in all areas of health care.

Frailty

In normal day-to-day circumstances, ageing organs are able to maintain normal metabolic function. However, when stressors are experienced, as in acute illness, functional capacity is exceeded and rapid clinical deterioration may occur. By definition, the frailer the person, the greater the deterioration and the more likely that deterioration will occur in the context of a relatively minor stressor. The frail person has a lower physiological reserve in response to any insult and will take longer to return to their previous level of functioning, if at all. This person may be old but younger people can be frail if they have a combination of disability and morbidity, which has an impact on their ability to

Table 7.1 Normal ageing and changes in body systems

System	Normal ageing	Pathophysiological changes common in older age
Cardiovascular	Slight increase in heart size Normal stroke volume and left ventricular ejection fraction Exertional oxygen consumption declines 7.5–10% per decade; thus exercise tolerance is reduced	Ischaemic heart disease Heart failure Valvular heart disease Peripheral vascular disease Aneurysms
Respiratory	Vital capacity: 40% reduction by age 70 FEV_1 and FVC: 30% reduction by age 80 Progressive reduction in PEFR after age 30	Haemoptysis Chronic obstructive pulmonary disease (COPD) Lung fibrosis Lung cancers
Alimentary	Reduced and abnormal peristalsis: 'grey-oesophagus' Slower colonic transit Reduced absorption of some nutrients; reduced energy requirements	Weight loss Dysphagia Change in bowel habits Bleeding from the upper or lower GI tract
Hepatobiliary	Reduced hepatic mass and metabolic reserve, but maintenance of normal function	Jaundice Deranged liver function tests, including abnormal clotting
Renal	Reduced GFR and numbers of functional tubules and glomeruli Reduced serum creatinine owing to loss of muscle mass	Renal impairment with raised serum creatinine Haematuria
Genitourinary	Men: Reduced testosterone Normal FSH/LH 50% of men over 70 have 'abundant spermatogenesis' Women: Postmenopausal low oestradiol; raised FSH and LH Loss of female reproductive capability Atrophic vaginitis owing to low oestrogen levels Loss of sexual interest may also occur, but this is complex and multifactorial	Erectile dysfunction Prostatic enlargement Bladder outflow tract symptoms Postmenopausal bleeding (PMB) Urinary incontinence Painful intercourse
Nervous system, including higher senses	High-frequency hearing loss Vision: close focusing declines from age 40 Distinguishing fine detail (reduced acuity) declines after 70 years Loss of muscle mass leads to decline in strength Reduced mental agility and minor loss of mental ability	Deafness, tinnitus and vertigo Glaucoma, macular degeneration Cataracts Dementia and delirium Hemiparesis, paraparesis Many other factors, including reduced distal sensation, vascular disease, poor balance
Endocrine	Pituitary dysfunction Abnormal thyroid function Abnormal pancreatic function Reduced adrenal response to stress	Hyponatraemia Hypothyroidism Impaired glucose tolerance and frank diabetes mellitus
Musculoskeletal	Increased body fat and loss of muscle mass (although this may be retarded with exercise)	Osteoarthritis and vertebral spondylosis Osteoporosis
Dermatological	Loss of collagen in the skin leads to thin, papyraceous skin Ecchymoses and senile purpura	Basal and squamous cell carcinoma Solar keratoses Malignant melanoma

Haematological and immune system	Loss of T-cell function with age may be associated with late-onset autoimmune disease
	Possible link between changes in immune system and:
	  • age-related cancers
	  • response to disease
		Anaemia
		Myelodysplasia
		Haematological malignancies
		Chronic lymphatic lymphoma and myeloma

FEV_1, forced expiratory volume in 1 second; FSH, follicle stimulating hormone; FVC, forced vital capacity; GI, gastrointestinal; GFR, glomerular filtration rate; LH, luteinizing hormone; PEFR, peak expiratory flow rate.

- The introduction: observation as they enter; greeting
- Cadence and interest
- Position and comfort of patient
- Vision, hearing, cognition
- Environment
- Autonomy and respect
- Use of multiple sources of information
- Interview versus interrogation

| Box 7.2 | Observations during the introduction |

- Can the patient see and hear you?
- Is behaviour normal?
- Is language normal?
- Does the patient understand your role as a doctor?
- Is the patient at ease, or in pain?
- Is there evidence of support from family or friends?

| Box 7.3 | Comprehensive geriatric assessment |

Physical and mental assessment key areas:

- Sleep
- Falls and mobility
- Appetite and weight
- Continence
- Skin
- Pain
- Memory
- Mood and energy levels
- Medication
- Vision, hearing and dentition

live independently and lowers their physiological reserve. Frailty can be measured formally using a variety of scales, which take into account day-to-day functioning, energy levels and need for support. A clear correlation exists between increasing frailty and increasing mortality, which makes it a more useful indicator of prognosis than chronological age alone.

History

Taking a good history is always essential, but it requires particular sensitivity in older people. The practical aspects of ensuring that patients have their hearing aids and glasses and teeth in are essential to optimizing the history-taking process. Sitting on the same level as the patient will support a patient who may also lip read. Some patients may need written questions. Frailer patients may not tolerate lengthy histories or being bombarded with questions and they may tire easily.

Some patients may rely on a carer or family member to support with communication but ensure that everyone is involved in the conversation. Ask the patient's permission to clarify something with a carer and by positioning yourself closer to the patient physically so that they feel involved. Some patients with cognitive problems may not remember much about their medical history, but they may still be able to tell you what matters most to them, how they spend their day and who is important to them.

It is useful to establish what the patient likes to be called because this is often not what is written on their record. Most of the communication skills required to support history taking in older people are transferable to ALL patients and will hone history-taking skills generally (Boxes 7.1 and 7.2)

Comprehensive geriatric assessment

This is an assessment tool used by the MDT to ensure that all aspects of a person's life have been assessed and that management plans reflect the outcome of this assessment and are patient focused. Geriatricians work closely with all members of the MDT, which incorporates nurses, physiotherapists, occupational therapists, pharmacists, speech and language therapists, dieticians and social workers. The assessment may take place over a number of ward rounds or days as it involves collating a lot of information.

The comprehensive geriatric assessment (CGA) tool is an evidenced-based and well-validated intervention for older and frailer people. At its core are five main areas of focus:

1. Physical health assessment.
2. Mental health assessment.
3. Functional assessment.
4. Social assessment.
5. Environmental assessment.

Each member of the team can contribute to any of the key areas, but doctors and nurses generally focus on the physical and mental health assessments. Physiotherapists and occupational therapists will assess the functional and environmental issues and a social worker will be involved in the social assessment. Combining information from the full team ensures that appropriate medical and social care can be implemented.

The physical and mental health assessment will need to ensure that the key 'geriatric giants' (immobility and falls, pressure ulcers, cognitive problems and incontinence) are assessed. Getting into the habit of doing this at an early stage in your career is essential to the future care of older and/or more frail patients (Box 7.3).

Older patients should be examined in the same way as younger patients, but there are some key additional areas to focus on to ensure a robust assessment has been completed and these are highlighted in each section.

Comprehensive geriatric assessment—physical health

Sleep

It is worth noting how well a patient feels he sleeps. What time does he go to sleep and how long does he sleep? Is his sleep interrupted or does he sleep 'badly'? Does he have frequent nightmares or terrors? Is his sleep disturbed by pain or needing to go to the toilet?

Good sleep is increasingly recognized as an important contributor to optimal physical and mental wellbeing. Disturbances in sleep can have an impact on concurrent medical issues, mood, energy levels and even memory. The link between poor sleep and poor cognition is gaining evidence, but being sleep deprived will have an impact on concentration and thinking in any person.

Nightmares and night terrors may be associated with Parkinson's disease and Lewy body dementia. Overnight pain must be explored and addressed. Frequent nocturia can be a sign of prostatism in men or may represent bladder instability, overflow or infection in either sex, all of which may be alleviated by advice around drinking habits, further physical assessment and medication, as needed. A person who gets up at night may be at increased risk of falling, so the assessment and management of simple issues like pain and continence may reduce the risk of falls and their associated complications.

Falls and bone health

Entire clinics are now devoted to assessing patients who 'fall', such is the impact of this seemingly simple event on morbidity and mortality. It is therefore important to ask if a person has fallen in the last year and how many times? Information about the pattern of any previous falls can be helpful: frequency, relationship to posture, activity or time of day, pre-warning and residual symptoms following the fall, and any avoiding steps taken by the patient should be ascertained. The absence of any warning implies a sudden event, usually neurological or cardiovascular in nature.

Sinister symptoms associated with falling include loss of consciousness (although, notoriously, this is poorly reported), focal neurological deficit, features of seizure, chest pain, palpitations or other cardiorespiratory symptoms. The most useful clinical investigation in 'older fallers' is to watch them walking; however, they may also need medical investigations to exclude cardiovascular problems such as a 24-hour ECG tape or a tilt test and brain imaging if a neurological cause is suspected.

It is also important to establish any previous injuries from a fall, especially any broken bones. Any patient who has had a previous fracture from a fall will need an assessment of bone health, including an assessment of vitamin D and calcium and potentially bone mineral density analysis.

Falls prevention programmes constitute a key part of local public health initiatives and entail education around falls, trip hazards and exercise programmes.

Key areas of examination

A focus on the cardiovascular and neurological systems and observation of the person walking are both aspects of any falls assessment (Box 7.4).

Cardiovascular examination in older patients does not differ from that in younger adults, but a number of important factors need to be taken into account. Brady-arrhythmias and tachy-arrhythmias are common in sick, older patients and may lead to cardiovascular collapse, despite similar heart rates being well tolerated in the young. The increase in heart rate in response to stress (e.g. exercise, illness or pyrexia) is reduced in advanced old age, and this may be exacerbated by medications such as β-blockers and other anti-arrhythmics. Pauses in heart rhythm caused by combinations of anti-arrythmic drugs and underlying ischaemic changes may result in sudden collapse and syncope.

A lying and standing (or sitting) blood pressure is extremely useful but may not be obtainable in the more disabled patient. Postural hypotension, defined as a drop in systolic blood pressure of more than 20 mmHg on standing, is a considerable cause of morbidity in old age; often it is caused or exacerbated by medications. The sitting or standing blood pressure should be measured immediately prior to and then 1, 3 and 5 minutes after changing position. The guidelines for managing blood pressure in older people now reflect the increased morbidity associated with hypotension and postural hypotension and a more relaxed approach to blood pressure management might be the less risky option in very frail or very elderly patients (a systolic blood pressure of up to 160 might be more tolerable than repeated falls or impacts on cerebral blood flow resulting from significant postural hypotension).

Heart valves, especially the aortic valve, can become less mobile, exacerbated by calcification. Known as aortic sclerosis, this is characterized by a non-radiating ejection systolic murmur, heard loudest in the aortic area. Some patients may present with aortic stenosis as a cause of their fall and this may be amenable to surgical intervention, depending on their overall general health. Degeneration and calcification of the mitral valve can result in either apical ejection murmurs or the more common pansystolic mitral regurgitant murmur (see Chapter 13).

The formal assessment of the peripheral nervous system by examining muscle bulk, tone, power, sensation and tendon reflexes is something the inexperienced clinician often finds difficult. In older, disabled patients, about whom judgements concerning normality and abnormality may be

Box 7.4   The causes of falls in elderly people

Premonitory

- Forerunner of acute, usually infectious, illness

Medication

- Multiple drug therapy
- Psychotropic drugs
- L-dopa
- Antihypertensives

Postural hypotension

- Drugs
- Alcohol
- Cardiac disease
- Autonomic failure/dysfunction

Neurological disease

- Neurocardiogenic syncope
- Multiple strokes
- Transient ischaemic attack
- Parkinson's disease
- Cerebellar disease
- Epilepsy
- Age-related loss of postural reflexes
- Spastic paraparesis (usually owing to cervical spondylosis)
- Peripheral sensory or motor neuropathy
- Situational and postprandial syncope

Cardiovascular disease

- Carotid sinus syndrome
- Brady- and tachyarrhythmia: second-degree and complete heart block, sick sinus syndrome, atrial and ventricular tachyarrhythmias
- Structural abnormalities: valvular stenosis and regurgitation, hypertrophic obstructive cardiomyopathy
- Myocardial infarction and ischaemia

Musculoskeletal disease

- General muscle weakness (e.g. owing to systemic malignancy)
- Muscular wasting caused by arthritis
- Unstable knee joints
- Myopathy (e.g. osteomalacia)

Miscellaneous

- Drop attacks
- Hypoglycaemia
- Cervical spondylosis
- Alcohol
- Elder abuse (e.g. physical mistreatment)
- Poor vision
- Multisensory deprivation:
  - deafness
  - poor vision
  - labyrinthine disorder
  - peripheral neuropathy

more subjective, this can be especially difficult. As with all clinical skills, such judgement is acquired only with practice. As part of this assessment, it is useful to ask the patient to hold his upper limbs fully extended and supinated, at shoulder height, with his eyes closed. Observe for pronator drift, which is a sign of pyramidal weakness. The reflexes should be examined in the normal manner. It is not uncommon for the ankle jerks to be diminished or hard to elicit in very old people but, as with all clinical signs, this should be viewed in the context of other findings and not in isolation.

It is essential to observe the walking or gait pattern wherever possible in someone who has fallen over. This may reveal subtle evidence of hemiparesis, poor balance or the furniture-clutching gait of the patient with long-standing mobility problems. When observing the gait, always have someone walk alongside the patient to offer a helping hand in case he stumbles or falls. Occasionally patients claim that they are capable of carrying out activities when in reality they cannot. Always check the feet for chiropody problems (e.g. onychogryphosis), which cause a 'painful' or antalgic gait.

Further tests of balance are often carried out by physiotherapists and, combined with the physical examination, creates a picture as to the most likely cause of the fall and stratifies the risk of a person falling again. Balance tests such as the Tinetti test (a person is assessed standing and sitting from a chair and then walking a set distance whilst gait is observed) and the 'Timed Up And Go' (TUAG test—a person is asked to stand from a chair, walk 3 metres and sit back down again) provide objective evidence that can be used to create a management plan for falls prevention. These tests can be reassessed to show improvement and progress. Strength and balance exercises are a key intervention in any falls prevention programme and there is good evidence to show that this intervention has a positive impact.

Appetite and weight

Does the person enjoy his food? Does he eat a varied diet? Is food provided by an outside agency and delivered to the door ('meals on wheels') or made by carers during the day? Has he lost weight?

Like sleep, food and nourishment form an essential part of human survival. People who rely on food being provided may not like what is served and people with absent teeth or dentures may manage only softer diets. Taste and smell may change as we age and this may impact on how much food is enjoyed. Loss of weight occurring in the presence of good oral intake should prompt a thorough investigation for an underlying cause, such as a malignancy. Loss of weight may have an impact on muscle bulk and therefore balance, which in turn may increase the risk of fall. Low sun exposure from being housebound may have an impact on vitamin D levels and, combined with a diet low in calcium, this also increases the risk of fall and fracture.

Key areas for examination

The older patient should be weighed at every visit. As in younger patients, nutritional assessment includes estimation of the body mass index (BMI): weight (kg)/height (m^2). Because of osteoporotic vertebral collapse and other age-related changes, height may reduce in the old and so trends in weight are a more useful benchmark. The 'Malnutrition Universal Screening Tool' or 'MUST' is used to screen for nutritional status in the acute care setting and ensures that anyone who requires nutritional support can be identified in a timely manner. It incorporates BMI, disproportionate weight loss and the presence of acute illness to establish a risk score, which can then trigger further dietetic review.

Abdominal examination may be limited by patients' orthopnoea, kyphoscoliosis or other disabilities. However, always try to perform an appropriate assessment. If abdominal examination is limited by such disabilities, the patient will also find it difficult to lie supine for investigations, such as computed tomography (CT) scanning or colonoscopy.

Continence

Sensitive questioning of bowel and bladder habits is an important skill to learn and may take some practice. Ask whether the person has to go to the toilet frequently during the day or night? Does he ever have accidents and leak urine or does he wear a pad to support this? Can he tell when he needs to go to the toilet? Does he have to rush before it comes out? Are his bowels regular? Is the stool sometimes too hard to come out or like rabbit pellets? Again, these build up a picture of whether someone can control his bowel and bladder and whether there may be potentially reversible pathology.

Incontinence should not be regarded as a normal part of ageing and is more specifically associated with sphincteric damage, loss of neurological control mechanisms, especially in dementia or stroke, and with severe disability, chronic illness and frailty. Amongst the institutionalized older population, as many as 50% may suffer urinary and/or faecal incontinence.

When taking a history of urinary or faecal incontinence, try to differentiate between loss of ability to control voiding and failure to identify or reach an acceptable place for elimination. Find out how socially disabling the incontinence has become: many patients become isolated or afraid to go out because of the associated anxiety and potential embarrassment.

Faecal incontinence is relatively rare in well, older men but is principally associated with severe chronic disability or cognitive impairment. In women, it is relatively more frequent but still rare. It may result from pelvic floor weakness. In both sexes, it may occur with carcinoma of the rectum, diverticular

---

Box 7.5	Faecal impaction may cause

- Faecal incontinence (ball-valve effect, with spurious diarrhoea)
- Intestinal obstruction
- Restlessness and agitation in the confused (but faecal impaction never causes confusion)
- Retention of urine
- Rectal bleeding
- Bowel perforation (termed 'stercoral perforation', rare)

Box 7.6	Common causes of urinary incontinence in the older person

- Pelvic floor weakness
- Sphincter defects from injury in childbirth
- Pelvic floor neuropathy
- Urinary tract infections
- Bedridden state with immobility
- Dementia and delirium
- Neurological disease, e.g. stroke, myelopathy
- Autonomic neuropathy

---

disease, laxative abuse and excess, faecal overloading with impaction and neurogenic bowel. Constipation severe enough to cause faecal impaction is not uncommon and may have serious consequences (Box 7.5). This is often iatrogenic caused by the use of opiate analgesia, iron supplements or calcium channel blockers; if of recent onset, it should be investigated appropriately.

Key areas for examination

The indications for digital rectal examination are the same as for younger patients, but this may not be feasible or appropriate, particularly in the very disabled or frail, older patient.

As part of the examination there should be an assessment of the prostate gland, evaluation of the pelvic floor muscles and culture of a mid-stream specimen of urine. An incontinence chart kept for a few days may suggest a recognizable pattern of urinary and/or faecal incontinence. The specialist help of a continence adviser is often useful. Causes of urinary incontinence are shown in Box 7.6. It is rarely useful to dip a urine sample to look for infection. If a urinary infection is suspected from symptoms and examination, then a culture should be taken and antibiotics commenced as appropriate. Urine dips should be reserved in the context of acute kidney injury and to check for hematuria and proteinuria. Older people frequently have 'positive' urine dips with asymptomatic bacteria and are treated with antibiotics erroneously.

Skin

Older skin is thinner, less elastic, bruises more easily and takes longer to heal. As such, multiple attempts

Figure 7.1 Superficial pressure ulcers.

Figure 7.2 Deep pressure ulcers.

at phlebotomy may cause considerable distress. Most patients and families will tell you about any 'sores'. It is worth checking how frequently the nurses attend to dress any skin lesions. Ask about painful sores, which may keep a person awake all night. Ask him if he thinks the sore has changed, become smelly or started leaking?

Skin breakdown in the form of pressure ulcers is a surrogate marker of inadequate support and care because this reflects that a person is not being provided with enough care to ensure clean, dry and pressure-free skin. New pressure ulcers should prompt safeguarding procedures to investigate how better to support this person's care.

About 80% of pressure ulcers are superficial (Fig. 7.1). They occur mainly in dehydrated, immobile and incontinent patients exposed to sustained pressure. People with impaired sensation or with diabetes are especially vulnerable. Decubitus ulcers are always potentially preventable but will occur in any setting if skin care is disregarded. Any superficial ulcer will deepen if the pressure is not relieved. Deep ulcers (Fig. 7.2) are formed when localized high pressure applied to the skin cuts off a wedge-shaped area of tissue, usually adjacent to a bony prominence.

Older people can frequently develop leg ulcers as a result of poor venous return or poor arterial blood supply (50% are owing to venous stasis (Fig. 7.3), 10% to arterial disease and 30% to 40% are of mixed origin). Some of these can be very resistant to healing and this can then have an impact on mobility, pain and sleep. Prolonged sitting in a chair with infrequent exercise can exacerbate skin breakdown, which may have originally been caused by a relatively minor insult. Pressure bandaging can be used to support venous return, but only in the presence of an adequate arterial blood supply.

Good skin care depends on fastidious nursing and close observation. Healthy skin requires good nutrition, careful positioning, alertness to potential pressure burdens as well as careful

Figure 7.3 Leg ulcers.

cleaning and drying routines. An alternating-pressure air mattress (APAM) in which horizontal air cells (Fig. 7.4) inflate and deflate over a short cycle, constantly supporting the patient, provides periods of low pressure at all pressure sites, and good protection.

Key areas for examination

A general assessment of a person's skin can reveal a host of clues to his general health. Wrinkles are mainly owing to past exposure to ultraviolet light and hence are not usually seen in covered areas. The skin of the elderly bruises easily (senile purpura); some people have skin like transparent tissue paper, described as papyraceous, especially

Figure 7.4 An alternating-pressure air mattress (APAM).

Figure 7.5 Transparent 'papyraceous' skin. The surface has been broken by trivial trauma.

on the backs of the hands and the forearms (Fig. 7.5). The skin around the eyes may show yellow plaques—Dubreuilh's elastoma. Some solar-induced changes to be aware of include keratoacanthoma, basal cell carcinoma, squamous cell carcinoma and malignant melanoma. The most common skin lesion noted is the small red Campbell de Morgan spot, a benign lesion seen most often on the trunk and abdomen.

Examination should include sensory (neuropathic ulcers) and vascular (ischaemia and varicose veins) examinations of the lower limbs. Measure the ankle and brachial blood pressures using a Doppler meter and sphygmomanometer cuff, the Doppler meter being used instead of a stethoscope at the feet. The ankle–brachial pressure index (ABPI) is calculated using the formula:

$$\mathrm{ABPI} = \frac{\text{Ankle systolic pressure}}{\text{Brachial systolic pressure}}$$

An ABPI of 1.0 is normal; an ABPI below 1.0 may indicate arterial disease. An ABPI <0.8 indicates a compromised distal circulation, and so pressure bandaging for leg ulceration should be avoided.

Pain

Concerns about pain may have been explored within other topics. Older people may normalize pain or regularly medicate it and therefore not think it relevant. When asking about pain it is worth checking when a person last felt 'pain free' and how effective any painkillers are at reducing or clearing pain completely. This might be an opportunity to establish if he uses alcohol to medicate pain or whether he uses other over-the-counter (OTC) medications or topical agents.

Musculoskeletal pain is common amongst older patients and may represent underlying osteoarthritis or other inflammatory arthropathies. A multidisciplinary approach to managing this type of pain may allow for the use of non-pharmacological agents, assessment of joint mobility and supportive measures, such as exercises and orthotic appliances.

Many people have a complex relationship with pain and trying to alleviate years of pain is a significant challenge. The role of patient-driven goals and wishes allows some focus on the management plan, e.g. 'I want to be able to sleep better' or 'I want to be able to see my family for the day'.

Key areas for examination

An examination of the large joints, shoulders, hips and knees to look for acute or chronic changes is required to establish the cause of any potential musculoskeletal pain. Older people may present with acute pain on chronic changes and acute inflammatory arthropathies, which can have a significant impact on mobility and functioning. Again the physiotherapists may be able to support some of this examination and suggest some non-pharmacological treatment for it. Exercise, good positioning and use of ultrasound can have a significant impact on the experience of musculoskeletal pain and reduce tablet burden.

Memory, mood and energy

Dementia

Cognitive problems are not a part of normal ageing. Our memory and our capacity for learning changes over the years, but dementia is a pathological process producing a clinical syndrome. In the UK currently, one-third of all persons over 65 years of age will die with a dementia diagnosis and 20% of all over 80 years of age have dementia (meaning 80% do not).

People with dementia are disproportionately represented in health care settings. At any one time in the UK, 25% of all hospital beds nationally are occupied by a person with dementia. Good knowledge around the assessment and care of people with dementia is essential if high-quality care is to be provided to this group of patients.

Not all patients will remember or know that they have dementia, but it is important to ask a person for a view on their memory. They may understand that other people are bothered about their memory even if they are not. It is important to establish the type of dementia a person has. It would not be acceptable to document a general 'cancer' diagnosis. The length of history and any behavioural or psychological symptoms, such as hallucinations, agitation and day/night reversal, are important as they often incur a significant burden on carers.

Delirium

The old terminology of 'acute confusional state' is now obsolete and a focus on correct diagnosis and treatment of patients presenting with cognitive problems is essential.

Delirium is an acute neuropsychiatric disorder occurring in response to a wide range of biological and environmental insults. It is a lot more common in people with dementia and is therefore often overlooked or considered as part of the normal progression of a dementia diagnosis. Delirium is extremely common in older patients presenting to hospitals acutely and is associated with a high mortality rate.

Delirium causes an acute change in cognition associated with clouding of consciousness and changes in attention. A person may present as **hyper**-alert and **over** attentive to surroundings or **hypo**-alert and **under** attentive to surroundings. People can often swing between the two states of arousal. Patients with delirium can be difficult to care for on an acute hospital ward and this can lead to negative perceptions around caring for this group of patients. However, delirium can be a deeply distressing experience and all health care staff should be trained to advocate and support this very vulnerable group of patients.

Delirium is rarely caused by a single pathology and half of all patients will have multiple triggers for their delirium, which can occur more commonly in the context of cognitive frailty (previous delirium, known dementia, cerebrovascular pathology). Triggers may be apparently minor, such as a new environment, unfamiliar routines, sleep deprivation, pain and constipation (Box 7.7). Good delirium management relies on early recognition, identifying those at most risk and addressing potential causes in turn. Simple interventions, such as ensuring good sleep hygiene and allowing a familiar carer to stay in the hospital, can make a big difference on the impact of delirium on a person.

Mood/mental state

Some questions about mood are also important. Do you feel down or sad about life? Do you have things to look forward to in life? What does the future look like? Do you ever get lonely at home?

Loneliness amongst older people is common and associated with poorer outcomes across the physical and mental health spectrum. Increasingly

Box 7.7	Causes of delirium

- Changes in environment
- Sleep deprivation
- Pain
- Constipation
- Medication (new or stopped)
- Infection
- Ischaemia
- Electrolyte abnormalities
- Urethral catheter insertion
- (50% have multiple causes; 20% no cause is found)

the pressure of jobs, childcare and housing means that many older people no longer have the support of their wider family members to keep them busy and supported. Some older people view a trip to the hospital or clinic as a social event and may be reluctant to go home. Establishing this as a key concern can trigger local befriending services and social prescribing to increase contact with other people and groups, which may in turn improve mood and health generally.

Asking about a person's perception of his energy levels can provide some insight into his level of frailty. Higher levels of frailty are associated with low perceived energy levels and fatigue. People may describe themselves as having no 'get up and go' which may be physical (deconditioned weaker muscles, after acute illness) or mental (low mood and lack of motivation, cognitive problems). With experience, these conversations can dovetail into more detailed exploration of a patient's expectations and wishes around his health and an opportunity to document this more formally as an advanced care plan.

Key areas for examination

All older patients attending a hospital or acute health care setting should have some form of screen for memory problems and cognitive testing. Nowadays the 4AT has largely superseded the use of the abbreviated mental test score because it is able to pick up both likely dementia and delirium. The 4AT is a well-validated tool for initial cognitive assessment that also tests for conscious level and alertness and is a more robust test of attention (using the months of the year backwards) (Table 7.2). It can be performed by any health care staff and is short enough to do during ward rounds.

If the initial screening indicates that longer-term cognitive problems may be present, then more formal cognitive assessments should be undertaken. This is rarely useful to do in an acute hospital setting and may be done better in a follow-up clinic.

The 'clock test' can be used as an indicator of underlying cognitive problem in the ward environment. A single fault in this test alone is

Table 7.2 The 'Four As' Test (4AT) for delirium and cognitive impairment. AMT4, Abbreviated Mental Test with four questions

[1] Alertness

This includes patients who may be markedly drowsy (e.g. difficult to rouse and/or obviously sleepy during assessment) or agitated/hyperactive. Observe the patient. If asleep, attempt to wake with speech or gentle touch on shoulder. Ask the patient to state his name and address to assist rating.

Normal (fully alert, but not agitated, throughout testing)	0
Mild sleepiness for <10 seconds after waking, then normal	0
Clearly abnormal	4

[2] AMT4

Age, date of birth, place (name of the hospital or building), current year.

No mistakes	0
1 mistake	1
2 or more mistakes/untestable	2

[3] Attention

Ask the patient: 'Please tell me the months of the year in backwards order, starting at December'. To assist initial understanding one prompt of 'what is the month before December?' is permitted.

Achieves 7 months or more correctly	0
Starts but scores <7 months/refuses to start	1
Untestable (cannot start because unwell, drowsy, inattentive)	2

[4] Acute change or fluctuating course

Evidence of significant change or fluctuation in: alertness, cognition, other mental function (e.g. paranoia, hallucinations) arising over the last 2 weeks and still evident in last 24 hrs.

No	0
Yes	4
4AT score	

Source: www.the4AT.com © MacLullich A, Ryan T, Cash H.

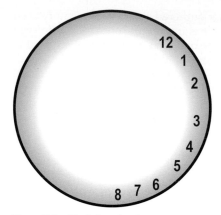

Figure 7.6 Clock-face drawing.

associated with an increase in mortality at 1 year. The patient is presented with a drawn circle, about 10–15 cm in diameter, and asked to fill in the numbers of a clock face (Fig. 7.6). Abnormalities may be caused by visual impairment, agnosia (owing to right parietal lobe lesions) or cognitive impairment. This test is easily reproducible and less influenced by cultural and language problems than the abbreviated mental test score (AMTS) or mini-mental test examination (MMSE). There are many more comprehensive tests of cognition, all of which can be equally useful, provided they cover the key areas of cognitive function, short-term memory, long-term memory, attention, language, higher executive function and orientation. It is useful to practise with some of these tests because they can initially appear long and cumbersome, but with time will become easier to perform.

One of the key issues that people with dementia and delirium have problems with is communication. Communication is a two-way process that involves understanding and comprehension as well as the production of appropriate speech. Difficulties with either or both of these processes can mean that a person may not be able to make his needs heard or met which, in turn, can lead to considerable frustration. Communication problems can be considered in terms of:

- disorders of language (dysphasia)
- disorders of articulation (dyspraxia, dysarthria)
- disorders of voice (dysphonia) or of fluency (dysfluency)

Dysphasia, that is difficulty in encoding and decoding language, is usually associated with a left hemisphere lesion (see Chapter 16). Dyspraxia is difficulty initiating and carrying out voluntary movements, for example of the tongue, and hence can affect speech. Dysarthria has many causes, including local factors in the mouth and dentition, stroke, Parkinson's disease and other neurological disorders. Dysphonia, an abnormality of the quality of the voice (e.g. hoarseness), can be owing to anxiety, vocal abuse, local disease of the larynx and pharynx or hypothyroidism. It is common after throat surgery and intubation. Dysfluency (stammer) is found in people of all ages.

Careful assessment of language and cognition should provide some pointers as to cause. Ensuring that all staff are able to identify and optimize communication with this person is everyone's duty and this can be supported with input from the speech and language therapists and specialist dementia and delirium nurses.

Medication

The number of comorbid conditions that many older people now accumulate over a lifetime means that the old saying 'a pill for every ill' now incurs

| Box 7.8 | Areas to cover in a treatment history |

- Current medications
- Previous hospital and family doctor medications
- Treatment from 'alternative' practitioners
- Self-medication
- Past bad experiences with medicines
- Other non-drug treatments
- Medicines kept in the home
- Compliance and help: dosette box; nurses; carers

| Box 7.9 | Common causes of acute and chronic loss of vision |

Acute

- Retinal detachment
- Vascular (central retinal artery/vein thrombosis)
- Angle-closure glaucoma

Chronic

- Cataract
- Macular degeneration
- Open-angle glaucoma
- Diabetic retinopathy

a considerable tablet burden. Asking people about their medicines may reveal those that they place faith in and those that they may admit to skipping on occasion. It is worth checking what medication has been started recently and what medication they have been unable to tolerate (this may differ from a true allergy to the drug). Some medications are started to alleviate the side effects of other drugs (anti-platelet agents and gastric protection, for example) and it is important to establish the use of OTC medication and topical agents, such as transdermal non-steroidal analgesia as there will still be some central absorption of these drugs (Box 7.8).

'Polypharmacy' is the term used to describe the use of multiple medications in one person. It is associated with an increase in falls risk as well as other impacts on appetite, sleep and functioning. The antidote to this is 'rationalizing medication', a key process during CGA. Rationalizing is not simply the removal of drugs but rather a careful assessment of each drug's impact, risks and benefits ensuring that older people are on the most effective combination of drugs conducive to a good quality of life.

Key areas for examination

Some drug side effects will become apparent during general examination, e.g. thin, papery, easily bruised skin of long-term steroid use or gynaecomastia seen in men taking spironolactone. A close inspection of tablet boxes, the date of issue and a pill count will also provide an insight into concordance. The same can be done for medication aids in which daily doses of tablets are provided in pre-filled, weekly packs (dosette boxes).

Vision, hearing and teeth

Changes in vision are inevitable with advancing age and most people will become long-sighted from middle age onwards as the muscles of the eye and lens shape change. Cataracts are also seen in all ageing lenses to a greater or lesser extent and can have an impact on the quality of vision. These changes will occur earlier in patients with diabetes. Not being able to see to read or distinguish faces can be a lonely place.

Hearing loss of higher frequencies is almost inevitable owing to presbycusis, an age-related degeneration of the cochlear hair cells. Hearing

aid batteries last less than a week so will have run out by the end of the average hospital stay. Many people do not like wearing their hearing aids because of discomfort and feedback and the use of 'hearing loops' or headsets may be more acceptable.

Few elderly people have their original dentition and many rely on the use of 'false plates'. These require considerable care to ensure they are clean and infection free. Any weight loss may render plates loose, which can cause pain and ulceration within the mouth. All of these issues may affect the types of food a person enjoys and sometimes the inventive use of blended and fortified foods is required to ensure that all nutritional components are included in a person's diet. A dietician can support this process.

Glasses, false teeth and hearing aids are easily lost in the hustle and bustle of busy hospitals. These seemingly minor irritants can have disastrous consequences for the patient who may now not be able to see his meals, hear staff asking him questions or chew the food provided.

Key areas for examination

Check what type of glasses a person is wearing, their condition and when he wears them. Visual acuity should be assessed and any loss of vision noted, together with the history of development of the visual disorder. Acute and chronic causes of loss of vision should be considered during the examination (Box 7.9).

Age-related loss of periorbital fat may give the eyes a sunken appearance; this may be severe enough to cause drooping of the upper lid (ptosis) and redundant skin at the lateral borders. The loss of fat can also cause the lower eyelid to curl in (entropion) and irritate the cornea, causing redness and watering (epiphora) or to fall outwards slightly (ectropion). A whitish rim around the iris (arcus senilis) is a zone of lipid deposition around the periphery of the cornea.

The visual fields should always be assessed. It is common to see irregular, asymmetrical pupils owing to previous iridotomy. Pupillary responses are normal in the well, older patient, but stroke and medication may cause abnormal size and responses. Abnormalities, such as Horner's syndrome, and palsies of the third, fourth and sixth cranial nerves are relatively common in the elderly, related to stroke and neoplastic disease. Funduscopy should be attempted wherever necessary but may be difficult in the presence of cataracts.

Look in the ears for wax or evidence of infection (an easily missed source) and ensure hearing aids are clean and not blocked and have fresh batteries.

Look in the mouth for moisture and the condition of the tongue. There are classic signs seen in tongues, such as the beefy red tongue of vitamin B_{12} deficiency or the white plaques of candidiasis infection, but the tongue may also be coated and dry. Check dentition and note the state of dentures. A dry, coated tongue is not conducive to the enjoyment of food and simple measures such as cleaning the tongue, mouth and dentures can lead to improved oral intake.

Social history

Although the multidisciplinary team will build a detailed picture of 'normal life' for the person being assessed, it is important that a social history is taken to support this.

Ask what type of housing a person lives in and whether he owns it. Who else is in the property? Does he ever leave the house and when? Does he have to navigate stairs? Does he have a downstairs toilet? Getting up and down stairs can be a precarious exercise for someone who is frail and lacking in muscle strength.

Activities of daily living can be subdivided into personal (washing, grooming, toileting, dressing, feeding and continence) and domestic (shopping, cooking, laundry, housework). Many people will still participate in 'extended' activities, such as using a mobile phone, getting on public transport, managing finances, etc. This can be formally recorded using The Barthel index (Table 7.3).

Support networks may be formal, provided through social care, or paid for privately; or informal, through family, friends and neighbours. When someone depends on the arrival of another person to get washed and dressed or to be provided with a drink and meal it is easy to understand how precarious this arrangement might be and how vulnerable this person is to even a minor change in the timetable (a late carer, a forgotten drink or insufficient time to provide the full meal). Some hospital admissions are described as purely 'social,' but it is always important to find out what has broken down in the support to cause admission. It might be that a change in someone's underlying health condition means that a fragile arrangement is no longer sufficient.

Review of systems

The use of the comprehensive geriatric assessment means that there is usually little left to be explored on review of systems. The only notable omission

Table 7.3 The Barthel ADL Index (total score 20)

Item	Categories
Bowels	0 = incontinent (or needs to be given an enema)
	1 = occasional accident (once per week)
	2 = continent
Bladder	0 = incontinent/catheterized, unable to manage
	1 = occasional accident (max once every 24 hr)
	2 = continent (for over 7 days)
Grooming	0 = needs help with personal care
	1 = independent face/hair/teeth/shaving (implements provided)
Toilet use	0 = dependent
	1 = needs some help but can do something alone
	2 = independent (on and off, dressing, wiping)
Feeding	0 = unable
	1 = needs help cutting, spreading butter, etc.
	2 = independent (food provided in reach)
Transfer	0 = unable—no sitting balance
	1 = major help (one or two people, physical), can sit
	2 = minor help (verbal or physical)
	3 = independent
Mobility	0 = immobile
	1 = wheelchair independent (includes corners)
	2 = walks with help of one (verbal/physical)
	3 = independent (may use any aid, e.g. stick)
Dressing	0 = dependent
	1 = needs help, does about half unaided
	2 = independent, includes buttons, zips, shoes
Stairs	0 = unable
	1 = needs help (verbal, physical), carrying aid
	2 = independent
Bathing	0 = dependent
	1 = independent (may use shower)

The Barthel Index should be used as a record of what a patient does, not as a record of what he was able to do previously. The main aim is to establish the degree of independence from any help, physical or verbal, however minor and for whatever reason. The need for supervision means the patient is not independent. Performance over the preceding 24–48 hours is important, but longer periods are relevant. A patient's performance should be established using the best available evidence. Ask the patient or carer, but also observe what the patient can do. Direct testing is not needed. Unconscious patients score 0 throughout. Middle categories imply that the patient supplies over 50% effort. Use of aids to be independent is allowed.

may be questions around respiratory symptoms. This might also be the opportunity to ask about what bothers a person most and what he expects or hopes to happen. Given that older people frequently have many pathologies, it is useful to establish what their priority is. What input would he most value? It may not necessarily align with that of their health care practitioners and finding this out can lead to more satisfying patient interactions.

Ethics, capacity and the law

Given the vulnerability of this group of patients, it is clear that a sound understanding of key ethical considerations and the law around consent and decision-making is vital. Clinicians are frequently asked to support decision-making during discharge arrangements, advanced care planning and treatment escalation plans.

Assessing capacity to make a decision is subject in the UK to the Mental Capacity Act 2005 (full information about this at legislation.gov.uk) The key principles guiding this are that a person is presumed to have capacity until proven otherwise, that he is entitled to make an 'unwise' decision if he has capacity and that, in the absence of capacity, a best interests decision will be made that encompasses the 'least restrictive option'.

The first principle of assessing capacity is that it can be done only in the event that a person has a disorder or impairment of mind or brain. Without this premise, capacity has to be assumed to be intact. The disorder may be temporary, such as during an episode of delirium, but it must be diagnosed.

It is not correct to say that a patient 'lacks capacity'. Capacity is decision- specific and even the most cognitively impaired person may have the ability to decide what he wears or whether he takes sugar in his tea today. The more complex the decision, the more complex the capacity assessment.

Any member of the MDT may perform a capacity assessment and, in fact, the person who knows the person best is likely to be best placed to do this. A person is deemed to have capacity if he can understand and retain the information required, can communicate this well and is not being coerced to a specific outcome (this may occur when there are financial implications, such as a move to a new home, etc.). There should be consistency in his decision and an ability to justify a potentially 'unwise' decision (Box 7.10).

In the absence of capacity a team must meet and make a 'best interests' decision on behalf of the patient. This team will consist of the health and social care staff looking after the patient and should also involve the next of kin. If no next of kin is available, then the team have to appoint an IMCA (an Independent Mental Capacity Advocate) who will advocate on behalf of the patient. The more life changing the decision is, such as a decision around discharge destination on leaving hospital, the more careful the members of the team should be selected. The team must make a decision on behalf of the patient ensuring that it most closely aligns with his preferred option (the least restrictive option).

Some people choose to designate a specific person to make decisions about their health and welfare should they lose the capacity to make their own decisions. This process is known as Power of Attorney (PoA). It is a formal, legally driven arrangement. In the event that a relative or carer has been registered

| Box 7.10 | The principles of capacity |

Persons are deemed to have capacity if they are able to demonstrate the following during decision-making
- understand the information relevant to the decision
- retain that information
- use or weigh that information as part of the process of making the decision, or
- communicate their decision (whether by talking, sign language or any other means)

as a PoA for health and welfare then he must make a decision 'as if he were the patient' but it will still be done within the context of the MDT.

Ethnic elders

Ethnic minority elders form a small but significant proportion of the older population in many contemporary societies. Older ethnic populations may have a racial predisposition to certain conditions, but often develop diseases similar to those of the indigenous population within one to two generations. Indeed, environmental excesses, such as the Western diet, alcohol and cigarettes, may contribute to an increased incidence of premature death compared with their own indigenous population. The availability of health services for this group is often inadequate and insensitive to their specific needs. Any health care professional must always try to understand and respect the cultural background of the patient and his family.

Inadequate care and elder abuse

There are many types of abuse of which any older person can be a victim. About 5% of older people suffer abuse. The most vulnerable are female partners, those living with adult children, perhaps because of financial difficulties or unemployment, and older people in poorly run institutional care homes.

Abuse can take the form of physical or verbal abuse, sexual abuse, financial abuse, psychological abuse and neglect. The 'abuser' may also be vulnerable, struggling with a caring role, have health and financial problems, have alcohol or psychological difficulties, and the relationship with the patient may have been dysfunctional for a long time. In institutions, inadequate staffing levels, poor staff training, repeated complaints and poor client and environmental hygiene are all indicators of potential abuse.

Recognition of elder abuse is made more difficult by the physiological and the pathological changes that occur with ageing (e.g. senile purpura). However, abrasions, pressure ulcers and poor nutrition should raise the possibility of abuse or inadequate care provision. Assessment requires a history that includes open questions about the possibility of aggressive behaviour, both verbal and physical, fear towards an abuser or a reluctance to report abuse. Enquiry regarding the full social background is important, including a sympathetic description of the carer's role. A thorough physical examination should be made and the patient's mental state assessed and recorded. If abuse is suspected, expert help from senior colleagues, social services, psychiatrists or clinical psychologists may be necessary for recognition, disclosure and management.

In the event of suspected abuse, any member of the health care team can now raise a safeguarding alert, which triggers a formal review of the person's welfare. This is usually led by a dedicated social services team and, from this, an action plan is generated to ensure any highlighted issues are appropriately managed and resolved. The action plan may involve increased carer support or respite care, or may require moving a person to a place of safety. A person with capacity must consent to safeguarding procedures before they can be triggered.

Death and dying

No chapter on older people should be complete without the mention of death and dying. There is only one certainty in life and that is that we die. Increasingly, society views conversations about death as distasteful and the pressure to provide medical intervention at any cost means that older people can be subjected to complex and invasive procedures right up until their death.

Death is not a failure of medicine, but a natural process. Many older people have very strong views about the end of their lives and if this is not explored it cannot be honoured. Time spent observing senior and experienced clinicians having conversations about end of life care and wishes and preferences of the patient are precious and require appropriate reflection afterwards. Trying out some of these conversations during training will help to build confidence. It is often staff rather than patients that recoil from these insights.

Some of these conversations can go on to form part of an 'Advanced Care Plan'. This is a documentation of a person's wishes in the event that he becomes seriously ill and at the end of his life. It may include preferred place of death, wishes around 'Do Not Attempt Resuscitation Order' and people he would like to be present. It is not legally binding, but rather an exploration of what medical care may be acceptable and what a 'good death' would look like for him. Current UK law states that someone cannot request a specific medical intervention but he can decline it. A legally binding form of this nature is known as an 'Advanced Decision to Refuse Treatment' and must be very specific to the situation. This form must be completed when the person has the capacity to do so and be countersigned by a legal representative.

It is hoped that this chapter has demonstrated how fulfilling and rewarding it can be to look after older and frailer people. Geriatric medicine now provides one of the few opportunities to provide holistic care within the framework of the MDT and all its expertise. Keen attention to detail is needed, but the impact of small, simple interventions cannot be overemphasized and has the potential to lead to many benefits. Older people are entitled to appropriate resources and care according to their need and in order to promote an optimal quality of life.

Psychiatric assessment | 8

Peter Byrne and Nicola Byrne

Introduction

Psychiatry is the ultimate clinical speciality. At one level, it is about one unique organ—the brain. Unlike other organs, our brains can argue, change jobs, vote and perform many other things. However, the practice of psychiatry is concerned with more than the brain, or even the mind; when the ways we think/feel/behave/interact go wrong, clinical psychiatry interrogates, formulates and treats. We rely on what people tell us (and do not mention or conceal); a unique mental state examination (MSE), evaluating this information in relation to different versions of the history given by a person's close friends and relatives; and reading medical notes from mental health professionals, general practitioners and other sources. This chapter will teach you how to take a comprehensive history and complete an MSE in situations in which you may be pressed for time, your patient is distressed, or the setting (emergency department, busy clinic, hospital ward lacking privacy) works against your objectives. More specialist assessments are listed at the end; no matter where your career takes you, you will encounter these complex patients.

Thoughtful planning, careful timing and good technique will increase the reliability of your psychiatric interview (i.e. the chance that another clinician would have/will produce the same history, MSE findings and formulation as this interview). Involved in this branch of medicine, psychiatrists produce more reliable findings than many other medical and surgical specialities. The absence of specific laboratory or radiological tests to 'prove' a diagnosis should not be seen as a disadvantage; it makes the interview process more important and gives clinicians the responsibility of getting it right the first time. If you are new to this, talk through your first assessments, before and after, with your supervising clinician. The potential areas to question are vast, so a helpful steer from someone experienced will hasten your acquisition of competencies, case by case. At first attempts, many students feel exhausted after completing a detailed psychiatric assessment; learning how to enquire for maximum yield will be time well invested for your future career. If you specialize as a primary care/family physician, you will see more cases of depression than most busy psychiatrists in theirs. If your destination is surgery or interventional medicine, the skills you learn in psychiatry will save some of your patients from unnecessary medical investigations, even treatments. For every completed assessment, with competent record keeping, the patient will benefit from your efforts well into the future.

Preparation

Preparation may be less important if you are a medical/nursing/other student or junior trainee; your trainers will not want you to approach a new patient (meaning new to you) with pre-read assessments and pre-conceived ideas. In emergency rooms, you do need to read something about the patient to determine if you need to take steps to protect your safety or his; a history of violence is a strong predictor of future violence, just as a history of self-harm predicts subsequent self-harm and suicide. Take time to search electronic notes for past safety concerns and evaluate if there were assaults on health professionals, perhaps in circumstances similar to your current setting. Risk varies with circumstances, and some patients may have particular triggers (become stimulated during lengthy interviews, resent being challenged on detail, do not like being interviewed by men, etc.) or have had prior difficulties in some settings (one-to-one meetings, crisis interviews). You need to commit at least 1 hour face-to-face time (longer for children and for people with intellectual disability), during which you are unlikely to be interrupted. In general hospitals, the demand for interviews is invariably 'right now', but few psychiatrists would wake a patient to interview unless absolutely necessary.

Some patients may be sedated (medication overdoses, either self-administered or iatrogenic) and it may be better to wait until their minds are clearer. If your patient is drunk, intoxicated on other substances or withdrawing from these, there are two reasons to delay the interview. First, the MSE is not reliable in this patient group; people are disinhibited, angry, volatile (elated or dysphoric) or mixtures of these and more likely to talk down (and up) their difficulties.

The second reason is your safety; assaults in mental health care are not common, but one assault is one too many. Remember that you are much more likely to be assaulted by an intoxicated person than by a sober patient with severe mental illness (SMI).

Plan and be practical. Decide how you will record key dates and other details (important for individual patients, but easy for us to forget) and direct speech (see later for the value of direct quotations). Even in this digital age, pen and paper are more efficient and sensitive to patients' needs. Think about what the likely outcomes of assessment will be; there are circumstances in which a collateral history before the history and MSE will yield more reliable information, such as suspected prodrome or negative symptoms in schizophrenia and cognitive decline in older people. Whilst, legally, you do not need someone's permission to receive information, it is standard to ask permission from the patient for this (ask for seniors' advice). It is defensible in law to seek information, but not to share it without consent. There are exceptions where the doctor may overrule confidentiality (e.g. significant potential risk of adverse outcomes in untreated psychosis or dementia—including situations in which exploitation by others is suspected).

Think also about who needs to be in the room with you; younger people, until mid-teens, have a parent or guardian present (this has advantages and disadvantages), and some adults ask for a partner or friend to sit in (usually more disadvantages than advantages). If your assessment of an adult patient has another adult insisting on joining the interview for reasons that are not clear, always consider *why* that might be the case (e.g. an abusive controlling partner, lack of boundaries within a family, other secrets). Referring clinicians will tell you if an interpreter is required, or if there are communication challenges (hearing difficulties, dysphasias, intellectual disability or cognitive decline); these can be mitigated with planning (amplification devices, picture cards, *Yes* or *No* options written out to point to answers, etc.). A familiar interpreter is useful, but be aware if the interpreter is leading your interview, perhaps by adding more questions to yours or 'interpreting' answers rather than translating them. If you are concerned about this, ask the interpreter to turn away from the patient and face you; this makes your eye contact the main non-verbal communication with the patient, and the interpreter's role is limited to translating. As a rule, using family members as interpreters for a first interview, or when sensitive information might be revealed, is discouraged.

Circumstances of the interview

Clarify who is asking for this assessment. Even if this interview was requested by the patient, you need to make clear to him your role, and the limits of confidentiality before you begin. No patient has a right to complete confidentiality; if you discover details of (for example) suicidal intent and plans, then you have a responsibility to share that information with others, and act to reduce the risks that this patient will end his life. The same principle applies to stated threats or ideas of harm to others (including children); share and act. Patients will often ask for some information not to be shared, for various reasons. Try to respect that wish, although record the nature of any objections. Discuss the specifics with your supervisor; in England Caldicott Guardians are appointed for each locality to assist with difficult decisions on confidentiality.

Introduce yourself by name, and make clear how junior/senior you are in the service: 'I am a student here and Dr X suggested we speak for about an hour so I can discuss your case with Dr X later'. If you think it will help, offer a handshake, although recently introduced social distancing measures currently make this less practical. Do not overthink it; if the person (for whatever reasons, some are cultural including a male-female dynamic, other reasons reflect infection control and an elbow bump establishes your professional relationship) does not shake your hand, smile, sit down and begin the interview. If the patient recoils from you, make a factual note of this ('he was not pleased to see me and turned away as I approached') as this is a positive finding that might indicate paranoia or past negative experiences with clinicians. Be open and honest at the start of your interview: 'Doctor X has asked me to assess your difficulties to see if there are psychological aspects we can identify and help you with' or 'I understand you have taken an overdose of tablets (or harmed yourself), and a psychiatric interview is a necessary part of our assessment and treatment'. If there is potential bias in the interview (e.g. you are admitting him to hospital following the completion of a legal involuntary committal by others, assessing him following a disagreement with another professional or you are preparing a court report), say this and record these circumstances at the start of your notes.

Keeping patients safe is the primary objective. Even a busy emergency department must provide a safe room for patients who have attended as a result of self-harm. These rooms are private, quiet, free from ligature points or equipment that could be used to injure, and have more than one door. Speedy exit is important if the interview overstimulates the patient and the interviewer (you) needs to leave quickly to protect your safety. This said, the vast majority of non-intoxicated emergency room patients welcome the time to talk about what led them here, and to explore solutions to their difficulties. Wanting to 'talk about it' in a crisis or at a low point is a universal human experience; this is true even for patients who did not choose to come for psychiatric evaluation.

Crisis interviewees show a range of behaviours, from people who freely communicate distressing emotions to those who will seek to conceal them. Suicidal ideas evoke shame and guilt; speaking about them is usually a great relief. However, some patients may choose a junior member of the team (e.g. a student [you]), to whom they disclose distressing suicide plans. This might be because they do not want anything done about it or to reflect other mixed, strong feelings. The important point is that you have already had an explicit conversation about the limits of confidentiality, and that you act professionally to share this new risk information with others.

Six-point checklist *before* your assessment begins:

- Time and place: when? For how long? And where will you interview?
- Safety: yours then his. Think through what you now know about this patient. Have you read about past safety concerns? Have you had a conversation with a senior colleague about risks, and what you need to do to mitigate these? What are the means by which you will get help if needed quickly?
- Preparation: available past notes. Decide whether you want to get a collateral history after or before your interview. Who else will be in the room?
- Dignity and privacy: ensure the interviewee feels comfortable, safe and respected. Acknowledge the disruption of a long interview.
- Record keeping during interview (pen and paper): write down key names, dates and some quotations as they are said. In your first attempts at psychiatric interview, write out some history and MSE headings as prompts.
- If the room has a computer, avoid staring at the screen when you could be interacting with your patient.

It is strongly recommended that you adhere closely to the structure of an interview outlined here as you learn how to complete a psychiatric evaluation; this improves the written records and reduces the chance you will forget a major component of either the history or the MSE.

History

History will comprise the bulk of your efforts in completing and recording the interview. The key headings are set out in Box 8.1. These are similar to medical and surgical history taking, but pay particular attention to the extra elements now (Box 8.2). It is human nature to minimize some behaviours (alcohol use, frequent changes of job, violence by/to others) and gloss over others ('I had a very happy childhood… I am a great parent') so record the details of what you are told with any inconsistencies, and add your impressions later. To learn how to interview, take the history in sequence, but be prepared to divert as long as you cover the ground needed. Sometimes more useful information is gathered by being flexible in how the history

is sequenced: you might return to difficult areas (childhood adversity, relationships (Box 8.3) later in the interview, as trust builds.

Students who are new to the 'twice as long' history-taking process (see Box 8.2) can rush in with checklists and find out very little. Empathic listening is non-judgemental, but it is not about agreeing with everything your patient says ('*yes, your mother was a terrible mother*'). Empathy is the human response to the experiences people relate: '*This must have been a tough time for you… this sounds very difficult for you, even now*'. At this point, reserve judgements: for example, even if the referrer identified this patient as a heavy drinker (Box 8.4), do not start now linking low mood episodes to heavy drinking—even though this is a common experience. As you gather information, you can move from the open '*How was your mood at that time?*' to less open '*Were you happy at that time?*' and then to closed (but neutral) '*If your mood was low, can you place a score out of 10, where 8 is average good mood, 0 is the lowest possible and 10 is the happiest ever?*' This scoring system is a useful way to quantify the degree of low mood from the patient's perspective. Correct them if they give a 'minus number', noting the dates of lowest mood (*their* choice of 1/10 or 0/10, etc.) and link these to any contemporaneous changes in suicidal ideation (Box 8.5). If you worry you are 'leading the witness' (inviting or forcing positive answers), ask someone to observe you interviewing and to provide feedback. You are new to this and do not want to pick up bad habits, such as: '*You must have been very depressed when your partner left you, reminding you of your dad's departure when you were nine.*'

The presenting complaint/history should use the patient's own words to describe his problems (e.g. '*I just feel sad all the time*'), not our technical labels for them. Presenting complaint is hard in psychiatry. Sometimes it is given to us by the referrer ('*overdose; looked sad on the ward; investigation of chest pain found no physical cause*'); less often, the patient supplies this as a symptom (or set thereof) that has bothered him. When they do not fit neatly into the seven categories of Box 8.2, record his difficulties as he recounts them, then try to frame the presenting complaints within the headings of mood symptoms, anxiety or psychotic symptoms and so forth. Psychosis, with less than 2% prevalence in the community, is very common on psychiatric wards so you should lead with psychosis headings in these patients. You can always add other presenting complaints as you proceed; for example one in four people with schizophrenia also have depressive symptoms. When a patient is vague about any presenting complaint, ask the open question: '*When were you last well and happy in yourself?*' and the less open '*You seem to be having a hard time right now, when did things change for you?*' Perhaps you can find out more by clarifying the behaviours that led others to request this assessment, and frame the presenting

Box 8.1   Psychiatric history

Background to assessment

- Basic demographics: name, age, gender, ethnic background, marital status, children, type of employment and if currently unemployed, for how long?
- Current treatment status: any established diagnosis; nature of current involvement with psychiatric services; if an inpatient, voluntary or involuntary admission
- Context of your interview: who referred the patient, where you saw that patient

Presenting complaint

- In the patient's own words (e.g. 'There's nothing wrong with me. I've no idea why I'm in hospital')
  - Cognitive or substance misuse or mood or anxiety or psychotic or eating disorders symptoms; personality disorder is not likely among the primary complaints

History of presenting complaint

- What is the problem? When did it start? How did it develop: onset/progress/severity/consequent impairment (e.g. unable to work, end of a relationship)?
- What makes it better or worse; what is its relationship to other problems?
- Relevant negative findings
- Collateral history from informants (e.g. friends, family, general practitioner (GP), work colleagues). Note any contradictions

Family history

- Family structure describes biological/adoptive/stepparents and siblings: age, state of health or cause and age of death, occupations, quality of relationships. Currently, who supports the patient and who exacerbates their problems?
- Family history of mental disorder includes alcoholism, substance misuse, bipolar disorder and suicide.

Personal history

- Obstetric and birth: conception planned/unplanned, wanted/unwanted; maternal physical and mental health during pregnancy and postnatally, any prescribed medication or substance misuse; birth full-term/premature, obstetric events and complications, low birth weight, congenital abnormalities, neonatal illness, maternal separation and bonding
- Development and milestones: delays in interaction with others, speech; motor control, walking, toilet training; sleep difficulties; emotional or behavioural difficulties; hyperactivity; physical illness
- Family atmosphere and stability: for example, warm and caring; abusive; emotionally impoverished or volatile; material circumstances; periods of separation from caregivers (e.g. in hospital because of childhood illness; in foster care owing to parental difficulties)
- Social development: establishment of friendships, imaginative play, experience of bullying, any juvenile delinquency
- Educational attainment: specific learning difficulties, school refusal, age left education and qualifications
- Occupation: periods of employment, nature of work/skills
- Psychosexual: age of first sexual experience, sexual orientation, number, length and quality of significant relationships, marriage(s), children from all previous relationships

Social circumstances

- Housing situation (e.g. renting, numbers of people in the house), employment, finances, benefits, debts
- Daily activities: **leisure** interests (hobbies); **spirituality** and religious affiliation;
- Sources of family and social support

Substance misuse history

- Alcohol use, amounts (in units)
- Illicit substance use: type, pattern of use, including frequency, **dependency**; associated problems—occupational, social, relationship, health and criminal activity
- Abuse of any prescribed or over-the-counter medications

Medical history

- Past and current physical illness and treatment, allergies
- Current medication, including any over-the-counter drugs taken regularly; any drug can be purchased online or acquired.
  - ALLERGY: list what happened (unwell, rash, severe anaphylaxis) with what substance

Past psychiatric history

- Age of onset of symptoms and first contact with services (there is always a time gap); nature and progression of difficulties; diagnoses
- Hospital admissions: when, length, voluntary or under section
- Past treatment: medication, psychological, electroconvulsive therapy. Electroconvulsive therapy (ECT): what has helped in the past, what has not, medication type, doses prescribed and actual doses taken (i.e. concordance with prescription); history of side effects?

Risk history

- Risk episodes: previous self-harm and suicide attempts; self-neglect and exploitation by others (financial, sexual), thoughts of and actual harm to others
- Context of episodes, worst harm resulting

Forensic history (always try for a second source)

- Arrests, charges and convictions: nature of offences, outcome (custodial sentence, community service, probation); you MUST ask about violent actions
- Include criminal activities where patient was not arrested, crime not detected

Premorbid personality

- When did they last—or have they ever—felt 'normal': What is normal for them, how is that different to now?
- General: how would they describe themselves, how would friends/family describe them? (use quotation marks)
- Specific character traits: 'How would you describe yourself as a person?' Then move from open questions (e.g. anxious, sensitive, suspicious, dramatic)
- **Prevailing mood** and **stability of mood; impulse control; nature of relationships with others**: partners, friends, colleagues (e.g. close and confiding, casual only)
- **Tolerance of stress** and coping style, including use of substances to manage stress, modify mood or facilitate social interaction

(Source: Peter Byrne and Nicola Byrne. In *Psychiatry: Clinical Cases Uncovered*. Wiley-Blackwell, Oxford, UK. 2008: page 2, Table 1.)

Box 8.2	Some differences between psychiatric history and medicine-surgery-ob/gyn	

Psychiatry	*Section*	Medicine/surgery/obstetrics
Must include circumstances, including the legal basis of admission (Box 8.1); demographics are about social context and more than a collection of risk factors.	*Background to this presentation*	The focus is on disease: 'emergency admission to CCU with chest pain; elective admission for hip replacement, etc'
There is seldom ONE reason a patient has presented: think first of major groups. These are composed of **seven** major diagnostic categories of confusion (acute, chronic, acute on chronic), substance misuse, mood disorders, anxiety (trait or state, with many subsets of the latter), psychosis, eating and personality disorders.	*Presenting complaint*	A short list of physical systems (in one system) that led to this presentation, at this time You already know the common presenting symptoms for cardiac, respiratory, gastrointestinal, etc; in psychiatry, there are **seven** common categories opposite to explore.
Genetics are important for autism and dementia, bipolar and addictions but not much else; this is a description of their experience of family life, the person's status in his family of origin, current family relationships; for personality, a useful question is 'among your close family, who are you like the most?'	*Family history*	Screening for genetic disorders that are relevant to this presentation: in many circumstances, we construct a genetic family tree of grandparents, parents and their siblings, then patient and all siblings and half-siblings, with their children and grandchildren below. Then indicate who has been affected by disorder.
(See text for details of personal and social histories), home '*who's at home with you?*' and work education	*Personal and social*	Not usually useful; orthopaedics will need to know occupation, hobbies; occupational illnesses too.
What substances used, how often and in what circumstances? (see Box 8.4) Note dependence. In MSE, record motivation.	*Substance misuse history*	Should NOT be neglected: details predict withdrawals from alcohol substances during admission.
Similar to medical colleagues, this is about safety and holistic care. Current medications and known allergies. Make sure your patient is physically well: record pain in any system, breathing difficulties, tiredness, etc, plus red flags (of possible cancer diagnosis) and any recent changes in physical health.	*Medical, surgical and obstetric history*	To document multimorbidity and link diseases to optimize treatments; in obstetric history, note number of pregnancies (not just children) as this includes terminations, miscarriages, etc. This is the area most likely to be neglected by psychiatrists.
Previous assessments: medications, therapy, admissions. For severe depression, patient may have had electroconvulsive therapy (ECT) in the past.	*Psychiatric history*	Usually ignored: depression is both a cause and effect of many medical diseases (cardiac, diabetes, chest).
Your assessment is fact collecting, supplemented from other sources, to identify the potential for self-harm or harm/violence to others (see details of Box 8.1).	*Risk and forensic history*	Usually ignored by non-psychiatric clinicians despite high predictive value of a past history of self-harm or violence to others in predicting similar acts.
Often the most challenging part of psychiatric interview. Questions asked at this stage of the history—after difficult questions about harm and violence—will achieve useful background information: see text.	*Premorbid personality*	Never the focus of routine medical contacts, although personality and coping styles are highly predictive of outcomes of medical and surgical interventions.

CCU, coronary care unit.

complaint as these behaviours, with his version of events ('*patient says he did not hear voices but resents his mother's accusations of voice hearing…*') and then set out how all this led to this presentation.

There are several circumstances (cognitive impairment, severe depression, paranoia) in which patients will deny any current difficulties. In this case, record that '*The patient denied the problems reported by his family and had no presenting complaint, but during the interview it became apparent that there were difficulties in cognition/mood/anxiety/psychotic*

symptoms, etc.' Because you will detail these domains later within MSE (see Box 8.5), provide only an outline of key symptoms here and record timing and durations in each case. In broad terms, you might focus presenting complaint on one or more of the following:

1. **Cognition**: subjective memory and concentration; record likely time frames.
2. **Alcohol and substances**: in most circumstances patients will tell you openly what has happened as they realize these activities have led to this

Box 8.3	Six principles of trauma-informed care for all clinical contacts	
1	Safety	This is about creating the physical and emotional space where people can disclose difficult personal information.
2	Trustworthiness and transparency	People need to know they can trust the recipient of this information. Make clear from the onset that there may be circumstances when you will need to disclose some information to others (e.g. to protect children).
3	Peer support	This may come late after disclosure: knowing that others have had similar experiences and good outcomes.
4	Collaboration and mutuality	We cannot normalize traumatic experiences, but we can explain how common they have become, and that many groups and institutions (schools, prisons) want to learn how to support people better than they have done.
5	Empowerment and choice	Almost universally, traumatized people have had choice taken away during the event. So even small choices here (asking for a female clinician) are important.
6	Cultural, historical and gender issues	There are wider societal forces here, and these change over time: xenophobia, racism, #BLM, homophobia, sexism and #MeToo are all culturally determined.

Based on the principles of Centre for Disease Control (CDC).

Box 8.4	Misuse of alcohol and substances

Screening questions, for example CAGE (see text), alert to excess use.

Alcohol history

- Amount consumed weekly in units: 1 unit = half a pint of regular strength beer, a small glass of wine (125 ml), a small (liqueur) glass of fortified wine (e.g. sherry) or a single measure of spirits. One bottle of wine is 10 units; fortified wines are higher. Many popular beers in the UK are stronger and wine is served in larger glasses. One bottle of spirits contains 30 units.
- Pattern of use: binges, steady intake over the week, sometimes throughout the day; define 'special occasions for drinking'. Friday is not one.
- Features of dependency: compulsion to consume; increased salience of drinking; difficulties controlling use despite harm; tolerance (needing to consume more for the same effect); physiological withdrawal as blood alcohol levels fall. Withdrawal manifests as a range of symptoms:
  - **mild**: tremor, nausea or retching, mood changes, sleep disturbance
  - **moderate**: perceptual distortions and hallucinations, usually visual
  - **severe** and potentially life-threatening: full-blown **delirium tremens** (confusion, terror, severe tremor, and seizures, leading to coma and death)
- Harm from use: physical, mental, relational, occupational (missing work or training, cautions by employer, fired from work) and trouble with the law: fights, drink driving, etc.

presentation. You might record quantity later in the history, but physical dependency (present or absent) and the effects of consumption fit well here.

3. **Mood**: decreased energy, low mood and reduced interest in things (in elevated mood, hypomania, all three parameters are increased, and elevated mood might manifest as irritability). Important quantitative measures are useful here: reduced hours' sleep; weight loss; days lost from work or education; and reduction in frequency of social activities. Establish time lines for when the mood declined and for how long. With elevated mood, sleep is usually impaired and many have a subjective feeling that less sleep is needed.

4. **Anxiety**: record subjective feelings of being tense; psychological and somatic anxiety symptoms (Box 8.6); sleep difficulties; and subtypes of anxiety syndromes (phobias, obsessive compulsive disorder (OCD), episodes of panic, post-traumatic stress disorder (PTSD): see later for definitions).

5. **Psychosis**: delusions, hallucinations and thought difficulties; some patients will describe any/ all of these three positive symptoms, but few

identify negative symptoms/deficit states of schizophrenia as actual complaints.

6. **Eating disorders**: intentional weight loss (define weights or changes to clothing sizes, over time), restriction of food intake or measures to reduce weight, such as excess exercise, misuse of laxatives, diuretics, etc. Anorexia nervosa is mostly a disorder of females (although not exclusively): ask about menarche, normal menstrual cycle and any current interruptions to these. A related group, people with disordered eating, is rising in prevalence: record unusual aspects of diet, food avoidance and specific food phobias, especially how his diet has changed over time. A subset of this latter group may be overweight (body mass index (BMI) > 25) or obese (BMI > 30)).

7. **Personality difficulties**: behaviours indicating emotional turmoil (other than depressive episodes or anxiety symptoms), impulsivity and more, that bring patients into conflict with others or (at the other extreme) isolation from others. These are unlikely to be the focus of the presenting complaint, and as complex adult lifetime disorders, will be described later.

| Box 8.5 | Components of mental state examination (MSE) |

Appearance and behaviour

General appearance, physical state, abnormal movements, behaviour and rapport

- Style and manner of dress, hygiene: self-neglect
- Physical state: signs of physical illness, drug/alcohol withdrawal, self-harm scars
- Manner of engagement during interview (e.g. suspicious/guarded/relaxed). Quality of eye contact (e.g. fixed stare, avoidant). Distractibility and preoccupation with internal world (e.g. appearing to respond to auditory hallucinations)
- Motor movements: involuntary tics, chorea, tremor, tardive dyskinesia (repetitive movements, typically orofacial, owing to high-dose antipsychotics) and akathisia (external manifestation of internal sense of restlessness, again a side effect of antipsychotics). Motor stereotypies are regular repetitive non-goal directed movements (e.g. rocking). Mannerisms are idiosyncratic goal-directed behaviours (e.g. style of walking). Catatonic symptoms include 'automatic behaviours', such as echopraxia and echolalia (imitation of interviewer's movements and speech, respectively), perseveration (repetition of a movement, words/syllables or maintenance of a posture once context has passed), forced (automatic) grasping of objects offered. Catatonia is a rare motor manifestation of schizophrenia or frontal lobe lesions.
- Hyper-/hypoactivity: relevant in delirium and mood states

Speech

Rate, amount, form and coherence

- Increased/decreased; fast/slow; loud/soft
- Verbal stereotypy: repetition of irrelevant words or phrases
- Formal thought disorder disruption to the continuity of thought. Answers initially may be appropriate, but circumstantial, straying far from the topic before returning or tangential, where they do not return. The latter represents mild derailment, with more severe forms seeing the juxtaposition of completely irrelevant ideas, also known as loosening of associations. The most extreme form of thought disorder is known as word salad where meaning is indecipherable. Flight of ideas in hypomanic/manic states is the rapid transition between topics via internal links (connected words, themes, rhyming, alliteration (e.g. 'Black cats scare me, I've a black bag'), or the inclusion of external distractions into the train of thought (e.g. subsequent comments on interviewer's black shoes)
- Poverty of thought describes insubstantial speech that conveys little meaning.
- Neologisms: words or phrases invented or used idiosyncratically to denote new meaning ('I don't like my boss: he's a bosstard').

Mood

Subjective mood, objective affect; thoughts of self-harm and of harming others

- Subjectively patient description of his current mood: rated out of 10, with 0 lowest; it is useful to rate his 'usual' mood as 8/10 and do NOT accept a negative number for worst.

- Objectively, interviewer's appraisal of the patient's affect (external manifestation of emotional state) and emotional range during interview, euthymic (within normal range) and normal reactivity/incongruous affect given context/perplexed/blunted emotional range
- Note FIVE biological or neurovegetative symptoms of depression that are associated with increased depression severity:
  - Diurnal variation of mood during day: typically worse in the mornings but recovers partly later
  - Late insomnia: early morning wakening (patient is unable to get back to sleep in the time before he needs to get up)
  - Loss of appetite and (consequent) loss of weight
  - Anhedonia: loss of pleasure and interest in life
  - Motor changes: agitation or psychomotor retardation (may lead to stupor)
- Presence or absence of thoughts of self-harm: state any plans and degree of intent (record the spectrum from passive death wish, through suicidal ideation and suicidal intent, to suicide plan, and actions (these are frequently concealed—always ask).

Thought content

Morbid preoccupations (i.e. ruminations), obsessions, overvalued ideas, delusions

- Obsessions: repetitive, intrusive, unwanted, stereotyped thoughts or images
- Overvalued ideas: those held with a morbid intensity, but without fulfilling the criteria for a delusion. They are not argued beyond the bounds of reason (e.g. patients with anorexia nervosa are not deluded, but have overvalued ideas about their weight).
- A delusion is a fixed (usually false) belief held without evidence that is out of keeping with an individual's sociocultural background. Delusions may be primary or secondary. Primary (delusional mood, perception and autochthonous delusions) occur out of the blue (i.e. without prior morbid experience). Delusional mood is an unpleasant sense that surrounding events refer to oneself. As the mind abhors a vacuum, delusional mood is usually resolved by the formation of an explanatory sudden delusional idea (an 'autochthonous' delusion): delusional mood is unlikely in a current MSE, but may be recalled retrospectively.

Delusional perception is the sudden attribution of self-referential meaning to a normally perceived object (e.g. 'The position of that cup on the table means I will be famous'). Secondary delusions (usually) evolve from pre-existing morbid psychological processes (altered mood, hallucinations, other delusions). They include delusions of persecution, grandiosity, reference, guilt, poverty, nihilism (i.e. extreme negation of self or world; e.g. believing part of the body has died). Passivity describes the experience that one's mind (thought passivity), emotions, actions, will or body (somatic passivity) is not under one's control. They include thought insertion, withdrawal and thought broadcast (loss of the sense of barrier between one's mind and the external world). Passivity is usually linked with a delusional explanation (e.g. thoughts removed by the government).

Box 8.5 Components of Mental State Examination (MSE)—cont'd

Perception

Sensory distortions, sensory deceptions (illusions, hallucinations)

- Distortions are changes in intensity or quality of real sensory phenomena (e.g. micropsia in a temporal lobe seizure).
- Deceptions are either illusions (i.e. misinterpretations of real stimuli), often in altered mood states or consciousness (e.g. hearing an innocuous noise as a sinister footstep when anxious) or hallucinations, which are internally generated perceptions in the absence of an external stimulus. Auditory hallucinations include noises and voices. Second-person auditory hallucinations talk to the patient, including giving commands. Third-person auditory hallucinations discuss the patient, sometimes in a running commentary on his actions. Thought echo is hearing one's thoughts repeated aloud after one thinks them. Other hallucinations include visual, somatic, olfactory, taste, sexual and touch. 'Formication' describes hallucinations of touch where small animals/insects are felt to be crawling all over the body, classically seen in organic disorders such as cocaine psychosis. Reflex hallucinations are triggered by an external stimulus in another modality (e.g. seeing a bus triggering a somatic hallucination of electric shocks). Functional hallucinations are triggered by an external stimulus and are experienced at the same time as the stimulus (e.g. auditory hallucinations associated with the sound of running water).

Extracampine hallucinations are experienced as outside of the sensory field (e.g. voices heard from another country).

Hypnagogic and hypnopompic hallucinations occur with reduced levels of consciousness when drifting off to sleep and on waking, respectively.

- Pseudohallucinations are experienced as arising from within the patient (e.g. 'voices in my head') rather than the external world, but they are beyond conscious control. In contrast to hallucinations, they are not experienced as having a material reality. They occur in normal grief (seeing or hearing the deceased) as well as a range of disorders, including post-traumatic stress ('flashbacks') and emotionally unstable personality disorder.

Cognition

Global, dominant and non-dominant hemispheres, frontal lobe function

- Global: level of consciousness (if abnormal, use the Glasgow Coma Scale), orientation in time, place and person, attention and concentration (e.g. test naming months of the year backwards), memory: anterograde short-term ('working') memory tested by immediate recall of three given items; long-term tested by their recall 5 minutes later. Retrograde memory includes public (e.g. 'Who is the prime minister?') and personal ('Where were you born?') information, semantic (e.g. 'How to use a fork?') and episodic memory (e.g. 'What happened yesterday?'). Global cognition includes IQ (usually estimated rather than formally tested; e.g. 'high', 'low normal').
- Dominant hemisphere tests: language (naming of objects, repetition of a phrase, comprehension of commands, reading and writing), calculation and praxis (limb apraxia, e.g. 'Show how you wave goodbye'; finger agnosia, e.g. Put pen in patient's hand with eyes closed—'What's this?'; conceptual apraxia, e.g. show toothbrush—'What's this used for?') and awareness of details.

Draw a clock at 3.45 (see text)

- Non-dominant hemisphere tests: neglect (hemispatial rather than sensory), construction and visuospatial ability
- Frontal lobes tests: verbal fluency (e.g. 'Name as many animals as you can in a minute': tests fluency plus strategy, e.g. listing farm animals first), similarities and proverb interpretation (i.e. conceptual thinking, e.g. 'What do a table and chair have in common?'; 'What is the difference between a mistake and a lie?'), estimates ('How fast can a leopard run?': frontal lobe lesions typically grossly overestimate) and alternating sequences (copying of alternating hand sequence, which tests sequential motor activity dependent on dorsolateral prefrontal cortex function)

Insight

Understanding of illness and its treatment

- Do they think there is anything wrong with them?
- If there is something wrong, do they think it is a physical or psychological problem, or both?
- How do they describe the problem and what caused it?
- Do they think they need treatment, if so what?
- What do they think of treatment offered?

Extend these questions to ask about motivation (to quit) in dependent and harmful use patients: see text for motivational interview stages under referral to psychotherapy.

One efficient way of asking for the high level of detail of Box 8.1 is to see this as a journey in time from mother's pregnancy and the patient's birth to now: How did your parents meet? (what sort of people are they?) → where do you come in your family? what age were they when you were conceived? → how was the pregnancy for your mother? → any difficulties (that you were told about) with your birth? → early milestones/development → who raised you? (one/two parents, grandparents, others) → primary school experiences → early experience of medical problems? Were other family members ill? → moving to 'big school': friends, learning, bullying → the bullying question is a useful entry to more difficult questions about abuse/neglect of any kind (see Box 8.3) → (in women) menarche → (in boys and girls) missing school, truancy, early trouble with the law → experiences of friendships then intimate relationships → (difficult questions must be asked) any abuse, threats or violence within those relationships → questions about sexuality or gender dysphoria → use of alcohol and substances? (At what

| Box 8.6 | Anxiety patterns and discrete anxiety syndromes |

Psychological anxiety symptoms

Subjective feeling of worry, sometimes specific concerns (e.g. health), often nonspecific anxieties—worrying about worrying or that something bad (unspecified) will happen; psychological restlessness; hypervigilant with exaggerated startle response (e.g. to noise); poor concentration; insomnia, especially initial insomnia—getting to sleep; depersonalization (feelings that he is not the same person) and derealization (feeling that the world around him is not real).

Try to get subjective measures of stress levels: if 0/10 is no anxiety and 10/10 is the highest possible level, how do you rate your anxiety level now? During your panics? Worst ever?

Somatic anxiety features (these are adrenalin-based, part of fight or flight)

GI	Dry mouth, lump in throat, swallowing sensations, nausea, vomiting, abdominal discomfort (especially in children as 'hurty tummies'), diarrhoea
CNS	Headaches, feeling light-headed or faints, perioral numbness, sweating, tremor, muscle pains (with hypocapnia), tetany of hands
Respiratory	Fast shallow breathing, subjective breathlessness, chest tightness
Cardiac	Chest discomfort or catch, palpitations, tachycardia
Genitourinary	Urinary frequency (nocturia unusual), failure of erection, premature ejaculation, amenorrhoea

Circumstances of anxiety (see Table 8.2).

age? With whom? Triggers to excessive use, etc: see Box 8.4) → transitions to work or further education → educational achievements and vocational history → current status: living circumstances, employment, income, etc. These final areas will guide you into the nature of this person's home life, financial status (income, ask about debts), social supports and key confidante(s) and what he likes about his life, right now. These are essential structures upon which your formulation and treatment plans will be built. In our experience, patients enjoy telling a version of their 'Life Story' as long as they feel respected and listened to. You will learn much from your patient with empathetic listening and eye contact: this is one more reason not to tap away on a keyboard during face-to-face interviews.

Two areas, sometimes related, may manifest at this point: past traumatic experiences and/or addiction. Adverse childhood experiences (ACEs) were originally described by paediatricians as a method to identify risk factors for later obesity. It is now becoming apparent that they have a high predictive value across a range of psychiatric and medical conditions, misuse of substances, accidents and even future criminal victimhood or criminal activity. The common ACEs are physical, emotional and sexual abuse by another, usually a family member. Childhood neglect is also a key ACE and reminds us to ask in general terms about the patient's parents, whether they perpetrated or knew of the abusive act(s) and what they did about it. Trauma can also occur in older children and adults. A useful understanding is that trauma is Event(s) → Experienced as physically/emotionally threatening/harmful → Effects subsequently that are physical, emotional, social and more. Box 8.3 sets out the principles of trauma-informed care. Sensitivity and a 'caring awareness' are key to all interactions with people who are living with past trauma. As part of your general approach here (Box 8.3), you might make clear that this section of the interview will be available to a few key people (on a 'need to know' basis), and would not be printed in a hospital report or letter for general practitioner (that is copied by default to a patient's home). Knowing about trauma early in the interview changes how we ask about historical details and the emphases within MSE: mood and anxiety levels, dissociation (see later), and belief systems (lower self-esteem, loss of trust of others).

Asking about alcohol use can be difficult in some people. In most countries, alcohol is legal, inexpensive and available in multiple outlets. Its excess consumption above recommended levels for health of 14 units weekly is encouraged by poorly regulated advertising, and a societal dialogue that normalizes heavy drinking to celebrate, commiserate and much else. Just as you list current medication doses and allergies, recording accurate alcohol consumed weekly is an essential part of your assessment. Practice your form of words: '*I need to ask you some questions about alcohol*' and then '*What types of alcohol do you usually drink?*' Sometimes a screening question helps to start the alcohol history, for example the CAGE:

Have you ever
felt you needed to **C**ut down your drinking?
felt **A**nnoyed by others criticizing your drinking?
felt **G**uilty about your drinking? and/or
needed an **E**ye-opener in the morning to steady your nerves?

Two or more 'Yes' answers suggest a significant problem, and merit full enquiry. Try to get an indication of habits (e.g. Friday night binges, drinking subcultures after work [hospitality industry, health care, students and many sports]), drinking at home, whether the person thinks it is acceptable to drink alone. Record the age of first alcohol (young age is a good predictor of future misuse), and whether he drank differently to, or more than, his peers. Most clinicians record both the units consumed in the past week, and what the patient describes as average weekly consumption (see Box 8.4). There are no safe alcohol levels, and health (physical and psychological) is impaired when people consume more than 14 units weekly. The essential task in heavy drinkers is to rule out alcohol dependence, as defined by five core features (Box 8.4), and hinted at in the fourth CAGE question. As with selective disclosure of suicidality (to some but not others), when a patient identifies physical dependence, you must share and act; for example, discuss the need for benzodiazepine detoxification in an alcohol-dependent person being admitted to any hospital, where withdrawals are likely. Previous withdrawals (delirium tremens, see Box 8.4) predict more severe symptoms (seizures, for example) provoked by the next planned or unplanned cessation of alcohol. Some vulnerable patients who withdraw are not eating, have poor nutrition, or vomiting; even without cognitive changes (signs of Wernicke's encephalopathy come too late to reverse them), they also will need intravenous B vitamin prescription.

If alcohol use is an extension of asking to list current medications, consider asking about *any* substance use as an extension of the mandatory cigarette smoking question. Cannabis misuse is usually coincident with tobacco smoking; a minority of people who vape (electronic cigarettes) also inhale cannabis oils and other substances. The key questions are which substances, an idea of quantity (usually the weekly spend), age at first use (young age, meaning ≤14 years, of cannabis use predicts subsequent psychosis) and any features of dependency. These are exactly the same five features listed in Box 8.4. Relief of physiological withdrawals is achieved by taking the substance itself or similar drugs (nicotine replacement for tobacco, methadone for heroin use, sedatives for stimulant drugs, etc). The best way to achieve a full drug history is direct questioning: *'Have you bought any legal or illegal compounds over the counter, online, on the street... or got these from others?'* Even specialists in addictions cannot keep pace with new 'designer' drugs, and a host of street names for substances. It is not unusual for drug suppliers to add other substances to popular compounds to achieve greater addiction (and higher sales). You can integrate answers into an immediate plan (e.g. will this patient need to receive a prescribed detoxification programme?) and a record of possible health sequelae of inhaled or injected substances. As with alcohol misuse, detail the social consequences (Box 8.4) of substance misuse, as well as any criminal convictions.

The later portions of history (see Box 8.1) cover the medical and psychiatric treatments to date (essential for your patient's safety and to achieve the best future treatment for him), forensic history and a preliminary assessment of his personality. Practice how you introduce neutral questions about forensic history: *'You told me about your teenage years living in _____ near a group of friends who _____. I wonder if you ever deliberately missed school. Did you ever get into trouble, or get warnings, from school or the police?'* As

with substances, you are asking if these things EVER happened—as reliable predictors of future risk. By necessity, these are closed questions. Patients will not easily forget a court conviction or prison sentence: if they deny these but other informants or documents contradict this account, this is an important finding. As described above and in Boxes 8.1 and 8.2, key questions are about violence to others. Protecting yourself, other health care staff, others living with the patient (children, elders, pets) and beyond, starts with these important enquiries.

As you gain more experience, you will know which aspects of personality might be different or exaggerated in the person you are interviewing. You have already asked a range of (often very personal) questions and gathered much information. An important rule applies here: one may highlight personality difficulties, but a personality disorder is not diagnosed at first interview. You are seeing someone at his low point if not actually in crisis, and this 'brings out the worst' in most of us. This section tries to answer the questions *'What is this person like? What are his prominent character traits?'* In practice, combine what you hear (history) and how you interact (MSE findings) with a reliable collaborative (parent or partner) to establish personality difficulties and their severity (see later and Box 8.10). In this, you might usefully identify the patient as someone who tends to worry excessively (trait anxiety), perhaps is overly perfectionistic (anakastic) by nature or has difficulty starting and maintaining friendships (interpersonal problems). Many sudden step changes in the life history suggest a character trait of impulsivity: multiple changes in jobs/residences/relationships, and if comorbid mood changes are present, there may be impulsive self-harm acts or overdoses. Some personality components are more common in women and men, respectively, overdependence on others being on a spectrum with 'loner' personalities, who are low on trust of others.

Mental state examination

Box 8.5 lists the seven essential components of MSE. General appearance and behaviour set down a description of what you observe over the course of your assessment. Speech records the content of what is said, and its highlights (quote your patient's speech segments directly at times for positive findings) may indicate underlying psychological processes. Mood comprises the subjective (score out of 10, as above), and your objective assessment; note any of five biological symptoms of depression (Box 8.5) and **always record suicidal thoughts** (on a spectrum), **an essential component of every MSE;** *thought content* will have positive findings in patients with psychosis, but so too in people with anxiety disorders such as OCD, obsessions or somatoform disorders (overvalued ideas); abnormalities in *perception* are characteristic of psychoses, but positive findings are common in acute confusional states (typically *visual* hallucinations) and some personality disorders too; *cognition* is impaired in confused patients; for example, delirium always shows abnormalities in concentration and memory, even in patients apparently orientated by day, month and year; lastly you need to record *insight*, which this gives an indication of how the patient understands his difficulties and symptoms.

At the beginning and end of the MSE, record mostly factual information: in general appearance and behaviour, '*She was brightly dressed, sitting comfortably and gave details in a relaxed manner*'. Into insight comes a clinician's perspective in evaluating answers to yes/no questions (Box 8.5): '*While she agreed that her insomnia, loss of pleasure, anxious thoughts and low mood could be explained by clinical depression, she did not see any link between low mood/increased anxiety and her recurrent abdominal pain*'. Insight is not merely a measure of agreement with the attending psychiatrist; large gaps between what doctors decide are 'best for someone' and what they seek will be problematic. In people with cognitive impairment, we prioritize facts (he knew the day, month but not the year) over interpretations. Where there are clear cognitive deficits, this section of MSE is paired later to a mental capacity assessment: see detailed cognitive assessment. Linked to insight in addicts, we record an assessment of their motivation to quit (Box 8.5 and referral for therapy below).

There are several challenges in examining other aspects of MSE. Comorbidity, which is common, may be one of many episodes of poor mental health and there are interactions between individual components of MSE. Mood exerts a strong influence over how we think, and thereby a person's speech—how that person's thoughts are expressed. Similarly, very high levels of anxiety change speech (too loud, too fast… or hesitations) via underlying thought processes. Worry can overwhelm; patients return to the same source of worry ('*It's my tummy pains doctor*'), or are anxious to the point of distraction (they cannot focus on answers). Anxiety–depression is the most common comorbidity in psychiatry, but try to separate these out during MSE. In general, anxiety is about fear of the future: patients with long '*I have to…*' lists of activities; depression is (literally or metaphorically) about past losses, and we put pressure on ourselves with '*should and should have*' statements. By this stage, you have set out the symptoms severity and subtype of anxiety (Box 8.6). When you observe low mood, try to place these symptoms in the context of past episodes: Box 8.7 shows different patterns of low mood on a spectrum. In describing mood, comparison with previous episodes is the best approach. Dysthymia is low mood that does not meet the criteria for a depressive episode; typically, this low mood lasts

2 years or more. Discrete episodes of depression (by definition, they must last 2 weeks or more) can occur during dysthymia—so called 'double depression'. Cyclothymia is a pattern of bouts of depression, sometimes seasonal, alternating with elevated mood that does not meet criteria for hypomania. Hypomania describes 'high' mood episodes without psychotic features. The presence of any psychotic features (delusions or hallucinations) achieves a mania diagnosis. Classic mania (type 1 bipolar) frequently has a family history; these patients achieve best outcomes from mood stabilizers such as lithium. Type 2 bipolar is a less severe variant in which, for example, mood becomes high in the context of antidepressant medication (that is then discontinued).

Psychiatry enhances each clinical interview with its focus on content (what was said) and form (how the belief or experience is constructed). In studying form, we take the same phenomenological approach as Karl Jaspers in his seminal psychopathology work (1913) and many who followed him. To diagnose psychosis we must examine form and content. *A man believes his thoughts and bodily functions are being controlled from outer space.* The 'contents' here are beliefs in extra-terrestrial life, that aliens have taken an interest in him, and that they are actively harming him. A scientist might rebut these beliefs in the absence of proof for any of the three, although clinicians might point to the third belief as subjectively self-evident; he believes this and has demonstrable symptoms. The 'form' however is composed of a false, fixed belief, based on illogical information ('*The idea of alien control of my body first came to me when I was playing cards*'), and it is argued beyond the bounds of reason (put simply, he cannot show or provide any reasoned evidence for this). For his bodily control, the form is a delusion of somatic passivity. When the aliens force their thoughts inside his head, this is a delusion of thought interference, namely thought insertion. The manifest content is paranoid: '*They are doing these things to ME… when I tell doctors or the police, no one believes me because they (aliens) have got to them too*'; this is secondary elaboration of his primary delusion. Delusions can have many themes, such as reference (random events even news items refer back to the patient), persecution, surveillance, control (as with aliens above), grandeur (special powers, special mission), guilt (common in severe depression), infestation (Ekbom's syndrome), love (erotomania), jealousy or catastrophe even nihilism, at its most extreme, that he is a person who is already dead and rotting from the inside (Cotard delusion). We have heard it said '*If you have seen one schizophrenic* (note the stigmatizing choice of language) *you've seen them all*'. Nothing could be further from the truth.

Disorders of perception also require exploration of form and content. An illusion is a precept that arises from a normal stimulus, such as hearing a crying

Box 8.7	Diagnostic criteria for depression (ICD10) and mood patterns

In typical depressive episodes of all three varieties described below (mild (F32.0), moderate (F32.1), and severe (F32.2 and F32.3)), the individual usually suffers from depressed mood, loss of interest and enjoyment, and reduced energy leading to increased fatiguability and diminished activity. Marked tiredness after only slight effort is common.

Other common symptoms are:
(a) Reduced concentration and attention
(b) Reduced self-esteem and self-confidence
(c) Ideas of guilt and unworthiness (even in a mild type of episode)
(d) Bleak and pessimistic views of the future
(e) **Ideas or acts of self-harm or suicide**
(f) Disturbed sleep
(g) Diminished appetite

Mild depressive episode (F32.0)

Depressed mood, loss of interest and enjoyment, and increased fatiguability are usually regarded as the most typical symptoms of depression. At least two of these, **plus at least two of the other symptoms** (a to g), usually should be present for a definite diagnosis. None of the symptoms should be present to an intense degree. Minimum duration of the whole episode is about 2 weeks.

Moderate depressive episode (F32.1)

At least two of the three most typical symptoms noted for mild depressive episode (F32.0) should be present, **plus at least three (and preferably four) of the other symptoms**. Several symptoms are likely to be present to a marked degree, but this is not essential if a particularly wide variety of symptoms is present overall. Minimum duration of the whole episode is about 2 weeks.

Severe depressive episode without psychotic symptoms (F32.2)

In a severe depressive episode, the sufferer usually shows considerable distress or agitation, unless retardation is a marked feature. Loss of self-esteem or feelings of uselessness or guilt are likely to be prominent, and suicide is a distinct danger in particularly severe cases.

Severe depressive episode with psychotic symptoms (F32.3)

A severe depressive episode that meets the criteria given for F32.2 above and in which delusions, hallucinations or depressive stupor are present. The delusions usually involve ideas of sin, poverty or imminent disasters, responsibility for which may be assumed by the patient. Auditory or olfactory hallucinations are usually of defamatory or accusatory voices or of rotting filth or decomposing flesh. Severe psychomotor retardation may progress to stupor.

The affective spectrum*

Dysthymia

Single episode of depression

Chronic episode of depression

Atypical depression

Psychotic depression

Recurrent depressive disorder

Cyclothymia

Hypomania + depression
(bipolar II disorder in DSM-IV)

Mania + depression
(bipolar I disorder in DMS-IV)

(*Source: Smith, Daniel and Blackwood, Douglas. (2004). Depression in young adults. Advances in Psychiatric Treatment. 10. 4–12. 10.1192/apt.10.1.4.)

voice as we listen to a kettle boiling. Hallucinations are precepts without a stimulus. A simple visual hallucination might be a flash of light; complex hallucinations usually involve objects or living things. Seeing things in a confused, fearful patient is invariably related to alcohol or other withdrawals. Some hallucinations, for example hypnoPompic (waking uP) and hypnoGogic (Going to sleep), in any modality (we *see* or *hear* things that are not real) are part of normal experience. Common in emotional turmoil are pseudohallucinations; patients hear or see something that is not there and perceive this as arising from their mind (inner space) not from the world (outside space). True auditory hallucinations have no external stimulus, do not come from that inner space (the mind) and are perceived as 'real' by the person. In active psychosis, these are voices, usually in the mother tongue, composed of men or women speaking. Content (what the voices say) is less important than form. Both content and form support a diagnosis of psychosis. In abnormal perceptions (Box 8.5), descriptive psychopathology describes content ('*I can hear two men talking about what I am doing 24/7—even when I am on my own*') and form (third-person auditory hallucination, running commentary). Variations in psychotic phenomena are probably the hardest concepts to master in psychiatry; try to learn them 'from' patients you encounter and think through the array of findings (see Box 8.7). Second-person auditory hallucinations (voices speaking to the person) are common in depression and tend to be derogatory, even abusive. A subset of these, command hallucinations, where patients are instructed to act ('*Stand up now and leave the room*') are well described in schizophrenia and it is important to assess any insight so as to evaluate whether there is a risk the person will obey these commands. None of these experiences are pleasant and patients usually will share descriptions of delusions and hallucinations, even ones that happened years ago. Additionally, and more in observation than communication, describe how he interacted with you as his affect (inappropriate, flat, depressed, etc.) and think too about other negative symptoms of schizophrenia (Box 8.8) when completing your MSE.

For completeness, dissociation experience is another symptom type not included in the common seven presenting complaint headings. It is a normal experience to 'switch off' at periods in the day and become 'lost in thought', unaware of our surroundings, for example during a familiar commute. Afterwards, we do not recall specific components of the journey as our mind activated autopilot settings. During this 'off period', we cycled or drove safely and did not forget how to operate these machines or obey the rules of the road. When pathological, dissociation can be anxiety-provoking but is not an anxiety symptom, nor is it a mood variant. Dissociation is a partial or complete loss of the normal integration between past memories, identity and immediate awareness—usually accompanied by bodily sensations. In emotionally unstable personality disorder, most usually during a crisis, people may experience unreality and features that are perceived as 'mental breakdown', for example hearing voices as pseudohallucinations. In what Freud called hysteria, a patient (who has no obvious personality difficulties) dissociates to a severe degree and a bodily function is suddenly lost (e.g. paralysis of a limb, loss of voice (or weakened voice)), an apparent stroke, seizure (nonepileptic attack), amnesia and more. These dramatic presentations have exercised physicians for centuries because the symptom bearer has (crudely) broken connections with identify-experience and current situation; his affect may seem inappropriate. This is the so-called *belle indifference* in which a patient seems unperturbed that he can no longer walk or speak or has lost a bodily function. Some have had a history of trauma (see Box 8.3) although may have 'sealed over' the distress generated. In some, there are current 'unfixable' personal dilemmas in their lives, usually relationships, and it is conjectured that these stresses have caused an unconscious switch into what the patient thinks of as physical or psychiatric disorders. Perhaps this reminds us that 'flight or flight' (see Box 8.6) is not the binary choice when we face threat; some vulnerable people respond as 'freeze or dissociate'. For example, we see dissociative freezing in a fugue state, with parallels to psychogenic amnesia. Extreme fatigue and withdrawal, neurasthenia, is currently considered unhelpfully alongside the dissociation spectrum; many would diagnose this as chronic fatigue syndrome, but current International Statistical Classification of Diseases and Related Health Problems-10 (ICD10) criteria require the exclusion of 'post viral fatigue' to diagnose neurasthenia. For one final dissociation variant, the iatrogenic and highly suggestible multiple personality disorder, current classifications (ICD10 and Diagnostic and Statistical Manual of Mental Disorders-5 (DSM5)) are wholly inadequate.

By the time you have moved from history to MSE, you should have a clearer indication of where this patient's difficulties lie. You have allowed the patient to talk, using open questions, and MSE is the opportunity to list the supporting evidence for your differential diagnosis. Drawing on the seven diagnostic headings of page 7, you will highlight *cognition* findings for confused patients, *mood* for depressed patients, *perception* and *thoughts* for psychosis, etc. When you present your MSE findings to others, some areas are less important; 'Cognition was intact in this adult patient', or '*There were no perception abnormalities in this depressed/anxious patient*'. That said, *appearance*, *mood* and *insight* are important in every psychiatric disorder. Insight will predict engagement with treatment; for addicts, it is necessary to define their motivation to quit right now (see Box 8.5, and referral for psychotherapy). Do not see the closed questions of MSE as a checklist, but as a structured series of exchanges on which you build

| Box 8.8 | Making the diagnosis of schizophrenia with ICD10 criteria |

Diagnosis of schizophrenia (ICD10)

At least one clear symptom, or two or more 'less clear' positive symptoms, or two or more negative symptoms must be present for at least 2 months.

Positive psychotic symptoms

'Clear' symptoms

- *Delusions* that are culturally inappropriate and completely impossible (e.g. being able to control the weather)
- *Hallucinatory voices* giving a running commentary on the patient's actions or discussing the patient amongst themselves, or voices coming from another part of the body
- *Delusions of reference:* beliefs that random external events in his/her life or wider society (details from a news item, song or television programme) relate in a special way to him/her
- *Delusions of thought interference:* others can hear, read, insert or steal their thoughts
- *Passivity phenomena:* beliefs and/or perceptions that others are able to control his/her will, limb movements, bodily functions or feelings
- *Thought echo:* hearing one's own thoughts spoken aloud
- *Hallucinations* other than the above, when accompanied by delusions or persistent overvalued ideas. In the paranoid subtype of schizophrenia these are the prominent symptoms
- *Thought disorder:* breaks in the train of thought (thought block), over indecisive and concrete thinking, neologisms
- *Catatonic behaviour* (p. 5)

Negative psychotic symptoms (by definition, these are 'less clear' symptoms)

- *Apathy:* (disinterest) manifest as blunted affect
- *Flat affect:* emotional withdrawal
- *Odd or incongruous affect* (e.g. smiles when recounting sad events, and vice versa)
- *Lack of attention* to appearance or personal hygiene
- *Poor rapport:* reduced verbal and non-verbal communication (e.g. eye contact)
- *Lack of spontaneity* and flow of conversation
- Difficulties in *abstract thinking* (e.g. explaining proverbs or common sayings)

(Source: The current diagnostic criteria for schizophrenia. https://www.who.int/classifications/icd/en/GRNBOOK.pdf)

your hypotheses. Some negative findings are just as important to record as physical observations: normal findings for mood/psychotic features, such as blood pressure, will be important in future assessments. Get into the habit of good MSE documentation; a failure to record your finding that '*He had no suicidal ideation or intent*' might have consequences later on, for both you and the patient.

Physical examination and investigations

Do not let the jargon 'routine physical' of psychiatric inpatient admission allow you to switch off your brain. This is about admitting someone to hospital and making sure he is medically safe to stay on a psychiatric inpatient ward, where nurses may not have trained in physical care nursing, and psychiatry trainees and consultants have 'forgotten their medicine'. In broad terms, you are also looking for physical illnesses that may have caused or are contributing to this presentation, and to multi-morbidity, including currently known, new or neglected disease manifestations. Be guided by what you have learned so far and direct your physical examination accordingly. Here are some key components of physical examination:

- Five 'routine' observations; make these or find where they have been documented. (1) High blood pressure needs observation, sometimes treatment, but low blood pressure alerts to overmedication, blood loss or sepsis. (2) Tachycardia might indicate pain, the anticholinergic effects of medication, anaemia, shock or other physical abnormalities; it could be withdrawals, mania or 'just anxiety' so follow this up to make sure pulse restores to normal. (3) Fever may indicate infection or a rare (potentially fatal) reaction to antipsychotic medications called neuroleptic malignant syndrome, NMS. (4) Tachypnoea may indicate chest or cardiac disease, anaemia or rarely (in the absence of other features) active anxiety variants (see Box 8.6). (5) Weight is the single most omitted physical examination finding. Is this patient's weight low? Adults' height is measured once, and this allows calculation of body mass index (BMI), as weight (kg) divided by height (metres) squared. The healthy range is 18.5–25, but values below this should raise the possibility of an eating disorder, even in 'athletic' types. For low weight, look for signs of weight loss and malnutrition, and document the skin changes of acute weight loss, noting hand signs of bulimia (Russel's sign of tooth marks on knuckles). Lanugo (excess fine bodily hair) is a very late sign in anorexia nervosa. In Western society, two of three people are overweight; this may

Box 8.9	Eating disorders and disordered eating

Diagnostic criteria for bulimia nervosa (1–3 all required). From ICD10

Domain	Mental state examination	Behaviour
1 Food	Preoccupation with eating Craving for food, typically carbohydrates	Episodes (binges) where large amounts of food are consumed in short periods of time
2 Solution	Overvalued ideas/concerns that food consumed is 'fattening' and needs to be removed from their body	Action to reduce food effects: self-induced vomiting; periods of restriction of food; abuse of purgatives/appetite suppressants/diuretics/thyroxine, etc.
3 Belief	Morbid fear of fatness: a belief, held to the intensity of an overvalued idea, but not delusional, that they will become fat with regular eating	Sets a carefully defined weight as target: this is usually below healthy BMI (18.5–25). There may have been a short history of anorexia nervosa and/or transient amenorrhoea
Atypical bulimia nervosa Food solution belief	Lack one or more MSE findings	Patient is overweight (BMI 25–30) or obese (BMI above 30)

BMI, body mass index; MSE, mental state examination.
(Source: https://www.who.int/classifications/icd/en/GRNBOOK.pdf)

Diagnostic criteria for anorexia nervosa (1–4 all required). From ICD10

Core symptoms and signs	Criteria	Unusual patient groups
1 Actual weight	BMI of 17.5 or less Weight at least 15% below expected weight	Children fail to achieve expected weight on centile charts
2 Self-induced weight loss	Food restriction and one of: excessive exercise; self-induced vomiting; purging (laxative use); appetite suppressants/diuretics	Diabetic patients may use insulin to excess in an effort to reduce body weight
3 Disorders of thinking (overvalued ideas)	Body image distortion (perceives self as heavier than objective evidence shows) Morbid fear of fatness	
4 Endocrine disorder	Amenorrhoea; in prepubertal patients, puberty is delayed or arrested	In men, loss of sexual interest and potency
	Laboratory findings: low levels of gonadal hormones; elevated levels of growth, cortisol, and thyroid hormones	
Atypical anorexia nervosa	Lacks one or more of 1–4 criteria	

(Source: https://www.who.int/classifications/icd/en/GRNBOOK.pdf)

ARFID (avoidant or restrictive food intake disorder)*

'These include having little interest in eating and/or avoidance of multiple types of food. The avoidance of specific types of food may be based on specific sensory properties (e.g. colour, appearance, texture, taste, temperature or smell) or on perceived adverse consequences of eating such food (to include, e.g. feared health problems, vomiting or choking). Avoidances of this nature typically result in acceptance of a diet that is not sufficient to provide the energy and nutrients for healthy development and functioning.' But without core symptoms numbers 2 and 3 from ICD-10 anorexia nervosa diagnostic criteria, as listed above.

*Al-Adawi S, Bax B, Bryant-Waugh R et al. Advances in Eating Disorders: Theory, Research and Practice, 2013: Vol. 1, 10–20.

have psychological sequelae (low self-esteem) but look also for signs of locomotor disease and diabetes.

- For cognitive impairment, depression and anxiety look for physical disorders as antecedents: gait/balance problems, focal neurology, liver/renal disease, signs of low or high thyroid, effects of poorly controlled diabetes or immunological disorders (rheumatoid arthritis, systemic lupus).
- Patients with psychosis (schizophrenia and bipolar) lose on average 17 years of their life expectancy, and those final years are spent in very poor physical health. Premature mortality is even worse for

people with intellectual disability, addictions and personality disorders. Regardless of their current age or duration of mental disorder, examine the patient for the effects of smoking, obesity-diabetes, alcohol and substance misuse, polypharmacy including prescribed opioid medication and some infectious diseases (hepatitis and HIV, both treatable). Physical examination at these opportunities is an ideal time to document disease progression or useful baseline measures, such as weight and blood pressure.

- Examination for the effects of alcohol and substance misuse essentially focuses on signs of possible liver disease, but consider how substances are taken (intravenous, nasal ingestion, inhalation) too. Palpate for liver tenderness or enlargement in alcohol excess; there may be epigastric tenderness of pancreatitis. Advanced alcoholic liver disease may lead to ascites, bruises (low platelets and prolonged clotting time), engorged superficial veins (plethoric facies, spider naevi) and epigastric veins at the umbilicus: caput medusae. For people who misuse substances, skin examination might reveal plethoric facies, excoriation around the nose (typically cocaine), arm/leg track marks or even skin abscesses from intravenous drugs. Novel psychoactive substances cause bodily damage too long to list here, for example the unstable, neuropathic bladder of ketamine misuse.

- In patients with impulsive personality difficulties or borderline traits (see Box 8.10), there may be old scars of self-harm (arms, thighs, abdomen, neck) that need to be documented in case new circumstances lead to a return of harmful behaviours. Tattoos are now common and, as with body piercings, record anything out of the ordinary.
- Patients rarely require a full neurological examination. Can he stand and walk? If he is having difficulties, observe for facies of Parkinsonism and test for cerebellar ataxia, suggesting demyelination but common in severe alcohol misuse. Speech has already been covered in MSE; you might ask patients to smile broadly to show teeth (a test for facial asymmetry) and to mime playing the piano with both hands outstretched as a very broad screen for major neurological deficit. Tremor should be noted; then test for increased tone of Parkinson's disease or antipsychotic medication excess (both cause cog wheel rigidity). Finally, and this is worth noting as an early *reversible* sign of alcohol excess, record signs of peripheral neuropathy of arms or legs, to motivate your patient to quit.

Box 8.10	ICD11 reconceptualization of personality

Trait domain qualifiers that contribute to the expression of personality dysfunction

Trait domain	Core definition	Specific features
Negative affectivity	A tendency to experience a broad range of negative emotions with a frequency and intensity out of proportion to the situation	Anxiety, anger, worry, fear, vulnerability, hostility, shame, depression, pessimism guilt, low self-esteem and mistrustfulness. For example, once upset, such individuals have difficulty regaining their composure and must rely on others or on leaving the situation to calm down.
Detachment	A tendency to maintain interpersonal distance (social detachment) and emotional distance (emotional detachment)	*Social detachment*, inducing avoidance of social interactions, lack of friendships and avoidance of intimacy. *Emotional detachment*: inducing being reserved, aloofness and limited emotional expression and experience. For example, such individuals seek out employment that does not involve interactions with others.
Dissociality	Disregard for the rights and feelings of others, encompassing both self-centredness and lack of empathy	*Self-centredness*: inducing entitlement, grandiosity, expectation of others' admiration and attention-seeking. *Lack of empathy*: inducing being deceptive, manipulative exploiting, ruthless, mean, callous and physically aggressive while sometimes taking pleasure in others' suffering. For example, such individuals respond with anger or denigration of others when they are not granted admiration.
Disinhibition	A tendency to act rashly based on immediate external or internal stimuli (i.e. sensations, emotions, thoughts), without consideration of potential negative consequences.	Impulsivity, distractibility, irresponsibility, recklessness and lack of planning. For example, such individuals may be engaged in reckless driving, dangerous sports, substance use, gambling and unplanned sexual activity.
Anankastia	A narrow focus on one's rigid standard of perfection and of right and wrong and on controlling one's own and others' behaviour and controlling situations to ensure conformity to these standards	*Perfectionism*: inducing concern with rules, norms of right and wrong, details, hyper-scheduling, orderliness and nearness. *Emotional and behavioural constraint*: including rigid control over emotional expression, stubbornness, risk-avoidance, perseveration and deliberativeness.
		For example, such individuals may stubbornly redo the work of others because it does not meet their standards.

(Adapted from the ICD11 Clinical Descriptions and Diagnostic Guidelines for Personality Disorder, which include a more detailed description of the trait domain qualifiers.)

Box 8.10	ICD11 reconceptualization of personality—cont'd

Borderline pattern qualifier

The borderline pattern qualifier may be applied to individuals whose pattern of personality disturbance is characterized by a pervasive pattern of instability of interpersonal relationships, self-image and affects, and marked impulsivity, as indicated by five (or more) of the following:

- Frantic efforts to avoid real or imagined abandonment
- A pattern of unstable and intense interpersonal relationships, typically characterized by alternating between extremes of idealization and devaluation
- Identity disturbance, manifested in markedly and persistently unstable self-image or sense of self
- Impulsivity manifested in potentially self-damaging behaviours (e.g. risky sexual behaviour, reckless driving, excessive alcohol or substance use, binge eating)
- Recurrent episodes of self-harm (e.g. suicide attempts or gestures, self-mutilation)
- Emotional instability owing to marked reactivity of mood. Fluctuations of mood may be triggered either internally (e.g. by one's own thoughts) or by external events. As a consequence, the individual experiences intense dysphoric mood states, which typically last for a few hours but may last for up to several days.
- Chronic feelings of emptiness
- Inappropriate intense anger or difficulty controlling anger manifested in frequent displays of temper (e.g. yelling or screaming, throwing or breaking things, getting into physical fights)
- Transient dissociative symptoms or psychotic-like features (e.g. brief hallucinations, paranoia) in situations of high affective arousal.
- Other manifestations of borderline pattern, not all of which may be present in a given individual at a given time, include the following:
  - A view of the self as inadequate, bad, guilty, disgusting and contemptible
  - An experience of the self as profoundly different and isolated from other people; a painful sense of alienation and pervasive loneliness
  - Proneness to rejection hypersensitivity; problems in establishing and maintaining consistent and appropriate levels of trust in interpersonal relationships; frequent misinterpretation of social signals

Adapted from the ICD11 Clinical Descriptions and Diagnostic Guidelines for Personality Disorder.
(Source: Bach, B., First, M.B. Application of the ICD11 classification of personality disorders. *BMC Psychiatry* 2018;**18**:351. https://doi.org/10.1186/s12888-018-1908-3)

Collateral history

Collateral history is all about the opportunities you make (asking a partner to attend, based on their availability; failing this, phone them) and your listening skills. Whether this is a parent or partner, friend or acquaintance, each collateral historian will want you to give details, rather than impart information to you. If there are areas of the history (see Box 8.1) for which there are gaps or inconsistencies, clarify these. Explore your working hypothesis, for example, in an anxious patient, is this *state* (collateral confirms recent stresses, important events) or *trait* (the patient has frequently been outwardly anxious, even in early childhood). Collateral history is often about unusual behaviours; they might be avoiding activities or people they usually enjoy (the core depressive feature of anhedonia), or perhaps avoiding eating or meal times (suggestive of an eating disorder). For psychosis and substance misuse, *'behaving strangely'* covers a multitude; document what people mean by this, as there may be cognitive deficits. If the referral is from a clinician who has barely met this patient, get in touch with the doctor who knows the patient best—usually the family doctor. Think through patients who (understandably) minimize their difficulties:

- Cognitive impairment: a family member will describe a decline in executive function, such as events forgotten, appointments missed or inability to manage shopping.
- Substance misuse without insight: 'I don't have a problem with my drinking but *my wife* has problems with my drinking'. Find out what is happening.
- Many patients hide or 'mask' their depression with a happy face, especially men; look for evidence of (undisclosed) suicidal behaviours, for example completion activities. These can include cancelling future trips, failing to book an annual holiday, paying off debts to friends or making a will.
- Paranoid patients might include hospital staff (you) in their delusional system. Some experience voices instructing them to silence: 'don't tell the doctors'.
- Obsessive compulsive disorder has rituals that the person recognizes as 'silly and unnecessary' and therefore will make efforts to hide them from others. Mostly, cohabitants will describe these OCD behaviours, but a close friend or partner

who does not reside with the patient might have accounts of appointments agreed then missed, or long delays in leaving home owing to rituals.

- Eating disorder presents other challenges, and experienced doctors can be distracted from making this important diagnosis. A parent or current cohabitating informant is essential (Box 8.9) and later.
- Self-harm and crisis; some patients brought to the Emergency Department may have a 'flight into health' and insist everything is somehow better, even though they might still be depressed and/or returning to the same adverse social setting that led to this crisis.
- Personality disorder: although this diagnosis is openly shared with patients, many resent it as a diagnosis of despair. In a recent example from our practice, it was difficult to identify diagnoses in a plausible patient with an acute self-harm presentation until her husband gave the collateral: 'My wife is the life and soul of every party, but when the party is over, it's hard to be around her' (Box 8.10).

Collateral history from the parent(s) or guardian(s) who has raised the patient is invaluable for more challenging diagnoses—right up until working age adults. Re-take parts of the life story progression of Pages 7–8 (Box 8.1 personal history to medical /psychiatric history): where do the two accounts (patient versus mother) diverge? When did things change? Has patient overlooked some protective factors?

- Ask the parent what he thinks is going on. This is just one opinion (about which you remain neutral), but you will feel very silly if he knew the diagnosis, but you struggled to join the dots.
- List the fact of ACEs (what? when? who?) and the family's response to them.
- To differentiate the onset of schizophrenia (as opposed to schizoid personality disorder or autism spectrum), define that normal personality was established by late teens, but then deteriorated in early 20s (or whenever).
- Record any parental concerns with the child's eating habits, use of alcohol and substances, school performance or contact with police in teenage years.
- Character descriptions (Who in the family is he most like? And why?) and life events during life course. Descriptions of important relationships—peers, teachers and intimate partners. Box 8.10 summarizes a rethinking of personality disorder, abandoning decades of pejorative terms. There are five trail domain qualifiers and these align to existing disorders; in addition, we describe severity (mild, moderate or severe), based on their impact on relationships and behaviours. A separate borderline diagnosis is set out.
- Record professional medical contacts throughout the lifespan in persistent physical symptoms; these can have a familial subcultural context and reinforce health anxiety (see later). Take a note of any parental resentment at doctors, and 'missed' or late diagnoses.

Formulation

At this point, resist the temptation to say 'time's up' and retreat to write up the diagnosis. Endings are important; start with two useful habits. First, no matter how long your interview and how experienced you become, have the humility to think you might have missed something; 'I must have asked you hundreds of questions. Have I left out anything (or skipped through something) that *you* think is important?' If the answer is at variance with your interview, record this verbatim. For traumatized patients (see Box 8.3), this is what matters to them, rather than 'what is the matter'. Second, and an excellent way to achieve closure of an interview, test your formulation in broad terms. You would not do this if you were uncertain (and needed to consult) or had an insightless patient with (say) cognitive impairment or psychosis. You are 'road testing' your conclusions, so invite feedback: 'I am not the expert here (remind the patient of your student or junior status) but, from this discussion, I think that this is…' In this, we suggest you give the early portions only of the five-part formulation. Finally, think about how this patient made you feel and specify which exchanges/topics drew out these feelings. Mental disorders are not infectious, but it is normal to feel anxious if we spend an hour in the company of someone who is very anxious, repeatedly seeking our reassurance (to no effect). With schizophrenia, we may feel a mercurial sense of that person—that we could not pin him down or identify much of his personality. Patients who are overfamiliar, perhaps even flirtatious, are pointing to emotionally unstable traits or attachment difficulties; transference describes the feelings patients develop for professionals (at extremes, enmeshed and unhealthy attachments) and countertransference defines our feelings for them. Discuss with seniors if your responses are extreme in either a positive or negative way.

Formulation is the integration of history, direct and collateral, with MSE and interacting biopsychosocial data to determine diagnoses, their antecedents and the best management plan. It has five components:

1. **Narrative summary** is a headlined introduction to assist others with the *what?* and the *why now?* of this presentation: 'Mary is a 28-year-old unemployed divorced woman, living with her older sister, self-presenting to emergency department with 10 days of escalating suicidal thoughts in the context of 2 weeks' heavy drinking that followed her grandfather's funeral earlier this month'.
2. **Aetiology** of single cause (and many) is a challenge in psychiatry, with the exception

Table 8.1 4 × 3 framework

Factors\dimension	Biological	Psychological	Social
Precipitating	Alcohol excess	Losses: g/father; over 2 years, also lost job and home	↓Contacts after funeral; argued with her sister
Predisposing	Family history of alcoholism; female gender doubles rates of depression after menarche	Father drank to excess during her childhood; divorce (no children) owing to husband's drinking	Isolated: lost friends when fired from her job; during same period, her marriage failed
Maintaining	Refused GP prescription of antidepressant	Sense of failure over her job, marriage, drinking	On own by day; lives 30 km from usual supports
Protective	She is not alcohol dependent	Links alcohol misuse to her low mood	Some local links; sister is supportive

of PTSD, although even this diagnosis is constructed on a vulnerable predisposing personality. We might use 4 × 3 framework for 'Mary' as illustrated in Table 8.1. Aetiology is more difficult with disorders that are predominantly psychosocial (e.g. eating disorders and psychoses) and do not have clear biological antecedents. Both, however, have physical sequelae (weight loss and gain, respectively) that can become biologically maintaining factors. Even that most medical (biological) of diagnoses, delirium, has psychosocial maintaining factors and psychosocial treatments.

3. **Differential diagnoses**: by convention, we list the likely diagnosis (diagnoses) first, and give an indication of severity. Then we open a discussion during formulation on a differential. When we find evidence that falls short of establishing an alternative diagnosis, we might say 'I considered X but I out ruled it owing to Y, as she had only two associated factors present'. Thinking about other diagnoses are part of this (Box 8.11). Comorbid conditions are common, and interlinked: formulation seeks to clarify their importance, for example primary depression example above (Mary), made worse by alcohol.

4. **Investigations**: many physical health test results will return the same day to reassure or point to pathology (full blood count, biochemistry of kidney and liver); others (thyroid, cortisol, hepatitis screen, HIV, autoimmune encephalitis screen) can take longer. One test is immediate—a urine test. A urine drugs screen is mandatory in new psychosis presentations, HCG necessary in young women who might be pregnant, and urinalysis rules out urinary tract infection in confused older people. Specific pathology (central nervous system [CNS]) may require brain scans and other testing, such as an electroencephalogram (EEG). We rely too on psychological testing batteries that build on the findings of this interview, which often lead to better psychotherapy choices.

5. **Management plan**: is the whole point of formulation. Interventions are *biological*, such as stopping or starting medications, reducing

Table 8.2 The anxiety and depression detector

Question: 'In the past 3 months…'	Disorder uncovered by question
1. 'Did you ever have a spell or an attack when all of a sudden you felt frightened, anxious or very uneasy?'	Panic disorder
2. 'Would you say that you have been bothered by 'nerves', feeling anxious or on edge?'	Generalized anxiety disorder
3. 'Would you say that being anxious or uncomfortable around other people is a problem for you in your life?'	Social phobia
4. 'Did you have a period of 1 week or more when you lost interest in most things you usually enjoyed?'	Depression
5a. 'Some people have terrible experiences happen to them (give examples of personal trauma, sexual assault or seeing someone badly injured or killed). Has anything like this ever happened to you?' If the answer is yes	Post-traumatic stress disorder
5b. 'Have you had recurrent dreams or nightmares about this experience, or recurrent thoughts or flashbacks?'	

(Source: Means-Christensen, AJ., Sherbourne, CD., Roy-Byrne, PP., et al (2006). Using five questions to screen for five common mental disorders in primary care: diagnostic accuracy of the Anxiety and Depression Detector. *General Hospital Psychiatry, 28*(2), 108–118.)

alcohol, improving sleep, taking regular exercise; *psychological*, such as problem-solving therapy to reduce self-harm recurrence, or more complex psychological therapies (see later); and *social*, such as leaving the house each day, joining a group, (re) connecting with friendship networks. Without the history and MSE, we would not be in any position to make these recommendations. Ideally, the person who shares the plan with the patient is the person who explored these details: this will achieve 'sign up'. If risks have been identified, you need to set out the short-term management of these: actions to protect children at risk; home

Box 8.11	Diagnostic hierarchy in Psychiatry – diagnoses higher up this list take priority over lower ones

Physical illness that manifests as psychiatric symptoms: 'organic psychiatry'

Cognitive deficits: chronic (dementia), acute (delirium), acute on chronic… or congenital as intellectual disability

Alcohol or substances: misuse, intoxication, dependence and withdrawals

Mood disorders   or   Psychosis: e.g. delusional disorder, schizophrenia (see Box 8.8)

(features of both) Schizoaffective disorder

Anxiety disorders: (see Box 8.7 and Table 8.2) plus others, e.g. acute stress reaction, prolonged grief disorder, complex post-traumatic stress disorder (PTSD) and obsessive-compulsive disorder (OCD)

Somatoform disorders (medically unexplained symptoms/functional somatic symptoms; see Boxes 8.15 and 8.16)

Dissociative (conversion) disorders (see MSE) and neurasthenia

Eating disorders (see Box 8.9)   Non-organic sleep disorders

ARFID: see text   Sexual dysfunction, non-organic

Gender identify disorders

Disorders of sexual preference

Psychosexual development disorders

Disorders of adult personality and behaviour: personality disorders

Factitious illness (malingering) is a diagnosis of exclusion.

ARFID, avoidant or restrictive food intake disorder.

treatment team or admission, etc. These plans need contingencies if the patient fails to sustain an improvement, or deteriorates. It is good practice to share widely the drivers of named risks with other professionals to encourage their vigilance for changes, if the plan needs to be escalated in the short or medium term.

Specialist presentations require a thorough history and MSE plus the following.

Detailed cognitive examination (neuropsychiatric assessment)

Cognitive impairment will be flagged in the referral or assessment process. We are accustomed to this approach in people over 65 years of age given their dementia prevalence of 5%, but consider this in some other groups: head injury and loss of consciousness, systemic illnesses with CNS manifestations (HIV, systemic lupus erythematosus [SLE], Covid-19, thyroid, sarcoid, paraneoplastic syndromes) and rare dementias in younger groups. Some impaired patients, especially those with advanced education, can hide their deficits in social exchanges, and (owing to their design) score better than their abilities on formal cognitive testing. Most of your assessment is contained in standard history and MSE, but even on initial assessment, you need to test mental capacity. Here, we evaluate urgent and immediate questions: does this patient understand and retain the (broad) reasons why he is in hospital? Does he understand the treatments on offer and the effects of those treatments? If his capacity is impaired, we then need to comment on and make a recommendation if this patient refused to stay in the current hospital setting. Does he understand the consequences of stopping treatments? Does he also understand the risks of attempting to 'go home' (he may not know where he lives despite his wish to go there), the hazards of travelling there and how others might take advantage of him in that process. The law assumes capacity and our due diligence (communication aids, multiple assessments, sometimes multiple assessors) to establish its absence. It is decision-specific and, for example, a patient could lack capacity for immediate care decisions, but be capacitous to decide longer term choices—last will and testament or power of attorney. Box 8.12 sets out six common instances where patients benefit from detailed neuropsychiatric assessment. This is not a complete list, omitting for example post-stroke depression (incidence approximately 50%), many require specialist teams and some are strong risk factors for completed suicide.

Children and young people

As standard, children have a parent present at interview, and there are several other differences from adult interviews. The doctor must rely on several interdisciplinary assessments, understanding the child's home life as a system (he is a symptom of family-based problems, not the problem child with symptoms), specific developmentally aware psychological testing and collateral history from schools (requires parental permission). A subset of children may have started out in abusive domestic settings, and may have lived in institutional care. The diagnostic categories are also different, with diagnoses of conduct and emotional disorder that are unique to children: 6% and 4% community prevalence, respectively. Some assessments are highly specific to the child's age, such as a mother–infant interaction observed by perinatal teams (whose initial focus is the mother's mental disorder); play therapy/assessment in very young children; educational psychology assessment (measuring intelligence quotient (IQ)) is just one aspect of psychometric testing) that may be linked to evaluation for attention deficit disorder and many others. The last 20 years has seen rising rates of mental disorders and self-harm in children, and

Box 8.12	Neuropsychiatry: six common clinical presentations	
Working clinical diagnosis	**Approach/likely findings**	**Instruments/course**
Dementia	Chronic course of global cognitive impairment	Addenbrooke's Cognitive Examination (ACE) III; full battery of testing from Memory Clinic to time interventions over decline
Age-associated cognitive decline	Age over 50, gradual onset and >6 months; subjective difficulties, but not global cognitive impairment	ACE, MOCA: usually normal in non-memory domains; depression is common and treatable
Traumatic brain injury (TBI)	Initial post-traumatic amnesia, then behavioural changes, low mood comes later; apathy and abnormal premorbid personality indicate poorer prognosis	EEG useful in prolonged confusion to identify limbic or other seizures; scanning may show specific damage associated with (e.g. affective or paranoid psychosis)
Functional cognitive disorders	Common: memory problems in depression Often: memory problems as a functional disorder, or as part of health anxiety Rare: psychogenic amnesia	Subset of depression has cognitive deficits that persist when mood lifts; with functional (as with memory lapses), there are inconsistencies; treat dissociation for amnesia
Epilepsy: Prodrome ± aura Seizure ± loss of consciousness (LOC) Seizure: partial or general. **Nonepileptic attacks** last longer (5–30 min) than seizures, and patient can remember events during apparent LOC.	One-third of epileptic seizures have psychiatric manifestations and comorbidities, higher in temporal lobe epilepsy (TLE); frequency of diagnoses: anxiety, NEAs (up to one-third of seizure presentations); depression, then psychosis	Psychometric tests help identify cognitive deficits; radiology to exclude structural pathology; video EEG to define actual seizure activity; tracing (not visuals) is normal in NEAs. Both epilepsy and NEAs run a chronic course, and often co-occur.
Frontal lobe syndrome/symptoms	Changes to personality, mood, social awareness and behaviours: *new onset* impulsivity/disinhibition; MSE shows attention and memory problems but collateral history key.	Generic psychometric tests often in normal range; show inflexibility within testing— Wisconsin Card Sorting Test; become 'impulsive rule breakers', aggression hard to manage.

EEG, electroencephalogram; MOCA, Montreal cognitive assessment; NEA, non-epileptic attacks.
(Source: Daniel David, Simon Fleming, Michael Kopelman, Simon Lodestone, John Millers. Lishman's Organic Psychiatry: A Textbook of Neuropsychiatry, 4th Edition. Wiley-Blackwell, 2012.)

the figures cited here may be an underestimate. Up to 10% of children have an anxiety disorder, mostly social phobia, specific phobias, panics or general anxiety. A 2% prevalence of hyperkinetic disorders is generally accepted, but United States diagnostic rates are higher than the rest of the world. Around 1% of children have eating disorders, and a smaller proportion have some of the other disorders listed in Box 8.11.

People with intellectual disabilities and/or on the autism spectrum

Collateral history from multiple sources guides the approach here. There may be locations that suit the patient better, perhaps seeing him in his own home, or favourite toys and objects to bring into the interview to improve rapport. In general, shorter, low-intensity multiple interviews work well. Up to 2% of the population have intellectual disability (ID), to varying degrees (Box 8.13), and only some will need psychiatric support. Mental disorders are up to five times more prevalent in people with ID,

and they also have higher alcohol misuse. Depending on diagnostic criteria for autism (Box 8.14), 75% people on the autism spectrum also have ID, and therefore a more thorough cognitive assessment will be required. In some groups, typically Down's syndrome, there may be a loss of social functioning in early adult life indicating Alzheimer's and other dementias.

Autism spectrum disorder (ASD) has a 1% prevalence in the child population, with a male-to-female ration of 3:1. Many good sources previously have cited this ratio as higher, leading to ASD being under diagnosed in females. The history and MSE, together with parents' collateral, will raise the suspicion of adult ASD; school difficulties, especially adjusting to new schools or new teachers, problems making new friends and challenges with independent living. Your enquiries may provoke anxiety in the patient—even for factual answers. Note these and try to formulate other information indicating social and communication difficulties. Back up clinical impressions with intelligence testing and educational assessments. Most

Box 8.13	ICD10 classification of intellectual disability

Clinical features of learning disability

Category	IQ level	Features	'Mental age' (years)
Borderline learning disability	70–84	Live independently as adults, difficulty sustaining employment. More vulnerable to exploitation	11
Mild learning disability	50–69	Superficially normal social and language skills; appear normal (people with lower IQ tend to be dysmorphic) with minimal deficits in motor skills; may require additional social supports during crises	9–10
Moderate learning disability	35–49	Can learn social and communication skills; self-care with supervision; a minority can lead independent lives	6–8
Severe learning disability	20–34	Very poor social and communication skills; require daily supervision and the provision of structure. Associations with genetic conditions—with reduced life expectancy. Frequent central nervous system pathology: cerebral palsy, epilepsy, hydrocephalus and autism	3–5
Profound learning disability	<20	Sometimes no social or language skills; require full-time, often institutional, care	<3

ASD teams use validated assessment interviews to confirm or rule out autism. Once ASD has been agreed as a diagnosis, work to create the best support system for patient and carers (this can be low level, low intensity but with contingencies) and treat mental disorder comorbidity in the usual ways in these contexts.

Patients with eating disorders/disordered eating

Patients with eating disorders/disordered eating are not a different species. However, achieving a diagnosis and thereby the best treatment has become more difficult in the digital age where patients are aware of the criteria used to diagnose eating disorders (see Box 8.9); they engage with others on social media who have made efforts to conceal both symptoms and the effects of their mental disorder. Drivers of concealment are the cognitive distortions of anorexia (low weight of itself makes these overvalued ideas stronger as weight reduces) and the stigma of an eating disorder. Above many other 'unpopular' groups who have mental disorders (including self-harm and addictive behaviours), many health professionals have negative attitudes about eating disorders. The disorders are seen (wrongly) as self-inflicted, a 'lifestyle choice' or rooted in excessive self-absorption. It may not be conscious to either professional or patient, but the patient is also expecting a negative reaction to disclosure of eating problems. Untreated, these disorders have the worst outcomes of any mental disorders, except dementia, through suicide and the physical sequelae of starvation. In acute settings, there are frequent interdisciplinary disputes; the disorder is psychological, but emergency medical treatment (perhaps forced feeding under mental health legislation) is necessary. Positive developments, such as the integration of physical and mental health information records, may help in identifying and supporting these patients earlier. One useful practice is to weigh all patients at medical contacts, and share results with other health professionals. There are emerging screening tools, but again, they depend on self-disclosure. Treatment is complex, but the best outcomes are seen from flexible, outreach eating disorders services over long-term engagement.

Persistent physical symptoms (PPS)/Medically unexplained symptoms (MUS)

Illness gives us biological disadvantages, and doctors find it hard to understand that someone might apparently 'choose' to become or remain ill. People do not usually get ill to benefit from illness (often called secondary gain; primary gain is the direct relief from symptoms). Illness roles might reflect a familial response (although well-intentioned) that maintains some behaviours and symptoms (in that order). In some cases, the symptoms have been encouraged by excessive medical investigations (Box 8.15), and these may have been arranged by doctors for financial gain. The term MUS was coined by, then later abandoned by, psychiatrist David Goldberg as a way of stating that current science cannot find (or explain) objective pathology, but the patient still has 'symptoms' from which he seeks relief. The term incorporates situations in which there is no identified pathological disease process but sometimes exaggerated or abnormal physiology; examples here might be lowered pain threshold, delayed gastric emptying, visceral hypersensitivity, etc. The cycle that begins at the clinic is one of a patient's search for more investigations, disappointment at negative (normal) results, rising physician frustration, further maladaptation (avoidance primarily) and 'doctor shopping' for different opinions to repeat the cycle (see Box 8.15). The interview is a standard psychiatric interview, but with direct conversations with the referring clinician and primary care physician, very

Box 8.14	Garland summary of changes to autism diagnosis

Links between signs and symptoms of autism spectrum disorders and ICD10 diagnostic criteria

Domain	ICD diagnostic criteria	Clues from history/examination
Development: required only for a diagnosis of childhood autism	Abnormal or impaired development before the age of 3 years in at least one of the following: (a) Receptive or expressive language in social communication (b) Development of selective social attachments or reciprocal social interaction (c) Functional or symbolic play	Clear delay in use of speech to communicate. No single words by 2 years of age. No phrase speech by 3 years of age.
Social	Qualitative abnormalities in at least two of the following: (a) Failure to adequately use eye-to-eye gaze, facial expression, body posture and gesture to regulate social interaction (b) Failure to develop peer relationships that involve a mutual sharing of interests, activities and emotions (c) Lack of socioemotionalal reciprocity or lack of modulation of behaviour according to social context or a weak integration of social, emotional and communicative behaviours (d) Lack of spontaneous seeking to share enjoyment, interests or achievements with other people	Lack of direct eye contact and poor modulation of eye contact to regulate social interactions Restricted or inappropriate range of facial expression Lack of emotional expression Absence of dose-sharing friendships or relationships Dislike of physical contact and impaired ability to comfort others Lack of social chit-chat or 'small tat' when in company Abnormal play: dislike of shared play, lack of symbolic use of toys in childhood
Communication	Qualitative abnormalities in at least one of the following: (a) Delay or total lack of spoken language, not accompanied by an attempt to compensate through the use of gesture or mime (childhood autism only) (b) Relative failure to initiate or sustain conversational interchange with reciprocal responsiveness (c) Stereotyped and repetitive use of language or idiosyncratic use of words or phrases (d) Lack of varied, spontaneous make-believe or social imitative play	Poor flexibility in language expression Lack of descriptive, conventional or informative gestures Lack of creativity and fantasy in thought processes Lack of emotional response to another's verbal and non-verbal overtures Impaired use of cadence of speech to reflect communicative intent Use of echolalia, neologisms and pronoun reversal Lack of spontaneous conversation or sharing of personal information
Behaviour	Restricted, repetitive and stereotyped patterns of behaviour, interests and activities in at least one of the following: (a) An encompassing preoccupation with at least one stereotyped and restricted interest which is abnormal in content or focus, or at least one interest which is abnormal in intensity and circumscribed nature (b) Apparently compulsive adherence to specific, non-functional routines or rituals (c) Stereotyped and repetitive motor mannerisms, such as hand/finger flapping or twisting or complex whole-body movements (d) Preoccupations with part-objects or non-functional elements of play materials	Imposition of non-functional rigidity and routine on everyday and novel experiences Resistance to change in routine or environment Abnormal play: preoccupation with parts of objects Lack of spontaneity, initiative and creativity Lack of spontaneous imitation/mirroring of others Unusual sensory-seeking or sensory-avoidance behaviours Increased sensitivity to noise Temper/outbursts Aggression Self-injury Anxiety symptoms Difficulties in the educational or occupational environment Sleep difficulties Eating disturbances

Garland, J., O'Rourke, L., & Robertson, D. (2013). Autism spectrum disorder in adults: Clinical features and the role of the psychiatrist. *Advances in Psychiatric Treatment, 19*(5), 378-391. doi:10.1192/apt.bp.112.010439.
(Sources: Lord 1989.1994; World Health Organization 1992: Fitzgerald 2001.)

Box 8.15	Persistent physical symptoms (medically unexplained symptoms)			
Early experience →	**Predisposing factors** →	**Thinking styles** →	**Health anxiety**
Difficult pregnancy/ birth; low birth weight Infant special care unit	Parental anxiety Attachment issues Family illness	All or nothing 'worst case scenarios' Family culture	Excessive focus on ill health

Genetic links for minority: chronic fatigue syndrome
Variation (between one, the expected rate and six-fold increases) in reporting childhood sexual abuse, or other traumas
Common story of recent precipitant of symptoms: stress, infection

---

Excessive health preoccupations: these are *overvalued ideas*, not delusions
Physiology (e.g. borborygmi or flatus per rectum) interpreted as symptoms
Significant time reading about health; searching online for 'symptom' explanations
Worst case scenario planning: *what if* questions, assumption 'this could be serious'
Joins online discussions or social media forum to discuss health and diseases
Focus on biomedical (rather than psychosocial): wish for complex investigations
Looking for cure through medication and (less commonly) surgical procedures
Disagreement with doctors* (almost universal) leading to doctor shopping
Language of disability with secondary withdrawal (leaves job or training, inactivity, refusal of social opportunities, becomes housebound)—reinforced by family

*Good evidence that for some patients, there are iatrogenic harms as part of the process: the doctor pushes for investigations and prescribes something, anything (because that is what doctors do), then gets frustrated with or loses interest in the patient when symptoms persist and the results are (inevitably) 'negative'.

---

careful reading of all medical sources and particular attention to the system from which persistent physical symptoms arise (Box 8.16). If you can strike a balance between acknowledgement of symptoms (that are real despite negative tests), sharing your understanding of medical investigations and systems, while opening up psychosocial explanations, then this will be a therapeutic assessment. MSE findings may differ from other mental disorders:

- Thoughts show abnormal belief systems—about where organs are located, how the body works (and breaks down) and overvalued ideas about the salience of some bodily sensations that have been upgraded or labelled as symptoms. Record the intrusion of the patient's opinions about 'diagnosis' and his interpretation of what other doctors have said; these answers usually intrude even when your questions are open ones to establish the physical symptoms.
- Try to characterize the nature of anxiety (about which symptoms? What might this be? Concerns that 'they have missed' cancer), its degree and a summary of dates of onset and progression.
- Depression is very common in PPS/MUS, but easily missed owing to the emphasis on physical symptoms, investigations and other doctors' actions. It is also treatable (usually cognitive behavioural therapy [CBT] plus antidepressants), allowing for relief of symptoms and progress.

- When MUS symptoms run a chronic course, cluster into systems (see Box 8.16), and polypharmacy gets established, sleep is a key outcome measure. Ask about its lack, or excessive daytime sleep in the housebound patient, and link this to questioning about suicidal ideas. A subset of these patients become desperate when hospital clinics discharge them; as a rule, they communicate distress to others as physical symptoms or not at all, plus they have supplies of lethal prescribed medication.
- Perceptions of bodily touch/movement/pain may be independent of any stimulant. Sequences, such as eating, can have conditioned responses, such as an expectation of nausea or vomiting based on past experience.
- Insight: this is frequently absent even if insight is defined that psychosocial stressors are driving and maintaining these symptoms.
- In the collaborative history, describe the current social setting in full: what supports might be put at risk if the patient recovered from these symptoms (people including regular contacts with health professionals, family and professional carers, financial benefits, housing, disability status)?

Assessing forensic risk

Consider this scenario: a prisoner is transferred to your unit, and you need to assess his safety, potential risks to others and make contingency plans. You need to know the offence that led to conviction, and all previous crimes. Breaking societal rules covers a multitude of issues. The main concerns are violence to others, but even a history of acquisitive crime (stealing without threat of violence) also predicts

Box 8.16	Functional somatic syndromes
System/specialty	**Common, named syndromes**
Cardiology	Noncardiac chest pain (Da Costa's syndrome)
Respiratory	Hyperventilation syndrome
Gastrointestinal	Globus hystericus
	Nonulcer dyspepsia/functional abdominal pain
	Irritable bowel syndrome
Neurology	Chronic headaches (tension headaches)
	Nonepileptic attacks (pseudoseizures)
Infectious disease	Chronic fatigue syndrome/myalgic encephalomyelitis. Long COVID
Rheumatology	Fibromyalgia
Orthopaedic	Chronic low back pain with no physical abnormality
Ear, nose and throat	Globus syndromes (subjective obstruction)
	Functional dysphonia
Gynaecology	Chronic pelvic pain
Dental	Temporomandibular joint dysfunction
	Atypical facial pain, burning mouth syndrome
Pain/any system	Somatoform pain disorder
Multiple systems	Somatization disorder (Briquet's syndrome)

increased future violence. Most people on a custodial sentence have personality difficulties (see Box 8.10), of which impulsivity is central to understanding their risks to others. Neither an actuarial assessment (calculating the odds, with reference to demographics and previous behaviours) nor unstructured clinical interviews are sufficient in this situation, even with maximum information gathering. Structured interviews, such as the historical clinical risk (HCR-20, management), are used to integrate our diagnoses (personality, substances, psychosis) with these factors, and to anticipate settings in which violence is more likely to occur. Box 8.17 summarizes similar, collaborative approaches to risk formulation. As with general formulations, the patient needs to hear the conclusions and the basis for any decisions that have an impact on his liberty. Some traits are less amenable to interventions, for example dissociality and detachment (see Box 8.10), and transfer to long-term facilities (such as prison or treatment units) is decided by specialists to contain these behaviours in the medium term. When a patient engages with this process to ameliorate treatable components, re-evaluation will be key to moving him on.

Referring someone for psychotherapy

Most aspects of formulation link to any potential benefits of psychotherapy. In essence, build on the insight and motivation that you find to allow discussion of the best therapy modality for this patient. Therapy must have an evidence base (CBT works better than antidepressants in the short- and long-term in people with mild to moderate depression), and your formulation must be a coherent account of this person, highlighting potential focus points for therapy. The main determinants of choice are what is available locally, waiting times, affordability (if the patient is to pay for this) and the commitment needed

Box 8.17	The five key elements of a risk formulation

Predisposing factors
These are social or environmental experiences or biological aspects of a person's history that are associated with problems in later life; examples include poor attachments, early emotional trauma or head injury.

Precipitating factors
These can be immediate triggers to an event, such as an argument, or more general circumstances in a person's life, such as stress. They also include destabilizing experiences, such as a deterioration in mental health, and disinhibiting factors, such as intoxication.

Motivating factors
In terms of motivation, it is important to consider the relative roles of intrinsic influences and circumstances. Generally, the former give rise to greater concern than the latter. For example, consider the difference between a violent offender who deliberately harms people he believes to have wronged him and another violent offender who once lost his temper in a particularly heated situation.

Perpetuating factors
These are characteristics of offenders or their circumstances that mean they continue to be risky. An example would be unhealthy relationships or poor engagement with treatment.

Protective factors
These are strengths within the person or external factors that reduce risk. An example would be effective coping skills or a supportive family.

(Source: Baird J, Stocks R. Risk assessment and management: forensic methods, human results. *Advances in Psychiatric Treatment*. [Online] Cambridge University Press; 2013;19(5): 358–365. DOI:10.1192/apt.bp.111.009407.)

to attend and practice its recommendations. Try to see therapy beyond the one-to-one 'on the couch' stereotype; social prescribing (short of formal therapy), peer support, couples and family therapy are all proven interventions. People with a personality disorder (see Box 8.10) do well in group therapy as they learn to mentalize their interactions with others, although a relationship with a care coordinator for frequent reviews is part of this. Most treatment programmes for addictions are based on motivational interviewing that divides patients into different stages on their journey. Stage 1 is the *Precontemplation Stage* in which the person does not intend to change behaviours as he does not view himself as having a problem. Stage 2 is the *Contemplation Stage* in which at times the patient might have made links between substance use and consequences but have not made efforts to change. Stage 3, *Preparation*, weighs up the positives and negatives of continuing to consume versus cessation, perhaps towards a plan, on which he has not yet acted. Stage 4 is the *Action Stage* in which attempts to cut down, even stop, are made. Often, asking and getting help is central to this. Stage 5, the *Maintenance Stage*, must have lasted for a minimum of 6 months; behaviours have changed with a sense there is 'no going back', even if the patient has not achieved complete abstinence. Last in, Stage 6, *Termination Stage*, the person has achieved abstinence and put measures in place to reduce lapses and relapses.

Patients presenting as emergencies | 9

Geraint Morris

Introduction

A medical emergency requires swift recognition and prompt action. Recognition of urgency does not necessarily require a precise diagnosis; the fact that the patient is dangerously unwell is usually obvious owing to an abnormality revealed by the internationally recognized assessment system for critically ill people of Airway, Breathing, Circulation, Disability and Exposure of the patient (ABCD and E). When an abnormality is found it should be acted upon and followed by a reassessment to establish if the intervention was useful. The clinician simultaneously needs to decide during this time as to whether and when summon help if available.

The importance of clinical assessment

High-quality history taking and clinical examination will usually identify a diagnosis in a timely fashion and enable the initiation of appropriate investigation and management plans. In modern medicine, much has been made of the awareness of 'vital observations' or 'vital signs', which are often recorded by nursing staff and are usually available prior to a doctor's clinical assessment. It should be remembered that observations support clinical diagnosis and management and do not replace them.

The relationship between good history taking, sound examination skills and the ordering of appropriate investigations is as important in an emergency situation as in any other clinical setting. Many could try to argue that with the advancement of science, history taking and clinical examination should be superseded by simple awareness of available investigations. A poorly taken and rushed history, followed by numerous irrelevant investigations, is poor-quality medicine. Such an approach often leads to a wrong or missed diagnosis and some abnormal results of uncertain significance. Investigations are not always risk free, and patients should not be exposed unnecessarily to interventions, such as ionizing radiation, without serious thought.

This chapter deals with conditions requiring assessment and management within the first hour and focuses on the presenting complaint. Recognizing the nature of an emergency presentation begins with how the patient comes to medical attention. This may be from information provided by the patient himself or witnesses such as paramedical (e.g. ambulance) staff, friends, family or concerned members of the public. The clinician will make an initial assessment by simply observing the patient; no apparent signs of life should initiate a life support response. If the patient is alive, then the general impression of how sick a patient appears is a reasonably accurate judgement of urgency. The experienced clinician will make these decisions in seconds. A particular clue will be in the respiratory rate and effort. An increased respiratory rate and work of breathing are the first physiological parameters to be altered in the shocked state and are often the subtle clues that alert a clinician to an unwell patient even from the end of the bed. Observing and recording this parameter for all patients is a fundamental part of developing a sound clinical method in emergency situations.

Urgency of response depends on the patient's responses when you are using the ABCD and E system of assessment. A talking patient has a patent airway, can maintain sufficient respiratory effort to make the vocal cords vibrate and move enough air to allow gas exchange. Similarly, if the patient is talking he must be perfusing his brain with sufficient oxygen to undertake the processes of speech as well as being responsive enough to do so. The clinician therefore has a degree of time with which to make further assessments and management decisions in this situation.

It should be stressed that the aim of this chapter is to help the reader develop a logical method for the clinical assessment of the acutely presenting patient. Although the topics covered here relate to common acute presentations, greater detail relevant to these presentations has not been provided, because much of this will be dealt with elsewhere in this book. It is also hoped that the reader will not look on this chapter as an amalgamation of lists, but rather as an approach to logical thinking.

Diagnosis versus resuscitation

Sometimes, the severity of illness dictates that life-saving resuscitative treatment should begin before any diagnosis is reached, especially in acutely ill patients with problems such as shock or breathlessness. However, it should be possible to make an underlying diagnosis (or a differential diagnosis) in the majority of cases; an acutely ill patient may not clinically improve until the treatment based on the correct diagnosis is provided. Acute resuscitation and the formulation of diagnoses will often be performed successfully in tandem.

The pyrexial and septic patient

Patients frequently present to emergency departments with signs and symptoms of infection, as do existing inpatients, irrespective of the cause for initial hospital admission. Severe infections have the potential for significant morbidity and mortality, and it is vital that they are identified and diagnosed promptly. Although the majority of patients presenting with fever will have an infective cause that can be easily elicited from the history and examination, it is also well recognized that there are many non-infective inflammatory causes (Table 9.1).

Infection with evidence of life-threatening organ dysfunction is now defined as sepsis. Patients with suspected sepsis who do not respond to immediate resuscitative measures are considered to be in septic shock. Delays in initiating treatment for sepsis, in particular the correct antibiotics, have consistently been shown to lead to a worse prognosis. Screening for evidence of organ dysfunction initially revolves around physiological parameters and historical details, such as reduced urine output and, most important, episodes of confusion or drowsiness. The brain is the organ most sensitive to metabolic derangements and any evidence of impairment from baseline should be taken seriously. Sepsis can be further broken down into amber and red flag sepsis owing to risk factors (immunosuppression), recent historical events (recent surgery), physiological changes and the need for additional oxygen.

The history will often suggest the source of infection (cough, abdominal pain, dysuria, headache). Other important features include details of any recent travel (country and duration of residence), a drug and lifestyle history (including any recreational drug use), weight loss, chronic illness and any risk factors for immunosuppression, such as recent chemotherapy, steroid therapy and the possibility of human immunodeficiency virus (HIV) infection.

Initially, the examination should focus on critical issues that need immediate action. If the patient has a raised pulse, heart rate or respiratory rate, prolonged capillary refill, hypoxia or hypotension, then oxygen, intravenous fluids and appropriate antibiotics should be administered urgently before embarking on a detailed examination (if possible and time allows, take blood cultures before administering antibiotics, because this may be the only opportunity for some time during what may be a long and severe illness to obtain cultures that are completely free of antibiotics). In searching for a source, look for exudate or pus at the back of the throat. Lung auscultation may reveal features of acute bronchitis (wheeze) or consolidation. Heart murmurs in the presence of fever may indicate infective endocarditis. The abdominal examination should identify any tenderness (e.g. right upper quadrant in cholecystitis, loin in pyelonephritis). If the patient complains of headache, look for features of meningism. Lymphadenopathy and superficial or skin abscesses should be noted as part of a thorough 'top-to-toe' examination. Less obvious sites should not be missed, especially cavities (e.g. a retained vaginal tampon leading to toxic shock), skin folds and the perineum.

Immediate investigations may include those which lend support to an inflammatory process (white cell count, C-reactive protein), severity of infection (blood lactate), consequences such as volume depletion (urea and electrolytes), underlying predisposition (blood sugar) and source (urinalysis, urine culture, blood culture, chest X-ray). In response to the history and examination, one may proceed to throat swab, blood films for malaria, faeces analysis (toxin or culture), lumbar puncture, transthoracic echocardiogram or abdominal imaging (ultrasound or computed tomography (CT) scan).

Table 9.1 Logical thinking for patients presenting with fever

Mechanism	Common or important examples
Infection	Viral (upper respiratory, lower respiratory (Covid-19), infectious mononucleosis, hepatitis A); bacterial (less-common causes include infective endocarditis, meningitis, tuberculosis, spontaneous bacterial peritonitis, pleural empyema, cholangitis); parasitic (malaria, schistosomiasis); fungal
Systemic inflammation	Rheumatoid arthritis; systemic lupus erythematosus (SLE); polymyalgia rheumatica; Wegener's granulomatosis; inflammatory bowel disease; malignant neuroleptic syndrome; blood transfusion reaction
Malignancy and granulomatous disease	Solid tumours; lymphoma; leukaemia; amyloidosis; sarcoidosis
Drugs	Prescription; recreational (e.g. ecstasy)

The patient with chest pain

Although most patients who present with chest pain will not have clinically significant coronary

Table 9.2 Logical thinking for patients presenting with chest pain

Potentially life-threatening conditions—all usually causing central chest pain	Other causes of central chest pain	Causes of pleuritic chest pain
Coronary artery disease (myocardial infarction or acute coronary syndrome)	Pericarditis	Pericarditis
Massive pulmonary embolus (PE)	Gastro-oesophageal reflux disease (GORD)	PE (more likely to be smaller and more peripheral)
Thoracic aortic dissection: severe, tearing in nature, radiating to interscapular area	Muscular or skeletal	Pneumothorax
Pneumothorax (particularly tension)	Anxiety	Pneumonia (reactive pleuritis)
Oesophageal rupture		Empyema
		Viral pleuritis
		Malignant involvement of chest wall (including mesothelioma)
		Rib trauma, fracture or metastases
		Inflammatory pleuritis (e.g. rheumatoid arthritis, systemic lupus erythematosus)

artery disease, it is this potential diagnosis that often dominates the initial thoughts of the assessing doctor. This is why patients presenting with chest pain who appear unwell or in need of immediate resuscitation should have an electrocardiogram (ECG) recorded before the initial history and examination are complete. The outcome from attempts to open an occluded coronary artery depends on the speed with which arrangements can be made for either thrombolysis or angioplasty, so little is to be gained (and much to be lost) from a prolonged assessment. However, in some patients with critical coronary artery disease the initial ECG recording may be normal, so it is essential that a careful history and examination are performed on all patients with chest pain not obviously in immediate need of resuscitation or intervention. Patients with chest pain are, understandably, often anxious about the possibility of underlying serious heart disease and an important part of the doctor's role is to project calm reassurance.

Chest pain that has a life-threatening cause (Table 9.2) is usually central and of sudden/rapid onset. Certain features may be diagnostically helpful; these include radiation of the pain to the left arm and/or jaw (myocardial ischaemia) or the interscapular area (aortic dissection); accompanying breathlessness (massive pulmonary embolus or pneumothorax); or a clear temporal association with prolonged vomiting (oesophageal rupture). In pericarditis, the pain may be 'classic' (central pain relieved by sitting forward) or pleuritic. The features of chest infections and viral infections should be obvious. Pneumonias not infrequently are associated with headache. Important examination features to note during the initial, rapid assessment of an ill patient with chest pain include the fine crepitations of pulmonary oedema, the hyper-resonant percussion and tracheal deviation of pneumothorax or the asymmetric blood pressure readings consistent with thoracic aortic dissection.

Box 9.1 Risk factors for coronary heart disease

- Age
- Blood pressure
- Smoking
- Cholesterol
- Diabetes
- Racial grouping
- Family history of coronary artery disease or stroke before the age of 60
- Girth (obesity)

If 'ABC' interventions are not required for resuscitation, if the patient is stable and no other features are requiring immediate action (e.g. peripheral cyanosis), then a more considered assessment is appropriate. In addition to the history, the risk factors for coronary artery disease and pulmonary embolism (PE) may be factored into the diagnostic process (Box 9.1 and Table 9.3). The blood pressure should be taken in both arms, particularly if the arm pulses feel unequal. Unequal blood pressure measurements in the arms raise the possibility of aortic dissection and serious consideration should be given to appropriate urgent imaging (usually thoracic CT scanning). A raised jugular venous pressure may suggest early heart failure. Precordial auscultation may reveal a pericardial rub. There may be classic signs of pneumonia. It can be difficult to differentiate between pleuritic and musculoskeletal chest pain from the history, but pain exacerbated by palpation and posture changes more than by inspiration is more likely to be musculoskeletal. Signs of deep venous thrombosis automatically raise the clinical suspicion of a PE.

The serious nature of many of the diagnoses of patients who present with chest pain dictates that the threshold for certain investigations is often low. In addition to being a crucial test at the moment of

Table 9.3 Modified Wells criteria for assessing the risk of pulmonary embolism (PE) in a patient with symptoms consistent with pulmonary embolism

Clinical parameter	Score
Clinical evidence of deep vein thrombosis (DVT)	3
No alternative diagnosis likely other than PE	3
Heart rate greater than 100 per minute	1.5
Surgery or immobility in preceding 4 weeks	1.5
Previous confirmed DVT or PE	1.5
Haemoptysis	1
Active malignancy	1
Total score	**Risk**
> 6	High
2–6	Moderate
2	Low

Table 9.4 Potentially life-threatening conditions presenting as breathlessness

Clinical assessment	Potentially life-threatening conditions
Stridor (may be mistaken for wheeze)	Partial obstruction of trachea or major airway
Audible wheeze (one should listen very carefully, as it may be very quiet)	Severe asthma Anaphylaxis Acute bronchitis Pulmonary oedema
Diffuse features	Pneumonitis Widespread pneumonia Pulmonary oedema
Significant asymmetry of findings in a whole lung on percussion and/or auscultation	Pneumothorax Massive pleural effusion Total lung collapse
Focal features of consolidation	Lobar collapse from tumour, foreign body or mucus plug Pneumonia
No obvious abnormality	Pulmonary embolism (hypoxia often present) Metabolic acidosis (hypoxia often absent)

initial assessment, the ECG has additional value when it is repeated over a period of time, looking for any evolution in its appearance (often called 'dynamic changes'). Detailed description and explanations of the possible ECG features of myocardial infarction and pulmonary embolism are given elsewhere. The chest X-ray may show features of pneumothorax, pneumomediastinum (from oesophageal rupture), heart failure, widened mediastinum (often seen in thoracic aortic dissection), pneumonia, rib fractures/destruction and pleural effusions. In the emergency unit, measurement of troponin in blood (a protein released when cardiac myocytes undergo ischaemic necrosis) is performed on many patients with chest pain. It is not a diagnostic test of cardiac chest pain, but 'negative' results (below a certain threshold) indicate that the risk of a serious acute cardiac event in the ensuing 30 days is extremely low. A negative troponin test does not obviate the need to make a detailed clinical assessment; a patient with a typical history of 'crescendo angina' (worsening in severity and/or frequency, occurring at rest or on minimal exertion over days to weeks) should still be treated as an emergency even if the troponin result is reassuring.

The breathless patient

When life-threatening conditions present with breathlessness, it should be rapidly established whether immediate and resuscitative interventions are required whilst simultaneously making a clinical assessment to establish the cause (Table 9.4). The patient should be placed in a safe, monitored (ECG and pulse oximetry) environment and clinicians should act quickly if there is evidence of visible distress, the usage of accessory muscles of respiration, high respiratory rate, high pulse rate, cyanosis or observable low oxygen saturations. The

immediate response should be to administer high-flow oxygen to the patient with any of the above findings, unless there is good evidence that this has on this occasion, or previous occasions, caused breathing difficulties (most commonly patients with chronic obstructive pulmonary disease, COPD). In the majority of cases, arrangements for urgent ECG and chest X-ray (CXR) will be made immediately, before the initial clinical assessment is complete. There may even be certain clinical scenarios (e.g. upper airway obstruction, tension pneumothorax) in which immediate clinical intervention is necessary.

General principles

A rapid clinical assessment will establish if detailed history taking is going to be realistic. A conscious, alert patient who is able to speak in full sentences is reassuring. Features suggestive of an obstructed airway include complete absence of airway sounds (complete obstruction) or added sounds of laboured breathing where air entry is diminished (partial obstruction). Tachycardia and tachypnoea may reflect respiratory distress. Use of accessory muscles of respiration is typical in the partially obstructed airway, and signs include a tracheal tug (a slight downward movement of the trachea with each inspiratory effort), paradoxical chest and abdominal movement ('see-sawing'—the chest wall moves inwards during inspiration and outwards in expiration and there is dyssynchrony between the rib cage and the abdomen), with supraclavicular and intercostal 'in-drawing'. Irritability, agitation and a reduced consciousness level may reflect hypoxaemia and carbon dioxide retention. Do not rely on cyanosis as a feature in identifying an obstructed airway as this is a very late preterminal sign. Observe or ask about 'best breathing position'. Be aware that the patient may have positioned himself for optimal airflow in the setting of airway obstruction; moving the patient into a supine position may precipitate loss of the airway altogether. Low pulse oximetry readings (SpO_2) reflect inadequacy of oxygenation, which is not the same as ventilation. Arterial blood gas sampling may be helpful but should not delay treatment. Respiratory acidosis, with a high carbon dioxide tension ($PaCO_2$) and reduced pH, reflects alveolar hypoventilation. When assessing patients, look carefully for these signs and symptoms and always call for help early from an anaesthetist if airway compromise is suspected. The young can compensate well initially, masking impending desaturation and hypoxaemia. Be mindful of injuries that will compromise the airway, such as facial burns, bleeding and foreign bodies obstructing the airway. Always provide high flow oxygen with a reservoir bag at 15 litres/minute, and reassess frequently, looking for signs of deterioration, which may be caused by deterioration of the underlying condition, or excess oxygen in a patient with chronic CO_2 retention.

In the emergency situation of the acutely breathless patient it is helpful to consider the potential problem in one of two 'groupings': upper airway obstruction and cardiopulmonary pathologies that affect ventilation and/or gas exchange (Table 9.5).

Airway obstruction

Most commonly, airway obstruction occurs in a patient with a decreased level of consciousness with resultant loss of the cough reflex used to clear normal bronchial secretions. Such patients are also at risk of aspiration of gastric contents because of depression of other reflexes that control the competence of the tracheo-oesophageal junction. Pragmatically, this can be easily inferred by the patient's response to insertion of an adjunct, such as an oropharyngeal (Guedel) airway. Fully conscious patients, in whom laryngeal reflexes are present, will not tolerate this airway and inserting one may precipitate gagging, vomiting and laryngospasm. In a patient with reduced consciousness and a threatened airway, the adjunct is tolerated, with consequent relief of backward tongue displacement and soft palate obstruction. Insertion of a Guedel airway usually should be combined with manoeuvring the patient into the recovery (lateral) position (the effect of which is to push the tongue and jaw forward under gravity, thereby improving the airway) (Fig. 9.1).

The second, less common scenario of airway obstruction is the patient presenting with stridor—the term used to describe the harsh, high-pitched musical breathing noise caused by narrowing of the upper airways with impending complete obstruction. It may be inspiratory, expiratory or biphasic, although it is most commonly heard just during inspiration. Inspiratory stridor indicates laryngeal obstruction, because the negative intrathoracic pressures exacerbate extrathoracic obstruction during inspiration. Intrathoracic obstruction may cause expiratory stridor, as the airways are compressed during expiration. Common causes of stridor include tumours (usually laryngeal/tracheal, but also mediastinal and oesophageal), peritonsillar and retropharyngeal abscesses, inhalation of a foreign body and laryngotracheobronchitis ('croup'). Children are more susceptible to the latter two causes owing to the narrower diameter of their airway and the fact that normal inquisitive behaviour often leads to objects being inserted into their mouths. In developed countries, vaccination programmes that include *Haemophilus influenzae* type B vaccine have led to a sharp reduction in the incidence of acute epiglottitis—an important cause of stridor in children in which infection by this organism of the valve at the tracheo-oesophageal junction causes fever, dysphagia, sore throat and (classically) drooling of saliva as the pain of swallowing dictates that the child will try to avoid doing this. If stridor, as opposed to wheeze, is considered, the cause may be evident from the history (airway cancer, foreign body exposure or anaphylaxis). The examiner's ear should be placed carefully close to the mouth of the patient to try to establish the source of airflow limitation. Stridor of any cause in any age group is frightening to patients; the attending doctor's demeanor needs to be calm and gentle whilst simultaneously arranging emergency assistance. Acute stridor is an airway emergency, and the teams of intensive care, anaesthesia and ear, nose and throat specialists should be mobilized as quickly as possible to establish a secure airway.

Specific mention should be made of burn victims in whom inhalation of superheated gases and toxins of combustion causes swelling of the lining of the tracheobronchial tree with consequent obstruction. The history will usually be obvious, but important clinical signs that suggest airway injury include a hoarse voice, singed hairs of the nasal passages and soot and erythema in the upper airway. Recognizing this promptly should initiate measures to secure the airway early with an endotracheal tube. The stridor associated with the severe upper airway oedema of anaphylaxis will be dealt with later in this chapter.

The importance of recognizing airway obstruction as the cause of acute breathlessness is self-evident; although provision of supplemental oxygen is a crucial therapeutic intervention, it will not resolve the underlying problem of hypercapnia associated with hypoventilation.

Table 9.5 Logical thinking for conditions causing breathlessness, including the emergency conditions

Clinical assessment	Classification	Condition
Stridor	Large airway disease	Partial obstruction of trachea or major airway
Bilateral or diffuse wheeze	Small airway disease	Asthma
		Acute bronchitis (including bronchitic component to chronic obstructive pulmonary disease)
		Anaphylaxis
		Pulmonary oedema (presenting as bronchial oedema)
		Obesity hypoventilation syndrome (although often the wheeze from obesity-related airflow limitation is not heard)
Asymmetric features in whole lung field (tracheal deviation, hyper-resonance to percussion and diminished breath sounds)	Pleural disease	Pneumothorax
Asymmetric features in whole lung field (tracheal deviation, stony dullness to percussion and diminished breath sounds)	Pleural disease	Massive pleural effusion
Asymmetric features in whole lung field (tracheal deviation, dullness to percussion and diminished breath sounds)	Large airway disease	Total lung collapse (tumour, foreign body, mucus plug)
Diffuse bilateral abnormalities (crepitations)	Diffuse parenchymal disease	Pneumonitis
		Pulmonary oedema
		Pulmonary fibrosis
Diffuse bilateral abnormalities (bronchial breathing)	Diffuse parenchymal disease	Multilobar or bronchopneumonia
Focal abnormality (bronchial breathing)	Focal parenchymal disease	Pneumonia
		Lobar collapse
		Bronchiectasis
Focal abnormality (dullness to percussion and diminished breath sounds)	Pleural disease	Pleural effusion
Bilateral, focal abnormalities (basal stony dullness and diminished breath sounds)	Pleural disease	Bilateral pleural effusions
Bilateral, focal abnormalities (bronchial breath sounds)	Parenchymal disease	Bilateral pneumonia (e.g. bibasal pneumonia)
Thoracic deformity	Chest wall skeletal disease	Scoliosis
		Thoracic surgery
No obvious abnormality	Pulmonary vascular disease	Pulmonary embolism
		Pulmonary hypertension
	Respiratory muscle weakness	Diaphragm paralysis
		Neuromuscular disease
	Compensatory effort	Metabolic acidosis
		Anaemia
	Psychogenic	Psychogenic hyperventilation

This table is not intended to be an exhaustive list. It is aimed at assisting logical thought, particularly with regard to clinical features.

Acute breathlessness owing to ventilatory and/or oxygenation defects

The sensation of breathlessness is poorly understood. In normal respiration active inspiration is followed by passive expiration, but in breathlessness of any cause there is active expiration and a change in the normal inspiration:expiration time ratio. The diaphragm works at a mechanical disadvantage when this ratio changes and hypoxia added to this situation may contribute further to the discomfort of breathlessness. The usual cause is loss of lung compliance/elastic recoil, which requires active expiration to compensate. This is seen either with

Figure 9.1 The recovery position.

chronic damage to lung parenchyma or acutely when the alveolar spaces are filled with material that is less compressible than aerated lung, such as interstitial fluid, pus or blood. In some conditions (classically acute asthma) severe overinflation of the lungs reduces their ability to expire effectively. Finally, the sensation of breathlessness may occur with conditions completely unrelated to the heart or lungs, such as diabetic ketoacidosis. Here, a change in blood pH is sensed by chemoreceptors in the brainstem leading to Kussmaul's breathing ('air hunger') as an attempt is made to hyperventilate and blow off carbon dioxide, thereby improving the acidosis.

History taking is often limited in breathless patients. Accompanying friends, relatives or carers may be able to provide collateral information and it may be possible to elicit certain key features by asking simple 'yes/no' questions ('Do you have asthma? Have you eaten something you are allergic to?'). It may be impossible to differentiate between the wheeze of acute asthma, anaphylaxis, bronchitis or, rarely, pulmonary oedema, but a history of previous asthma and atopy, fever or chest pain may help direct the clinician to a working diagnosis. If asthma is suspected, then early administration of a beta-2-adrenergic agonist can be lifesaving and will rarely cause harm. The ability to administer this medication, either via nebulizer or metered dose inhaler and spacer device, is a fundamental skill that should be familiar to all clinicians. If it is ineffective owing to severe bronchoconstriction, then intravenous administration can be considered by experienced clinicians.

Clinical examination of the breathless patient may reveal significant asymmetry in chest expansion, percussion and/or auscultation. In general, the side that moves less has the pathology within it. The deviated trachea will be ipsilateral to the side of lung collapse or focal fibrosis and contralateral to a tension pneumothorax or very large pleural effusion. These are differentiated by the percussion note, which will be hyper-resonant in tension pneumothorax and dull (some say 'stony dull') in

the presence a massive effusion. Breath sounds may be absent or poorly heard in the affected lung in all of these conditions. Relief may be immediate with minimal aspiration of either air (tension pneumothorax) or fluid (pleural effusion) prior to formal drainage.

Diffuse polyphonic wheeze or indistinct widespread coarse crackles with acute on chronic shortness of breath is typical of an exacerbation of COPD. Widespread bilateral unchanging fine crepitations are most often heard with acute pulmonary oedema. Focal features, such as tactile fremitus, dullness to percussion, increased vocal resonance and bronchial breathing, provide evidence of consolidation and/or collapse and can usually be confirmed by an urgent chest X-ray.

If there are no obvious examination abnormalities in the acutely breathless patient, then the history will need further clarification. Chest pain and/or breathlessness in the presence of relevant risk factors raise the possibility of a PE (see Table 9.3). Investigation with an arterial blood gas is useful in determining oxygen and carbon dioxide exchange alongside any disturbances in pH. Most conditions causing breathlessness are exacerbated by lying flat and relieved by sitting up, although this 'orthopnoea' is most obvious with pulmonary oedema and respiratory muscle weakness. Breathlessness relieved by lying flat (platypnoea) is relatively rare and is most often associated with PE; in this case, the supine posture improves pulmonary perfusion and provides relief. A cough acutely productive of purulent sputum may support a working diagnosis of pneumonia. Longer-standing cough may be associated with non-purulent sputum production (asthma, chronic COPD and bronchiectasis) or non-production (interstitial lung disease and lung cancer). An absent or weak cough may suggest respiratory muscle disease. Acute, frothy sputum (occasionally tinged with blood) may be seen in pulmonary oedema. Frank haemoptysis may occur in PE, lung cancer, pulmonary vasculitis, pneumonia, tuberculosis and acute bronchitis.

The patient with hypotension or shock

There are numerous definitions for 'shock' but a useful one may be considered to be 'a failure of blood flow to provide sufficient perfusion of the major organs'. It is often associated with hypotension. Hypotension and shock are clinical emergencies and require appropriate and immediate intervention. Hypotension may be defined as 'abnormally low blood pressure for that given patient', which means interpreting the documented blood pressure in context. For one patient, a 'normal' recorded blood pressure may be 'abnormal for him' as it is significantly lower compared with previous readings. In another, a 'low' blood pressure may be entirely normal for that specific patient. If in doubt, a low blood pressure should always be acted upon. For the purposes of this chapter, it will be accepted that hypotension and shock encompass similar pathologies and belong on the same spectrum. Severe hypotension may lead to shock. It is essential, therefore, that, irrespective of aetiology, this is seen as a medical emergency, and a joint effort is made simultaneously to initiate resuscitative treatment and make a diagnosis. This involves administering intravenous fluids while other clinical features and vital observations are elicited. The fluids may be subsequently stopped if pulmonary oedema becomes evident. The organ that is most sensitive to under perfusion is the brain; confusion and decreased levels of consciousness in the context of shock indicate poor cerebral oxygenation, so patients should usually be nursed lying flat to promote cerebral perfusion.

Teamwork is paramount. If more than one clinician is available, one may focus on taking a history while another may take responsibility for examination and institution of treatment. Examination findings, irrespective of the cause, may include a rapid pulse and heart rate and a third heart sound. It should be noted that in otherwise fit individuals, in the face of severe hypovolaemia, there may be a prolonged period of 'compensation', in which the healthy heart maintains cardiac output and a normal blood pressure by increasing the heart rate and the force of contraction. Therefore, the patient with unexplained tachycardia should be examined and investigated thoroughly, and impending shock should not be missed.

During resuscitation, a quick starting point is needed when assessing the causes of shock, because a correct diagnosis will dictate the most appropriate intervention. One way to categorize shock is to differentiate causes into those with a wide or a narrow pulse pressure ('pulse pressure' is the difference between systolic and diastolic blood pressure) (Table 9.6). As a general rule, patients with widened pulse pressure will present with warmer peripheries, and the palpable peripheral pulse may be more 'bounding' in nature. Patients with narrowed pulse

Table 9.6 Logical thinking in shock

Mechanism	Common or important examples
Narrow pulse pressure	Hypovolaemic shock (haemorrhage, fluid losses from enteral tract, fluid losses from renal tract, fluid losses from skin [burns]); cardiogenic shock from myocardial failure (coronary ischaemia, acute myocarditis)
Widened pulse pressure	Septic shock; anaphylactic shock; neurogenic shock (all can also be known as distributive shock)

Box 9.2 Types of shock

1. Hypovolaemic
2. Cardiogenic
3. Distributive
4. Obstructive

pressure often have cooler peripheries, with weak, 'thready' peripheral pulses. Although 'normal' pulse pressure is often quoted as 40 mmHg, it should be noted that during hypotension this figure should be interpreted with caution. For example, a blood pressure of 75/40 mmHg could be interpreted as having a widened pulse pressure of 35 mmHg, as this is in the context of a low systolic blood pressure.

There are varying types of shock, which need general discrimination to apply definitive treatment (Box 9.2). One type of shock may evolve into another, leading to a mixed clinical picture requiring more than one treatment strategy. For example, it is not uncommon for septic shock (ordinarily presenting with a widened pulse pressure) to lead rapidly to cardiogenic shock (usually characterized by a narrow pulse pressure) in patients with coexisting heart disease. Septic shock is also often associated with hypovolaemic shock. It is not uncommon for cardiogenic shock to improve with treatment, but then be superseded by infection and septic shock. If it is not possible to categorize a pulse pressure into narrow or wide, other features described below may help identify the cause of shock.

Narrow pulse pressure associated with shock is almost always a consequence of cardiac failure ('cardiogenic shock') or hypovolaemia ('hypovolaemic shock'). Examination findings, in addition to specific features described below, may include cold and pale limb peripheries. Although there are many general causes of widened pulse pressure (including aortic regurgitation, thyrotoxicosis, fever, anaemia, pregnancy, patent ductus arteriosus, aortic dissection, raised intracranial pressure, vasodilating drugs, Beriberi heart disease and old age), wide pulse pressure *with shock* is almost always a consequence of profound vasodilatation, usually with warm limb peripheries. The most common cause is infection ('septic shock'); less common causes include

Table 9.7 Classes of haemorrhage

	Class I	Class II	Class III	Class IV
Blood loss (ml)	Up to 750	750–1500	1500–2000	>2000
Blood loss (% Blood volume)	Up to 15%	15%–30%	30%–40%	>40%
Pulse rate	<100	>100	>120	>140
Blood pressure	Normal	Normal	Decreased	Decreased
Pulse pressure (mmHg)	Normal or increased	Decreased	Decreased	Decreased
Respiratory rate	14–20	20–30	30–40	>35
Urine output (ml/hr)	>30	20–30	5–15	Negligible
CNS/mental status	Slightly anxious	Mildly anxious	Anxious, confused	Confused, lethargic

anaphylaxis ('anaphylactic shock') and loss of neurogenic vasomotor tone ('neurogenic shock').

Hypovolaemic shock

Conceptually, hypovolaemic shock is the easiest to understand as simply insufficient circulating volume to provide for the oxygen demands of the organs. Typically, this is caused by haemorrhage and may be divided into four classes (Table 9.7). External haemorrhage is usually clinically obvious, either from the history or from visual evidence of blood loss. The source of internal bleeding may be more difficult to diagnose, although the prevailing clinical picture is common to both (Table 9.8). Cool peripheries and corresponding changes in heart rate, blood pressure and respiratory rate are key indicators. Simple assessment through testing the capillary refill time and provocative testing, such as a postural blood pressure, is useful in unmasking compensated shock. In the initial period following a haemorrhage, it should be remembered that the blood haemoglobin concentration may be preserved. Once bleeding is suspected as the cause of hypovolaemic shock, the clinical approach is straightforward and intuitive; replace the blood that has been lost (as it is the best resuscitative fluid) and stop the bleeding. External bleeding can be controlled in most situations by locally applied pressure. Internal bleeding often necessitates surgical or endoscopic intervention, and interventional radiology techniques are increasingly being applied in a number of situations and specialist institutions.

Although external and internal bleeding are the most common causes of hypovolaemic shock, non-haemorrhagic causes also exist. In developing countries gastrointestinal fluid loss (e.g. caused by cholera) is a leading cause of death, especially in children. Other volume-losing conditions include salt-wasting renal conditions, burns, sequestration of fluid into the bowel and adrenal insufficiency. As a rule, hypovolaemic shock in the context of these conditions takes longer to develop than, for example, acute intra-abdominal blood loss, so a carefully taken history is likely to be diagnostically informative. Replacement of fluid with crystalloid in the first instance is the most important intervention.

Table 9.8 Internal bleeding sites

Pelvis	Pelvic fracture
	Ectopic pregnancy
Abdomen	Liver
	Spleen
	Kidney
Thorax	Massive haemothorax
Gastrointestinal	Oesophageal and/or gastric varices
	Duodenal ulcer
Retroperitoneal	Ruptured abdominal aortic aneurysm
Peripheries	Long bone fractures

Cardiogenic shock

Cardiogenic shock refers to a failure of the heart to pump blood effectively to meet peripheral oxygen demands. It is most frequently caused by a large myocardial infarction but may also be owing to cardiac dysrhythmias, other causes of cardiac muscle pump failure (e.g. myocarditis, cardiomyopathy) or acute cardiac valve problems. In this situation, as with hypovolaemic shock, there will usually be a narrow pulse pressure. Cardiogenic shock may be associated with a preceding history of chest pain, palpitations or breathlessness (in particular orthopnoea). There are frequently auscultatory features of pulmonary oedema. Patients with brittle cardiac function may present with cardiogenic shock irrespective of the initial trigger. An ECG is often informative and may show changes of recent infarction, dysrhythmia and non-specific changes of pericarditis, myocarditis and cardiomyopathy. Treatment will largely depend on the cause; inotropic support and invasive measures are frequently required.

Distributive shock

Distributive shock is owing to inappropriate distribution of a normal or elevated cardiac output. Invariably there is profound vasodilatation with associated capillary leakage. The most common cause is severe sepsis, in which an overwhelming cascade of inflammatory mediators causes distribution of blood to inappropriate areas. The clinical history may suggest an obvious source of infection and examination findings may include a fever, observed rigors, auscultatory features of lung consolidation or abdominal features of peritonitis.

Anaphylactic shock is usually clinically easily apparent (respiratory distress, agitation, urticarial rash, face, mouth, tongue and orbital swelling and wheeze), but there may not be a history of allergy or hypersensitivity. Accompanying hypotension is frequent, owing to marked vasodilatation, pooling of blood and a consequent reduction in venous return to the heart. Knowing the common causes of the allergy and the ability to recognize urticaria are important. Once recognized, detailed clinical assessment is inappropriate; immediate resuscitation is required with intramuscular adrenaline (epinephrine) and intravenous fluids.

Neurogenic shock, another form of distributive shock, is very rare. It is caused by disruption of the vasomotor tone of blood vessels causing inappropriate dilatation and pooling of blood with a marked reduction in venous return and, consequently, cardiac output. A history of either spinal trauma or medical intervention (e.g. epidural anaesthesia or autonomic blocking agents) usually prompts its consideration as a diagnosis.

Obstructive shock

Most commonly, obstructive shock occurs with massive pulmonary embolism in which obstruction to blood flow through the pulmonary circulation reduces venous return to the left atrium and ventricle so markedly that cardiac output into the systemic circulation falls and hypotension develops. Patients will be breathless and usually have chest pain. The combination of clinical signs of right-side heart strain with hypotension and hypoxia should prompt consideration of massive pulmonary embolism. Obstruction to the outflow of the left ventricle occurs with severe aortic stenosis, although usually this condition develops over a prolonged period of time.

The patient with diminished consciousness

The definition of 'consciousness' may be the (waking) state of awareness of oneself and environment. The absence of awareness, therefore, even when one is stimulated, may implicate diffuse or multifocal brain dysfunction and may be defined as 'coma' or 'diminished consciousness'. Although the last two terms may be seen as synonymous, the term 'coma' may have widespread and conflicting implications. In these situations, ambiguity should be avoided, and the patient should be described as having 'diminished consciousness'.

Consciousness is controlled by the brainstem through a system of nerve cells and fibres known as the 'reticular activating system' or the 'ascending arousal system'. The cerebrum helps maintain consciousness and alertness and at least one hemisphere, as well as the reticular activating system, must be functioning normally to maintain consciousness. The brain's ability to adjust its activity and consciousness levels can therefore be impaired in several ways, particularly when both cerebral hemispheres are suddenly and severely damaged, when the reticular activating system malfunctions, when blood flow or the amount of nutrients (such as oxygen or sugar) supplying the brain decreases or when toxic substances impair brain function.

There are several ways to describe the conscious state objectively, although perhaps the two best-known 'scores' are the Glasgow Coma Scale (GCS) and the 'AVPU' (*a*lert, *v*erbal, *p*ain, *u*nresponsive) score (Tables 9.9 and 9.10). The GCS attributes a score, ranging from 3 to 15. It was originally devised to assess the level of consciousness after head injury, although now is used for almost all acutely presenting patients. The GCS has the advantage of being easily and reliably administered by a range of different health professionals. When faced with a poorly conscious patient, the usual pairing of resuscitation and diagnostics should be followed. Severe neurological conditions may affect upper airway tone, respiratory drive (e.g. Cheyne–Stokes respiration), vasomotor tone and cardiac rhythm. Also, if the cause of the brain dysfunction is systemic (see Table 9.11),

Table 9.9 The Glasgow Coma Scale						
	1	**2**	**3**	**4**	**5**	**6**
Eyes	Does not open eyes	Opens eyes in response to painful stimuli	Opens eyes in response to voice	Opens eyes spontaneously	N/A	N/A
Verbal	Makes no sounds	Incomprehensible sounds	Inappropriate words	Confused, disoriented	Orientated, converses normally	N/A
Motor	Makes no movements	Extension to painful stimuli (decerebrate response)	Abnormal flexion to painful stimuli (decorticate response)	Flexion or withdrawal to painful stimuli	Localizes painful stimuli	Obeys commands

Table 9.10 The 'AVPU' score (a simplification of the Glasgow Coma Scale)*

Alert	Verbal	Pain	Unresponsive
A fully awake (although not necessarily oriented) patient. This patient will spontaneously open eyes, will respond to voice (although may be confused) and will possess motor function	The patient makes some kind of response (eyes or voice or motor) when prompted by questions, e.g. 'Are you ok?' The patient's eyes may open, or the response may simply be a moan or slight movement of a limb	The patient makes some kind of response (eyes or voice or motor) when pain stimulus is used on them	No response to voice or pain

*APVU, alert, verbal, pain, unresponsive.

this will need to be dealt with. Therefore, it is paramount that the 'airway, breathing, circulation' (ABC) algorithm is given due respect. The airway should be supported appropriately (if necessary with endotracheal intubation), the 'recovery' lateral position may be required in the unintubated patient to prevent aspiration, hypotension may require vigorous intravenous fluids and monitoring will be required for hypertension and cardiac dysrhythmias.

After resuscitation, one should focus on rapidly identifying the cause of brain dysfunction (see Table 9.11). If a systemic cause is obvious, it should already have been dealt with. A brief history from witnesses may reveal preceding hemiparesis, headache, trauma, fit, recreational drug or alcohol intake, or a history of cancer, diabetes, liver or renal disease. Examination should include a full body inspection for features of trauma, fundoscopy, cranial nerves and motor function (including power, tone and reflexes). The power, sensory, cerebellar and visual assessments may not be possible owing to a lack of cooperation. One should attempt to examine for meningism by assessing nuchal rigidity (diminished neck flexion with otherwise retained neck movements) and knee extension with the patient supine, with the hip and knee preflexed (pain on knee extension is Kernig's sign).

A very brief description of common pathologies leading to changes in conscious level includes the following:

- Vascular lesions include cerebral arterial or venous thromboses leading to infarcts. Intracranial haemorrhages may be subarachnoid or intracerebral. Relevant cases should be referred early to stroke units or neurosurgeons.
- Primary cranial infections may manifest as meningitis, encephalitis or meningoencephalitis. One may also become acutely encephalopathic from widespread non-infective inflammatory vascular lesions. With infective and inflammatory pathologies, changes may or may not be evident on cranial imaging. Treatment with antibiotics and/or antiviral agents will be empirical initially, and should not be withheld in favour of preceding lumbar puncture, especially if the patient is critically unwell.
- After trauma, extradural and subdural haematomata may be suspected, as may

Table 9.11 Logical thinking in the poorly conscious patient

Primary cranial diffuse or multifocal disease, where structural lesions will be obvious on imaging	Primary cranial diffuse disease where no structural lesions will be obvious on imaging
Vascular	Infection
Infection	Inflammation
Inflammation	Trauma ('concussion')
Tumours	Non-convulsive status epilepticus or postictal state
Trauma	Psychiatric (conversion, stupor)

Secondary cranial disease: systemic	Secondary cranial disease: metabolic
Hypoxia/anoxia	Alcohol
Hypotension	Drugs
Hypothermia	Hypoglycaemia
	Endocrine disturbance (sodium balance, thyroid disturbance)
	Liver
	Renal
	Non-cranial infection

subarachnoid and intracerebral haemorrhages. The condition known as 'diffuse axonal injury' (DAI) refers to extensive lesions in white matter tracts and is one of the major causes of unconsciousness after head trauma. 'Concussion' is the most common type of traumatic brain injury, where there is temporary loss of brain function with a variety of subsequent physical, cognitive and emotional symptoms. Usually no changes are visible on imaging, and symptoms usually resolve spontaneously over days or weeks. Relevant cases should be referred early to the neurosurgical unit.

- Non-convulsive status epilepticus as a cause of altered consciousness is often overlooked. There will often be no obvious clinical clues other than eye deviation or involuntary eye movements. Often, the unconscious patient who has been intensely investigated in the emergency

Table 9.12 Relationship of pupillary changes to site of anatomical damage

Unilateral pathological dilatation (mydriasis)	Unilateral pathological constriction (miosis)	Mid-point pupil
Pupillary fibres close to the origin of the third cranial nerve are especially susceptible when uncal herniation or a posterior communicating aneurysm compresses the nerve. This mydriasis is usually accompanied with sparing of oculomotor function. When pupillary fibres more distal in the third cranial nerve are affected, the mydriasis usually occurs together with oculomotor dysfunction.	Hypothalamic damage may lead to ipsilateral Horner's syndrome. Pontine damage may lead to bilateral miosis. Lateral medullary and ventrolateral cervical cord lesions may lead to ipsilateral Horner's syndrome.	Mid-brain damage: the mid-point pupil shows no reaction to light.

department, and who spontaneously becomes more alert over the subsequent hours, will have had an unwitnessed seizure.

- If opioid overdose is suspected, one may consider administering the opioid antagonist naloxone. This may be essential if the unconscious state is affecting the airway. If the vital observations are stable, however, the benefit of rapid opioid reversal should be weighed against the disadvantages (e.g. disorientation, aggression, vomiting, removal of analgesia).
- The psychiatric patient (with or without a known past history) may have a poor consciousness level from conversion disorder, or stupor secondary to depression or schizophrenia. Often, the diagnosis will be made after preceding exhaustive negative tests and will need an expert assessment by the psychiatrist.

Pupillary examination deserves special mention. As pupillary pathways are resistant to metabolic insult, the identification of absent pupillary reflexes usually implies structural pathology. The brainstem areas governing conscious level are anatomically close to the areas controlling the pupils and so pupillary changes help to identify brainstem pathology causing altered conscious level (Table 9.12).

Investigations, as always, should be targeted to the index of suspicion from clinical assessment. Those pertaining to resuscitation, including CXR, ECG and blood sugar, should be performed on initial encounter. Cranial imaging (usually a cranial CT scan) will be indicated if there is a significant possibility of structural lesions. It should be remembered, however, that the transfer of the patient to the radiology department may carry major risk, particularly if the patient requires general anaesthesia for intubation. Therefore, the advantages of performing neuroradiology should always be measured against risk. A lumbar puncture may be required; contraindications according to existing national and local guidelines should be referred to and, if present, the procedure should be deferred. An electroencephalogram (EEG) may reveal abnormalities consistent with a seizure disorder.

Plasma alcohol may easily be measured and may lend support to a clinical diagnosis of alcohol toxicity. Some, although not all, hospitals are able to perform urine toxicology analyses for recreational and other drugs. Plasma levels for paracetamol, salicylates and anticonvulsant medications are also easily available. These may be relevant in cases of deliberate or inadvertent self-harm. Some plasma levels for drugs are only available in specialist 'poisons' units. It is therefore often good practice to have a saved sample of serum, which may subsequently be transported, if required. Tests of renal function and liver function (including blood clotting) should be included in the context of altered conscious level.

The syncopal patient

Syncope is a frequent cause of presentation to hospital and the emergency department. It may be defined as temporary loss of consciousness with rapid onset and spontaneous recovery. The implication is that there is temporary, global hypoperfusion to the brain. The brevity of the event is mostly limited to a few minutes. Although the causes of syncope are often not sinister (the most common cause is a vasovagal episode), the consequences may be catastrophic if, for instance, the onset occurs while driving. The condition should therefore always be taken seriously (Table 9.13).

When the duration of the loss of consciousness is unknown or thought to be prolonged, the possibility of seizures should be considered. This impression may be reinforced by the presence of tongue biting, urinary incontinence, preceding aura or unusual behaviour, ongoing drowsiness, confusion or headache or a collateral history of involuntary movements during the episode. The approach to patients with seizures is discussed elsewhere in this chapter.

The history of the syncopal event will not be complete when told by the patient, although events preceding and following it may be recounted. It is important, therefore, that any witnesses of the event

Table 9.13 Logical thinking for conditions causing syncope

Mechanism	Common or important examples
Cardiac structural disease	Valvular heart disease
	Obstructive cardiomyopathy
	Atrial myxoma
	Severe systolic dysfunction
Cardiac dysrhythmia	Any dysrhythmia
Pulmonary hypertension (poor left atrial filling)	Acute pulmonary embolism
	Any cause of chronic pulmonary hypertension
'Steal' syndromes	Subclavian 'steal'
Nervous system mediated	'Vasovagal'
	Carotid sinus disease
	Autonomic nerve dysfunction (e.g. secondary to alcohol, antihypertensive drugs, hypoglycaemia and diabetes mellitus)
Hypovolaemia	Blood loss
	Diarrhoea
	Vomiting

Table 9.14 Simple terminology for seizures

Term	Description
Generalized seizure	Involvement of the whole cerebral cortex and therefore abnormalities (e.g. convulsions) may be seen in the whole of the body.
	Consciousness is always impaired.
Focal (partial) seizure	Involvement of a focus in the cerebral cortex and therefore abnormalities (e.g. convulsions) may be seen in one part of the body.
	Consciousness may be retained (simple partial seizure) or impaired (complex partial seizure).
	There may be secondary generalization (i.e. a focal seizure leading on to a generalized seizure).
Convulsive seizure	For example, tonic-clonic, tonic and clonic.
Non-convulsive seizure	The term 'absence seizure' should generally be avoided unless a specific syndromic diagnosis is being made by a clinician experienced in epilepsy.
Status epilepticus	A single seizure for more than 5 minutes or two or more seizures within a 5-minute period without fully recovering between seizures.

are available to give a collateral history. Dramatic sequelae, such as motor vehicle accidents or personal injury, will prompt urgent investigations. The history should explore any relationship between syncope and exertion, chest pain, palpitations, dyspnoea, posture changes, body fluid losses and overt bleeding. A careful drug and alcohol history should be taken and a past history of heart and lung disease or diabetes noted. A family history of sudden death should be taken very seriously.

One should examine for an implanted cardiac device (such as a pacemaker), irregular or rapid heart rate and heart murmurs. Measurement of lying and standing blood pressure is mandatory unless there is a clear alternative cause. Investigations could initially include full blood count, ECG, echocardiography and 24-hour ECG monitoring. Formal autonomic function testing may be needed.

The patient with seizures

One definition of 'seizure' is the 'uncontrolled electrical activity in the brain, which may produce a physical convulsion, minor physical signs, thought disturbances or a combination of symptoms'. 'Epilepsy' is a pattern of repeated seizures. The occurrence of a seizure or 'fit' is a common mode of presentation to the emergency department. In most cases, the final diagnosis will not be epilepsy.

If the patient is actively having a seizure, the 'ABC' of resuscitation should be meticulously followed. Intravenous anticonvulsant agents should be administered promptly, within the constraints of

formulary guidelines. The aim should be to suppress the seizure as quickly as possible. If unsuccessful with standard anticonvulsants, the administration of a general anaesthetic (together with intubation, ventilation and admission to intensive care) should be considered. The definition of 'status epilepticus' is under continuous scrutiny (Table 9.14).

If the patient is not actively having a seizure at the time of clinical assessment, the task is to identify whether the episode preceding admission was a seizure or not. It should be remembered that a diagnosis of seizures may lead to social and employment consequences (including the ability to drive), so it is crucial to establish a credible collateral history together with a detailed history from the patient. Tongue biting and post-event drowsiness, headache or confusion may help lend support to a diagnosis of seizures. Although urinary and faecal incontinence is often quoted, it is not a strong differentiating feature between seizures and non-seizures.

The diagnosis of non-convulsive status epilepticus may be missed unless specifically thought of. The patient may present with non-specific features, such as prolonged confusion or drowsiness. On occasions there may be clinical features to arouse suspicion, such as nystagmoid eye movements or repetitive (often stereotypic for the patient) movements of the tongue, jaw or limbs.

Some conditions are commonly misdiagnosed as seizures. Severe exacerbation of extrapyramidal disease may mimic myoclonus. Vasovagal episodes may, on occasions, be followed by jerking of the limbs. Dissociative seizures (previously called pseudoseizures and which occur in patients for psychological and other complex reasons) are often difficult to differentiate from genuine seizures, even for many experienced neurologists (Table 9.15).

In history taking, there is considerable overlap with the principles described for the patient with syncope. It is essential that witnesses are available to give a collateral history, because the seizure itself will not be recalled by the patient. However, on recovery, the events preceding and following the seizure may be recounted by the patient. As with syncope, dramatic sequelae such as motor vehicle accidents or personal injury should be taken seriously. It should be established whether there is a known history of epilepsy. In patients with known epilepsy, a history should be taken for compliance, anticonvulsant changes, concurrent illnesses, alcohol intake and lifestyle issues. In other cases, specifically ask about alcohol intake, recreational drug usage, diabetes, head injury, foreign travel and pregnancy.

General examination will include the assessment of features of infection. Mild, transient, fever is a common phenomenon after seizures from muscle contractions. Persistent fever together with other abnormal observation, such as tachycardia and raised respiratory rate, may suggest the presence of an infection. If there is genuine doubt as to whether the fever is related to the seizure or an infection, look vigorously for a source of infection (including performing a lumbar puncture) and consider administering empirical intravenous antibiotics (after taking blood cultures) while awaiting investigations. One should examine for evidence of cranial trauma, alcoholic foetor and severe hypertension.

In the drowsy postictal patient, some aspects of neurological examination, such as visual fields, voluntary eye movements, cerebellar function, power and sensory deficits, will be difficult or impossible to ascertain. However, the following should be performed to a high standard: fundoscopy; pupillary, corneal and gag reflexes; limb tone; limb reflexes; and spontaneous limb movement. Any asymmetry should be noted and it may prompt urgent investigations.

Testing for blood sugar level should be performed urgently, because hypoglycaemia may be quickly reversed and brain injury prevented. Plasma biochemistry and liver function tests will identify reversible electrolyte deficiencies and features of liver disease. Possible infections should be identified with the help of white cell count, blood culture and urinalysis. Toxicology tests may include blood alcohol and urine drug analysis. Women of childbearing age should have a pregnancy test. Patients with unexplained seizures and a history of travel abroad

Table 9.15 Awareness of conditions commonly misdiagnosed as seizures	
Condition	**Awareness**
Dissociative seizure (pseudoseizure)	The reasons for patients presenting with contrived movements mimicking seizures are complex. They often occur in known epileptics. The risk of death is significantly higher in epileptic patients with dissociative seizures, and so the latter needs to be taken seriously and not merely dismissed as a non-organic event. Many epilepsy experts maintain that with increasing clinical experience, there is increased awareness of the difficulty in the differentiation of seizures from dissociative seizures. There are, however, some features which may lend support to the diagnosis of dissociative seizures: resistance to attempted eye opening by the clinician, limb thrashing and pelvic thrusting, full alertness immediately after the event (i.e. lack of postictal drowsiness) and down-going plantar responses during attack.
Vasovagal episode	Prolonged vasovagal episodes may lead to cerebral hypoperfusion and brief, self-limiting convulsive-type movements.
Cranial trauma	This is particularly seen in sports events, where cranial trauma may lead to brief, self-limiting convulsive-type movements, similar to those seen in vasovagal episodes.
Extrapyramidal disease	Patients may present with worsening or poorly controlled Parkinson's disease, manifested as severe coarse tremor which, to the untrained eye, may resemble myoclonus.

should have parasite analysis. If the patient has no known identity and therefore no known past history, plasma anticonvulsant analysis may lend support to recent ingestion and therefore the possibility of previously diagnosed epilepsy.

A cranial CT scan will be required if one or more of the following are present: the seizure is unexplained, there are features of cranial trauma, there are focal or lateralizing features, there are fundoscopic features of raised intracranial pressure and there are features of infection. The gross features uncovered by a cranial CT scan may include intracranial haemorrhage or space-occupying lesions. Although it is a misconception that a CT scan is always required prior to lumbar puncture, it is overwhelmingly recognized that lumbar puncture to investigate for meningitis in the patient with seizures should always be preceded by a cranial CT scan. The cerebrospinal fluid from the lumbar puncture should be analysed for meningitis and for subarachnoid haemorrhage. An EEG may be performed acutely to lend support to the diagnosis of a postictal state and occasionally to identify features of herpes encephalitis.

Once a seizure is diagnosed, the clinician should advise the patient of his duty to contact the driving licensing authority, who in turn will issue guidelines for cessation of driving for a defined period. The diagnosis of epilepsy should be made by an expert in epilepsy, because this diagnosis will have social and drug-therapy implications. The epilepsy expert will also decide, together with the patient, on the clinical value of prescription of anticonvulsants after a first seizure.

The patient with delirium (acute confusion)

Patients with delirium (previously termed acute confusion) are often seen in the emergency setting. Often, the patient will have pre-existing cognitive dysfunction, which may have been present for weeks, months or years. It is important in this scenario to investigate both the acute confusion and the pre-existing pathology. Remember that those with longer-standing cognitive dysfunction (e.g. consequent upon cerebrovascular pathology) will be more susceptible to episodes of delirium when affected by minor pathology, such as infection and metabolic derangement. In elderly patients, particularly, systemic problems, such as infections or cardiac disease, may not lead to any symptoms other than acute confusion.

The causes and mechanisms of confusion should be logically arranged in the mind of the clinician (Table 9.16). Toxaemia from infections, inflammation and drugs will lead to varying degrees of cerebral dysfunction, as will metabolic derangements. Any episode of acute pain or anxiety affects intellectual function. Poor cerebral oxygenation will occur with episodes of hypoxia and diminished cerebral perfusion from circulatory impairment. Any brain pathology may cause cerebral dysfunction; one should be aware that, in these cases, confusion may progress to a diminished consciousness level. The possibility of underlying psychiatric disorder should be borne in mind, particularly in the younger patient.

The history, as in cases of altered conscious level, syncope and seizures, will often not be meaningful when given by the patient. The collateral history from relatives and other sources is therefore paramount. The presence of any long-standing cognitive issues should be established. Specific, directed questioning should deal with the presence of head injury, pain (including chest pain), breathlessness, light-headedness, headache and features of infection. A meticulous history should be taken for drugs and alcohol. Nutritional history should be explored because malnourished patients may present with Wernicke's encephalopathy even if they are not

Table 9.16 Logical thinking for conditions causing acute confusion

Mechanism	Common or important examples
Infection	Urine, chest
Inflammatory	Acute pancreatitis, vasculitis, ischaemic bowel, myocardial ischaemia
Drugs and external toxins	Prescription drugs, recreational drug usage, alcohol (toxicity or withdrawal)
	The most severe form of alcohol withdrawal is 'delirium tremens', a condition that traditionally starts up to 3 days after cessation of heavy alcohol consumption.
Metabolic derangement	Hypoglycaemia, hyperglycaemia, hyponatraemia, hypernatraemia, hypercalcaemia, liver dysfunction (synthetic or cholestasis), uraemia, thyroid dysfunction, nutritional deficiency (particularly vitamin B_{12}, thiamine and niacin)
Acute pain or anxiety	Urinary retention, severe constipation
Psychiatric issues	Depression, schizophrenia
Hypoxaemia	Chest infection, pulmonary oedema, pulmonary embolism
Circulatory impairment	Cardiac disease (dysrhythmia, systolic dysfunction), sepsis, haemorrhage, prolonged vagal episode
Brain pathology	Haemorrhage, ischaemia, seizure disorder, infection (encephalitis and meningoencephalitis), head injury, cerebral vasculitis

excessive alcohol users. The presence of established chronic diseases, such as diabetes, seizure disorders, liver, kidney or thyroid disease, must be documented. Previous psychiatric illness and long-standing mood changes should be noted.

The examination should be targeted, because the patient most likely will not be able to comply with the complicated directions required in neurological and other assessments. Start with the 'vital' observations: oxygen saturation, respiratory rate, blood pressure (erect and supine) and heart rate. Look for pyrexia, features of head injury, smell of alcohol, cachexia and features of jaundice or uraemia. There may be obvious features of a thyroid disorder. The presence of pain on palpation and abnormalities on chest examination should be identified. Neurological examination will elicit any gross focal or lateralizing features and also features of meningism. The examination should also include an abbreviated mental test (see Chapter 7, Elderly Medicine). The latter will objectively document the confusion and help track any progress.

Unless the diagnosis is absolutely clear, investigations may commence with full blood count, C-reactive protein, standard electrolytes, urea and creatinine, liver function, thyroid function, vitamin B_{12}, urinalysis, urine and blood cultures, CXR, toxicology, blood alcohol (to help differentiate alcohol withdrawal from toxicity), ECG and arterial blood gases (if low oxygen saturation is identified). With evidence of focal or lateralizing features, meningism, altered conscious level or unexplained headache, a cranial CT scan should be considered. A lumbar puncture should be performed if meningitis remains a consideration.

The patient with acute headache

Many patients present to the emergency department with severe acute headache. This will either be a 'worst ever' exacerbation in the context of chronic, long-term headache or a first presentation of headache.

On initial presentation, it should be established whether there have been any additional features that may suggest sinister pathology, often referred to as 'red flags'. One should specifically enquire about severity (is this the 'worst ever'?); rapidity of onset (implying vascular pathology, such as subarachnoid haemorrhage); recent head injury; loss of consciousness; altered intellect; features of sepsis; features of meningism (photophobia and neck stiffness); features of raised intracranial pressure (headache exacerbated by straining, coughing and lying flat); asymmetry (consistent with temporal arteritis and glaucoma, as well as migraine and sinusitis); and blurred visual disturbance (consistent with raised intracranial pressure, glaucoma and temporal arteritis).

Additional features need clarification. A past history and temporal patterns of long-standing headache need to be established, as does the presence of coexisting illness. Viral infections and pneumonia are not uncommonly associated with headache. Foreign travel may be relevant as well as the drug history.

It is important to be aware of some distinctive features of the more common causes of headache (Table 9.17). Distinctive features in the history of a patient with a subarachnoid haemorrhage include a sudden-onset, occipital 'worst ever' headache (classically described as like being kicked on the back of the head). There may have been an episode of loss of consciousness (this may be seen in up to half of all patients presenting with subarachnoid haemorrhage). Features of meningism and raised intracranial pressure are not uncommon. Urgent investigations (cranial CT scan, with targeted lumbar puncture) and specialist referral are paramount. Bacterial meningitis may be rapidly fatal, and treatment with intravenous antibiotics must commence as soon as the diagnosis is suspected. Viral meningitis is usually less dramatic, although this is not inevitably the case.

Table 9.17 Logical thinking for conditions causing acute headache

Mechanism	Common or important examples
Vascular: haemorrhage	Subarachnoid, intracerebral, subdural, extradural
Vascular: occlusive	Migraine, temporal arteritis, carotid artery dissection
Muscular	Tension-type headache
Meningeal irritation	Meningitis (bacterial, viral), subarachnoid haemorrhage
Raised intracranial pressure	Space-occupying lesion (tumour, abscess, localized haemorrhage), malignant hypertension, benign intracranial hypertension
Drugs and toxins	Oral or sublingual nitrates, carbon monoxide
Carbon dioxide retention from respiratory failure	Obstructive sleep apnoea, obesity hypoventilation syndrome
Tropical disease	Malaria, any one of the tropical endemic encephalitides
Upper respiratory tract infections	Influenza, sinusitis
Intraocular pressure	Glaucoma
Neuralgia	Trigeminal neuralgia, cluster headache

The headache of meningitis is of acute onset and severe. There are accompanying features of photophobia and neck stiffness. In severe cases, there may be features of raised intracranial pressure. Although pure encephalitis does not produce features of meningism, meningoencephalitis does. Temporal arteritis is a form of vasculitis in which the temporal arteries are inflamed and tender. The headache is usually asymmetrical. There may be pain in the jaw with chewing ('jaw claudication'). Vision changes (blurred vision) should prompt urgent treatment with steroids (to prevent complete loss of vision), followed by specialist referral or a very likely diagnosis and confirmation of the diagnosis with a temporal artery biopsy. The migrainous headache is typically unilateral and pulsating. The acute period often lasts between 4 and 72 hours; there may be accompanying nausea, vomiting, photophobia, phonophobia (increased sensitivity to sound) or osmophobia (sensitivity to pungent smells).

The examination should include identification of general and specific features of sepsis, such as pyrexia, tachycardia and signs of lung consolidation. Altered consciousness level should have been detected on initial encounter and immediately acted upon. Altered intellectual function and disorientation, though, may only be apparent later in more detailed conversation. A history of neck stiffness should prompt an examination of nuchal rigidity in which there is a painful deficit of neck flexion with relative preservation of all other neck movements. When meningism is suspected, both legs should also be examined where each leg in turn is bent at the hip and knee at 90° angles; if subsequent further extension in the knee is painful (leading to resistance), this should be described as a 'Kernig's positive' sign, which in turn suggests that there is significant inflammation of the meninges. Positive features of meningism should prompt the clinician to search for a non-blanching purpuric rash, which may lend support to a diagnosis of meningococcal meningitis. A full neurological examination should identify any focal or lateralizing motor or sensory abnormalities, and also any cranial nerve or cerebellar deficits. One should look for papilloedema on fundoscopy. Additional areas of clinical examination may include palpation of the temporal arteries or the sinuses, looking for tenderness in these areas; examination of the scalp, looking for herpetic lesions; and inspection of the sclerae, looking for the acute red eye of glaucoma.

In cases of suspected subarachnoid haemorrhage, a cranial CT scan is not diagnostic in all cases, particularly more than 24 hours after the acute event. If the diagnosis is suspected and the CT scan is normal, a lumbar puncture is mandatory to exclude the diagnosis and is best done more than 12 hours after the onset of symptoms. If encephalitis is suspected, a magnetic resonance image (MRI) should be considered. Lumbar puncture for cerebrospinal fluid analysis should be performed when meningitis is suspected. Antibiotics should never be withheld while waiting for the lumbar puncture. Other investigations that may help identify or support a diagnosis are CXR, white cell count, blood culture, parasite analysis for malaria and viral serology. In unexplained headache, particularly in the presence of drowsiness, plasma carboxyhaemoglobin may support a diagnosis of carbon monoxide poisoning.

The acutely weak patient

The term 'weakness' will often be used by patients for a variety of complaints. Although the term should be reserved for the original definition of 'reduced motor power', many patients will confess to 'weakness' when in fact they are 'fatigued' or 'lethargic'. It is reasonable to infer reduced motor power when weakness is present without significant tiredness. This should be contrasted with fatigue and lethargy, where the diminished power is generalized, commensurate with and caused by significant tiredness. This should form the basis of initial questioning. ('Do you feel weak because you are tired, or do you think that you have specifically lost muscle power?'). Sometimes, even with an experienced history taker and a cooperative patient it may not be possible to differentiate between weakness, fatigue and lethargy. The term 'fatigue', which is used here synonymously with the term 'lethargy', should not be confused with the neurological term 'fatiguability' (Table 9.18).

When assessing the patient, it is also helpful to differentiate between lesions of the 'upper motor neuron' (lesions of the motor cortex or pyramidal tracts) from the 'lower motor neuron' (lesions of the 'motor unit', that is the anterior horn cell, axon, neuromuscular junction or muscle). This differentiation is important in order to help direct investigations.

Acute quadriparesis and paraparesis deserve special mention. It should be assumed that the cause is external cord compression until proven otherwise. As recovery from the latter depends on speedy decompression, one should urgently organize imaging and specialty assessment. Any delay in imaging should not lead to a delay in specialty assessment.

The history should establish the speed of onset and distribution of weakness. Rapid onset of weakness over minutes suggests a vascular pathology, whereas an onset over hours or days is more indicative of an infective, inflammatory or malignant condition. Associated pain is most often a consequence of nerve root or peripheral nerve involvement and it also occurs with acute myopathy, in which there may be muscle tenderness. A careful drug history should be taken to identify agents, such as chemotherapy drugs which may cause peripheral neuropathy, and a family history enquiry may uncover inherited muscle disorders. Risk factors for stroke, such as hypertension, hyperlipidaemia, diabetes mellitus, alcohol intake and smoking history, should be documented.

On general inspection, look for gait disturbance, facial palsy, muscle wasting and fasciculation. Test for tone and reflexes before testing power, as muscle tone may be affected by recent muscle contraction. Diminished tone and diminished reflexes are seen in lower motor neuron conditions. In addition to formally testing power, a quick functional test for power is to ask the patient to stand from a sitting position, testing hip and knee extension; walk on his heels, to test ankle dorsiflexion; and walk on his toes, to test ankle plantarflexion. Coordination should be tested in the upper limbs (finger-to-nose tests) and lower limbs (heel-to-knee-to-toe), although one should be aware that weakness in itself will affect coordination. Sensory examination, testing for sensory loss, paraesthesiae, hyperaesthesiae and pain, will be meaningful only in cooperative and coherent patients. This should not prevent the clinician from attempting to establish sensory deficits consistent with nerve, nerve root or central pathology.

Timely cranial CT scans are essential in stroke, whereas MR scans are useful in a variety of cranial and spinal cord lesions. The spinal cord MR scan should be booked as an emergency when cord compression is suspected. Nerve conduction studies

Table 9.18 Logical thinking for conditions causing acute weakness

Scenario	Common or important examples
Fatigue or lethargy leading to generalized weakness	Chronic heart failure, chronic lung disease, sleep disorders, anaemia, chronic kidney disease, diabetes mellitus, chronic infection, malignancy, depression
Loss of motor power leading to generalized weakness	Myasthenia gravis (crisis), post-infectious inflammatory polyneuropathy ('Guillain-Barré syndrome'), acute myopathy (myositis, rhabdomyolysis)
Hemiparesis or hemiplegia (weakness or total paralysis of one side of body)	Lesion in contralateral cerebral motor cortex or contralateral brainstem
	Lesion in ipsilateral high cervical cord (often with ipsilateral dorsal column, i.e. proprioception deficit, and contralateral spinothalamic tract deficit, i.e. pain and temperature)
Monoparesis or monoplegia (weakness or total paralysis of single limb)	Lesion in contralateral cerebral motor cortex, contralateral brainstem
	Lesion in ipsilateral spinal cord (often with ipsilateral dorsal column, i.e. proprioception deficit, and contralateral spinothalamic tract deficit, i.e. pain and temperature)
	Lesion of nerve roots
	Mononeuropathy or mononeuritis multiplex
Paraparesis or paraplegia (weakness or total paralysis of both legs)	Lesion in parasagittal cerebral motor cortex
	Lesion in spinal cord (external compression, ischaemia, inflammation, e.g. transverse myelitis, infection, intramedullary space-occupying lesion)
	Post-infectious inflammatory polyneuropathy ('Guillain-Barré syndrome'), acute myopathy (myositis, rhabdomyolysis)
	Lesion of nerve roots and cauda equina lesions; usually affects one leg more than the other
	Mononeuropathy or mononeuritis multiplex; usually affects one leg more than the other
Quadriparesis and quadriplegia (weakness or total paralysis of both arms and both legs)	Lesion in brainstem
	Lesion in upper cervical cord (external compression, ischaemia, inflammation, e.g. transverse myelitis, infection, intramedullary space-occupying lesion)
	Post-infectious inflammatory polyneuropathy ('Guillain-Barré syndrome'), acute myopathy (myositis, rhabdomyolysis)

and electromyography (EMG) are useful to confirm the diagnosis of Guillain-Barré syndrome and, on occasion, will help differentiate peripheral nerve from nerve-root pathology.

The patient with acute abdominal pain

It is important to be familiar with some principles governing the location of pain. Oesophageal, gastric or duodenal pain may be evident over the lower chest or epigastrium (and oesophageal pain may radiate to the arms); gallbladder pain usually commences in the right upper quadrant and often radiates around the right chest wall to the right dorsal area; pancreatic pain usually localizes over the epigastrium and radiates through to the back; pain from the small bowel is often manifested diffusely or over the periumbilical area, whereas large bowel pain is usually found over the site of the pathology or lesion (e.g. splenic flexure); pain from the distal colon may be referred to the lumbar area; any pathology affecting or irritating the diaphragm (e.g. a subphrenic abscess) may present with referred pain in the shoulder; ureteric colic usually radiates from the flank to the inguinal area on the affected side ('loin to groin') (Table 9.19).

In contrast, pathology in areas distant to the abdomen may present with referred or radiated

Table 9.19 Logical thinking for conditions causing acute abdominal pain

Mechanism	Common or important examples
Enteral visceral pain (usually colicky pain)	Oesophageal spasm or oesophagitis, duodenal ulcer, small bowel enteritis or ischaemia, colitis, colonic obstruction, or ischaemia, complex gut perfusion deficit (diabetic ketoacidosis, sickle crisis)
Non-enteral visceral pain	Gallbladder pain from cholecystitis, pancreatic pain from pancreatitis or malignancy
Peritoneal pain (exacerbated by any changes in intra-abdominal pressure such as coughing, moving)	Perforated enteral viscus (gastric, duodenal, small bowel, appendix, large bowel), perforated non-enteral viscus (gallbladder, spleen, ruptured ectopic pregnancy), inflamed organ (pancreatitis), spontaneous bacterial peritonitis, malignant infiltration, bleeding vessel
Non-visceral pain	Aortic aneurysm, renal colic, referred pain

pain in the abdomen. For example, pneumonia, pleuritis and pleural effusions may manifest as upper quadrant pain on the affected side, and pain caused by myocardial ischaemia may be felt most in the epigastrium. When taking a history,

Table 9.20 Logical thinking for conditions causing haematemesis or melaena

Mechanism	Common or important examples
Peptic ulcer disease	Gastric or duodenal (with or without *Helicobacter pylori* colonization)
Inflammation of upper gastrointestinal tract	Reflux oesophagitis, gastritis, duodenitis (the latter two often occur secondary to excess alcohol intake or usage of non-steroidal anti-inflammatory drugs)
Oesophageal and/or gastric varices, or portal hypertensive gastropathy	Portal hypertension from chronic liver disease
Coagulopathy or increased bleeding tendency	Liver synthetic dysfunction, altered warfarin metabolism (infection, antibiotics), clotting factor deficiencies, thrombocytopenia, anti-platelet drug usage (aspirin, clopidogrel), recent thrombolytic therapy; note: over-anticoagulation may reveal bleeding from specific pathology previously unknown
Upper gastrointestinal malignancy or malformation	Oesophageal carcinoma, gastric carcinoma, upper gastrointestinal angiodysplasia (vascular malformation)
Mallory–Weiss tear	Tear of lower oesophagus or upper stomach from recurrent vomiting
Nose bleeds (epistaxis)	A large amount of swallowed blood may lead to melaena

establishing the abdominal location of pain will help identify the affected organ, using the principles outlined above. The speed of onset of pain is also relevant; rapid onset may be associated with vascular catastrophes and rupture. The timing of the last menstrual period and the possibility of pregnancy should be considered in women of child-bearing age. There may be an association between eating and abdominal pain: exacerbation by food may indicate gastritis, intestinal obstruction or gut ischaemia, whereas rapid relief upon eating may be suggestive of peptic ulceration. The presence of diarrhoea with or without blood may be suggestive of gut infection, inflammatory bowel disease or gut ischaemia.

The examination should focus initially on general features, such as hydration and cachexia, and vital parameters including respiratory rate, peripheral pulses, heart rate and blood pressure. Peritonitis may particularly be associated with severe hypotension or shock. Abdominal distension consistent with intestinal obstruction should be noted. Initial palpation may reveal diffuse, severe tenderness consistent with peritoneal inflammation, or localized tenderness. Rectal examination should be performed as a matter of routine; rectal masses and evidence of bleeding per rectum should be identified. If there is any suspicion of pelvic pathology in women, a gynaecological assessment is necessary.

General investigations that may help include full white cell count, haemoglobin, urea and electrolytes, liver function tests, amylase and pregnancy test (for the appropriate age group), or lipase. Samples of diarrhoea should be sent for *Clostridium difficile* toxin analysis and also culture. An erect CXR may demonstrate a perforated viscus or primary chest pathology and supine abdominal films may show features of obstruction. Abdominal ultrasound may demonstrate biliary tract dilatation or ureteric stones. Abdominal CT scans may reveal free fluid, the site of intestinal obstruction, pancreatic structure, evidence of ruptured aortic aneurysm or some detail with regard to intra-abdominal masses. Sigmoidoscopy may be useful if inflammatory bowel disease is suspected.

The patient with haematemesis and/or melaena

Haematemesis and melaena are common causes of presentation to the emergency department. The term 'haematemesis' describes the vomiting of blood, which may be bright red and fresh or altered/partly digested (commonly described as 'coffee grounds'). The presence of haematemesis almost always means acute bleeding from a source above the duodenojejunal flexure. 'Melaena' is faeces containing digested blood; they have a black (often described as 'jet black') tarry appearance and a characteristic and offensive smell. Although its presence may suggest acute bleeding from any source proximal to the ascending colon, the most common source is in the upper gastrointestinal tract (Table 9.20).

The passing of fresh blood per rectum (as opposed to melaena) usually means that the source of bleeding is in the large or small bowel. However, it is possible for very rapid upper gastrointestinal bleeding to lead to fresh blood per rectum because there is insufficient time for melaena to develop. Patients who incidentally describe dark stools without the characteristic appearance and smell of melaena do not usually have gastrointestinal bleeding. Iron-stained stool is black, but usually solid and formed.

In taking the history enquire about epistaxis, alcohol intake, pre-existing liver disease and both prescription and over-the-counter drugs. One severe or several episodes of vomiting before the onset of haematemesis may suggest a Mallory-Weiss tear. Epigastric pain may suggest peptic ulcer disease, and unexplained weight loss and anorexia is suggestive of malignancy.

The initial examination should focus on identifying if the patient is in shock and acting accordingly (see above). Young, otherwise fit hypovolaemic individuals may compensate with raised cardiac output and remain normotensive for some considerable time but exhibit a fall in blood pressure when changing posture from supine to erect. Features of malignancy (cachexia, supraclavicular lymphadenopathy, abdominal mass) and chronic liver disease (spider naevi, palmar erythema, jaundice, splenomegaly, ascites) should be noted. The clinical features of anaemia could suggest that there has been a period of occult bleeding before the acute bleed. Rectal examination is mandatory to see if there is objective evidence of melaena or fresh blood.

The initial investigations should include full blood count, clotting screen, urea, electrolytes and liver function tests. Blood should be 'grouped and saved', unless the patient is in shock, in which case, for example, four units of blood should be 'cross-matched' immediately. Blood is the best replacement fluid for a patient in shock with gastrointestinal bleeding, but should not necessarily be given immediately for the stable patient who is anaemic.

The availability of urgent upper gastrointestinal endoscopy varies widely among hospitals and different health care systems. Whatever the local provision, it follows, rather than replaces, prompt and effective resuscitation for the patient in shock.

Summary

Emergencies, by their very nature, require swift action. The initial approach consistently relics on implementing the ABCD and E methodology. Initial investigations are similarly repetitive, consisting of readily available blood tests, urinalysis, X-rays and ECGs as directed by the initial presentation. Monitoring response to interventions and planning further courses of action are the key skills of a clinician caring for patients who are dangerously unwell. Doing the basics well and reacting to unexpected responses or unsuccessful interventions with a logical approach will ensure that the clinician delivers the best care possible.

Patients with a fever | 10

Caryn Rosmarin and Ali Jawad

Introduction

Fever is one of the most common presenting features in the practice of any doctor who sees patients with acute illness. It is the hallmark of the body's response to infection or inflammation. Before looking at the causes of fevers it is important to understand what we mean by that term and how the reaction to it is generated in the body.

Fever is an increase in the core body temperature (the temperature within the deep tissues of the body) above the daily range for an individual. The daily range of core body temperature is between 35.6°C and 37.8°C (97.0°F and 100.4°F). The closest to core body temperature we can measure is rectal temperature. Because this is usually not easily performed and is less acceptable to patients, the next best is ear (tympanic) temperature. This requires a specific device that can be inserted into the ear using disposable covers. Oral temperature is about 0.5°C less than ear temperature and axillary temperature a further 0.5°C lower than oral temperature.

The normal core temperature of any individual does not remain static but varies according to certain rhythms and characteristics. It is affected by time of the day (known as diurnal variation), age, gender, height, time in the menstrual cycle, as well as with exercise and meals.

The diurnal variation of core body temperature is usually up to 0.6°C, but can be exaggerated with a variation of 2°C to 3°C. Core body temperature is at its highest in the late afternoon and evening, with lowest point in the early hours of the morning (Fig. 10.1).

How is normal core body temperature regulated?

Control of body temperature is termed thermoregulation. Under normal circumstances the body temperature will be in a state of stable internal temperature, or in homeostasis.

The temperature of the body depends on the balance between heat production and heat loss. Core body temperature is regulated by a system of control mechanisms affecting heat generation and heat loss. These include the autonomic nervous system, the endocrine system, musculoskeletal system and behavioural responses. The centre of this mechanism is called the thermoregulatory centre. It lies in the hypothalamus and acts like a thermostat in controlling the systems to produce the right balance of heat production and loss. The thermoregulatory centre has heat-sensitive receptors that respond to changes in body temperature by switching on and off systems to keep the balance within normal range. The range of temperature considered normal by the hypothalamus is termed the set point (Fig. 10.2). Damage to the hypothalamus can lead to loss of its thermostat control and result in very high or low core body temperatures.

Heat is gained and lost by the body through normal body functioning. Heat is produced all the time in the tissues of the body as a product of their metabolic processes. Heat is also produced by increased activity of skeletal muscles, such as during exercise or when shivering.

Normally, this heat is lost to the environment through transfer from deep tissues, via the blood stream, to body areas in contact with the outside. This is mostly through the skin, but also occurs through the lungs. Heat loss occurs through four main mechanisms called evaporation, convection, conduction and radiation as described in Box 10.1.

The amount of heat lost from the skin via the above mechanisms depends on environmental conditions, with more heat loss occurring in cold, dry and windy environments. When the temperature of the environment is higher than body temperature or when there is a lot of humidity, heat cannot easily be lost, leading to a rise in body temperature (Fig. 10.3).

What effects on thermoregulation lead to fever?

Despite fever being an indicator of an abnormal clinical finding, it is a normal physiological response. Although fever is an increase above normal in the core body temperature, it is not an indicator that the thermoregulatory system has lost control of its thermostatic function. It is rather a function of the up-regulating or resetting of the set point of the thermoregulatory centre to a higher level, much like

Figure 10.1 Diurnal variation of core body temperature.

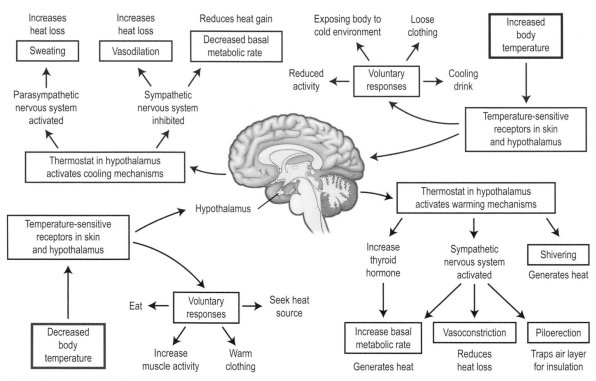

Figure 10.2 Regulation of core body temperature.

turning up the thermostat to a higher temperature. So long as the reset temperature remains below the range of the normal function of the thermoregulatory centre (<41.5°C) it will function to keep the body at this higher temperature. Above this temperature, the centre can no longer function to control body temperature and the fever is termed hyperpyrexia, a medical emergency requiring immediate and rapid cooling of the body.

Hyperthermia, on the other hand, is an example of a high temperature that is not a fever. It differs from a fever in that it is not associated with a change in the set

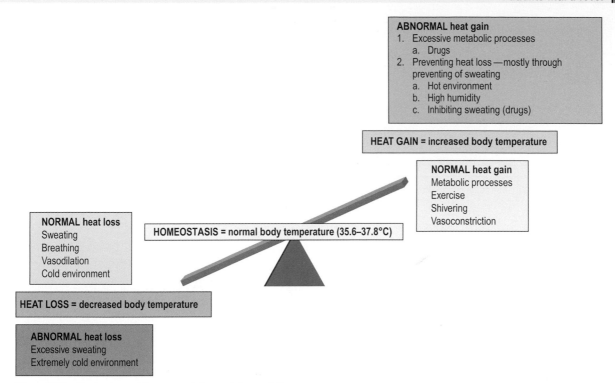

Figure 10.3   Mechanisms of thermoregulation and dysregulation.

point of the thermoregulatory centre, but occurs owing to raising the body temperature above the normal set point. It can be caused by heatstroke, neuroleptic malignant syndrome, malignant hyperthermia and stimulants such as amphetamines and cocaine.

Fever is produced when a stimulus from either outside (external) or inside (internal) the body is detected by the body's immune system as foreign, and a host of immune responses occur. External stimuli are usually in the form of infectious agents or drugs, whereas internal stimuli may be in the form of antibodies or damaged tissue. These (perceived) foreign objects activate the cells of the immune system to release chemical mediators called cytokines, including tumour necrosis factor alpha (TNF-α), interferon, IL-1 and IL-6. These cytokines act on the hypothalamus to reset the set point to a higher temperature or to 'turn up the thermostat'. Some bacterial proteins can act directly on the thermoregulatory centre in the hypothalamus to cause the same effect.

Elevation of the internal set point results in a higher core body temperature and causes the individual to feel cold. This leads to increased generation of heat and reduction of heat loss in the form of peripheral vasoconstriction and shivering. Rigors are a form of severe shivering.

Should you always treat a fever?

Because fever is a physiological response of the body, it must have some inherent value, and so is

there always a need to be so quick to reduce it? Benefits of having a high temperature include an increase in the phagocytic and bactericidal activity of neutrophils and the cytotoxic effects of lymphocytes, impairment of the growth and virulence of bacteria and evidence of survival benefit for individuals with an elevated body temperature in response to infection.

On the other hand, there are negative effects of a raised body temperature. Oxygen consumption and fluid and calorie requirements increase; increased metabolic activity can increase stress if organs are failing; inflammatory cytokines increase muscle breakdown; and fever can reduce mental acuity, cause delirium and trigger convulsions, especially in children.

Therefore, there is an indication to treat fever in those who are pregnant, in children, in those with impaired organ function or those with a very high temperature of >41.5°C.

Fever can be treated by increasing heat loss through physical cooling or by resetting the upregulated hypothalamic set point using antipyretics.

The patterns of fever

Fever can reveal a characteristic pattern in some diseases and this pattern of rise and fall of temperature may be a clue for diagnosis (Fig. 10.4).

Sustained/continuous: Persistent rise in temperature with minimal (<1°C) diurnal variation.
   Causes: Pneumonia, meningitis, urinary tract infection, brucella

Sustained fever

Normal range

①

Step-ladder fever: A type of sustained fever where the temperature rises gradually to a higher level with every spike.
   Causes: Typhoid, typhus

Step-ladder fever

Normal range

②

Intermittent: Exaggeration of the normal circadian rhythm. If the variation between high and low is extremely large it is called *hectic*.
   Causes: Deep seated infection, abscesses, kala-azar, malignancy, drug fever

Intermittent fever

Normal range

③

Remittent: Temperature spikes fall daily with diurnal variation of >2°C, but don't go down to normal.
   Causes: Tuberculosis, infective endocarditis, many viral and bacterial infections

Remittent fever

Normal range

④

Relapsing: Febrile episodes are separated by intervals of normal temperature.
   Causes: Malaria, borrelia (relapsing fever), tuberculosis, lymphoma

Relapsing fever

Normal range

If this occurs daily, it is called *quotidian* fever.
   Causes: *Plasmodium falciparum*

A *double quotidian* fever occurs when there are two spikes of fever every day, generally once in the morning and once in the evening.
   Causes: Miliary tuberculosis

If it occurs every 48 hours it is called *tertian* fever.
   Causes: *Plasmodium falciparum, Plasmodium vivax, Plasmodium ovale*

If it occurs every 72 hours it is called *quartan* fever.
   Causes: *Plasmodium malariae*

Quartan fever

Normal range

⑤

Inverse fever: The temperature rises in the early hours of morning rather than in the evening
   Causes: Some cases of miliary tuberculosis

⑥

Night sweats: In some diseases, the rise in body temperature is evident only in the evening or late at night when the patient is woken up sweating. This pattern is seen when the mild rise in temperature is added to the normal diurnal evening rise leading to the body temperature rising beyond the normal level.
   Causes: Tuberculosis, leukaemia, lymphoma, autoimmune disorders

⑦

Temperature-pulse disparity: This is the counter-intuitive response of a slower pulse associated with a high fever, commonly associated with typhoid fever.

⑧

Figure 10.4   The patterns of fever.

Approach to a patient with a fever— causes of fever

Fever is one of the most common presenting features at acute medical facilities around the world. Although it is a characteristic sign of infection, not all fever has an associated infectious cause. It is also a feature of a number of non-infectious inflammatory diseases (autoimmune connective tissue and autoinflammatory disease and vasculitis) and neoplasms. It may also occur as a drug reaction. In a significant number of cases, the temperature

Box 10.2	Causes of fever

- Infections
- Non-infectious inflammatory diseases
  - Autoimmune inflammatory
  - Autoinflammatory
  - Vasculitis
- Malignancy
- Miscellaneous causes such as drug reactions
- Undiagnosed

subsides spontaneously and no cause is identified (Box 10.2).

The likelihood that fever is caused by an infection differs from one area of the world to another and reflects the burden of disease in the particular country (Fig. 10.5). It is also important to remember that the very young and the very old may have a serious infection without producing a fever.

History

As with any medical condition, the starting point of diagnosis is a detailed and meticulous history. The history taking should follow a logical scheme to ensure important questions are not missed; causes of fever have a broad aetiology and can present as multisystem diseases. Taking a 'fever history' is unlike most other history taking, as it does not focus on a particular body system. Aspects of the personal, general and specific histories of all other systems need to be explored.

All histories should begin with an introduction, stating clearly your designation as a trainee, student or observer. Ensure you have the correct patient and that the patient understands the language. If the patient is a minor or a guardian or parent is present, be aware that certain sensitive questions may have to be asked at a later time when you are alone with the patient.

Main presenting complaint

Patients presenting with fever will often have a raft of associated complaints, many or all of which may be perceived as the main problem to the patient. It is therefore prudent to refer to the fever as the main presenting complaint and the associated complaints as part of the systematic history.

History of the presenting complaint

Details of the fever itself should be taken and the pattern described as continuous, intermittent or recurrent as noted above. Ask whether the fever is worse in the morning or at night. Some open-ended questions should be followed by direct questions to elicit the finer distinguishing characteristics of the fever. Remember that the taking of antipyretics, anti-inflammatories or antibiotics can mask a fever, so ask the patient if he has taken any medication. Enquire as to the duration of fever, which should reflect when the patient first noticed having a fever. This differs from the onset of fever that may be sudden or gradual; the former more likely to represent a more virulent disease, whereas the latter suggests a more indolent one. A description of the fever should include the presence or absence of *rigors* (profound chills associated with exaggerated shivering and chattering of teeth), which usually indicates a rapidly rising temperature found in malaria or severe bacterial sepsis.

High fever of more than 39°C is the initial symptom in most patients with adult onset Still's disease (AOSD). The classic fever pattern is one or two daily febrile spikes exceeding 39°C, usually occurring late in the day. At times the fever is continuous or, less commonly, there is an early morning spike.

Personal history

Although the patient's name, age and date of birth are used as identifiers, the country of birth and countries of residence are the first questions of the infection history. These are important both in respect to disease exposures and disease protection in the form of childhood and other vaccinations. Rates of diseases such as tuberculosis (TB) are higher in people who were born or resided in a country with a high incidence of tuberculosis, even if they have left the country. Vaccination schedules differ among countries and because of this, immunity to certain childhood diseases may vary.

History of associated and constitutional symptoms

These include the presence of any of the following:

- **Headache** is a non-specific symptom and does not differentiate the cause of the fever. A severe headache associated with photophobia or vomiting could indicate meningitis. Vasculitides affecting the head and neck vessels may present with headache.
- **Muscle ache** (myalgia) is again a non-specific finding present in all causes of fever. If infectious, myalgia is more suggestive of infection with intracellular pathogens, particularly viral infections and malaria.
- **Joint pain** (arthralgia) is an additional non-specific symptom, which may be caused by multiple infectious and non-infectious aetiologies. In a patient complaining of arthralgia, one should distinguish between mono-arthralgia (single joint) and poly-arthralgia (multiple joint) involvement.
- Presence or absence of a **rash** is particularly important to enquire about, because many infections and autoimmune disorders are associated with a typical rash, both in pattern and evolution. The rash may not be present at the time of consultation or it may have changed

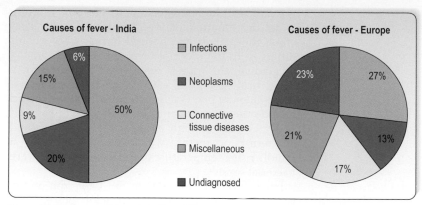

Figure 10.5 Causes of fever in India and Europe.

over the course of the illness. Ask details about the rash history, finding out where on the body it began, its associations, where it spread, whether the lesions changed over time and, if no longer present, how it resolved. Further details to help the diagnosis include details on the colour, type of lesion (e.g. vesicle, pustule, lacey) and whether it was pruritic, painful or neither. If the rash is intermittent, patients can be asked to photograph it with their mobile phone, and may have done so of their own accord.

- **Weight loss** in a patient with a fever suggests a more chronic process and is a classic feature of YB (consumption) or malignancy.
- A full systematic history should be included looking for a pattern of disease in systemic infectious or non-infectious disease, or a specific organ source of infection (e.g. cough, abdominal pain, dysuria, diarrhoea and redness or pain of skin or soft tissue).

History of behaviours and exposures are important in infectious diseases

- Contact with anyone having similar symptoms or living with someone who has been treated for an infection. It is also useful to know about close contacts who have not been ill.
- Living arrangements, including access to clean water and sanitation, proximity to animals or rodents. A history of insect or animal bite or scratches.
- Occupation, hobbies and sports, especially those involving exposure to water, animals or health care.
- Recreational habits, especially illicit drug use or tattoos.
- Sexual habits are vitally important and patients may need some encouragement to be open and honest about these risks. Unprotected sexual practices increase the risk of both sexually transmitted diseases and blood-borne viruses.
- Food habits, including ingestion of unpasteurized milk or cheese.

| Box 10.3 | Infections to consider if there is a history of travel |

Sub-Saharan Africa—malaria, reproductive tract infection (RTI), diarrhoeal illness, HIV, rickettsia, haemorrhagic fevers, TB, hepatitis

South East Asia—dengue, malaria, diarrhoeal illness

Sub-Continent Asia/India—enteric fever, dengue, malaria, diarrhoeal illness, hepatitis

South America—diarrhoeal illness, RTI, dengue, malaria, mosquito-borne viruses

Central America/Caribbean—diarrhoeal illness, RTI, dengue, malaria, mosquito-borne viruses

North America/Europe—influenza, HIV, Lyme, tick-borne viruses, TB (eastern Europe)

- Taking of appropriate prophylaxis, including vaccinations, either when travelling or at home.
- Travel is one of the most important histories to explore. Details of the destinations include whether the stay was in an urban or rural setting, stay was with family or friends, in a hotel or without facilities (Box 10.3).

Past medical and surgical history

Although all past history is important to obtain, certain aspects play a more important role as risks for infections.

- Infections are more frequent and more serious in patients with diabetes. A past history of rheumatic heart disease increases the risk for infective endocarditis. Previous TB assumes a risk of recurrence.
- Immune compromise increases the risk, severity and scope of infections. The patient's immune status should be determined, specifically by asking about underlying diseases, such as human immunodeficiency virus (HIV); medications, such as steroids or chemotherapy; or a history of a splenectomy.
- Recent hospitalization is associated with hospital-acquired multiresistant pathogens.

- Surgery, invasive procedures, medical devices, implants and transfusions all provide a means for introduction of infectious agents.
- Antibiotic use may select for more resistant pathogens and increases the risk of antibiotic-associated diarrhoea. Antibiotics may also provide protection against infection in certain groups of immune compromised patients.
- A history of immune compromise, radiation, toxin exposure or certain chronic infections may increase the risk of certain malignancies.
- A family history of non-infectious inflammatory diseases can indicate a genetic predisposition that may increase the risk of developing a non-infectious inflammatory disease.

Systematic history

Symptoms focusing on specific organ systems will provide direction towards the likely diagnosis when considering infectious causes of fever. Malignancies may also be found in any organ system. Non-infectious inflammatory diseases tend to affect multiple systems together, although a single system may predominate. The following detail focuses on infectious causes of fever.

Respiratory tract

- **Upper respiratory tract infection** is suggested by rhinorrhoea, nasal stuffiness, sneezing, sore throat, cough and a hoarse voice.
- **Sinusitis** is likely to cause facial pain and headache.
- **Otitis** is associated with ear pain, ear discharge with or without auditory symptoms such as deafness.
- **Lower respiratory tract infections** present with a cough, productive of purulent sputum, shortness of breath, wheeze or chest pain. Haemoptysis (coughing blood) suggests invasion of or damage to the blood vessels of the lung. This is present in TB, invasive fungal infection or non-infectious causes, such as lung cancer or vasculitis.

Genitourinary tract

- **Lower urinary tract infection** classically presents with a combination of dysuria, frequency, urgency and change in smell and colour of urine.
- **Upper urinary tract infection** may have the above (or a history of the above) with additional loin or back pain.
- **Sexually transmitted infections and pelvic inflammatory disease** can present with the same symptoms as a lower or upper urinary tract infection, but may have the additional symptoms of a vaginal or urethral discharge, dyspareunia (pain during intercourse), anogenital ulcers, genital warts, painful swelling of the scrotum, pubic itch or swelling of lymph glands in the groin.
- **Vaginal candidiasis** is not uncommon in women, particularly those who use vaginal douches or after a course of antibiotics. It may present as urinary tract infections do with a whitish vaginal discharge and vaginal itching.
- **Bacterial vaginosis** is not considered a true infection, but rather an imbalance of normal vaginal flora and overgrowth of anaerobes. It presents with watery, foul-smelling vaginal discharge.

Gastrointestinal tract

Abdominal pain may be present with almost all gastrointestinal causes of infections, but may be less prominent than pain caused by inflammatory or malignant gastrointestinal diseases. It is important to characterize the pain, including the site and radiation, associated abdominal symptoms and relieving and aggravating factors.

- **Gastroenteritis**, the most common gastrointestinal infection, is associated with abdominal pain and diarrhoea, with or without vomiting. Characterizing the diarrhoea may help in narrowing the aetiology owing to the characteristic pathogenesis of some of the gastrointestinal pathogens. Determining whether the diarrhoea is acute or chronic can distinguish infective from non-infective causes. Direct questions to ask about diarrhoea include frequency, colour and consistency, presence of mucus and/or blood in the stool (rather than just on the paper).
- **Hepatitis** is usually caused by viral agents, but can also occur as a complication of medications or other toxins. Jaundice is the classic sign of hepatitis, along with a history of exposure to risk factors involving contact with body fluids or excretions. Leptospirosis, a rare cause of jaundice, is caused by an organism that is carried by rats.
- **Cholecystitis and cholangitis** classically present with pain in the right upper quadrant of the abdomen associated with nausea with or without jaundice.
- **Other forms of intra-abdominal infection,** including bowel perforation and peritonitis, present with varying abdominal symptoms, including generalized or localized abdominal pain, bowel distension, diarrhoea, constipation or vomiting.

Nervous system

Headache, photophobia, vomiting, altered consciousness, fits, fainting, muscle weakness, numbness, paralysis, tremor, abnormal sensation and change of behaviour can all suggest an infection of the central nervous system. In neonates and young children the symptoms of infection are mostly non-specific.

Patients with multisystem non-infectious inflammatory diseases can have central and peripheral nervous system symptoms. A variety of neurological complications can be present, including spinal cord involvement in rheumatoid arthritis, neuropsychiatric involvement in systemic lupus erythematosus and neurological sequelae in vasculitic disorders.

Certain predisposing factors play a role in various forms of nervous system infection. A history of immune suppression, head injury and neurosurgery should be elicited.

- **Meningitis** is an inflammation of the subarachnoid space and meninges (membranes covering the brain and spinal cord) most often secondary to an infection. It classically presents with headache, vomiting, neck stiffness and fever. Depending on the duration of onset, meningitis can be classed as acute, subacute or chronic. Acute meningitis develops over hours to days; chronic meningitis over weeks or longer, and may last for months to years; subacute meningitis is in between the two, usually over weeks.
- Acute meningitis is most often bacterial, with the frequency of pathogens differing according to age group and immune status. Some forms of acute bacterial meningitis (meningococcal disease) can present with a typical purpuric non-blanching rash and may be associated with severe sepsis and shock. Viral meningitis is usually less severe and self-limiting and often begins with symptoms of a viral infection, such as fever, malaise, headache and muscle aches.
- Head injury increases the risk of meningitis by damaging the protective layer of meninges and allowing respiratory or skin flora into the protected subarachnoid space. Neurosurgery predisposes to infection with the above and also hospital-acquired pathogens.
- Chronic meningitis presents with the same symptoms as acute, only over a more prolonged period. Associated features should be sought for the more common causes of chronic meningitis, including tuberculosis, cryptococcus and Lyme disease.
- **Encephalitis** is inflammation of the brain tissue resulting in an altered level of consciousness, headache and fever. Additional symptoms may be present, depending on the site of infection, and they include seizures, tremors, stroke, hallucinations and abnormal behaviours. Encephalitis is usually viral in aetiology, but may also be bacterial (e.g. syphilis) or parasitic (e.g. toxoplasmosis).
- **Intracranial abscesses** are bacterial infections of the central nervous system (CNS); they include brain abscess, subdural or extradural empyema, classified according to their anatomic location. These abscesses occur secondary to seeding from a primary site, either from a contiguous one such as in otitis media, sinusitis, mastoiditis or dental infection; secondary to haematogenous spread from a remote site such as endocarditis; after a head injury or neurosurgery and, rarely, following meningitis.

Not all patients with nervous system symptoms and fever have a primary nervous system infection. Some systemic infections can cause neurological symptoms, such as severe or cerebral malaria, neurologic signs in severe typhoid fever and meningeal signs in HIV seroconversion illness.

Skin and soft tissue

A detailed history of any skin conditions should be sought, even if this is not present at the time of consultation. Many skin conditions and rashes have a characteristic course, may fluctuate or change over time and therefore a full 'progress report' of the condition can help to guide the diagnosis. The presence of a rash is more likely to suggest a systemic rather than a localized condition. Many multisystem non-infectious inflammatory diseases have an associated rash, such as the typical butterfly facial rash of systemic lupus erythematosus and petechial rash in vasculitic disorders.

Remember to ask about any insect or tick bites; rashes following a bite (including an eschar at the bite site) could indicate a vector-borne disease.

It is important to distinguish a generalized rash illness from a localized skin or soft tissue lesion. The latter is more likely to be asymmetrical or unilateral, involve tissues deeper than the skin, affect surrounding structures and be associated with localized enlarged lymph nodes.

Some examples of localized infections include:
- **Impetigo** is a contagious infection caused by staphylococci or, occasionally, streptococci, found mainly in preschool children or in other ages associated with playing contact sports. It usually starts as a small pustule around the nose or mouth which bursts, oozes fluid and leaves a golden crust. It characteristically occurs in groups of lesions.
- **Cellulitis** is a bacterial infection of the skin involving deeper structures most commonly affecting the leg. Other causes of a red or swollen leg should be excluded before the diagnosis is made. Cellulitis is rarely bilateral. Certain groups of people are at increased risk, including diabetics. It can affect any area of the body and facial cellulitis should be managed as a medical emergency.
- **Necrotizing fasciitis** is a severe and rapidly spreading form of cellulitis. It is a medical emergency and requires urgent surgical as well as antibiotic management. Pain that is disproportionate to the visible inflammation or swelling is an important clue to the presence of necrotizing fasciitis.
- **A history of human or animal bite or scratch** preceding the infection is important to elicit because specific pathogens are associated with these, including blood-borne virus transmission.

Musculoskeletal system

Bone, joint and muscle pain can form part of the constitutional symptoms of infectious and non-infectious diseases.

- **Joint infections** occur in both native and prosthetic joints. A history of joint replacement or joint procedure, such as arthroscopy, increases the risk of infection developing in the joint. In a patient complaining of arthralgia, one should distinguish between mono-arthralgia (single joint) and poly-arthralgia (multiple joint) involvement. Mono-arthralgia is more likely to be a septic arthritis in the affected joint whereas poly-arthralgia suggests a more systemic disease. Many viral infections and collagen vascular diseases present with poly-arthralgia.
- **Bone infection** (osteomyelitis) can occur in any bone in the body, either as a primary infection or secondary to an overlying skin or soft tissue infection or previous surgical procedure. Bone pain, swelling, deformities, pus draining through the skin overlying a bone or a persistent soft tissue infection close to a bone should alert you to the possibility of this diagnosis.
- **Adult onset Still's disease** presents with a classic triad of persistent high spiking fevers, joint pain and a distinctive evanescent salmon pink, macular or maculopapular rash that peaks with the rise in the temperature. The rash occurs mainly on the trunk and extremities, but rarely involves the palms of the hands, the soles of the feet or the face. Joint pains may range from arthralgia to a severe arthritis. Other features include lymphadenopathy, hepatomegaly and splenomegaly, sore throat and constitutional symptoms, such as anorexia, arthralgia, myalgia, fatigue and weight loss. The classic fever pattern is one or two daily febrile spikes exceeding 39°C, usually occurring late during the day. At times the fever is continuous or, less commonly, spikes in the early morning.
- Although fever and constitutional symptoms occur in around half the patients with **polymyalgia rheumatica,** they are rarely the dominating features.

Cardiovascular system

- **Infective endocarditis** is an infection of the endocardium or lining of the heart. The most common form of this infection is infection of the heart valves. Symptoms are usually non-specific and the diagnosis should be considered in patients with damaged or prosthetic heart valves or those patients with risk factors for recurrent bacteraemias (e.g. poor dentition, intravenous drug use, long-term use of a intravascular device or underlying bowel cancer).
- **Myocarditis**, an inflammation of the muscle of the heart, is usually caused by viral infections. Symptoms are non-specific and may include chest pain, shortness of breath or palpitations.
- **Vascular infection** can occur as primary vascular infection of the endothelium or secondary to damage caused by catheters or cannulas, trauma or surgery. Occasionally vascular grafts, such as for aortic aneurysm, can become infected.

Examination

General assessment

Examination should begin when you first make visual contact with the patient. Get a general impression of whether the patient looks well, unwell or severely ill. Summaries of the pertinent features are described in Table 10.1.

Systematic assessment

A systematic and thorough examination of all organ systems may be necessary to elicit the cause of the fever. Both autoimmune disorders and systemic infections may produce clinical findings in multiple organ systems, and the pattern and collection of signs should be able to be collated into a single cause most of the time. It is not unusual for those with compromised immune systems or those who have travelled to have more than one infection at a time.

Skin and mucous membranes

Rashes are of particular importance and many infectious diseases present with a rash. Describe the location of the rash. Is it generalized, localized, symmetrical or asymmetrical? Rashes may indicate either a localized or generalized infection. Some rashes are typical of the causative infection; a few examples are given in Table 10.2.

Fever and constitutional symptoms, although common in patients with antineutrophil cytoplasmic antibodies (ANCA)-associated vasculitis (AAV), rarely occur in isolation. Palpable (non-thrombocytopenic) purpura is present in half the patients. Erythematous cutaneous nodules, with or without superficial crusting, may occur on the scalp, elbows, hands and feet (cutaneous extravascular necrotizing granulomas or Churg-Strauss granulomas) in patients with granulocytosis with polyangiitis (GPA) and eosinophilic granulocytosis with polyangiitis (EGPA). Subcutaneous nodules, skin ulcers, subungual splinter haemorrhages, digital gangrene and livedo reticularis may be seen and, mainly in EGPA, urticarial rash (Box 10.4).

Mild fever may accompany around a fifth of patients with Behçet's syndrome (BS) with active lesions. Febrile attacks seem to be associated strongly with vascular, neurological or joint involvement. Other features of BS include mouth and genital ulcers, erythema nodosum-like lesions, pyoderma gangrenosum, folliculitis and uveitis.

Respiratory tract

Perform a full respiratory examination looking for signs of upper respiratory tract infection, such as pharyngitis, tonsillitis, tonsillar abscess (quinsy) or otitis.

Use palpation, percussion and auscultation to determine whether there is any suggestion of a

Table 10.1 General examination in patients with fever	
Temperature	Oral or ear temperature is preferred to axillary to give a closer indication of core temperature. Ear temperature is 0.5°C higher and axillary temperature is 0.5°C lower than oral temperature. Fever is defined as a core temperature above normal. In clinical practice this translates to an oral temperature of ≥38.3°C.
Pulse	Tachycardia is characteristic during fever. For every 1°C rise in temperature the pulse increases by 10 beats per minute. A pulse-temperature dissociation is characteristically seen in typhoid, brucellosis, leptospirosis and diphtheria.
Respiratory rate	For every 1°C rise in temperature the respiratory rate rises by 4 breaths per minute. Higher respiratory rates signify additional lung pathology such as pneumonia.
Blood pressure	Hypotension may signify severe sepsis or septic shock.
Lymph nodes	Note the pattern and groups involved. Check cervical, axillary and inguinal areas. Describe the consistency of the nodes. Are they firm, hard, regular, irregular, mobile or fixed? Are enlarged lymph nodes unilateral, bilateral, above and/or below the diaphragm? Note the size of the lymph nodes and whether a single or multiple lymph nodes are present. Significant lymphadenopathy is found in TB, brucellosis, toxoplasmosis, viral infections such as HIV or infectious mononucleosis. They are also a predominant feature of lymphoma and metastatic spread of malignancies.
Jaundice	Examine the conjunctivae, nail beds and skin for evidence of jaundice. This may indicate underlying either haemolysis, such as in malaria and haemorrhagic fevers, or liver disease as in viral hepatitis, cholangitis or liver abscess.
Eyes	Conjunctivitis may indicate a localized eye infection or be associated with a systemic infection such as measles. Roth's spots on the retina may be found in infective endocarditis. Tubercles of miliary TB may be found on the choroid.
Ears	Inflammation and redness of the external ear canal indicates otitis externa, whereas a bulging red eardrum suggests otitis media. If the eardrum has perforated, fluid or pus may be found in the external ear canal.
Mouth	Examination of the mouth may yield a host of information and should include visualization of the inner cheeks, palate, tongue, pharynx, tonsils, gums and teeth. General oral and dental hygiene should be noted. Lesions on the wall of the mouth or palate should be characterized as described for skin rashes below. White lesions may indicate oral thrush; the throat and tonsils should be examined for erythema and exudates; ulcers in or around the mouth may indicate oral herpes. Dry mouth is a feature of some non-infectious inflammatory diseases.
Skin	The entire surface of the skin should be examined, because a lesion or rash may be present only in an area hidden to view in a clothed individual. Describe and characterize any rash, petechiae and areas of redness or swelling. Determine if there are any open wounds, ulcers or bite marks, including an eschar. The presence of open wounds, intravascular devices or injection sites should be noted and closely examined for signs of erythema, swelling or tenderness. Intravascular devices may be the source of either localized skin or disseminated infections.
Hands and nails	Splinter haemorrhages on the palms and nail beds require further investigation for infective endocarditis. Scaly, itchy lesions between the fingers suggest the presence of scabies mites. Typical nail deformities of non-infectious inflammatory diseases, such as psoriasis, should be noticed.

Table 10.2 Examples of rashes in patients with fever	
Maculopapular	Scarlet fever, measles (look for conjunctivitis and white lesions in the mouth — Koplik's spots), rubella, erythema infectiosum, roseola, typhus, typhoid (rose spots), dengue, rickettsial infection
Vesicular	Herpes simplex, chicken pox, shingles, coxackie virus, allergy
Petechial, purpuric, haemorrhagic, vasculitic	Meningococcal (non-blanching), viral haemorrhagic fevers, dengue, splinter haemorrhages of infective endocarditis, non-infective vasculitis
Erythematous	Cellulitis, erysipelas, drug allergy
Pustular	Staphylococcal, disseminated gonococcal infection
Rash on palm and soles	Enteroviral infections, meningococcal infection, spotted fever, typhus, infective endocarditis, secondary syphilis, scabies (burrows between fingers and toes)
Nodular	Erythema nodosum, TB, leprosy, non-infective vasculitis, Behçet's syndrome

---

Box 10.4	ANCA-associated vasculitis

- Granulomatosis with polyangiitis (GPA) (Wegener's granulomatosis)
- Eosinophilic granulomatosis with polyangiitis (EGPA) (Churg–Strauss syndrome)
- Microscopic polyangiitis (PA)

---

lower respiratory tract infection such as bronchitis, pneumonia, pleural effusion or empyema, cavitation or lung abscess.

Palpate for tenderness over the sinuses or mastoids.

Harshening of normal breath sounds may indicate inflammation of the bronchi in bronchitis. The presence of consolidation in the lung indicating pneumonia can be determined by finding dullness to percussion along with increased vocal resonance of crepitation and/or bronchial breathing. Pleural effusion or empyema is suggested by dullness to percussion and decreased or absent vocal resonance. Cavitation or abscess formation suggesting TB produces an increase in resonance.

The presence of rhinorrhoea, nasal congestion, sneezing, cough and a hoarse voice suggest a viral upper respiratory tract infection.

Cardiovascular system

The diagnosis of infective endocarditis is based on the modified Duke's criteria. Although relying mainly on investigations for confirmation, certain clinical signs are suggestive and should be looked for in patients with risk factors. These include new valvular regurgitation, temperature more than 38°C, splinter and conjunctival haemorrhages, Janeway lesions (small, non-tender red lesions on the palms or soles) and Osler's nodes (painful, red raised lesions on hands and feet) (see Box 13.25.)

Infected thrombophlebitis or vasculitis may occur secondary to a cannula or catheter insertion into a vein or as a primary infection of the vessels by certain pathogens (*Campylobacter fetus*, non-typhi *Salmonellae*), usually in immunocompromised patients.

Genitourinary tract

Examine for suprapubic and renal angle tenderness in suspected cases of urinary tract infection. Note the presence or absence of a urinary catheter.

Genital examination should be performed with a chaperone present, if requested, or when a male clinician is examining a female patient.

Female genital examination is best performed in lithotomy position to enable ease of examination. External examination should note any evidence of redness, swelling, vaginal, urethral or anal discharge, vesicles, ulcers, warts or foreign bodies. Unilateral swelling of the labia may indicate an abscess of the Bartholin's gland, which can be palpated only when enlarged.

The groin should be examined for evidence of lymphadenopathy or diseases such as tinea, candida or pubic lice.

Speculum examination allows examination of the cervix as well as the vaginal vault. If a discharge is present, describe its consistency. Candidiasis is white and cheesy, whereas trichomonas infection gives a frothy greenish fish-smelling discharge. A purulent discharge coming from the cervix is suggestive of gonococcal infection, whereas chlamydia causes a more mucoid or mucopurulent discharge. Cervical warts may appear as flat or raised.

If anal lesions or symptoms are present, a proctoscope can be used to examine the rectal mucosa.

A bimanual examination is required for palpation of cervical excitation tenderness, fallopian or uterine tenderness in suspected pelvic inflammatory disease.

Male genital examination includes examination of the penis, scrotum, testes, epididymis, spermatic cord and anorectum. External examination should note the presence of any ulcers, warts, excoriations or rashes. Examine the urethral meatus for any discharge or ulcer not visible on external examination. Examine the scrotum for redness, swelling, ulcers or other lesions. Tenderness on palpation of the testes and/or epididymis may suggest epididymo-orchitis.

Gastrointestinal tract

Abdominal examination begins by inspection of the patient with an exposed abdomen between the xiphisternum and symphysis pubis (allowing for patient privacy).

Determine if ascites or abdominal swelling is present and whether the abdomen is tender. Palpate for the presence of hepatomegaly, splenomegaly or a distended gall bladder and whether any of these organs are tender.

Splenomegaly may be present in many diseases, caused by either an increase in its function or by direct infiltration. Infectious causes of increased function are owing to immune stimulation in response to the infection and include infectious mononucleosis, viral hepatitis, AIDS, typhoid, brucellosis, tuberculosis, histoplasmosis, infective endocarditis, leptospirosis, leishmaniasis and malaria.

Infective causes of hepatomegaly include infectious mononucleosis, liver abscess, amoebic infection, hydatid cyst, malaria, leptospirosis and actinomycosis. Viral hepatitis rarely causes an enlarged liver.

Nervous system

Global examination of the nervous system includes cognitive as well as physical function. The level of consciousness can be determined using the Glasgow Coma Score. Reduced, altered or fluctuating levels of consciousness may be present in any infection of the central nervous system, but is more likely in encephalitis and brain abscess than in meningitis.

The characteristic triad signs of meningitis include nuchal rigidity (neck stiffness), photophobia and headache. To detect neck stiffness, passively bend the patient's chin towards the chest. This will elicit pain by stretching the inflamed meninges leading to resistance in movement. Other signs caused by pain on stretching the inflamed meninges include Brudzinski's and Kernig's signs.

Kernig's sign is positive when the thigh is bent 90 degrees at both the hip and knee, and the knee is then straightened leading to pain and resistance. Brudzinski's sign is positive if the patient involuntary lifts his legs when the clinician lifts the patient's head off the examination bed.

Focal neurological signs could be suggestive of a space-occupying lesion, such as a brain abscess, tuberculoma or toxoplasmosis. Focal signs may also be present owing to cranial nerve involvement caused by meningitis.

Some forms of nervous system infection have associated features which should be noted. Meningococcal meningitis may occur with a typical purpuric non-blanching rash.

Musculoskeletal system

Joint infections occur in both native and prosthetic joints. A history of joint replacement or joint procedure, such as arthroscopy, increases the risk of infection developing in the joint. In a patient complaining of arthralgia one should distinguish between mono-arthralgia (single joint) and poly-arthralgia (multiple joint) involvement. Mono-arthralgia is more likely to be a septic arthritis in the affected joint whereas poly-arthralgia suggests a more systemic disease. Many viral infections and collagen vascular diseases present with poly-arthralgia. Septic arthritis with major pathogens, such as staphylococci, usually result in a joint that is extremely painful when movement is attempted.

Bone infection (osteomyelitis) can occur in any bone in the body, either as a primary infection or secondary to on overlying skin or soft tissue infection or previous surgical procedure. Bone pain, swelling, deformities or pus draining through the skin overlying a bone should alert you to the possibility of this diagnosis. Spinal infection can affect the bone itself, as in Pott's disease caused by tuberculosis or the intervertebral disc, most often caused by staphylococcal infection, when spinal percussion is often tender.

Rheumatic fever can occur in any age group, but is rare under the age of 3 and above 15 years. In Western countries, acute rheumatic fever is generally preceded 2 to 4 weeks by group A streptococcal (GAS) tonsillopharyngitis, but not by GAS skin infections. Fever is one of the four minor manifestations of rheumatic fever and may be high or low. The period between the GAS infection and the onset of rheumatic fever is free of clinical features and C-reactive protein is normal. The most common major manifestation of rheumatic fever is arthritis followed by pancarditis, chorea (Sydenham's), erythema marginatum and subcutaneous nodules.

Although fatigue is a prominent complaint in idiopathic inflammatory myositis, fever occurs mainly in patients with **juvenile dermatomyositis** and anti-synthetase syndrome. Other features include Raynaud's phenomenon, hyperkeratosis especially of the radial side of the index fingers (mechanic's hands), polyarthritis and interstitial lung disease. These patients have positive antiaminoacyl-tRNA synthetase antibodies such as Jo-1.

About one-fifth of patients with relapsing **polychondritis** present with fever and in the absence of chondritis of the external ear and the nose, the diagnosis may be difficult to make.

Multisystem diseases

Fever in autoinflammatory periodic syndromes

Apart from Familial Mediterranean Fever (FMF), the autoinflammatory periodic syndromes are rarely encountered in routine clinical practice (Box 10.5). Nearly 90% of patients with FMF become symptomatic before the age of 20 years. However, genetic testing has helped diagnose mild disease in adults. More males are affected than females. A typical acute attack, usually lasting 1 to 3 days, is characterized by fever, serositis and arthritis or skin rash. The attacks may recur every few weeks, but may be as infrequent as every few years. Acute abdominal pain, owing to acute sterile peritonitis, occurs in 90% of patients. Pleurisy is another clinical feature, but it mainly occurs in patients of Armenian origin. The term FMF is confusing because in a significant number of cases, there is no family history, no Mediterranean roots (Arabs, Armenians, Italians and Jews) and fever may be absent. The patient may present with acute arthritis or an erysipelas-like erythema (neutrophilic dermatosis) with mild or even absent fever. The arthritis may last up to a week.

Nearly two thirds of patients with polyarteritis nodosa develop fever and constitutional symptoms (arthralgia, myalgia, malaise and weight loss). Hypertension, usually mild, is present in up to half the patients, particularly in those with hepatitis B viral infection. Cutaneous lesions include livedo reticularis (Fig. 10.6), ischaemic changes in the digits (Fig. 10.7), subcutaneous nodules and ulcerations.

Fever and constitutional symptoms may be the main clinical features in patients with **Takayasu's arteritis**. In more than half the patients, peripheral pulse is decreased or absent. In a small number of patients, the inflammation of the wall of the carotid artery may cause local tenderness (carotidynia).

Fever in patients with systemic lupus erythematosus (SLE) can prove a challenging clinical problem. Fever may be a major feature in about two fifths of patients with active SLE. Infection is not easy to exclude and the fever may be drug induced. Very rarely the fever may be caused by lymphoma complicating lupus. The most challenging situation is when the patient

| Box 10.5 | The classic periodic fever syndromes (monogenic autoinflammatory diseases) |

- Familial Mediterranean fever (FMF)
- TNF receptor-associated periodic syndrome (TRAPS)
- Hyperimmunoglobulinemia D with periodic fever syndrome (HIDS)

Table 10.3 Mechanisms of drug fever

Mechanism	Examples
Hypersensitivity	Anticonvulsants, penicillin, minocycline, sulfonamide, allopurinol
Altered thermoregulatory mechanisms	Thyroxine, drugs with anticholinergic activity, amphetamine, cocaine
Directly related to administration of the drug	Paraldehyde, pentazocine, amphotericin B, bleomycin
Direct extension of the pharmacologic action of the drug	Chemotherapy
Idiosyncrasy	Succinylcholine, haloperidol, serotonin syndrome

Figure 10.6   Livedo reticularis in a 39-year-old woman with polyarteritis nodosa.

Figure 10.7   Ischaemic changes in the right second digit in a 39-year-old woman with polyarteritis nodosa.

with lupus presents with high fever, respiratory symptoms and radiographic changes. The difficulty is whether the radiographic changes are caused by complicating infection or organizing pneumonia.

Fever is not a feature in patients with uncomplicated scleroderma.

Drug fever

Drugs can cause fever via several mechanisms (Table 10.3). This is a diagnosis by exclusion. A rash is not always present nor is eosinophilia. By definition, the fever coincides with administration of the drug and disappears when the drug is discontinued. The risk of developing drug fever increases with the number of drugs prescribed, especially in elderly patients, patients with active HIV infection and patients with cystic fibrosis.

Investigations for infectious causes of fever

Testing for infectious disease should include both laboratory and radiological investigations.

Laboratory

Both routine and specialist tests should be performed in the haematology, chemistry, microbiology and virology laboratory where appropriate.

Full blood count with differential and film

White blood cell count is often raised in infection, although a low count may indicate specific pathogens or overwhelming infection. In patients on immune suppression or chemotherapy the white cell count should not be used as a marker of infection because it may be falsely raised or suppressed.

- **Neutrophilia** with band forms and toxic granulation suggest bacterial infection.
- **Neutropenia** may be seen post chemotherapy or with typhoid fever, brucellosis, severe sepsis or viral infection.
- A reactive **lymphocytosis** may be seen in acute viral illnesses, particularly infectious mononucleosis when atypical lymphocytes may be present. It may also occur in tuberculosis, brucellosis or in leukaemias and lymphomas.
- **Lymphopaenia** is common in viral infection (influenza, dengue, HIV) and typhoid fever.
- **Eosinophilia** is seen in hypersensitivity reactions, as well as in invasive parasitic infections.

Platelets

- **Thrombocytopaenia** may be seen in malaria, haemorrhagic fevers, meningococcal sepsis or disseminated intravascular coagulation (DIC) associated with overwhelming infection.

- **Thrombocytosis** may occur as an acute response to inflammation or can occur in chronic infections such as TB.

A **blood film** or smear is used to look for parasites that may be present in the blood. The most common of this is malaria, but can also be used to detect babesia, trypanosomiasis or microfilaria. It may suggest Epstein-Barr virus (EBV) if atypical lymphocytes are seen.

Inflammatory markers

Acute-phase reactants (APRs) are a heterogeneous group of plasma proteins that increase or decrease in response to inflammatory stimuli such as infections, trauma, arthritis, autoimmune disorders and malignancies. The levels of APRs rise and fall in response to the rise and fall of the inflammatory process. Common tests used for this purpose include C-reactive protein (CRP) and erythrocyte sedimentation rate (ESR) and, more recently, procalcitonin (PCT). ESR is an indirect APR because it measures the rate of movement of red blood cells, which is increased by binding of an APR. Most APRs are produced in the liver.

The ESR rises fairly rapidly (within 24–48 hours) from the onset of inflammation and is slow to fall once the cause of inflammation resolves. It has a low sensitivity for infection and is affected by many factors, including age, gender, weight and renal function. Despite this, an ESR over 100 mm/hour warrants further investigation.

CRP is a more sensitive marker of inflammation than ESR and is less affected by external factors such as age and gender. It rises more rapidly (within 6–24 hours) and is quicker to fall than ESR. Very high levels of CRP are more likely to be associated with bacterial infection than other causes of inflammation.

Procalcitonin has several advantages over both ESR and CRP. It rises within 3–4 hours, quicker than either ESR or CRP, and a result can be obtained in 30 minutes or less using a semiquantitative point-of-care test. It is a more sensitive marker of bacterial infection because raised PCT levels are not seen in other non-infectious inflammatory conditions, and viral infections tend to inhibit PCT rather than raise it. It can, however, be raised in invasive fungal infection, malaria, by massive trauma such as severe burns or major surgery, any therapy that stimulates cytokines such as T-cell antibody therapy, granulocyte transfusion or graft-versus-host disease.

The usefulness of the above tests may differ, depending on the situation and site of infection.

Basic biochemistry tests

Renal and liver function tests are useful in determining the presence of any renal or hepatic impairment, which may assist in determining severity of disease and affect antimicrobial dosing. Abnormal liver function tests may also assist in diagnosis of gastrointestinal infections such as hepatitis or cholecystitis. Serum ferritin is hugely raised in adult onset Still's disease.

Microbiology and virology tests

The type of samples sent will depend on the site of infection identified. A few examples are listed below.

Blood cultures should be taken if you suspect the patient may have bacteraemia from any source. The signs of sepsis, severe sepsis or septic shock should be used to indicate the need to take these cultures. If possible, two sets should be taken aseptically prior to any antibiotic therapy. There should be a low threshold for taking blood cultures, before antibiotics are given, so as not later to regret the missed opportunity to take antibiotic-free cultures.

Bone marrow cultures may be more useful than blood cultures for some intracellular pathogens.

Sample any fluid that represents the possible site of infection as follows:

1. Urine
   - Dip, culture and microscopy for lower or upper urinary tract infection and urogenital infections
   - Molecular tests for urogenital infections
   - Urine antigen testing for Legionella and *Streptococcus pneumoniae* in cases of community-acquired pneumonia
2. Urethral, vaginal and cervical swabs for urogenital infections
   - Culture and microscopy for lower or upper urinary tract infection and urogenital infections
   - Molecular tests for urogenital infections
3. Cerebrospinal, peritoneal, joint and pleural fluid, biopsy tissue, sputum and bronchoalveolar lavage
   - Microscopy, culture and sensitivity for bacterial and fungal infection
   - Ziehl-Neelsen (ZN) staining and culture for acid-fast bacilli for diagnosis of TB
   - Molecular tests for viral pathogens
4. Stool
   - Culture and sensitivity for bacterial infection
   - Microscopy for parasites
   - Molecular tests for viral pathogens
5. Pus and tissue samples from abscesses, surgical debridement, biopsies and wound infections
   - Microscopy, culture and sensitivity for bacterial and fungal infection
   - ZN staining and culture for acid-fast bacilli for diagnosis of TB

Serology

Serology is used mainly in the diagnosis of viral infections. A positive IgM usually indicates current or recent infection and a positive IgG indicates a previous infection or vaccination. The following are common serology tests used in the diagnosis of infectious diseases:

Rash diseases: Measles, rubella, parvovirus, varicella, rickettsia, typhus, syphilis

Gastrointestinal infection: Viral hepatitis, cytomegalovirus (CMV), amoebic liver abscess

Systemic infections: HIV, Lyme disease, dengue, brucellosis, leptospirosis

Molecular diagnostics

This diagnostic platform is used mainly in the diagnosis of viral infections, but is increasingly used for bacterial, fungal and parasitic infections. It is a rapid and sensitive technique and is not affected by previous antibiotic treatment or the inability to culture the pathogen. Most sample types can be used for molecular diagnostics. It is used routinely to diagnose viral infections, such as gastroenteritis, respiratory tract infections, central nervous system infections and viral haemorrhagic fevers. Bacterial infections commonly diagnosed in this way include pertussis, meningococcal disease and tuberculosis.

Immunological tests

Systemic lupus erythematosus is defined by the presence of autoantibodies. Antinuclear and double-stranded antibodies, antibodies to the extractable nuclear antigens and complement 3 and 4 need to be tested. The predictive value of ANCA testing depends on the clinical presentation of the patient and the laboratory performing the test. It is best that all reasonable attempts to confirm clinical suspicions of systemic vasculitis with histopathological proof should be undertaken before treating the patient with potentially toxic medications.

Histopathology

Biopsy and staining of lymph nodes, tissue, fluid or bone marrow may reveal infectious structures such as caseating granulomas, acid-fast bacilli, protozoal cysts, fungal hyphae or spores.

Radiology

Imaging studies may help to elucidate the source and extent of infection in those with a fever and localized site. All modalities of imaging have a role in diagnosis with the indications for X-rays, including ultrasound, computed tomography (CT) and magnetic resonance imaging (MRI) scanning, depending on the site of infection being investigated. Radionucleotide or PET scan may be more sensitive at defining foci of infection.

Pyrexia of unknown origin (PUO)

Despite an adequate history, examination and set of investigations, the cause of some fevers remains unknown. This is termed a PUO or pyrexia of unknown origin. The classic definition of a PUO is a fever of more than 38.3°C for more than 2 weeks during which time there has been at least:

- Three separate outpatient appointments, OR
- 3 days in hospital, OR
- 1 weeks' worth of appropriate and thorough investigation

Box 10.6	Common disease presenting atypically
Bacterial	

Abscesses (dental, subphrenic, liver, ovarian, prostate)
Vascular infections
Extrapulmonary TB, atypical mycobacteria
Protected sites
    – Sinuses/Ears
    – Heart
    – Prostate/Ovaries
    – Bone, joint, intervertebral disc
    – Thyroid
Partially treated infections

Viral

Immune compromised host
Partial immunity

Fungal

Immune compromised host

Protozoal and rickettsial

Travel history

Box 10.7	Uncommon disease presenting typically
Bacterial	

Brucella	HACEK organisms*
Bartonella	Leptospirosis
Atypical mycobacteria	Nocardia
Borrelia	Actinomycosis

Viral

HIV	EBV, CMV
Hepatitis D & E	Viral haemorrhagic fever

Fungal

Cryptococcus	Histoplasmosis

Protozoal

Malaria	Leishmaniasis
Amoebiasis	Schistosomiasis
Trypanosomiasis	Toxoplasmosis

Rickettsial

Q fever

Mycoplasmas

*HACEK includes *Haemophilus parainfluenzae, Haemophilus aphrophilus, Actinobacillus, actinomycetemcomitans, Cardiobacterium hominis, Eikenella corrodens,* and *Kingella kingae.*

Infections account for 40% of cases of PUO. Causes of a PUO often fall into one of two categories:
1. A common disease presenting in an atypical way
2. An uncommon disease presenting typically

A common disease presenting in an atypical way requires more thought about the less-common sites of infection, acquiring samples from more protected sites, consideration of testing in the immune compromised and the possibility of partially treated infections (see Boxes 10.6 and 10.7 for examples.)

An uncommon disease presenting in a typical manner requires thought about travel, occupation, pets, hobbies, habits and any other unusual activity that may present an infection risk.

Non-infectious causes of a PUO need to be considered; they include neoplasms, autoimmune syndromes, granulomatous diseases, drug fevers and other miscellaneous causes, such as haematomas, brain lesions, hyperthyroidism, tissue ischaemia or infarction.

A thorough history, examination and investigations, as described above, should be performed on all patients with pyrexia of unknown origin, and the examination repeated from time to time.

Patients in pain | 11

Shankar Ramaswamy

Introduction

Pain is a familiar phenomenon that is part of our everyday life and is a feature of various diseases. It most commonly accompanies an injury, where it serves its most important purpose, namely, to protect us, alert us and make us remove ourselves from danger. It can possibly trigger a spinal withdrawal reflex (Fig. 11.1). Both congenital insensitivity to pain and extreme sensitivity to pain (paroxysmal extreme pain disorder and erythromelalgia) are rare genetic conditions, which are disabling and shorten life span, highlighting the importance of pain to our welfare and survival. Pain severity and its impact on an individual ranges from a trivial occurrence, such as a needle-prick injury, to a sensation of such intensity that it induces thoughts of suicide.

Definition

The International Association for the Study of Pain (IASP) proposed the following definition (1979): 'Pain is an unpleasant sensory and emotional experience associated with actual or potential tissue damage or described in terms of damage'. This definition has important implications. Pain is not necessarily or always associated with ongoing tissue damage; rather, it is a subjective experience and has an emotional as well as a sensory component and is always unpleasant.

Pain is notoriously difficult to describe and even harder to assess and quantify. Nevertheless, pain assessment is crucial in order to evaluate its impact on the sufferer and also to plan a treatment strategy. It has been termed 'the 5th vital sign' and is mandated as part of routine assessment of patients in hospital. In 2004 the IASP declared that the relief of pain should be a human right.

Although pain is a major source of suffering and economic burden for patients, until recently, it was not considered as a separate condition and systematically classified. Recognizing this, the World Health Organisation (WHO), in their recent adoption of the International Classification of Diseases (ICD-11) in May 2019, for the first time included chronic or longstanding pain as an independent disease and paved the way for a systematic classification of the condition.

Classification of pain

There are many ways in which pain can be classified in order to formulate an optimal treatment strategy. Despite this, classifying a particular pain state can be challenging because the pain syndrome may be of mixed aetiology rather than fit into a single category.

Pain is commonly classified according to the following:
- Aetiology and underlying condition
- Mechanism
- Duration

Aetiology/underlying condition

- Trauma: an acute response to an injury
- Surgery
- Medical illness, such as myocardial infarction or appendicitis
- Physiological conditions, such as menstruation and labour
- Cancer

Mechanism

- Inflammatory/Nociceptive: Pain generated and maintained by inflammatory mediators (such as prostaglandin E_2), secondary to an ongoing disease process. Examples include inflammatory arthritis.
- Neuropathic: Neuropathic pain, which is generated in malfunctioning nerves, is defined as 'pain arising as a direct consequence of a lesion or disease affecting the somatosensory system'. This type of pain has special clinical features as described below and may arise from injury or dysfunction of the central or peripheral nervous system. Examples include painful diabetic neuropathy and post-stroke pain.
- Nociplastic: Nociplastic pain is a new terminology described in 2017. It is defined as pain that arises from altered nociception despite no clear evidence of actual or threatened tissue damage causing the activation of peripheral nociceptors or evidence for disease or lesion of the somatosensory system causing the pain. Examples include fibromyalgia, complex regional pain

Figure 11.1 Spinal withdrawal reflex with pain.

'Spinal withdrawal reflexes'
Rapid behavioural response

'Perceive unpleasant sensation'
Dominates attention

Modify behaviour

Pain 'warning system' essential for survival

syndrome (CRPS) type 1, some 'musculoskeletal' pain conditions, such as 'nonspecific' chronic low back pain, and 'functional' visceral pain disorders, such as irritable bowel syndrome, bladder pain syndrome.

- Mixed pain: This includes features of both nociceptive and neuropathic pain, such as back pain with radiculopathy (radiating leg pain caused by nerve irritation or compression).
- Psychosomatic: Pure psychosomatic pain is rare. However, pain, especially chronic pain, almost invariably has an emotional and behavioural component.

Duration

- Acute: Most commonly a physiological response to an injury. It resolves with the disappearance of a noxious stimulus or within the time frame of a normal healing process.
- Chronic: It can either be associated with an ongoing pathological process, such as rheumatoid arthritis or degenerative disc disease, or be present for longer than is consistent with a normal healing time. Pain is arbitrarily described as chronic if it persists for longer than 3 months. Chronic pain is often associated with disability, mood and sleep disturbance and a significant behavioural response.

Mechanisms of pain

At its simplest, pain is generated by a noxious stimulus that excites the central nervous system. This mechanism was first proposed by Descartes in the 16th century and conceptually still holds true. However, it is crucial to appreciate that the final subjective experience of pain is shaped by various modulatory factors (Fig. 11.2).

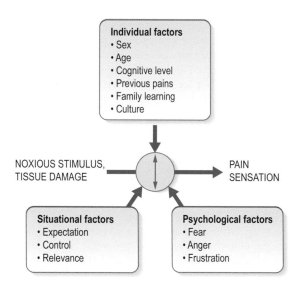

Figure 11.2 Biopsychosocial model of pain.

A stimulus (which can be thermal, pressure or chemical) excites nociceptors and the resulting impulse is then transmitted to the spinal cord by two different classes of nerve fibres, via the first-order neurons located in the dorsal root ganglion (Fig. 11.3): (i) faster, myelinated Aδ fibres and (ii) smaller, slower unmyelinated C fibres. They transmit the sensation to the dorsal horn of the spinal cord, where these primary afferents synapse in lamina I, lamina II (substantia gelatinosa), lamina IV and some in lamina V. All these afferent sensory fibres are excitatory. Second-order fibres are then carried in the spinothalamic and spinoreticular tracts to the thalamus, where they synapse. From the thalamus, third-order neurons project to the somatosensory cortex, anterior cingulate gyrus and the insular cortex, where they terminate. It is at this cortical level that a stimulus is perceived as pain (see Fig. 11.3).

Cingulate cortex

Somatosensory cortex

Thalamus

Insular cortex

Amygdala

Periaqueductal grey

Parabrachial nucleus

Rostral ventral medulla

Brain stem

Nociceptor

Spinal cord

Figure 11.3   Pain pathway.

However, it is now known that the noxious sensory input may be modulated at several levels in the spinal cord and brain, thus altering the final pain experience. The gate control theory proposed by Melzack and Wall in 1965 states that non-noxious stimulation of the large Aβ fibres inhibits the response to painful stimuli of neurons with wide dynamic range (WDR neurons, located primarily in lamina V of spinal cord), reducing the input of small fibres mediating the sensation of pain. A good example of this modulation at the spinal level is 'rubbing it better' i.e. rubbing a painful area can decrease the intensity or perception of pain. In addition, descending input from higher centres (periaqueductal grey matter and rostral ventral medulla) also modulates neural activity in the spinal cord, reducing or enhancing the pain sensation. Such descending input is one of the mechanisms by which emotional and cognitive factors modulate pain perception. Much remains to be understood about the central pathophysiology of pain.

In recent years, pain management has increasingly adopted a biopsychosocial model. This has highlighted the need to take into account the interactions between biological, psychological and social factors leading to an individual's emergent pain experience.

The patient in pain

As with any other branches of medicine, careful and meticulous assessment of a patient's symptoms and signs is fundamental. Two key questions should be considered when dealing with a patient in pain:

- Is the pain a symptom of ongoing tissue damage or of another condition that needs to be dealt with by another medical professional?
- What is the optimal treatment strategy: either to abolish the pain altogether or reduce it to a more bearable level?

History

Taking a history from a patient in pain is more complex than recording symptoms and making a diagnosis. Even in acute pain states, where pain represents a protective function and is a symptom of an injury, approaching the patient as a whole and bearing in mind the overall context, emotional, cognitive and behavioural aspects is crucial for optimizing the treatment strategy.

The first step is to evaluate the pain and thereby try to understand its underlying mechanisms. This process is described in Boxes 11.1 and 11.2 and Tables 11.1 and 11.2.

Examination

The purpose of examination as part of pain evaluation is described in Box 11.3.

Detailed examination will focus on different systems according to a particular pain condition. It may involve basic orthopaedic, neurological or surgical examination. Regardless of the approach, it should follow conventional basic methods: inspection, palpation and range of movement, where appropriate. For example, a patient who presents with back pain will require at least inspection to check for muscle spasm, posture, deformity, gait and use of aids, such as crutches, and evidence of previous surgery; palpation of paravertebral and bony areas; and range of movement to evaluate any restriction. The examination will also need to include a neurological examination looking at dermatomal sensory dysfunction (suggesting radiculopathy) and particular tests (depending on the region of the spine) to detect signs of nerve root irritation using stretch tests such as Lasègue's test (or straight leg raising test) for low back pain; and for the neck, the Spurling test (turning the patient's head to the affected side while extending and applying downward pressure to the top of the patient's head; a positive test is indicated by pain arising in the neck radiating in the direction of the ipsilateral corresponding dermatome). The examination should also assess glove and stocking sensory loss (characteristic of peripheral neuropathy), reflexes and plantar response, muscle power, sensation and reflexes.

As part of the clinical examination it is important to elicit features of neuropathic pain, such as allodynia (pain caused by a stimulus that does not usually provoke pain, for example a light touch using cotton wool eliciting pain), and hyperalgesia or hypoalgesia (increased or decreased pain, respectively, from a stimulus such as pressure or pinprick that usually provokes pain).

Investigation

Investigation of a patient in pain is tailored to the individual's presentation. It serves three important goals:
- To exclude more sinister pathology
- To provide diagnostic clues
- To arrive at an optimal management strategy

The most common investigation employed by pain specialists is imaging, for example using simple X-rays to exclude a pathological fracture, MRI

Box 11.1 Scheme for evaluating history associated with pain

- The site of pain: This may give a clue to the underlying pathology.
- Distribution: Pain may follow a dermatomal or peripheral nerve distribution or have no relation to anatomical patterns.
- Character of pain: Nociceptive (somatic or visceral) versus neuropathic (see Table 11.1).
- Duration of pain: This may have a bearing on the level of disability and psychosocial cost of the pain.
- Rapidity of onset and any precipitating factors: A rapid or relatively recent-onset pain syndrome is more likely to follow a conventional medical model, whereby it is appropriate to search for an underlying cause. Chronic pain requires a more biopsychosocial approach.
- Severity of pain and its change over time: This requires a consistent method for measuring pain (see below).
- Alleviating and exacerbating/aggravating factors: These may support a better understanding of mechanisms that sustain the pain.
- Exclusion of more sinister pathology: 'Red flags'. Important conditions not to be missed include pain related to underlying (or undiagnosed) cancer, pain related to inflammation (such as rheumatoid arthritis) and pain related to other serious medical/surgical conditions requiring emergency treatment such as cauda equina syndrome caused by spinal cord compression.
- Evaluation of psychosocial elements also known as 'yellow flags' (see Box 11.2): These are not life-threatening symptoms, but their presence means that the psychosocial history has special relevance. Major psychological illness should be addressed, along with symptomatic relief of the pain, in the interim.
- Previous and current treatments and their impact
- Past medical history: Taking a full medical history must not be overlooked. It may give invaluable clues as to the aetiology and pathogenesis of pain. For instance, history of recent herpes zoster (shingles) infection along with a dermatomal distribution of neuropathic-type pain (confirmed on examination with a residual, typical rash, allodynia and hypoalgesia/hyperalgesia) will suggest a diagnosis of postherpetic neuralgia. Certain common illnesses associated with neuropathic pain are listed in Table 11.2.
- Impact of pain: Consider the effect of pain on the patient's activity, ability to work, mood, sleep, relationships, etc.
- Psychosocial history: The psychosocial assessment of pain should be directed at finding the psychological setting of the pain, particularly mood. It should explore the patient's beliefs and expectations. Generally speaking, this is more relevant in chronic pain states, because acute pain usually resolves quickly.

to demonstrate changes within the central nervous system or an ultrasound examination of the abdomen or soft tissues and joints. Neurophysiological (EMG) studies are helpful to determine the presence and extent of any nerve damage, and various blood tests may be used to determine, for example, the activity of rheumatoid arthritis. Any test used must be considered only as a part of a more global approach, never in isolation. Some tests such as Quantitative Sensory Testing and functional imaging using PET-CT or fMRI are used in the research setting to understand more about the underlying pain mechanisms.

By the end of the assessment, any pathology that needs to be dealt with by the relevant medical professional should be identified, either for urgent management, if 'red flags' are elicited, or electively.

Difficult cases

As the history is the key to pain assessment and treatment, it is clear that communication is paramount. Difficulty arises if there is a language barrier between the physician and the patient, if the patient is a young

---

Box 11.2 Psychosocial aspects of pain

Pain is described as having at least five dimensions, each of which should be addressed:

- The sensation of pain — the subjective experience
- Suffering and distress — the emotional component
- Expectations and beliefs — the cognitive component
- Verbal (complaints) or non-verbal communication — the behavioural component (illness behaviour) is the way in which the patient responds to and expresses the sensation of pain, which is influenced by various cultural and social factors
- Impact of social environment

Table 11.1 Nociceptive versus neuropathic pain

	Nociceptive	Neuropathic
Description of pain	Aching, localized, toothache-like, sharp, squeezing	Shooting, radiating, stabbing, burning, electric shock-like
Movement impact	Associated with movement	Independent
Physical examination	Normal response	Allodynia, hyperalgesia, vasomotor changes
Examples	Injury, postoperative pain	Peripheral neuropathies, shingles, cancer pain
Treatment strategies	More classic approach, conventional analgesics	More biopsychological approach, conventional analgesics ± non-conventional (antidepressants, anticonvulsants, etc.)

Table 11.2 Common illnesses associated with chronic pain

Illness	Nature of pain disorder
Diabetes	Diabetic neuropathy: Commonly glove and stocking peripheral neuropathic pain
Connective tissue disorder	Variable presentation of accompanying neuropathy
HIV	Neuropathy owing to disease as well as to antiretroviral drugs
Trauma	Multifactorial aetiology: Associated nerve injury causing neuropathy and or complex regional pain syndrome
Herpes zoster infection	Post-herpetic neuralgia: Neuropathic pain with dermatomal distribution
Multiple sclerosis	Central neuropathic pain, including trigeminal neuralgia
Cerebrovascular accident	Post-stroke central neuropathic pain
Fibromyalgia	Nociplastic musculoskeletal pain, usually primary but could be secondary to other disorders, such as connective tissue disease
Complex regional pain syndrome	Most likely owing to previous injury: Usually has features of allodynia, hyperalgesia and vasomotor changes of the extremities, recently classified as nociplastic pain
Chronic post-surgical pain	Variable incidence following variety of surgeries causing neuropathic pain
Degenerative bone and joint disease	Variable sites: Mostly nociceptive, but with possible neuropathic component
Phantom limb pain	Neuropathic pain following amputation, most commonly of extremities
Cancer	Cancer and its treatment, such as radiotherapy and chemotherapy, cause chronic pain with neuropathic and/or nociceptive features

- To elucidate and evaluate any physical signs associated with a particular painful condition
- To reassure the patient that pain does not imply any ongoing damage
- To define baseline parameters and monitor their change over time
- To understand the mechanisms that generate and sustain the pain, in particular to identify neuropathic elements

child or has learning difficulties, confusion or dementia. It is important as a physician to understand that the pain a patient perceives could be influenced by social and cultural factors as well as past experience. The pain may prove refractory to treatment, with all treatment options already exhausted, which again can pose a challenging situation, necessitating a change in goal setting.

Measuring pain

Pain is a subjective experience and therefore difficult to quantify. However, being able to quantify pain will aid management by assessing severity and allowing the measurement of treatment or intervention effect and is crucial in research studies looking at new treatment modalities. Measurement tools may be unidimensional or multidimensional, with the latter being more useful in chronic pain conditions.

Unidimensional scales

Unidimensional scales are used very commonly, particularly in cases of acute pain. They are simple, sensitive, reproducible and quickly applied and give a numerical value to the pain severity. They can be either analogue or discrete. The latter may be numerical or verbal.

The most common of these scales is the Visual Analogue Scale (VAS): The patient is given a horizontal line 10 cm long with 'no pain' on the left-hand side and 'worst possible pain' on the right and is asked to mark the line according to the severity of the pain.

The numerical rating scale: The patient is asked to assign a number from 0 to 10 to his pain, 0 being no pain at all and 10 being the worst imaginable pain. In the verbal rating scale the patient rates his pain into one of the following categories: none, mild, moderate or severe.

Multidimensional (complex) scales

The development of multidimensional scales acknowledges the multidimensional impacts of pain on a

sufferer's life. Common scales used include the McGill Questionnaire and Brief Pain Inventory. The original McGill Questionnaire assesses various aspects of pain, including sensory qualities of pain, affective qualities (e.g. tension, fear) and has evaluative words that describe the subjective intensity of the total pain experienced. Various measurements are derived from the data, but a short form of the McGill Questionnaire is most often used (Fig. 11.4). It is easy to apply and is reproducible.

To build up a complete assessment of a patient with longstanding disabling pain, a battery of measurement tools may be required, which may include anxiety and depression measurement scales, catastrophizing scales and disability index.

To assess for neuropathic pain, recently introduced and validated tools such as the 'painDETECT' and 'LANSS' questionnaires are used to look for specific features pertaining to neuropathic pain.

Treatment strategies

Acute pain

Acute pain management should be directed to the treatment of the underlying cause as well as symptomatic pain relief itself. For example, fractures should be reduced and immobilized and infections treated with antibiotics. Pain in the acute setting as well as that caused by cancer is then treated symptomatically with analgesic drugs in accordance with the WHO pain ladder (Fig. 11.5). Pharmacological options include simple analgesics, such as paracetamol, non-steroidal anti-inflammatory drugs and opioids. There is also an option for considering local anaesthetic nerve blocks, especially for pain following surgery and trauma. It is increasingly recognized that poorly treated acute pain can result in a chronic pain state, which can become quite refractory to treatment.

Chronic pain

In chronic pain the emphasis shifts from management of the pain itself to addressing its psychosocial sequelae and improving the patient's function. This often involves a multimodal treatment approach under the umbrella of a biopsychosocial model. The pharmacological options include the same as that for acute pain, but medications can be less effective. In particular, there should be less emphasis on the use of strong opioids in chronic pain, because they become less effective and are associated with significant short-term as well as long-term side effects. The British Pain Society guidelines on the use of opioids for persistent pain recommend a maximum dose of 120 mg morphine-equivalent

I. Pain Rating Index (PRI):
The words below describe average pain. Place a check mark (✓) in the column that represents the degree to which you feel that type of pain. Please limit yourself to a description of the pain in your pelvic area only:

		None		Mild		Moderate		Severe
a	Throbbing	0		1		2		3
	Shooting	0		1		2		3
	Stabbing	0		1		2		3
	Sharp	0		1		2		3
	Cramping	0		1		2		3
	Gnawing	0		1		2		3
	Hot-Burning	0		1		2		3
	Aching	0		1		2		3
	Heavy	0		1		2		3
	Tender	0		1		2		3
	Splitting	0		1		2		3
b	Tiring-Exhausting	0		1		2		3
	Sickening	0		1		2		3
	Fearful	0		1		2		3
	Punishing-Cruel	0		1		2		3

II. Present Pain Intensity (PPI)–Visual Analog Scale (VAS). Tick along scale below for pelvic pain:

No pain   Worst possible pain

III. Evaluative overall intensity of total pain experience. Please limit yourself to a description of the pain in your pelvic area only. Place a check mark (✓) in the appropriate column:

Evaluation		
0	No pain	
1	Mild	
2	Discomforting	
3	Distressing	
4	Horrible	
5	Excruciating	

IV. Scoring

		Score
I-a	S-PRI (Sensory Pain Rating Index)	
I-b	A-PRI (Affective Pain Rating Index)	
I-a+b	T-PRI (Total Pain Rating Index)	
II	PPI-VAS (Present Pain Intensity-Visual Analog Scale)	
III	Evaluative overall intensity of total pain experience	

Figure 11.4 Short form McGill Pain Questionnaire.

dosage per 24 hours in the non-specialist setting. The Faculty of Pain Medicine, UK has developed an 'Opioid Aware' initiative to guide patients and health care professionals in the prescription of opioid medicines for pain. Chronic pain often has a neuropathic component, which is treated with antineuropathic agents, including antidepressants such as amitriptyline and anticonvulsants such as gabapentin and pregabalin.

Non-pharmacological options

The non-pharmacological management of chronic pain is multidisciplinary and is usually available only through specialized pain clinics. A detailed discussion is beyond the scope of this chapter, but pain management may include interventional techniques such as spinal injections (e.g. with steroids), radiofrequency therapy, neuromodulation, acupuncture and transcutaneous nerve stimulation and also involve physiotherapy, occupational therapy and psychological techniques. The aim is to provide physical and psychological rehabilitation leading, where possible, to patient self-management. As the presence of chronic pain can be considered a long-term illness or a disease, the goal for treatment is to attain a good functional outcome rather than being pain free.

Essential pain management approach

More recently, an 'Essential Pain Management' (EPM) programme has been developed with the aim of teaching a systematic approach to pain management. EPM uses the pneumonic 'RAT' (*r*ecognize, *a*ssess, *t*reat) in order to develop a structure (Fig. 11.6). As

Step 3
Strong opioid
e.g. morphine, hydromorphine, oxycodone, buprenorphine, fentanyl, methadone

Step 2
Weak opioid
e.g. codeine, dihydrocodeine, tramadol

Step 1
Non-opioid
e.g. aspirin, ibuprofen, diclofenac, COX-2 inhibitors, paracetamol

• The World Health Organization (WHO) guidelines advocate that when pain occurs, there should be prompt oral administration of drugs, administered in accordance with steps 1–3.

• To maintain freedom from pain, drugs should be taken 'by the clock' every 3–6 hours, rather than 'on demand' and each patient should receive tailored pain management.

• This 3-step approach of administering the right drug in the right dose at the right time is inexpensive and 80–90% effective.

Figure 11.5   WHO pain ladder.

Figure 11.6   Essential pain management (EPM). (A) A RAT: Like pain, a rat causes a lot of suffering, but is often hidden from view. (B) A core EPM framework.

Ⓐ

Recognize
● **Impact of pain**
  ○ patient and society
Assess
● **Type**
  ○ Acute/chronic
  ○ Nociceptive/neuropathic
  ○ Cancer/non-cancer
● **Intensity**
● **Other factors involved in presentation**
  ○ Psychology
Treat
● **Non-pharmacological**
● **Pharmacological, guided by pain type**

Ⓑ

an example, based on such a structured assessment, it can be concluded that:

The patient has mild/mod/severe (severity), acute/chronic (duration), nociceptive/neuropathic/mixed (mechanism) pain, owing to cancer/non-cancer (cause) aetiology, with (or without) a significant impact on physical and/or psychological function (other factors).

Further details on EPM can be obtained from: https://www.accs.ac.uk/faculty-of-pain-medicine/essential-pain-management/epm-uk and http://fpm.anzca.edu.au/fellows/essential-pain-management.

Conclusion

Pain is complex and essentially a patient-reported, subjective phenomenon. Pain assessment includes unidimensional and also multidimensional tools looking at its social and psychological consequences as well as its sensory characteristics. With wide inter-patient variability, perhaps more than with any other symptom, management must be individualized to the context and needs of each patient.

SECTION 3

BASIC SYSTEMS

Respiratory system | 12

Veronica L.C. White

Introduction

Diseases of the respiratory system account for up to a third of deaths in most countries and for a major proportion of visits to the doctor and time away from work or school. As with every aspect of diagnosis in medicine, the key to success is a clear and carefully recorded history; symptoms may be trivial or extremely distressing, but either may indicate serious and life-threatening disease.

The history

Most patients with respiratory disease will present with breathlessness, cough, excess sputum, haemoptysis, wheeze or chest pain.

Breathlessness

Everyone becomes breathless on strenuous exertion. Breathlessness inappropriate to the level of physical exertion, or even occurring at rest, is called dyspnoea. Its mechanisms are complex and not fully understood. It is not caused simply by a lowered blood oxygen tension (hypoxia) or a raised blood carbon dioxide tension (hypercapnia), although these may play a significant part. People with cardiac disease (see Chapter 13) and even non-cardiorespiratory conditions, such as anaemia, thyrotoxicosis or metabolic acidosis, may become dyspnoeic as well as those with primarily respiratory problems (Box 12.1).

An important assessment is whether the dyspnoea is related only to exertion and how far the patient can walk at a normal pace on the level (exercise tolerance). This may take some skill to elicit, because few people note their symptoms in this form, but a brief discussion about what they can do in their daily lives usually gives a good estimate of their mobility (Box 12.2).

Other clarifications will include whether the symptoms vary, whether there are good days and bad days and, very importantly, whether there are any times of day or night that are usually worse than others. Variable airways obstruction caused by asthma is very often worse at night and in the early morning. By contrast, people with predominantly irreversible airways obstruction owing to chronic obstructive pulmonary disease (COPD) will often say that as long as they are sitting in bed, they feel quite normal; it is exercise that troubles them.

Cough

The symptom of cough can be short-lived or last years; cough can be defined as acute (lasting fewer than 3 weeks) or chronic (lasting more than 8 weeks) (Box 12.3). A cough may be dry or it may produce sputum. Acute cough is most commonly caused by recent infection, either viral or bacterial; however, any cough that is associated with haemoptysis should be a cause for concern, prompt appropriate assessment and a baseline chest X-ray (CXR) at the very least. Any patient with a chronic cough (i.e. one that lasts more than 8 weeks) should also be sent for a CXR and spirometry as baseline investigations (Box 12.4). Discussion about cough should include:

- How long has the cough been present? A cough lasting a few days following a cold has less significance than one lasting several weeks in a middle-aged smoker, which may be the first sign of a malignancy.
- Is the cough worse at any time of day or night? A dry cough at night may be an early symptom of asthma, as may a cough that comes in spasms lasting several minutes.
- Is the cough aggravated by anything, for example allergic triggers such as dust, animals or pollen, or non-specific triggers such as exercise or cold air? The increased reactivity of the airways seen in asthma and in some normal people for several weeks after viral respiratory infections may present in this way. Severe coughing, whatever its cause, may be followed by vomiting (Box 12.5).

Sputum

- Is sputum produced?
- What does it look like? Children and some adults swallow sputum, but it is always worth asking for a description of its colour and consistency. Yellow or green sputum is usually purulent. People with

Box 12.1	Causes of breathlessness	
Acute	**Subacute**	**Chronic**
Airways obstruction	Pneumonia	COPD
Anaphylaxis	Exacerbation of COPD	Pleural effusion
Asthma	Angina	Malignancy
Pneumothorax	Cardiac tamponade	Chronic pulmonary emboli
Pulmonary embolus	Metabolic acidosis	Restrictive lung disorders, including interstitial lung disease
Myocardial infarction	Pain	Congestive cardiac failure
Pulmonary oedema	Pontine haemorrhage	Valvular dysfunction
Arrhythmias		Cardiomyopathy
Anxiety		Diastolic dysfunction
		Pulmonary hypertension
		Anaemia
		Neuromuscular disorders
		Deconditioning
		Obesity

COPD, chronic obstructive pulmonary disease.

Box 12.2	Medical Research Council grading of dyspnoea (breathlessness scale)

1. Not troubled by breathlessness except on strenuous exercise.
2. Short of breath when hurrying or walking up a slight hill.
3. Walks slower than contemporaries on the level because of breathlessness, or has to stop for breath when walking at own pace.
4. Stops for breath after about 100 m or after a few minutes on the level.
5. Too breathless to leave the house, or breathless when dressing or undressing.

Box 12.3	Causes of cough	
Causes of cough	**Examples**	
Respiratory	Viral or bacterial infection, bronchospasm, COPD, non-asthmatic eosinophilic asthma, bronchiolitis, malignancy, parenchymal disease (e.g. ILD, bronchiectasis, cystic fibrosis, sarcoidosis, pleural disease, aspiration)	
Upper airways disease	Post nasal drip, sinusitis, inhaled foreign body, tonsillar enlargement, laryngopharyngeal reflux (LPR)	
Cardiovascular disease	LVF, mitral stenosis	
Gastro-oesophageal disease	GORD	
Neurological disease	Aspiration	
Drugs and irritants	ACE inhibitors, cigarette smoke	

ACE, angiotensin converting enzyme; COPD, chronic obstructive pulmonary disease; ILD, interstitial lung disease; LVF, left ventricular failure; GORD, gastro-oesophageal reflux disease—also associated with laryngopharyngeal reflux (LPR).

Box 12.4	Five most common causes of chronic cough with a normal CXR

- Post viral upper respiratory tract infection (URTI)
- Smoking
- Asthma—including cough variant asthma and non-asthmatic eosinophilic asthma
- Post nasal drip (hay fever)
- Gastro-oesophageal reflux disease (GORD)

Box 12.5	Important questions in the history of chronic cough

- Have you had a recent cold, sore throat or viral infection?
- Do you have a history of asthma, nocturnal cough or wheeze?
- Do you experience nasal discharge, hay fever or sinusitis?
- Do you suffer from acid reflux, indigestion or coughing after meals?
- What time of day is the cough worse?
- Do you smoke?
- Are you breathless?
- Have you coughed up blood?
- Do you have a hoarse voice?
- Have you had fevers or night sweats?
- Have you lost weight?
- Are you getting chest pain?

asthma may produce small amounts of very thick or jelly-like sputum, sometimes in the shape of a cast of the airways. Eosinophils may accumulate in the sputum in asthma, causing a purulent appearance even when no infection is present.

- How much is produced? When severe lung damage in infancy and childhood was common, bronchiectasis was often found in adults. The amount of sputum produced daily often exceeded a cupful. Bronchiectasis is now rare, and chronic bronchitis causes the production of smaller amounts of sputum.

Haemoptysis

Haemoptysis is the coughing up of blood in the sputum. It should never be dismissed without very careful evaluation of the patient. The potentially serious significance of blood in the sputum is well

Box 12.6	Causes of haemoptysis

- Malignancy and benign lung tumours, including lung metastasis
- Pulmonary infection, including bacterial pneumonia, tuberculosis (TB), lung abscesses and fungal infection
- Bronchiectasis including cystic fibrosis
- Pulmonary emboli
- Congestive heart failure
- Pulmonary fibrosis
- Pulmonary vasculitis
- Severe pulmonary hypertension
- Arteriovenous malformation
- Chest trauma and foreign bodies
- Endometriosis
- Anticoagulation or coagulopathy
- Drugs (e.g. cocaine, thrombolytics)

known, and fear often leads patients not to mention it. A specific question is always necessary, as well as an attempt to decide if it is fresh or altered blood, how much is produced, when it started and how often it happens (Box 12.6).

Blood may be coughed up alone, or sputum may be bloodstained. It is sometimes difficult for the patient to describe whether the blood has originated from the chest or whether it comes from the gums or nose or even from the stomach. Always ask patients about associated conditions, such as epistaxis (nose bleeds) or the subsequent development of melaena (altered blood in the stool), which occurs in the case of upper gastrointestinal bleeding. Usually, however, it is clear that the blood originates from the chest, and this is an indication for further investigation.

Wheezing

Always ask whether the patient hears any noises coming from the chest. Even if a wheeze is not present when you examine the patient, it is useful to know that he has noticed it on occasions. Sometimes wheezing will have been noticed by others (especially by a partner at night, when asthma is worse) but not by the patient.

Sometimes stridor (see Chapter 22) may be mistaken for wheezing by both patient and doctor. This serious finding usually indicates narrowing of the larynx, trachea or main bronchi. Also, it is not unusual for patients with a pneumothorax to describe 'rubbing' or 'gurgling' sounds in their chest which may well be owing to the displaced lung.

Pain in the chest

Apart from musculoskeletal aches and pains consequent upon prolonged bouts of coughing, chest pain caused by lung disease usually arises from the pleura. Pleuritic pain is sharp and stabbing and is made worse by taking a deep breath or coughing. It occurs when the pleura is inflamed, most commonly by infection in the underlying lung. More constant pain, unrelated to breathing, may be caused by local invasion of the chest wall by a lung or pleural tumour.

A spontaneous pneumothorax causes pain which is worse on breathing, but which may have more of an aching character than the stabbing pain of pleurisy. If a pulmonary embolus causes infarction of the lung, pleurisy and hence pleuritic pain may occur, but an acute pulmonary embolus can also cause pain that is not stabbing in nature. A large pulmonary embolus causing haemodynamic disturbance may cause cardiac-type chest pain. Costocondritis and Tietze's syndrome can also cause acute pain and tenderness in the chest wall owing to inflammation around the chondrosternal joints.

Other symptoms

Quite apart from the common symptoms of respiratory disease, there are some other aspects of the history that are particularly relevant to the respiratory system.

Upper airway

Questions related to the ear, nose and throat are relevant. Rhinosinusitis often coexists with asthma or, less commonly, bronchiectasis and can be an aggravating factor. A common cause of chronic cough is postnasal drip secondary to rhinitis. A change in the voice may indicate involvement of the left recurrent laryngeal nerve by a carcinoma of the lung. Sometimes patients using inhaled corticosteroids for asthma develop oropharyngeal candidiasis or even hoarseness or weakness of the voice, which improves on changing the treatment. Laryngopharyngeal reflux (LPR) increasingly is recognized as a cause of hoarseness and chronic cough and can be diagnosed on direct visualization of the upper airway. However, do not ascribe hoarseness to these causes in older patients, because carcinoma of the vocal cords can also be present with hoarseness or a change in the quality of the voice. Laryngoscopy is always indicated if hoarseness persists for more than 4 weeks.

The smoking and recreational drug history

Always take a full smoking and recreational drug history. Do so in a sympathetic and non-judgemental way, or the detail is unlikely to be accurate. The time for advice about smoking cessation is after completion of your assessment, not at the outset. Simply asking 'Do you smoke?' is not enough. Novices will be astonished at how often closer probing of the answer 'no' reveals that the patient gave it up yesterday or that he states his intention of doing so from the time of your consultation. Age of starting and stopping, if an ex-smoker, and average consumption for both current and ex-smokers are the bare minimum information needed.

Identifying an individual as a current or ex-smoker will greatly influence the interpretation you place on your findings upon history and examination. Almost all cases of lung cancer and COPD occur in those who have smoked.

Recreational drug use tends to be more common in younger people, but do not assume that this is the case and ask all patients, of all ages, from all walks of life about such use. Again, sounding sympathetic rather than judgemental is crucial and a good opening line can be, 'If you don't mind me asking…'. Heroin, crack, cannabis and other drugs are smoked and, in some cases, cause more damage to the lungs than tobacco. Cannabis can cause severe emphysema in younger patients, who are often unaware of its effects. Use the consultation to discuss its long-term sequelae.

The family history

There is a strong inherited susceptibility to asthma. Associated atopic conditions, such as eczema and hay fever, may also be present in relatives of those with asthma, particularly in those who develop the condition when young.

The occupational history

No other organ is as susceptible to the working environment as are the lungs. Several hundred different substances have now been recognized as causing occupational asthma. Paint sprayers, workers in the electronics, rubber or plastics industries and woodworkers are relatively commonly affected (Box 12.7). Always ask about a relationship between symptoms and work.

Damage from inhalation of asbestos may take decades to become manifest, most seriously as malignant mesothelioma. In industrialized countries, this once extremely rare tumour of the pleura has become more common and will become even more so in the next 20 years. In middle-aged individuals who present with a pleural effusion (often the first sign of a mesothelioma) always ask about possible asbestos exposure in jobs back to the time of first employment (Box 12.8).

As far as the occupational history is concerned, the best way to proceed is chronologically. Most people cannot randomly remember, for example, what they might have been doing 20 years ago or indeed, if asked in isolation, when they worked in a particular job. However, if you start at the beginning of their life and work forward they find it much easier to remember (try it yourself starting with your school exams!)

Start by asking the patient how old he was when he left school, then what job or further education he had; then ask him to continue through his life to the present day. Particularly for those who went on to further education, ask about holiday jobs (you might be surprised at their responses!) and it might be worth asking if they travelled overseas with their

---

Box 12.7 List of common occupations that may be associated with asthma

- Car paint sprayers—isocyanates
- Electricians—colophony
- Woodworkers
- Rubber and plastic industries
- Bakers—flour dust and enzymes, e.g. amylase
- Working with animals—vets, zoo keepers, laboratory worker—rodent urinary proteins
- Working with agriculture—farmers, fish worker—salmon proteins
- Health care professionals—latex and diathermy
- Hairdressing—persulphate, henna
- Tea sifters and packers

Box 12.8 List of activities that may lead to asbestos exposure

- Mining and manufacture of asbestos
- Shipbuilding and aircraft manufacturing
- Dock and rail workers—unloading asbestos from ships/ trains
- Thermal and fire insulation—lagging
- Construction, building repair and demolition
- Plumbers and gas fitters
- Car mechanics (brake linings)
- Electricians, carpenters, upholsterers
- Manufacture of gas masks in World War II
- Teachers and health workers—old school buildings and hospitals as the source
- Family member of one of the above, and/or working or living near an asbestos source (particularly if asbestos fibres are taken home on workers' clothing)

---

employment, especially if they were in the armed forces. Do not assume that all 80-year-olds are retired or indeed that all young patients are employed.

The examination

General assessment

An examination of the respiratory system is incomplete without a simultaneous general assessment (Box 12.9). Watch the patient as he comes into the room, during your history taking and while he is undressing and climbing on to the couch. If this is a hospital inpatient, is there breathlessness just on moving in bed? Is he needing oxygen therapy? If so, at what flow rate and what is the mode of delivery—nasal cannula, Venturi mask, high flow? Look at the observation chart and review pulse, blood pressure, oxygen saturations and what is their early warning score (EWS)? A breathless patient may be using the accessory muscles of respiration (e.g. sternomastoid) and, in the presence of severe COPD, many patients find it easier to breathe out through pursed lips (Fig. 12.1).

Box 12.9	Points to note in a general assessment

- Physique and gait
- Voice
- Breathlessness
- Clubbing of the fingers
- Tobacco staining of fingers
- Bruising and/or thinness of skin
- Venous pulses
- Cyanosis or pallor
- Ptosis
- Swollen face
- Collateral vessels across anterior chest wall
- Intercostal recession
- Use of accessory respiratory muscles
- Lymph nodes

Box 12.10	Signs to look for in the hands

- Clubbing
- Pallor
- Warm, well-perfused palms (CO_2 retention)
- Cyanosis
- Flap
- Tremor
- Tobacco staining
- Bruising and/or thin skin
- Pulse rate and character

Box 12.11	Observing the chest

- Rate of respiration
- Rhythm of respiration
- Chest expansion
- Symmetry
- Shape of the chest—elliptical, barrel, funnel
- Surgical scars

Figure 12.1 Respiratory failure. The patient is breathless at rest and there is central cyanosis with blueness of the lips and face. The lips are pursed during expiration, a characteristic feature of COPD. This facial appearance is often accompanied by heart failure with peripheral oedema (cor pulmonale).

Is there an audible wheeze or stridor?
- Is the voice hoarse?
- Is the patient continually coughing? Dry or productive?
- Is the patient capable of producing a normal, explosive cough, or is the voice weak or non-existent even when he is asked to cough?
- Is the wheezing audible, usually loudest in expiration, or is there stridor, a high-pitched inspiratory noise?
- What is on the bedside table (e.g. inhalers, a peak flow meter, tissues, a sputum pot, an oxygen mask, nebulizer, continuous positive airway pressure (CPAP) machine)?

- What is the physique and state of general nourishment of the patient?

For the examination, the patient should be resting comfortably on a bed or couch, supported by pillows so that he can lean back comfortably at an angle of 45° (this is often more upright than patients choose for themselves).

Upper airways

A comprehensive account of examination of the upper airways is given in Chapter 22; a focused assessment should be included in the evaluation of all new patients or those with new upper airway symptoms.

Hands

The hands should be inspected for clubbing, pallor or cyanosis (Box 12.10). Tobacco-stained fingers may indicate a heavy smoker. Respiratory causes of clubbing include carcinoma of the bronchus, pulmonary fibrosis, bronchiectasis, lung abscess and pleural empyema. A fine tremor may indicate the use of inhaled β_2 agonists, such as salbutamol. A flap may indicate carbon dioxide retention or hypercapnia. Such patients are often drowsy, with warm hands and a bounding pulse. In a significant asthma attack, the pulse rate is usually raised. The systolic blood pressure also falls during the severe inspiratory effort of acute asthma, and the degree of this fall (the degree of pulsus paradoxus) can be used as a measure of asthma severity.

Respiratory rate and rhythm

The respiratory rate and pattern of respiration should be noted. The normal rate of respiration in a relaxed adult is about 14–16 breaths per minute (Box 12.11). Tachypnoea is an increased respiratory rate observed by the doctor, whereas dyspnoea is the symptom of breathlessness experienced by the patient. Apnoea means cessation of respiration.

Cheyne-Stokes breathing is the name given to a disturbance of respiratory rhythm in which there is cyclical deepening and quickening of respiration, followed by diminishing respiratory effort and rate, sometimes associated with a short period of complete apnoea, the cycle then being repeated. This is often observed in severely ill patients and particularly in severe cardiac failure, narcotic drug poisoning and neurological disorders. It is occasionally seen, especially during sleep, in elderly patients without any obvious serious disease.

Some patients may have apnoeic episodes during sleep owing to complete cessation of respiratory effort (central apnoea) or, much more commonly, apnoea despite continuation of respiratory effort. This, which is known as obstructive sleep apnoea, is caused by obstruction of the upper airways by soft tissues in the region of the pharynx and is most common in obese patients.

Venous pulses

The venous pulses in the neck (see Chapter 13) should be inspected. A raised jugular venous pressure (JVP) may be a sign of cor pulmonale, right heart failure caused by chronic pulmonary hypertension in severe lung disease, commonly COPD. Pitting oedema of the ankles and sacrum is usually present. However, engorged neck veins can be caused by superior vena cava obstruction (SVCO), usually because of malignancy in the upper mediastinum. SVCO can also be associated with facial swelling and plethora (redness) and collateral circulation across the anterior chest wall.

Head

Examination of the eyes may reveal anaemia or, rarely, Horner's syndrome, secondary to a cancer at the lung apex (Pancoast tumour) invading the cervical sympathetic chain. The lips and tongue should be inspected for central cyanosis, which almost always indicates poor oxygenation of the blood by the lungs, whereas peripheral cyanosis alone is usually owing to poor peripheral perfusion. Oral candida may indicate use of inhaled steroids or be a sign of debilitation or underlying immune suppression in the patient.

Examination of the chest

Relevant anatomy

The interpretation of signs in the chest often causes problems for the beginner. A review of the relevant anatomy may help.

The bifurcation of the trachea corresponds on the anterior chest wall with the sternal angle, the transverse bony ridge at the junction of the body of the sternum and the manubrium sterni. Posteriorly,

the level is at the disc between the fourth and fifth thoracic vertebrae. The ribs are most easily counted downwards from the second costal cartilage, which articulates with the sternum at the extremity of the sternal angle.

A line from the second thoracic spine to the sixth rib, in line with the nipple, corresponds to the upper border of the lower lobe (oblique or major interlobar fissure). On the right side, a horizontal line from the sternum at the level of the fourth costal cartilage, drawn to meet the line of the major interlobar fissure, marks the boundary between the upper and middle lobes (the horizontal or minor interlobar fissure). The greater part of each lung, as seen from behind, is composed of the lower lobe; only the apex belongs to the upper lobe. The middle and upper lobes on the right side and the upper lobe on the left side occupy most of the area in front (Fig. 12.2). This is most easily visualized if the lobes are thought of as two wedges fitting together, not as two cubes piled one on top of the other (Fig. 12.3).

The stethoscope is so much a part of the 'image' of a doctor that it is very easy for the student to forget that listening is only one part of the chest examination. Obtaining the maximum possible information from your examination requires you to look, then to feel and, only then, to listen.

Looking: inspection of the chest

Appearance of the chest

First, look for any obvious scars from previous surgery. Thoracotomy scars (from lobectomy or pneumonectomy (removal of the whole lung)) are usually visible running from below the scapula posteriorly, sweeping round the axilla to the anterior chest wall. Pleural procedures, such as intercostal drain insertion, biopsy or VATS (video-assisted thoracoscopic surgery), may be associated with small scars, often in the axilla or posteriorly. A small scar above the sternal notch indicates a previous tracheostomy. Older patients may have small scars in the midline below the clavicle indicative of a phrenic nerve crush (a previous treatment for TB). Look for any lumps visible beneath the skin or any lesions on the skin itself. If you are examining from the right of the patient, ensure that you thoroughly inspect the left side. It is easy to miss a lateral thoracotomy scar or one that is hidden in a skinfold.

Next, inspect the shape of the chest itself. The normal chest is bilaterally symmetrical and elliptical in horizontal cross-section, with the narrower diameter being anteroposterior. The chest may be distorted by disease of the ribs or spinal vertebrae as well as by underlying lung disease (Box 12.12). Lobar collapse produces characteristic changes on chest X-ray and they are shown in Figure 12.4.

Kyphosis (forward bending) or scoliosis (lateral bending) of the vertebral column will lead to asymmetry of the chest and, if severe, may significantly restrict lung movement. A normal chest X-ray is

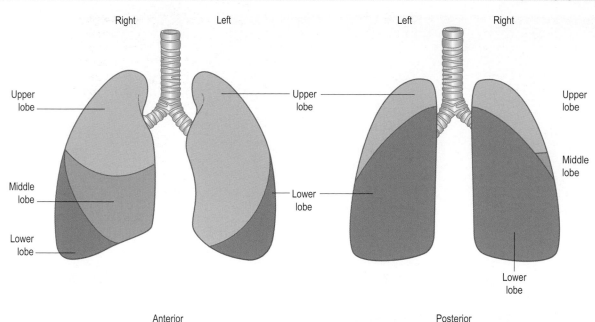

Figure 12.2 Anterior and posterior aspects of the lungs.

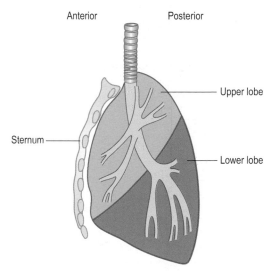

Figure 12.3 Lateral aspect of the left lung.

Box 12.12	Features to note in assessing the shape of the chest

- Kyphosis
- Scoliosis
- Flattening
- Pectus excavatum, pectus carinatum
- Overinflation
- Previous surgery causing asymmetry, such as thoracoplasty

airways obstruction, as in laryngeal disease or tumours of the trachea. In COPD, the lower ribs often move paradoxically inwards on inspiration instead of the normal outwards movement.

Feeling: palpation of the chest

Lymph nodes

The lymph nodes in the supraclavicular fossae, cervical regions and axillary regions should be palpated; do not forget to feel gently behind the sternocleidomastoid muscles. If they are enlarged, this may be secondary to the spread of malignant disease from the chest, and such findings will influence decisions regarding treatment. Lymph nodes in the neck are best felt by sitting the patient up and examining from behind.

Swellings and tenderness

It is useful to palpate any part of the chest that presents an obvious swelling or where the patient complains of pain (Box 12.13). Feel gently, because pressure may increase the pain. It is often important, particularly in the case of musculoskeletal pain, to identify a site of tenderness (Box 12.14). Surgical emphysema (air

seen in Figure 12.5. Severe airways obstruction, particularly long-term as in COPD (Fig. 12.6), may lead to overinflated lungs. On examination, the chest may be 'barrel shaped', most easily appreciated as an increased anteroposterior diameter, making the horizontal cross-section more circular. On X-ray, the hemidiaphragms appear lower than usual, and flattened.

Movement of the chest

Look to see if the chest movements are symmetrical. If they seem to be diminished on one side, then that is likely to be the side on which is an abnormality. Intercostal recession, a drawing-in of the intercostal spaces with inspiration, may indicate severe upper

Figure 12.4 Chest X-rays (CXR) showing lobar collapses. **(A)** CXR showing right upper lobe collapse; note the raised 'tented' right hemidiaphragm. **(B)** CXR showing right middle lobe collapse; the right heart border has become obscured. **(C)** CXR showing right lower lobe collapse, note the right hilum is lowered and now behind the right heart. **(D)** CXR showing left upper lobe collapse; note the 'veil-like' appearance over the left hemithorax with loss of the left heart border silhouette. **(E)** CXR showing left lower lobe collapse; also known as 'sail-sign' because the lobe collapses and sits behind the left side of the cardiac silhouette and obscures the medial hemidiaphragmatic silhouette. (Courtesy of Dr Stephen Ellis.)

Figure 12.5 Normal chest X-ray.

Figure 12.6 Chest X-ray in severe chronic obstructive pulmonary disease.

by putting the second and fourth fingers of the examining hand on each edge of the sternal notch and use the third finger to assess whether the trachea is central or deviated to one side. Warn the patient in advance what you are about to do and avoid heavy-handedness in this situation. Rough technique is uncomfortable for the patient who may feel like he is being choked. A slight deviation of the trachea to the right may be found in healthy people.

Displacement of the cardiac impulse without displacement of the trachea may be owing to scoliosis, to a congenital funnel depression of the sternum (pectus excavatum) or to enlargement of the left ventricle. In the absence of these conditions, a significant displacement of the cardiac impulse or trachea or of both together suggests that the position of the mediastinum has been altered by disease of the lungs or pleura. The mediastinum may be pushed away from the affected side (contralateral deviation) by a pleural effusion or pneumothorax. Fibrosis or collapse of the lung will pull the mediastinum towards the affected side (ipsilateral deviation).

Chest expansion

As well as by simple inspection, possible asymmetrical expansion of the chest may be explored further by palpation. Face the patient and place the fingertips of both hands on either side of the lower ribcage so that the tips of the thumbs meet in the midline in front of the chest but are not touching the skin. A deep breath by the patient will increase the distance between the thumbs and indicate the degree of expansion. If one thumb remains closer to the midline, this suggests diminished expansion on that side. Essentially the hands are being used like a pair of calipers to measure expansion in the lateral bases of the lungs where maximum expansion occurs.

in the tissues), which feels like popcorn or bubble paper underneath the skin, is caused by trauma, pneumothorax, pneumomediastinum and infection, as well as chest instrumentation following surgery or a chest drain.

Trachea and heart

The positions of the cardiac impulse and trachea should then be determined. Feel for the trachea

Tactile vocal fremitus is detected by palpation, but this is not a commonly used routine examination technique. It is discussed further under auscultation, below.

Feeling: percussion of the chest

The technique of percussion was probably developed as a way of ascertaining how much fluid remained in barrels of wine or other liquids. Auenbrugger applied percussion to the chest, having learned this method in his father's wine cellar. Effective percussion is a knack that requires consistent practice; do so upon yourself or on willing colleagues, because percussion can be uncomfortable for patients if performed repeatedly and inexpertly.

The middle finger of the left hand is placed on the part to be percussed and pressed firmly against it, with slight hyperextension of the distal interphalangeal joint. The back of this joint is then struck with the tip of the middle finger of the right hand (vice versa if you are left-handed). The movement should be at your wrist rather than at your elbow. The percussing finger is bent so that its terminal phalanx is at right angles and it strikes the other finger perpendicularly. As soon as the blow has been given, the striking finger is raised: the action is a tapping movement.

The two most common mistakes made by the beginner are first, failing to ensure that the finger of the left hand is applied flatly and firmly to the chest wall, with slight pressure, and second, striking the percussion blow from the elbow rather than from the wrist. The character of the sound produced varies both qualitatively and quantitatively (Box 12.15). When the air in a cavity of sufficient size and appropriate shape is set vibrating, a resonant sound is produced, and a characteristic sensation is also felt by the finger placed on the chest. Try tapping a hollow cupboard and then a solid wall. The feeling is different as well as the sound. The sound and feel of resonance over a healthy lung are learned by practice, and it is against this standard that possible abnormalities of percussion must be judged.

The normal degree of resonance varies between individuals and in different parts of the chest in the same individual, being most resonant below the clavicles anteriorly and the scapulae posteriorly where the muscles are relatively thin and least resonant over the scapulae. On the right side, there is loss of resonance inferiorly as the liver is encountered. On the left side, the lower border overlaps the stomach, so there is a transition from lung resonance to tympanitic stomach resonance.

Always systematically compare the percussion note on the two sides of the chest, moving backwards and forwards from one side to the other, not all the way down one side and then down the other. Percuss over the clavicles; traditionally, this is done without an intervening finger on the chest, but there is no

Box 12.15	Points to note on percussion of the chest

- Resonance
- Dullness
- Pain and tenderness

reason for this and it is more comfortable for the patient if the finger of the left hand is used in the usual way. Percuss three or four areas on the anterior chest wall, comparing left with right. Percuss the axillae, then three or four areas on the back of the chest.

Reduction of resonance (i.e. the percussion note is said to be dull) occurs in two important circumstances:
1. When the underlying lung is more solid than usual, usually because of consolidation or collapse
2. When the pleural cavity contains fluid (i.e. a pleural effusion is present).

Less commonly, a dull percussion note may be owing to thickened pleura. The percussion note is most dull when there is underlying fluid, as in a pleural effusion. Pleural effusion causes the sensation in the percussed finger to be similar to that felt when a solid wall is percussed. This is often called 'stony dullness'. By comparing side with side, it is usually easy to detect a unilateral pleural effusion. Pleural effusion usually leads to decreased chest wall movement. Effusions may occur bilaterally in some patients, and this may be more difficult to detect clinically.

An increase in resonance, or hyper-resonance, is more difficult to detect than dullness, and there is no absolute level of normal percussion against which extra resonance can be judged. It may be noticeable when the pleural cavity contains air, as in pneumothorax. Sometimes, however, in this situation one is tempted to think that the slightly duller side is the abnormal side. Further examination and chest X-ray will reveal the true situation, remembering that the side of the chest that expands less is usually the side with pathology.

Listening: auscultation of the chest

Listen to the chest with the diaphragm, not the bell, of the stethoscope (chest sounds are relatively high pitched, and therefore the diaphragm is more sensitive than the bell). Ask the patient to take deep breaths in and out through the mouth. Demonstrate what you would like the patient to do, and then check visually that he is doing it while you listen to the chest. If the patient has a tendency to cough, ask him to breathe more deeply than usual but not so much as to induce a cough with each breath. As with percussion, you should listen in comparable positions to each side alternately, switching back and forth from one side to the other to compare (Box 12.16).

- Vesicular breath sounds—normal breath sounds
- Bronchial breath sounds—consolidation
- Vocal fremitus and resonance:
  - whispering pectoriloquy—consolidation
  - aegophony—top of pleural effusion, consolidation
- Added sounds:
  - pleural rub—associated with infection
  - wheezes—asthma, chronic obstructive pulmonary disease (COPD), infection, cardiac failure
  - crackles—pulmonary fibrosis, cardiac failure, COPD

The breath sounds

Breath sounds have intensity and quality. The intensity (or loudness) of the sounds may be normal, reduced or increased. The quality of normal breath sounds is described as vesicular.

Breath sounds will be normal in intensity when the lung is inflating normally, but may be reduced if there is localized airway narrowing, if the lung is extensively damaged by a process such as emphysema or if there is intervening pleural thickening or pleural fluid. Breath sounds may be of increased intensity in very thin subjects.

Breath sounds probably originate from turbulent airflow in the larger airways. When you place your stethoscope upon the chest, you are listening to how those sounds have been changed on their journey from their site of origin to the position of your stethoscope diaphragm. Normal lung tissue makes the sound quieter and selectively filters out some of the higher frequencies. The resulting sound that you hear is called a vesicular breath sound. There is usually no distinct pause between the end of inspiration and the beginning of expiration.

When the area underlying the stethoscope is airless, as in consolidation, the sounds generated in the large airways are transmitted more efficiently, so they are louder and there is less filtering of the high frequencies. The resulting sounds heard by the stethoscope are termed bronchial breathing, classically heard over an area of consolidated lung in cases of pneumonia. The sound resembles that obtained by listening over the trachea, although the noise there is much louder. The quality of the sound is rather harsh, the higher frequencies being heard more clearly. The expiratory sound has a more sibilant (hissing) character than the inspiratory one and lasts for most of the expiratory phase.

The intensity and quality of all breath sounds is so variable from patient to patient and in different situations that it is only by repeated auscultation of the chests of many patients that one becomes familiar with the normal variations and learns to recognize the abnormalities.

Added sounds

Added sounds are abnormal sounds that arise in the lung itself or in the pleura. The added sounds most commonly arising in the lung are best referred to as wheezes and crackles. Older terms such as râles to describe coarse crackles, crepitations to describe fine crackles and rhonchi to describe wheezes are poorly defined, have led to confusion and are best avoided.

Wheezes are musical sounds associated with airway narrowing. Widespread polyphonic wheezes, particularly heard in expiration, are the most common ones; they are characteristic of diffuse airflow obstruction, especially in asthma and COPD. These wheezes are probably related to dynamic compression of the bronchi, which is accentuated in expiration when airway narrowing is present. A fixed monophonic wheeze can be generated by localized narrowing of a single bronchus, as may occur in the presence of a tumour or foreign body. It may be inspiratory or expiratory or both and may change its intensity in different positions.

Wheezing generated in smaller airways should not be mistaken for stridor associated with laryngeal disease or localized narrowing of the trachea or the large airways. Stridor almost always indicates a serious condition requiring urgent investigation and management. The noise is often both inspiratory and expiratory. It may be heard at the open mouth without the aid of the stethoscope. On auscultation of the chest, stridor is usually loudest over the trachea.

Crackles are short, explosive sounds often described as bubbling or clicking. When the large airways are full of sputum, a coarse, rattling sound may be heard even without the stethoscope. However, crackles are not usually produced by moistness in the lungs. It is more likely that they are produced by sudden changes in gas pressure related to the sudden opening of previously closed small airways. Crackles at the beginning of inspiration are common in patients with COPD. Localized loud and coarse crackles may indicate an area of bronchiectasis. Crackles are also heard in pulmonary oedema. In diffuse interstitial fibrosis, crackles are characteristically fine in character and late inspiratory in timing (and said to sound like rolling your fingers through your hair near your ear).

The pleural rub, which is characteristic of pleural inflammation, usually occurs in association with pleuritic pain. It has a creaking or rubbing characteristic (said to sound like a foot crunching through fresh-fallen snow) and, in some instances, can be felt with the palpating hand as well as being audible with the stethoscope.

Take care to exclude false added sounds. Sounds resembling pleural rubs may be produced by movement of the stethoscope on the patient's skin or of clothes against the stethoscope tubing. Sounds arising in the patient's muscles may resemble added sounds: in particular, the shivering of a cold patient makes any attempt at auscultation almost useless. The stethoscope rubbing over hairy skin may produce sounds that resemble fine crackles.

Vocal resonance

When listening to the breath sounds, you are detecting with the stethoscope vibrations that have been made in the large airways. Vocal resonance is the resonance within the chest of sounds made by the voice. Vocal resonance is the detection of vibrations transmitted to the chest from the vocal cords as the patient repeats a phrase, usually the words 'ninety-nine'. The ear perceives not the distinct syllables but a resonant sound, the intensity of which depends on the loudness and depth of the patient's voice and the conductivity of the lungs. As always in examining the chest, each point examined on one side should be compared at once with the corresponding point on the other side.

Not surprisingly, conditions that increase or reduce conduction of breath sounds to the stethoscope have similar effects on vocal resonance. Consolidated lung conducts sounds better than air-containing lung, so in consolidation the vocal resonance is increased and the sounds are louder and often clearer. In such circumstances, even when the patient whispers a phrase (e.g. 'one, two, three'), the sounds may be heard clearly; this is known as whispering pectoriloquy. Above the level of a pleural effusion, or in some cases over an area of consolidation, the voice may sound nasal or bleating; this is known as aegophony, but is an unusual physical finding.

Vocal fremitus

Vocal fremitus is detected with the hand on the chest wall. It should, therefore, perhaps be regarded as part of palpation, but it is usually carried out after auscultation (see below). As with vocal resonance, the patient is asked to repeat a phrase such as 'ninety-nine'. The examining hand feels distinct vibrations when this is done. Some examiners use the ulnar border of the hand, but there is no good reason for this; the flat of the hand, including the fingertips, is far more sensitive, but make sure the fingers are pressed firmly onto the chest wall.

From the above, it should be clear that listening to the breath sounds, listening to the vocal resonance and eliciting vocal fremitus that they are all doing essentially the same thing: they are investigating how vibrations generated in the larynx or large airways are transmitted to the examining instrument, the stethoscope in the first two cases and the fingers in the third. It follows that in the various pathological situations, all three physical signs should behave in similar ways. Where there is consolidation, the breath sounds are better transmitted to the stethoscope, so they are louder and there is less attenuation of the higher frequencies, that is, 'bronchial breathing' is heard. Similarly, the vocal resonance and the vocal fremitus are increased. Where there is a pleural effusion, the breath sounds are quieter or absent and the vocal resonance and vocal fremitus are reduced or absent.

The intelligent student should now ask: 'Why try to elicit all three signs?' The experienced physician will answer: 'Because it is often difficult to interpret the signs that have been elicited, and three pieces of information are more reliable than one'.

Putting it together: an examination of the chest

There is no single perfect way of examining the chest, and most doctors develop their own minor variations of order and procedure. The following is one scheme that combines efficiency with thoroughness:

- Observe the patient generally and the surroundings. Look for any medicine, sputum pots, inhalers, nebulizers or, for example, CPAP machine around the patient's bed. Look at the patient's observation chart. Is the patient using oxygen; if so, how much, what is the rate?
- Ask the patient's permission for the examination and ensure he is lying comfortably at 45°.
- Examine the hands and take the pulse.
- Count the respiratory rate.
- Assess the JVP.
- Check the face for signs of anaemia or cyanosis as well as evidence of ptosis and miosis.
- Inspect the chest movements and the anterior chest wall. What is the shape of the chest?
- Feel the position of the trachea and check for axillary lymphadenopathy.
- Feel the position of the apex beat.
- Check the symmetry of the chest movements by palpation.
- Percuss the anterior chest and axillae.
  Sit the patient forward:
- Inspect the posterior chest wall.
- Check for cervical and supraclavicular lymphadenopathy.
- Percuss the back of the chest.
- Listen to the breath sounds.
- Check the vocal resonance.
- Check the tactile vocal fremitus.
- Check for sacral oedema.

If you are examining a hospital inpatient, always take the opportunity to turn the pillow over before lying the patient back again; a cool, freshened pillow is a great comfort to an ill person.

- Listen to the breath sounds on the front of the chest.
- Check the vocal resonance.
- Check the tactile vocal fremitus.
- Check for pitting oedema of the ankles.

Stand back for a moment and reflect upon whether you have omitted anything or whether you need to check or repeat anything. Thank the patient and ensure he is dressed or appropriately covered.

Putting it together: interpreting the signs

Developing an appropriate differential diagnosis on the basis of the signs you have elicited requires thought and practice. Keeping the following in mind will help:

| Box 12.17 | Characteristics to note when assessing sputum |

- Mucoid
- Purulent
- Frothy
- Bloodstained
- Rusty
- Frank haemoptysis
- Casts

- If movements are diminished on one side, there is likely to be an abnormality on that side.
- The percussion note is dull over a pleural effusion and over an area of consolidation; the duller the note, the more likely it is to be a pleural effusion.
- The breath sounds, the vocal resonance and the tactile vocal fremitus are quieter or less obvious over a pleural effusion, and louder or more obvious over an area of consolidation.
- Over a pneumothorax, the percussion note is more resonant than normal, but the breath sounds, vocal resonance and tactile vocal fremitus are quieter or reduced. Pneumothorax is easily missed.

Other investigations

Sputum examination

At the bedside

Hospital inpatients should have a sputum pot which must be inspected (Box 12.17). Mucoid sputum is characteristic in patients with chronic bronchitis when there is no active infection. It is clear and sticky and not necessarily produced in a large volume. Sputum may become mucopurulent or purulent when bacterial infection is present in patients with bronchitis, pneumonia, bronchiectasis or a lung abscess. In these last two conditions, the quantities may be large and the sputum is often foul smelling.

Occasionally asthmatics have a yellow tinge to the sputum, owing to the presence of many eosinophils. People with asthma may also produce a particularly tenacious form of mucoid sputum, and sometimes they cough up casts of the bronchial tree, particularly after an attack. Patients with bronchopulmonary aspergillosis may bring up black sputum or sputum with black parts in it, which is the fungal element of the *Aspergillus*.

When sputum is particularly foul smelling, the presence of anaerobic organisms should be suspected. Very ill patients with pulmonary oedema may bring up pink or white frothy sputum. Rusty-coloured sputum is characteristic of pneumococcal lobar pneumonia. Blood may be coughed up alone or bloodstained sputum produced in bronchogenic carcinoma, pulmonary tuberculosis (TB), pulmonary embolism, bronchiectasis or pulmonary hypertension (e.g. with mitral stenosis) being possible causes.

In the laboratory

Sputum may be examined under the microscope in the laboratory for the presence of pus cells and organisms and may be cultured in an attempt to identify the causative agent of an infection and antibiotic resistance patterns. It is seldom practical to wait for the results of such examinations, and most clinical decisions have to be based on the clinical probability of a particular infection being present.

Do not forget to ask for sputum to be examined for acid-fast bacilli when appropriate; tuberculosis requires specialized techniques of laboratory microscopy and culture to identify the responsible organisms; if the diagnosis is suspected, these tests must be specifically requested. Non-tuberculous mycobacteria (NTN) can occur in patients with chronic underlying lung pathology such as COPD and bronchiectasis.

Lung function tests

Measurements of respiratory function may provide valuable information. First, in conjunction with the clinical assessment and other investigations, they may help establish a diagnosis. Second, they will help indicate the severity of the condition. Third, serial measurements over time will show changes indicating disease progression or, alternatively, a favourable response to treatment. Finally, regular monitoring of lung function in chronic diseases, such as idiopathic pulmonary fibrosis, cystic fibrosis or obstructive airways disease, may warn of deterioration.

Simple respiratory function tests fall into three main groups:
1. Measuring the size of the lungs
2. Measuring how easily air flows into and out of the airways
3. Measuring how efficient the lungs are in the process of gas exchange

A spirometer will measure how much air can be exhaled after a maximal inspiration: the patient breathes in as much as he can, then blows out into the spirometer until no more air at all can be breathed out. This volume is called the vital capacity (VC). The amount of air in the lungs at full inspiration is a measure of the total lung capacity and that still remaining after a full expiration is called the residual volume (RV).

The actual value of total lung capacity (TLC) cannot be measured with a spirometer. The simplest way of determining it is to get the patient to inspire a known volume of air containing a known concentration of helium. Measuring the new concentration of helium that exists after mixing with the air already in the lungs enables the total lung capacity (TLC) to be calculated. Subtraction of the VC from this value gives the RV.

Usually, vital capacity is measured after the patient has blown as hard and fast as possible into

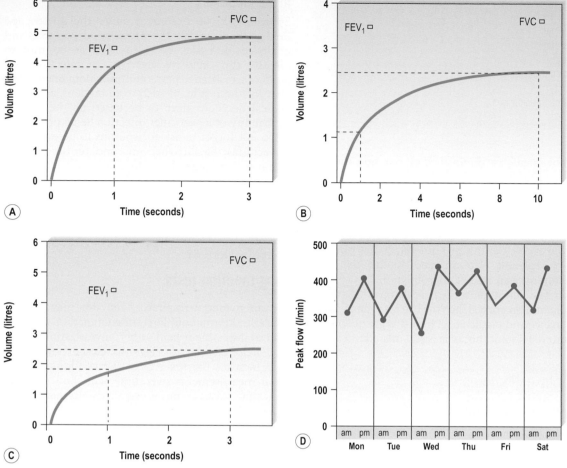

Figure 12.7 **(A)** Normal expiratory spirometer trace. **(B)** Spirometer trace showing an obstructive defect. Note the very prolonged (10-second) expiration. **(C)** Spirometer trace showing a restrictive defect. **(D)** Typical diurnal variation of peak flow, worse in the mornings, seen in a young asthmatic, during an exacerbation.

the spirometer, when the measurement is known as the forced vital capacity, or FVC. In normal lungs, VC and FVC are almost identical, but in COPD, compression of the airways during a forced expiration leads to closure of the airways earlier than usual, and FVC may be less than VC.

Figure 12.7A shows the trace produced by a spirometer. Time in seconds is on the x-axis and volume in litres is on the y-axis. Thus, the trace moves up during expiration assessing FVC and along the x-axis as time passes during expiration.

The volume of air breathed out in the first second of a forced expiration is known as the forced expiratory volume in the first second—almost always abbreviated to FEV_1. In normal lungs, the FEV_1 is more than 70% of FVC. When there is obstruction to airflow, as in COPD, the time taken to expire fully is prolonged and the ratio of FEV_1 to FVC is reduced. An example is shown in Figure 12.7B. A trace like this is described as showing an obstructive ventilatory defect. As noted above, the FVC may be reduced in severe airways obstruction but, in such

cases, the FEV_1 is reduced even more and the FEV_1-to-FVC ratio remains low.

Some lung conditions restrict expansion of the lungs but do not interfere with the airways. In such individuals, both FEV_1 and FVC are reduced in proportion to each other, so the ratio remains normal even though the absolute values are reduced. Figure 12.7C shows a trace of this kind, a restrictive ventilatory defect in a patient with diffuse pulmonary fibrosis.

Look again at the normal expiratory spirogram (Fig. 12.7A). The slope of the trace is steepest at the onset of expiration. The trace thus shows that the rate of volume change with time is greatest in early expiration; in other words, the rate of airflow is greatest then. This measurement, the peak expiratory flow rate (PEFR), can be measured easily with a peak flow meter. A simplified version of this device is shown in Figure 12.8. This mini-peak flow meter is light and inexpensive. People with asthma can use it to monitor themselves and alter their medication, as suggested by their doctor, at the first signs of any

Figure 12.8 A mini-peak flow meter.

fall in peak flow measurement, which indicates a deterioration in their condition (Fig. 12.7D).

Normal gas exchange consists of the uptake of oxygen into the pulmonary capillary blood and the release of carbon dioxide into the alveoli. For this to be achieved, the ventilation of the lungs by air and their perfusion by blood need to be matched anatomically. An approximation of the efficiency of the process of gas exchange may be obtained by measuring the pulmonary transfer factor for carbon monoxide. This is assessed with an apparatus similar to that used for the helium-dilution technique for measuring lung volumes. Instead of using helium, which does not easily enter the blood, a known and very low concentration of carbon monoxide is used. The haemoglobin in the pulmonary capillaries very readily binds this gas. The patient inspires to TLC, holds the breath for 10 seconds, then expires fully. The difference between the inspired carbon monoxide concentration and the expired concentration is a measure of the efficiency of gas exchange and can be expressed per unit lung volume if TLC is simultaneously measured by the helium-dilution technique.

The bronchial provocation test, which is useful in the diagnosis of asthma, assesses airway hyper-responsiveness. It uses increasing concentrations of histamine or methacholine whilst measuring spirometry, FEV_1 and FVC and produces transient airflow limitation in susceptible patients.

Arterial blood sampling

In a sample of arterial blood, the partial pressures of oxygen (PaO_2) and of carbon dioxide ($PaCO_2$) and the pH can be measured. The arterial $PaCO_2$ will reflect the effective ventilation of alveoli that are adequately perfused with blood so that efficient gas exchange can take place. Provided the rate of carbon dioxide production by the body remains constant, the $PaCO_2$ will be directly related to the level of alveolar ventilation. The normal range is 4.7–6.0 kPa (36–45 mmHg). When alveolar ventilation is reduced, the $PaCO_2$ will rise. A number of different

Box 12.18	Arterial blood gases

Type 1: Respiratory failure (on air)

- pH—7.43
- PCO_2—3.8
- PO_2—7.5
- HCO_3—22.0
- O_2 Sats—91%

Type 2: Decompensated respiratory failure (on air)

- pH—7.25
- PCO_2—9.3
- PO_2—7.5
- HCO_3—31.2
- O_2 Sats—92%

Type 2: Compensated respiratory failure (1 L O_2 and overnight bilevel positive airway pressure (BIPAP))

- pH—7.41
- PCO_2—6.3
- PO_2—8.3
- HCO_3—30.0
- O_2 Sats—94%

conditions may reduce alveolar ventilation. Alveolar ventilation rises and $PaCO_2$ may fall in response to metabolic acidosis, in very anxious individuals who hyperventilate and in many lung conditions that tend to reduce the oxygenation of the blood. The PaO_2 is normally in the range 11.3 to 14.0 kPa (80 100 mmHg). Any lung disease that interferes with gas exchange may reduce arterial PaO_2 (Box 12.18).

Exhaled nitric oxide

Nitric oxide (NO) is produced by the bronchial epithelium and its concentration is increased in asthma and other forms of airway inflammation; measurement can guide treatment in poorly controlled asthma.

Six-minute walking test

This validated test, which measures oxygen saturations, pulse rate and distance walked over a period of 6 minutes, is useful in measuring exercise tolerance in patients with chronic airway disease, heart failure and investigation of breathlessness.

Cardiopulmonary exercise testing (CPET)

A useful tool in the investigation of unexplained breathlessness, CPET provides an assessment of cardiopulmonary reserve. Together with cardiorespiratory and metabolic muscle function it measures oxygen consumption, CO_2 produced and ventilation whilst the patient uses a treadmill or a cycle ergometer.

Overnight oximetry and nocturnal polygraphy

Overnight oximetry measures the patient's O_2 saturations during sleep looking for evidence of

| Box 12.19 | Points to note when assessing the chest X-ray |

- Name, hospital number and date of birth of patient and date (and time) of X-ray
- Position of the patient
- Outline of heart and mediastinum
- Position of the trachea
- Diaphragm
- Lung fields
- Bony skeleton

nocturnal hypoventilation and hypoxia. Nocturnal polygraphy is a multichannel sleep study that records pulse, O_2 saturations, nasal flow, body position and thoracic and abdominal wall movement and is used to investigate sleep disordered breathing.

Imaging the lung and chest

The chest X-ray

The chest X-ray is an important extension of the clinical examination (Box 12.19). This is particularly so in patients with respiratory symptoms. A normal X-ray taken some time before the development of symptoms should therefore not be accepted as a reason for not taking an up-to-date film. In many instances, it is of great value to have previous X-rays for comparison but, if these are lacking, then careful follow up with subsequent films may provide the necessary information.

The standard chest X-ray is a posteroanterior (PA) view taken with the film against the front of the patient's chest and the X-ray source 2 m behind the patient (see Fig. 12.5). The X-ray is examined systematically on a viewing box or computer screen, according to the following plan and referring to the thoracic anatomy described at the beginning of this chapter (see Figs 12.14–12.16 for more X-rays.)

The position of the patient

Is the patient straight or rotated? If straight, the inner ends of the clavicles will be equidistant from the midline of the vertebral body. This is important because any rotation usually tends to alter the appearance of the mediastinum and the hilar shadows.

The outline of the heart and the mediastinum

Is this normal in size, shape and position?

The position of the trachea

The position of the trachea is seen as a dark column representing the air within the trachea. Is the trachea centrally placed or deviated to either side? Is there any evidence of tracheal narrowing?

The diaphragm

Can the diaphragm be seen on each side? Is it normal in shape and position? Normally, the anterior end of

the sixth or seventh rib crosses the mid-part of the diaphragm on each side, although the diaphragm on the right is usually a little higher than on the left. Are the cardiophrenic angles clearly seen?

The lung fields

For radiological purposes, the lung fields are divided into three zones:

1. The upper zone extends from the apex to a line drawn through the lower borders of the anterior ends of the second costal cartilages.
2. The mid-zone extends from this line to one drawn through the lower borders of the fourth costal cartilages.
3. The lower zone extends from this line to the bases of the lungs.

Each zone is systematically examined on both sides, and any area that appears abnormal is carefully compared with the corresponding area on the opposite side. The horizontal fissure, which separates the right upper and middle lobes, may sometimes be seen running horizontally in the third and fourth interspaces on the right side. Systematically compare not only the right and left lung fields, but also scan your eye up and down the chest film from top to bottom.

The bony skeleton

- Is the chest symmetrical?
- Is scoliosis present?
- Are the ribs unduly crowded or widely spaced in any area?
- Are cervical ribs present?
- Are any ribs eroded or absent?

As well as the standard PA view, lateral views are sometimes carried out to help localize any lesion that is seen. In examining a lateral view, as in Figure 12.9, follow this plan:

- Identify the sternum anteriorly and the vertebral bodies posteriorly. The cardiac shadow lies anteriorly and inferiorly.
- There should be a lucent (dark) area retrosternally that has approximately the same density as the area posterior to the heart and anterior to the vertebral bodies. Check for any difference between the two or for any discrete lesion in either area.
- Check for any collapsed vertebrae. The lowest vertebrae should appear darkest, becoming whiter as they progress superiorly. Interruption of this smooth gradation suggests an abnormality overlying the vertebral bodies involved.

The computed tomography (CT) scan

The routine chest X-ray consists of shadows from anatomical structures at all depths in the chest superimposed on one another. In computed tomography (CT) scanning, X-rays are passed through the body from many different positions around the body and capture on the other side, thereby recording the density of the tissues. The

Figure 12.9 A lateral chest X-ray.

resulting information is processed by a computer to generate a series of cross-sectional images that display the various tissues in a slice dependent on their density. A thoracic CT scan thus is composed of a series of cross-sectional 'slices' through the thorax either at intervals or much more commonly as a contiguous set of images.

The CT scan plays a vital part in the imaging of thoracic pathology. Thin sections aid in the diagnoses of diffuse/interstitial lung disease and airways disease, such as bronchiectasis. The investigation, diagnosis and staging of lung cancer are heavily reliant on CT imaging. The addition of intravenous contrast that opacifies the pulmonary arteries allows detection of emboli as filling defects and has advantages over isotope lung scanning (see below) in diagnosing pulmonary embolism in patients with pre-existing lung disease.

Similarly, opacification of the aorta permits identification of vascular abnormalities, such as dissection, and cardiac gating enables the capture of slices in diastole only allowing accurate pictures of the coronary arteries to be obtained without the degrading influence of cardiac motion. In many cases this technique has replaced conventional coronary angiography. Using helical CT technology, scanners capture large volumes of data from which contiguous thin sections may be reconstructed, followed by post-processing techniques such as 3D reconstructions and the more clinically useful multi-planar reconstructions (Fig. 12.10).

Radioisotope imaging

For the lungs, the most widely used radioisotope technique is combined ventilation and perfusion scanning, used to aid the diagnosis of pulmonary embolism.

The perfusion scan is performed by injecting intravenously a small dose of macroaggregated human albumin particles labelled with technetium-99m (^{99m}Tc). A gamma-camera image is then built up of the radioactive particles impacted in the pulmonary vasculature; the distribution of perfusion in the lung can then be seen. The ventilation scan is obtained by inhalation of a radioactive gas, such as krypton-81m (^{81m}Kr), again using scanning to identify the distribution of the radioactivity.

Blood is usually diverted away from areas of the lung that are unventilated, so a matched defect on both the ventilation and perfusion scans usually indicates parenchymal lung disease. If areas of ventilated lung are not perfused (i.e. an unmatched defect), this is evidence in support of an embolism to the nonperfused area. Figure 12.11 shows a ventilation-perfusion isotope scan. The unmatched defects (areas ventilated by the inspired air but not perfused by blood) suggest a high probability of pulmonary embolism.

Magnetic resonance imaging

Magnetic resonance imaging (MRI) is useful in demonstrating mediastinal abnormalities and can help evaluate invasion of the mediastinum and chest wall by tumour. Apart from the fact that it does not use ionizing radiation, currently it has few other advantages over CT in imaging the thorax. MRI is particularly degraded by movement artefact in imaging the chest because of the relatively long data acquisition time and therefore is not used for assessing the lung parenchyma, but faster scanners are beginning to overcome this drawback.

Ultrasound

Ultrasound reveals much less detail than CT scanning but has the advantages that it does not involve radiation and, as it gives 'real-time' images, the operator can visualize what is happening as it happens. It is used for examining diaphragmatic movement and, when available, it is recommended that ward-based pleural procedures, such as chest drain insertion and pleural aspiration or biopsy, be undertaken under ultrasound guidance.

A paralysed hemidiaphragm usually results from damage to the phrenic nerve by a mediastinal tumour. If the patient is asked to make a sudden inspiratory effort (e.g. sniffing), the non-paralysed side of the diaphragm moves down, so intrathoracic pressure drops, and the paralysed side moves up.

Ultrasound is also valuable in distinguishing pleural thickening from pleural fluid. With real-time imaging, the latter can be seen to move with changes in posture. When such fluid is present, ultrasound

Figure 12.10 Axial images from a CT scan demonstrating an endobronchial lesion in the right main bronchus (**A**). The contiguous nature of the thin axial slices enables the display of the same structures in multiple planes. The coronal (**B**) and sagittal planes (**C**) have been created, allowing the surgeon to accurately place the endobronchial lesion anatomically to aid the planning of the operative resection (Courtesy of Dr Stephen Ellis.)

may be used to aid placement of a catheter to drain the collection and also to steer a draining catheter accurately into an intrapulmonary abscess.

Positron emission tomography (PET) scanning

In this technique, a radiolabelled 18-flurodeoxyglucose (FDG) molecule is administered, which is taken up by metabolically active tissues, such as cancers, showing as 'hot spots' on the image. It is useful in detecting regional and mediastinal lymphadenopathy and is widely used in the staging of lung cancers and to assess suitability for surgery in patients with lung cancer.

Flexible bronchoscopy and endobronchial ultrasound (EBUS)

Bronchoscopy is an essential tool in the investigation of many forms of respiratory disease. For discrete abnormalities, such as a mass seen on chest X-ray and suspected to be a lung cancer, bronchoscopy is usually indicated to investigate its nature. Under local anaesthesia, the flexible bronchoscope is passed through the nose, pharynx and larynx, down the trachea, and the bronchial tree is then inspected. Figure 12.12 shows a lung cancer seen down the bronchoscope. Flexible biopsy forceps, which are

(A) Anterior ventilation

(B) Anterior perfusion

(C) Posterior ventilation

(D) Posterior perfusion

Figure 12.11   Ventilation/perfusion isotope scan of the lungs. Segmental and subsegmental loss of perfusion (**B and D**) can be seen with relatively normal ventilation (**A and C**). The clear, punched-out areas in the perfusion (**B and D**) scans indicate areas of reduced isotope concentration during the perfusion scan. Thus, these are areas of reduced blood flow. The ventilation scans show normal aeration of the lungs as depicted by the isotope distribution in the pulmonary airways. These sequences of scans are suggestive of pulmonary embolism because they show impaired perfusion with normal ventilation.

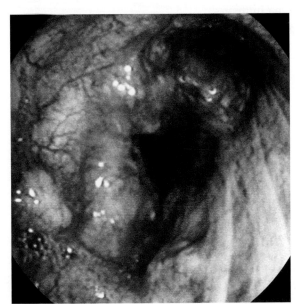

Figure 12.12   A lung cancer, seen down the bronchoscope.

passed down a channel inside the bronchoscope, are used to obtain tissue samples for histological examination. Similarly, aspirated bronchial secretions and brushings of any endobronchial abnormality can be sent to the laboratory for cytological examination.

At bronchoscopy, specimens are also taken for microbiological examination in order to determine the nature of any infecting organisms and should include samples for acid-fast bacilli (AFB). In diffuse interstitial lung disease, such as sarcoidosis or pulmonary fibrosis, the technique of transbronchial biopsy can be used to obtain small specimens of lung parenchyma for histological examination to help confirm the diagnosis.

Endobronchial ultrasound (EBUS) is gradually becoming more available. It involves a modified bronchoscope fitted with an ultrasound probe and a fine-gauge aspiration needle and is used to biopsy thoracic lymph nodes. The procedure is normally undertaken as a day case and under sedation. The scope is thicker than the average bronchoscope and is passed into the patient's airways via a plastic mouth guard rather than the nose. The ultrasound processor is able to image lymph nodes on the other side of the bronchial airways; the operator can then use the aspiration needle to puncture that bronchial wall and biopsy the lymph nodes. A similar procedure, endoscopic ultrasound (EUS), can be used via the oesophagus. Combining these two techniques allows all of the mediastinal lymph nodes to be biopsied. In the majority of cases, they have replaced mediastinoscopy as the biopsy technique of choice and are particularly useful in the diagnosis and staging of lung cancer, sarcoidosis and tuberculosis.

Navigational bronchoscopy is a developing specialist technique. It takes place with the anaesthetized patient lying on an electromagnetic table. This is linked to the patient's most up-to-date CT scan of the thorax via a computer using appropriate software to produce a 3D map of the thorax. It allows the operator, via a bronchoscope, to guide a probe into a diseased area of lung, either for biopsy to make a diagnosis or to deliver treatment, such as microwave ablation directly to a tumour.

Pleural aspiration and biopsy

A pleural effusion (Fig. 12.15) can give rise to diagnostic problems and, sometimes, management problems when the amount of fluid causes respiratory embarrassment. When a pleural effusion is seen as a presenting feature in a middle-aged or older patient, the most likely cause is a malignancy. Less commonly, particularly in younger patients, it may be owing to tuberculosis. In either case, the diagnosis is best obtained by both aspiration of the fluid and pleural biopsy. Aspiration alone has a lower diagnostic yield.

After anaesthetizing the skin, subcutaneous tissues and pleura, pleural fluid may be aspirated by syringe and needle for microbiological and cytological examination. Large pleural effusions may need to be drained by an indwelling catheter, left in situ until the fluid has been fully removed. As noted above, ultrasound guidance can be helpful, particularly if the fluid is loculated in various pockets, and should be used whenever equipment and trained personnel are available.

Cytological examination of pleural fluid may demonstrate the presence of malignant cells. Many polymorphs may be seen if the effusion is secondary to an underlying pneumonic infection. With tuberculosis, the fluid usually contains many lymphocytes, although tubercle bacilli are rarely seen. Therefore, all pleural fluid samples should be cultured for possible tuberculosis, because this infection can coexist with other pathologies and it is so important not to miss it. In empyema, pus is present in the pleural cavity. It has a characteristic appearance and is full of white cells and organisms. An indwelling catheter should be left in situ to drain an empyema when possible.

The pleural fluid should also be examined for protein content. A transudate (resulting from cardiac or renal failure) can be distinguished from an exudate (from pleural inflammation or malignancy) by its lower protein content (<30 g/l). Light's criteria may also be applied (Box 12.20). When infection is suspected, pleural fluid pH should be measured in non-purulent effusions and, if not available, pleural fluid glucose should be assessed. A pH < 7.2 strongly suggests the need for pleural drainage (pleural fluid glucose <3.4 mmol/l). Pleural fluid lactate dehydrogenase (LDH) is also raised in the presence of infection.

It is recommended that pleural biopsies are undertaken under CT or ultrasound guidance, where available, and whilst Abram's pleural biopsy needles continue to be used in some centres, they are no longer the first choice of technique. Samples should be sent for histological examination, microscopy, culture and sensitivity (MC&S) and, whenever TB is a possibility, for AFB staining and TB culture.

Box 12.20	Light's criteria for diagnosing a pleural effusion

An effusion is exudative if it meets one of the following criteria:

- Pleural fluid protein/serum protein > 0.5
- Pleural fluid lactate dehydrogenase (LDH)/serum LDH ratio > 0.6
- Pleural fluid LDH > two-thirds the upper limit of normal serum LDH

Ridge thoracoscopy and video-assisted thoracoscopic surgery (VATS)

These techniques enable the pleural cavity to be examined directly and biopsies taken; VATS is now becoming the procedure of choice. The ridge method is normally performed under a general anaesthetic by a surgeon who uses direct vision down a rigid thoracoscope after the lung has been deflated. Increasingly, however, more minimally invasive procedures using flexible thoracoscopes attached to cameras are being used—VATS, and are not only able to biopsy the pleura but also biopsy the lung, mediastinal nodes and tumours, decortication of empyemas, lobectomy and pneumonectomy, pleurodesis and endoscopic stapled bullectomy (lung volume reduction surgery).

Lung biopsy

As noted above, the technique of transbronchial biopsy can be used to obtain samples of lung parenchyma, but often samples are too small for diagnosis. In this circumstance, biopsies of the lung taken at thoracoscopy may be of value. Occasionally, a formal open lung biopsy obtained at thoracotomy may be necessary.

When there is a discrete, localized lesion, it may be possible to obtain a biopsy percutaneously with the aid of CT scanning to direct the insertion of the biopsy needle (Fig. 12.13). All samples should be sent for histology, microbiology and TB culture.

Immunological tests

Asthma attacks may be caused by type I immediate hypersensitivity reactions on exposure to common environmental proteins known as allergens. In such individuals, an inherited tendency to produce exaggerated levels of immunoglobulin E (IgE) against these allergens is responsible. Part of the assessment of such allergic patients might include skin-prick tests (see Chapter 20). Alternatively, serum levels of specific (individual) IgEs against allergens may be measured by blood tests (formerly known as radioallergosorbent (RAST) tests) to demonstrate sensitization. The total IgE level is often raised in patients with asthma, rhinitis or eczema. Delayed (type IV, cell-mediated) hypersensitivity is shown by the Mantoux and Heaf skin tests, used to detect the presence of sensitivity to tuberculin protein.

Figure 12.13 A CT-guided percutaneous biopsy in progress. The radiodense (*white*) structure penetrating the chest wall is the biopsy needle.

Figure 12.15 Chest X-ray showing a large left pleural effusion in a young man with a 4-month history of malaise, fever, night sweats and weight loss. The diagnosis of tuberculosis was confirmed on histology of a pleural biopsy and culture of the pleural fluid.

Figure 12.14 Chest X-ray showing right apical scarring and tracheal deviation (detectable clinically) from previous tuberculosis and hyperinflation of the lungs caused by chronic obstructive pulmonary disease in a 66-year-old long-term smoker with 5 years of increasing breathlessness.

Precipitating immunoglobulin G (IgG) antibodies in the circulating blood are present in patients with some fungal diseases, such as bronchopulmonary aspergillosis or aspergilloma. In patients suspected of having an allergic alveolitis, IgG antibodies may be demonstrated to the relevant antigens.

Tests for tuberculosis (TB)

Tuberculosis continues to be a worldwide problem, occurring most frequently as a pulmonary infection, but also commonly in the lymph nodes, as well as

Figure 12.16 Chest X-ray showing a right basal pneumonia in a previously fit 40-year-old man with fever, breathlessness, central cyanosis and pleuritic pain. Chest signs included bronchial breathing and a pleural rub in the right lower zone. The cyanosis was caused by the shunting of deoxygenated blood through the consolidated lung, the increased respiratory rate leading to a low $PaCO_2$ because of increased clearance of carbon dioxide by the unaffected alveoli. *Streptococcus pneumoniae* was grown on blood cultures.

being able to affect any organ of the body. As outlined above, sending relevant samples for smear and culture is essential and often forgotten in hospitals where TB is less common. Sputum can easily be tested by light microscopy using a Zeihl-Neelsen or auramine stain to look for the AFB. Where available, culture should be undertaken as drug monoresistance and multidrug-resistant TB (MDR TB) continue to be a major problem in the fight against the infection. Newer techniques help to diagnose active infection and drug resistance using molecular methods to detect *Mycobacterium tuberculosis* (MTB) complex DNA (e.g. the polymerase chain reaction (PCR)) assay Xpert® MTB/RIF (Cepheid, California, United States) and the line probe assay MTBDRplus® (Hain Lifescience, Nehren, Germany). More recently whole genome sequencing (WGS) is replacing routine culture and sensitivity testing to include different strains of mycobacterium and drug resistance.

Tests for latent TB and the Heaf and Mantoux skin tests are still widely used to look for evidence of previous TB exposure. In many centres, they are being superseded by blood tests that use the interferon gamma-releasing assay (IGRA), which measures interferon gamma released from T-cells activated by the presence of *Mycobacterium tuberculosis*. At the present time, the IGRA blood test does not differentiate between active and latent TB and should be used only to diagnosis latent disease. False-negative results can occur in disseminated and non-pulmonary active disease and can therefore be misleading when diagnosing active infection.

Cardiovascular system | 13

Andrew Archbold, Adam Timmis, and Ceri Davies

Introduction

Recent decades have seen major changes in patterns of cardiovascular disease. In the developed world, syphilitic and tuberculous involvement of the cardiovascular system has become rare, and the incidence of rheumatic disease has declined considerably. Myocardial and conducting tissue diseases are diagnosed with increasing frequency and the importance of arterial hypertension has become recognized. Coronary artery disease has emerged as the major cardiovascular disorder of the era, becoming the most common cause of premature death throughout Europe, North America and Australasia. In the last 30 years, there has been a steady fall in age-specific death rates from coronary artery disease in Western societies, but elsewhere its prevalence is increasing; in the underdeveloped world it now threatens to overtake malnutrition and infectious disease as the major cause of death.

As patterns of cardiovascular disease have changed, so have the cardiologist's diagnostic tools, although a good history and thorough clinical examination remain cornerstones of the assessment of patients with cardiovascular disease. A century that started with the stethoscope, the sphygmomanometer, the chest X-ray and a very rudimentary electrocardiogram saw the development of a variety of new imaging modalities, using ultrasound, radioisotopes, X-rays and magnetic resonance. This non-invasive capability was complemented by the introduction of the catheterization laboratory, permitting angiographic imaging, electrophysiological recording and tissue biopsy of the heart. Add to this the resources of the chemical pathology, bacteriology and molecular biology laboratories, and the array of diagnostic technology available to the modern cardiologist becomes almost overwhelming.

The cardiac history

The history should record details of presenting symptoms, of which the most common are chest pain, fatigue and dyspnoea, palpitations, and presyncope or syncope (see below and Box 13.1). Previous illness should also be recorded, as it may provide important clues about the cardiac diagnosis; thyroid, connective tissue and neoplastic disorders, for example, can all affect the heart. Rheumatic fever in childhood is important because of its association with valvular heart disease, and diabetes and dyslipidaemias because of their association with coronary artery disease. Smoking is a major risk factor for coronary artery disease. Alcohol abuse predisposes to cardiac arrhythmias and cardiomyopathy. The cardiac history should quantify both habits in terms of pack-years smoked and units of alcohol consumed. The use of other recreational drugs (in particular cocaine) can be associated with acute presentations of chest pain and intravenous drug use is an increasingly important cause of infective endocarditis.

The family history should always be documented because coronary artery disease and hypertension often run in families, as do some of the less common cardiovascular disorders, such as hypertrophic cardiomyopathy. Indeed, in patients with hypertrophic cardiomyopathy, a family history of sudden death is probably the single most important indicator of risk. Finally, the drug history should be recorded, because many commonly prescribed drugs are potentially cardiotoxic. β-Blockers and some calcium channel blockers (diltiazem, verapamil), for example, can cause symptomatic bradycardias, and tricyclic antidepressants and β agonists can cause tachyarrhythmias. Vasodilators cause variable reductions in blood pressure, which can lead to syncopal attacks, particularly in patients with aortic stenosis. The myocardial toxicity of certain cytotoxic drugs (notably doxorubicin and related compounds) is an important cause of cardiomyopathy.

Chest pain

Myocardial ischaemia, pericarditis, aortic dissection and pulmonary embolism are the most common causes of acute, severe chest pain. Chronic, recurrent chest pain is usually caused by angina, oesophageal reflux or musculoskeletal pain.

Myocardial ischaemia

Ischaemia of the heart results from an imbalance between myocardial oxygen supply and demand,

---

Box 13.1   Structure for the cardiac history

Presenting complaint (PC)

- The symptom that prompts the patient to seek medical attention—commonly chest pain, breathlessness (dyspnoea), palpitation, dizziness or blackouts (syncope)

History of presenting complaint (HPC)

- This should define the nature of the symptoms, initially through open questioning. Closed questions are used to elicit the presence or absence of features which help to differentiate between diagnoses:
  - Chest pain: site, radiation, character, duration, provoking and relieving factors, associated symptoms?
  - Breathlessness: orthopnoea, paroxysmal nocturnal dyspnoea, ankle swelling, cough, wheeze, haemoptysis?
  - Palpitation: sudden onset and offset, 'thumps' or 'pauses', presyncope or syncope?
  - Dizziness/syncope: provoking factors, warning, duration, recovery?

Risk factors for cardiovascular disease

- Smoking, hypertension, hypercholesterolaemia, diabetes, family history of premature vascular disease

Past medical history (PMH)

- Stroke or transient ischaemic attack (TIA), renal impairment, rheumatic fever, peripheral vascular disease, other
- Operations, hospital clinic attendances

Family history

- Cardiac disease, sudden death

Drug history

- Include quantification of alcohol intake
- If a patient with known cardiovascular disease is not taking the recognized standard treatment, the reason for this should be established. For example, why no statin treatment in a patient with previous myocardial infarction?—'Because it caused muscle pains'.

Box 13.2   Angina

Typical patient

- Middle-aged or elderly man or woman often with a family history of coronary heart disease and one or more of the major reversible risk factors (smoking, hypertension, hypercholesterolaemia, diabetes)

Major symptoms

- Exertional chest pain and shortness of breath. Pain often described as 'heaviness' or 'tightness', and may radiate into arms, neck or jaw. Pain comes predictably after exertion

Major signs

- None, although hypertension and signs of hyperlipidaemia (xanthelasmata, xanthomas) may be present
- Peripheral vascular disease, evidenced by absent pulses or arterial bruits, is commonly associated with coronary heart disease

Diagnosis

- Typical history is most important diagnostic tool
- Electrocardiogram (ECG): often normal; may show Q waves in patients with previous myocardial infarction
- Exercise ECG test: exertional ST depression
- Isotope or magnetic resonance perfusion scan: stress-induced perfusion defects
- Coronary angiogram: confirms coronary artery disease

Additional investigations

- Blood sugar and lipids to rule out diabetes and dyslipidaemia

Comments

- A careful history is the single most important means of diagnosing angina

---

Box 13.3   Causes of angina

Impaired myocardial oxygen supply

- Coronary artery disease:
  - atherosclerosis
  - arteritis in connective tissue disorders
  - diabetes mellitus
- Coronary artery spasm
- Congenital coronary artery disease:
  - arteriovenous fistula
  - anomalous origin from pulmonary artery
- Severe anaemia or hypoxia

Increased myocardial oxygen demand

- Left ventricular hypertrophy:
  - hypertension
  - aortic valve disease
  - hypertrophic cardiomyopathy
- Tachyarrhythmias

---

producing pain called angina (Boxes 13.2 and 13.3). Angina is usually a symptom of atherosclerotic coronary artery disease, which impedes myocardial oxygen supply. Other causes of coronary artery disease (Box 13.4) are rare. However, it is important to be vigilant for causes of angina owing to increased myocardial oxygen demand, such as aortic stenosis. The history is diagnostic for angina if the location of the pain, its character, its relation to exertion and its duration are typical. The patient describes retrosternal pain, which may radiate into the arms, the throat or the jaw. It has a constricting character, is provoked by exertion and relieved within minutes by rest. The patient's threshold for angina is typically reduced after eating or in cold weather owing to the diversion of blood to the gut and the increased myocardial work consequent upon peripheral vasoconstriction, respectively. Occasionally angina is

| Box 13.4 | Causes of coronary artery disease |

- Atherosclerosis
- Arteritis:
  - systemic lupus erythematosus
  - polyarteritis nodosa
  - rheumatoid arthritis
  - ankylosing spondylitis
  - syphilis
  - Takayasu's disease
- Coronary dissection:
  - spontaneous
  - catheter or angioplasty induced
- Embolism:
  - infective endocarditis
  - left atrial/ventricular thrombus
  - left atrial/ventricular tumour
  - prosthetic valve thrombus
  - paradoxical embolism
  - complication of cardiac catheterization
- Coronary mural thickening:
  - amyloidosis
  - radiation therapy
  - Hurler's disease
  - pseudoxanthoma elasticum
- Other causes of coronary luminal narrowing:
  - aortic dissection
  - coronary spasm
- Congenital coronary artery disease:
  - anomalous origin from pulmonary artery
  - arteriovenous fistula

| Box 13.5 | Acute coronary syndromes |

Typical patient

- Middle-aged (male) or elderly (either sex) patient, often with a family history of coronary artery disease and one or more of the major reversible risk factors (smoking, hypertension, hypercholesterolaemia, diabetes). Care must be taken in female patients: coronary artery disease occurs frequently and is often under-diagnosed.
- In many patients, there is no preceding history of angina.

Major symptoms

- Chest pain and shortness of breath. Pain usually prolonged and often described as 'heaviness' or 'tightness', with radiation into arms, neck or jaw. Alternative descriptions include 'congestion' or 'burning', which may be confused with indigestion.

Major signs

- Frequently none
- Autonomic disturbance, sweating, vomiting – implies myocardial infarction
- Tachycardia (anterior myocardial infarction), bradycardia (inferior myocardial infarction)
- Fourth heart sound, dyskinetic precordial impulse, pulmonary oedema with large infarcts

Diagnosis

(STEMI = ST elevation myocardial infarction)

	STEMI	Non-STEMI	Unstable angina
ECG	ST elevation	Normal, ST depression, T-wave inversion	Normal, ST depression, T-wave inversion
Cardiac biomarkers (e.g. troponin I or T)	Raised	Raised	Normal

Additional investigations

- Biochemistry: blood sugar and lipids to rule out diabetes and dyslipidaemia
- Risk stratification: echocardiogram (left ventricular function), coronary angiogram in high-risk patients, perfusion imaging in low-risk patients

Comments

- History and troponin testing most useful diagnostic tools in non-ST elevation acute coronary syndromes

provoked only by the first significant activity of the day, a phenomenon known as the 'warm-up effect', which is caused by myocardial preconditioning. Less commonly, myocardial ischaemia may manifest as breathlessness, fatigue or symptoms that the patient finds difficult to describe—'I just have to stop'—in which case the clues to the diagnosis are the relation of the symptoms to exertion, the presence of risk factors for coronary artery disease and the absence of an alternative explanation for the symptoms, such as heart failure.

Acute coronary syndromes

In acute coronary syndromes, which are life-threatening cardiac emergencies, the pain is similar in location and character to angina, but is usually more severe, more prolonged and unrelieved by rest (Box 13.5).

Pericarditis

Pericarditis causes central chest pain, which is sharp in character and aggravated by deep inspiration, cough or postural changes. Characteristically, the pain is exacerbated by lying recumbent and reduced by sitting forward. Pericarditis is usually idiopathic or caused by Coxsackie B infection. It may also

occur as a complication of myocardial infarction, but other causes are seen less commonly (Box 13.6). Myocardial involvement—myocarditis—is increasingly recognized. It is associated with the release of cardiac enzymes and abnormalities on the electrocardiogram (ECG) that can be indistinguishable from myocardial infarction.

Aortic dissection

Aortic dissection produces severe tearing pain in either the front or the back of the chest. The onset

Box 13.6	Causes of acute pericarditis

- Idiopathic
- Infective:
  - viral (Coxsackie B, influenza, herpes simplex)
  - bacterial (*Staphylococcus aureus*, *Mycobacterium tuberculosis*)
- Connective tissue disease:
  - systemic lupus erythematosus
  - rheumatoid arthritis
  - polyarteritis nodosa
- Uraemia
- Malignancy (e.g. breast, lung, lymphoma, leukaemia)
- Radiation therapy
- Acute myocardial infarction
- Post-myocardial infarction/cardiotomy (Dressler's syndrome)

Box 13.7	Aortic dissection

Typical patient

- Middle-aged or elderly patient with a history of hypertension or arteriosclerotic disease
- Occasionally younger patient with aortic root disease (e.g. Marfan's syndrome)

Major symptoms

- Chest pain, typically interscapular

Major signs

- Often none
- Sometimes regional arterial insufficiency (e.g. occlusions of coronary artery causing myocardial infarction, carotid or vertebral artery causing stroke, spinal artery causing hemi- or quadriplegia, renal artery causing renal failure); subclavian artery occlusion may cause differential blood pressure in either arm; aortic regurgitation; cardiac tamponade; sudden death.

Diagnosis

- Chest X-ray: widened mediastinum, occasionally with left pleural effusion
- Transoesophageal echocardiogram, computed tomography (CT) scan or magnetic resonance imaging (MRI) scan: confirms dissection

Comments

- Type A dissections involve the ascending aorta and are usually treated surgically. Type B dissections involve the arch and/or descending aorta and are usually managed medically or with an endovascular stent.

is abrupt, unlike the crescendo quality of ischaemic cardiac pain (Box 13.7).

Pulmonary embolism

Peripheral pulmonary embolism causes sudden-onset sharp, pleuritic chest pain, breathlessness and haemoptysis. Major, central pulmonary embolism

Box 13.8	Pulmonary embolism

Typical patient

- Recent surgery, lower limb fracture or long-distance air travel; obese; sedentary; heart failure; malignancy

Major symptoms

- Chest pain, dyspnoea, haemoptysis, syncope

Major signs

- Peripheral emboli: pleural rub
- Large, central emboli: tachycardia, hypotension, cyanosis, raised jugular venous pressure (JVP)

Diagnosis

- D-Dimer: a negative D-dimer in a low-risk patient makes pulmonary embolism very unlikely.
- ECG: sinus tachycardia; right bundle branch block (RBBB); classic 'S1, Q3, T3' pattern uncommon
- Chest X-ray: normal; wedge-shaped peripheral opacification; absent pulmonary vascular markings
- Echocardiogram: dilated right heart in some cases of large central pulmonary embolism
- CT pulmonary angiogram: has superseded V/Q scanning as the diagnostic test of choice.

Comments

- Suspect pulmonary embolism in patients with unexplained hypoxia. Thrombolytic therapy should be considered for patients with pulmonary embolism associated with shock and/or a dilated right heart on echo. Patients with no risk factors for pulmonary embolism should be investigated for prothrombotic states.

presents with breathlessness, chest pain that can be indistinguishable from ischaemic chest pains and syncope. Risk factors for pulmonary embolism should be sought in the history (Box 13.8).

Rare cardiovascular causes of chest pain include mitral valve disease associated with massive left atrial dilatation. This causes discomfort in the back, sometimes associated with dysphagia owing to oesophageal compression. Aortic aneurysms can also cause pain in the chest owing to local compression.

Dyspnoea

Dyspnoea is an abnormal awareness of breathing occurring either at rest or at an unexpectedly low level of exertion. It is a major symptom of many cardiac disorders, particularly left heart failure (Table 13.1), but its mechanisms are complex. In acute pulmonary oedema and orthopnoea, dyspnoea is caused mainly by elevated left atrial pressure that characterizes left heart failure (Box 13.9). This produces a corresponding elevation of the pulmonary capillary pressure and increases transudation into the lungs, which become oedematous and stiff. Oxygenation of blood in the pulmonary arterioles is reduced, causing hypoxaemia, and this, together

Table 13.1 Causes of heart failure

Ventricular pathophysiology	Clinical examples
Restricted filling	Mitral stenosis
	Constrictive pericarditis
	Restrictive cardiomyopathy
	Hypertrophic cardiomyopathy
Pressure loading	Hypertension
	Aortic stenosis
	Coarctation of the aorta
Volume loading	Mitral regurgitation
	Aortic regurgitation
Contractile impairment	Coronary artery disease
	Dilated cardiomyopathy
	Myocarditis
Arrhythmia	Severe bradycardia
	Severe tachycardia

Box 13.9 Acute left ventricular failure

Typical patient

- Patient with acute myocardial infarction or known left ventricular disease

Major symptoms

- Severe dyspnoea, orthopnoea, frothy sputum

Major signs

- Low-output state (hypotension, oliguria, cold periphery); tachycardia; S3; sweating; crackles at lung bases

Diagnosis

- Chest X-ray: bilateral air space consolidation with typical perihilar distribution
- Echocardiogram: usually confirms left ventricular disease

Additional investigations

- ECG: may show evidence of acute or previous myocardial infarction
- Blood gas analysis: shows variable hypoxaemia

Comments

- Although most cases are caused by acute myocardial infarction or advanced left ventricular disease, it is vital to exclude valvular disease, which is potentially correctable by surgery.

Box 13.10 Congestive heart failure

Typical patient

- Middle-aged (male) or elderly (either sex) patient with a history of myocardial infarction or longstanding hypertension
- In cases where there is no clear cause, always enquire about alcohol consumption.

Major symptoms

- Exertional fatigue and shortness of breath, with orthopnoea and paroxysmal nocturnal dyspnoea in advanced cases

Major signs

- Fluid retention: basal crackles, raised JVP, peripheral oedema
- Reduced cardiac output: cool skin, peripheral cyanosis
- Other findings: third heart sound

Diagnosis

- ECG: usually abnormal; often shows Q waves (previous myocardial infarction), left ventricular hypertrophy (hypertension), or left bundle branch block (LBBB)
- Chest X-ray: cardiac enlargement, congested lung fields
- Echocardiogram: left ventricular dilatation with regional (coronary artery disease) or global (cardiomyopathy) contractile impairment

Additional investigations

- Raised B-type natriuretic peptide useful in cases of diagnostic uncertainly
- Renal function as prelude to diuretic and angiotensin converting enzyme (ACE) inhibitor therapy
- Blood count to rule out anaemia

Comments

- The echocardiogram is the single most important diagnostic test in the patient with heart failure.

Table 13.2 NYHA classification

NYHA class	Description
I	Asymptomatic
II	Symptoms on normal exertion (e.g. walking up a flight of stairs)
III	Symptoms on minimal exertion, e.g. getting dressed
IV	Symptoms at rest

NYHA, New York Heart Association.

with the extra effort required to ventilate the stiff lungs, causes dyspnoea.

Exertional dyspnoea

Exertional dyspnoea is the most troublesome symptom in heart failure (Box 13.10). Exercise causes a sharp increase in left atrial pressure and this contributes to the pathogenesis of dyspnoea by causing pulmonary congestion (see above). However, the severity of dyspnoea does not correlate closely with exertional left atrial pressure, and other factors must therefore be important. These include respiratory muscle fatigue and the effects of exertional acidosis on peripheral chemoreceptors. As left heart failure worsens, exercise tolerance deteriorates. In advanced disease, the patient is dyspnoeic at rest.

Breathlessness in heart failure can be simply classified by use of the New York Heart Association Classification (Table 13.2). It is simple to acquire and despite poor reproducibility and its subjective nature provides powerful prognostic information. For example, patients with Class IV heart failure have a very poor outlook.

Orthopnoea

In patients with heart failure, lying flat causes a steep rise in left atrial and pulmonary capillary pressure, resulting in pulmonary congestion and severe dyspnoea. To obtain uninterrupted sleep, extra pillows are required, and in advanced disease, the patient may choose to sleep sitting in a chair.

Paroxysmal nocturnal dyspnoea

Frank pulmonary oedema on lying flat wakes the patient from sleep with distressing dyspnoea and fear of imminent death. The symptoms are corrected by standing upright, which allows gravitational pooling of blood to lower the left atrial and pulmonary capillary pressure, the patient often feeling the need to obtain air at an open window.

Fatigue

Exertional fatigue, an important symptom of heart failure, is particularly troublesome towards the end of the day. Its aetiology is complex but is caused partly by deconditioning and muscular atrophy.

Palpitation

Awareness of the heartbeat is common during exertion or heightened emotion. Under other circumstances it may be indicative of an abnormal cardiac rhythm. A description of the rate and rhythm of the palpitation is essential as are exacerbating behaviours—such as exercise, caffeine intake. Extrasystoles are common but rarely signify important heart disease. They usually are experienced as 'missed' or 'dropped' beats; the forceful beats that follow may also be noticed. Rapid irregular palpitation is typical of atrial fibrillation. Rapid regular palpitation of abrupt onset occurs in atrial, junctional and ventricular tachyarrhythmias.

Dizziness and syncope

Cardiovascular disorders produce dizziness and syncope by transient hypotension, resulting in abrupt cerebral hypoperfusion. For this reason, patients who experience cardiac syncope usually describe either brief lightheadedness or no warning symptoms at all prior to their syncopal attacks. Recovery is usually rapid, unlike with other common causes of syncope (e.g. stroke, epilepsy, overdose).

Postural hypotension

Syncope on standing upright reflects inadequate baroreceptor-mediated vasoconstriction. It is common in the elderly in whom it is frequently compounded by medication. Abrupt reductions in blood pressure and cerebral perfusion cause the patient to fall to the ground, whereupon the condition corrects itself.

Vasovagal syncope

Vasovagal syncope is caused by autonomic overactivity, usually provoked by emotional or painful stimuli, less commonly by coughing or micturition ('cough syncope' or 'micturition syncope'). Only rarely are syncopal attacks so frequent as to be significantly disabling ('malignant' vasovagal syndrome). Vasodilatation and inappropriate slowing of the pulse combine to reduce blood pressure and cerebral perfusion. Recovery is rapid if the patient lies down.

Carotid sinus hypersensitivity

Exaggerated vagal discharge following external stimulation of the carotid sinus (e.g. from shaving or a tight shirt collar) causes reflex vasodilatation and slowing of the pulse. These may combine to reduce blood pressure and cerebral perfusion in some elderly patients, causing loss of consciousness.

Valvular obstruction

Fixed valvular obstruction in aortic stenosis may prevent a normal rise in cardiac output during exertion, such that the physiological vasodilatation that occurs in exercising muscle produces an abrupt reduction in blood pressure and cerebral perfusion, resulting in syncope. Vasodilator therapy may cause syncope by a similar mechanism. Intermittent obstruction of the mitral valve by left atrial tumours (usually myxoma or thrombus) may also cause syncopal episodes (Fig. 13.1).

Stokes–Adams attacks

Stokes–Adams attacks are caused by self-limiting episodes of asystole (Fig. 13.2) or rapid tachyarrhythmias (including ventricular fibrillation). The loss of cardiac output causes syncope and striking pallor. Following restoration of normal rhythm, recovery is rapid and associated with flushing of the skin as flow through the dilated cutaneous bed is re-established.

The cardiac examination

A methodical approach is recommended, starting with inspection of the patient and proceeding to examination of the radial pulse, measurement of heart rate and blood pressure, examination of the neck (carotid pulse, jugular venous pulse), palpation of the anterior chest wall, auscultation of the heart, percussion and auscultation of the lung bases and, finally, examination of the peripheral pulses and auscultation for carotid and femoral arterial bruits (Box 13.11).

Figure 13.1   Left atrial myxoma: 2D echocardiogram (long-axis view). During diastole, the tumour (*arrowed*) prolapses through the mitral valve and obstructs left ventricular filling.

Figure 13.2   Prolonged sinus arrest. After the fifth sinus beat there is a pause of about 1.8 seconds terminated by a nodal escape beat (*arrowed*) before sinus rhythm resumes.

Box 13.11	Routine for the cardiovascular system examination

- Wash hands
- Introduce yourself to patient
- Recline patient at 45°
- Observe general appearance: comfortable, breathless, pale?
- Inspect the hands for clubbing, splinter haemorrhages, nicotine staining
- Examine the radial pulse(s) for symmetry, rate, rhythm, character (collapsing?)
- Measure the blood pressure
- Assess the height and waveform of the JVP
- Examine the carotid pulse character (slow rising?) and volume (Corrigan's sign?)
- Inspect the face, eyes and mucous membranes for xanthelasma, corneal arcus and anaemia, and cyanosis, respectively
- Inspect the chest for scars and pulsations
- Assess the position and character of the apex beat
- Palpate the praecordium for heaves and thrills
- Auscultate the heart
- Auscultate the lungs
- Examine the ankles and sacrum for oedema
- Examine the peripheral pulses

Inspection of the patient

Chest wall deformities, such as pectus excavatum, should be noted, because these may compress the heart and displace the apex, giving a spurious impression of cardiac enlargement. The presence of a median sternotomy scar usually indicates previous coronary artery bypass graft (CABG) and/or cardiac valve surgery. The long saphenous vein is the standard conduit for vein grafts so patients with prior CABG often also have a scar along the medial aspect of one or both legs. A lateral thoracotomy scar may indicate previous mitral valvotomy. Large ventricular or aortic aneurysms may cause visible pulsations. Superior vena caval obstruction is associated with prominent venous collaterals on the chest wall. Prominent venous collaterals around the shoulder occur in axillary or subclavian vein obstruction.

Hypercholesterolaemia may be suggested by the presence of tendon and ocular xanthelasma.

Evidence of device implantation (permanent pacemaker or implantable defibrillator) is seen with a scar usually under the left clavicle. In thin patients a bulge from the generator may also be seen.

Anaemia

This may exacerbate angina and heart failure. Pallor of the mucous membranes is a useful but sometimes misleading physical sign, and diagnosis requires laboratory measurement of the haemoglobin concentration.

Cyanosis

Cyanosis is a blue discolouration of the skin and mucous membranes caused by increased concentration of reduced haemoglobin in the superficial blood vessels. Peripheral cyanosis may result when cutaneous vasoconstriction slows the blood flow and increases oxygen extraction in the skin and the lips. It is physiological during cold exposure. It also occurs in heart failure, when reduced cardiac output produces reflex cutaneous vasoconstriction. In mitral stenosis, cyanosis over the malar area produces the characteristic mitral facies or malar flush.

Central cyanosis may result from the reduced arterial oxygen saturation caused by cardiac or pulmonary disease. It affects not only the skin and the lips but also the mucous membranes of the mouth. Cardiac causes include pulmonary oedema (which prevents adequate oxygenation of the blood) and congenital heart disease. Congenital defects associated with central cyanosis include those in which desaturated venous blood bypasses the lungs by ('reversed') shunting through septal defects or a patent ductus arteriosus (e.g. Eisenmenger's syndrome, Fallot's tetralogy).

The mouth should also be inspected for signs of poor dental hygiene.

Clubbing of the fingers and toes

In congenital cyanotic heart disease, clubbing is not present at birth but develops during infancy and may become very marked. Infective endocarditis is the other cardiac cause of clubbing.

Other cutaneous and ocular signs of infective endocarditis

Other cutaneous and ocular signs of infective endocarditis are caused by immune complex deposition in the capillary circulation. A vasculitic rash is common, as are splinter haemorrhages in the nail bed, although these are a very non-specific finding. Other 'classic' manifestations of endocarditis, including Osler's nodes (tender erythematous nodules in the pulps of the fingers), Janeway lesions (painless erythematous lesions on the palms) and Roth's spots (erythematous lesions in the optic fundi), are rarely seen now.

Coldness of the extremities

In patients hospitalized with severe heart failure, coldness of the extremities is an important sign of reduced cardiac output. It is caused by reflex vasoconstriction of the cutaneous bed.

Pyrexia

Infective endocarditis is invariably associated with pyrexia, which may be low grade or 'swinging' in nature if paravalvular abscess develops. Pyrexia also occurs for the first 3 days after myocardial infarction.

Oedema

Subcutaneous oedema that pits on digital pressure is a cardinal feature of congestive heart failure. Pressure should be applied over a bony prominence (tibia, lateral malleoli, sacrum) to provide effective compression. Oedema is caused by salt and water retention by the kidney. Two mechanisms are responsible:
1. Reduced sodium delivery to the nephron. This is caused by reduced glomerular filtration owing to constriction of the preglomerular arterioles in response to sympathetic activation and angiotensin II production.
2. Increased sodium reabsorption from the nephron. This is the more important mechanism. It occurs particularly in the proximal tubule early in heart failure but, as failure worsens, renin-angiotensin activation stimulates aldosterone release, which increases sodium reabsorption in the distal nephron.

Salt and water retention expands plasma volume and increases the capillary hydrostatic pressure. Hydrostatic forces driving fluid out of the capillary exceed the osmotic forces reabsorbing it, so that oedema fluid accumulates in the interstitial space. The effect of gravity on capillary hydrostatic pressure ensures that oedema is most prominent around the ankles in the ambulant patient and over the sacrum in the bedridden patient. In advanced heart failure, oedema may involve the legs, genitalia and trunk. Transudation into the peritoneal cavity (ascites), the pleural and pericardial spaces may also occur.

Arterial pulse

The arterial pulses should be palpated to evaluate rate, rhythm, character and symmetry.

Rate and rhythm

By convention, both rate and rhythm are assessed by palpating the right radial pulse. Rate, expressed in beats per minute (bpm), is measured by counting the number of beats in a timed period of 15 seconds and multiplying by four. Normal sinus rhythm is regular, but in young patients may show phasic variation in rate during respiration (sinus arrhythmia). An irregular rhythm usually indicates atrial fibrillation, but it may also be caused by frequent ectopic beats or self-limiting paroxysmal arrhythmias. In patients with atrial fibrillation, the rate should be measured by auscultation at the cardiac apex, because beats that follow very short diastolic intervals may create a 'pulse deficit' by not generating sufficient pressure to be palpable at the radial artery.

Character

Character is defined by the volume and waveform of the pulse and should be evaluated at the right carotid artery (i.e. the pulse closest to the heart and least subject to damping and distortion in the arterial tree). Pulse volume provides a crude indication of stroke volume, being small in heart failure and large in aortic regurgitation. The waveform of the pulse is of greater diagnostic importance (Fig. 13.3). Severe aortic stenosis produces a slow-rising carotid pulse; the fixed obstruction restricts the rate at which blood can be ejected from the left ventricle. In aortic regurgitation, in diastole, the left ventricle receives not only its normal pulmonary venous return but also a proportion of the blood ejected into the aorta during the previous systole as it flows back

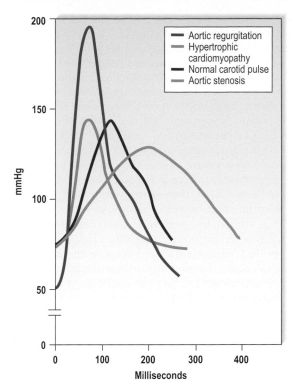

Figure 13.3 The waveform of the pulse is characterized by the rate of rise of the carotid upstroke. Note that in aortic regurgitation, the upstroke is rapid and followed by abrupt diastolic 'collapse'. In hypertrophic cardiomyopathy, the upstroke is also rapid and the pulse has a jerky character. In aortic stenosis, the upstroke is slow with a plateau.

Figure 13.4 Paradoxical pulse (radial artery pressure signal). The patient had severe tamponade. Note the exaggerated (>10 mmHg) decline in arterial pressure during inspiration.

through an incompetent valve. The resultant large stroke volume, vigorously ejected, produces a rapidly rising carotid pulse, which collapses in early diastole owing to backflow through the aortic valve. This collapsing pulse can be exaggerated at the radial artery by lifting the arm. In mixed aortic valve disease, a biphasic pulse with two systolic peaks is occasionally found. Alternating pulse—alternating high and low systolic peaks—occurs in severe left ventricular failure, but the mechanism for this is unknown.

Paradoxical pulse refers to an inspiratory decline in systolic pressure greater than 10 mmHg (Fig. 13.4). In normal circumstances, inspiration results in an increase in venous return as blood is 'sucked into' the thorax by the decline in intrathoracic pressure. This increases right ventricular stroke volume, but left ventricular stroke volume falls slightly (ventricular interdependence). When the heart is constrained in a 'fixed box' by a pericardial effusion (cardiac tamponade) or by thickened pericardium (pericardial constriction), the increased inspiratory right ventricular blood volume reduces left ventricular compliance, resulting in a more pronounced reduction in left ventricular filling, stroke volume and systolic blood pressure during inspiration. 'Pulsus paradoxus' therefore represents an exaggeration of the normal inspiratory decline in systolic pressure and is not truly paradoxical. Pulsus paradoxus in acute severe asthma is thought to be caused by negative pleural

pressure increasing afterload and thereby impedance to left ventricular emptying.

Blood pressure is measured by inflating a cuff until no sounds are heard. The pressure is then slowly decreased until systolic sounds are first heard during expiration but not during inspiration; note this reading. The pressure is slowly decreased further until sounds are heard throughout the respiratory cycle (inspiration and expiration); note this second reading. If the pressure difference between the two readings is above 10 mmHg, it can be classified as pulsus paradoxus.

Symmetry

Symmetry of the radial, brachial, carotid, femoral, popliteal and pedal pulses should be confirmed. A reduced or absent pulse indicates an obstruction more proximally in the arterial tree, caused usually by atherosclerosis or thromboembolism, less commonly by aortic dissection. Coarctation of the aorta causes symmetrical reduction and delay of the femoral pulses compared with the radial pulses ('radio-femoral delay'), a sign that should be looked for in younger patients with hypertension. Bruits from collateral vessels may also be heard over the back of such patients.

Measurement of blood pressure

Blood pressure is measured indirectly, traditionally by sphygmomanometry, but automated blood pressure monitors are being used increasingly in clinical practice. The principle of manual blood pressure measurement is that turbulent flow through a partially compressed artery (typically the brachial) creates noises that can be auscultated with a stethoscope and the points at which these noises (called Korotkoff sounds) change in intensity correlate with systemic arterial pressures. Accurate blood-pressure measurement requires careful technique; patients should be sitting or lying at ease because significant changes in arterial pressure occur with exertion, anxiety and changes in posture. The manometer should be at the same level of the cuff on the patient's arm and the observer's eye. For most adult patients, a standard cuff (12 cm width) is appropriate, but obese subjects require use of a wider (thigh) cuff of 15 cm or the blood pressure will be overestimated. For children, various sized cuffs are available; select the one that covers most of the upper arm leaving a gap of 1 cm or so below the axilla and above the antecubital fossa.

Palpate the radial pulse as the cuff is inflated to a pressure of 20 mmHg above the level at which radial pulsation can no longer be felt. Place the stethoscope lightly over the brachial artery and reduce the pressure in the cuff at a rate of 2–3 mmHg/second until the first sounds are heard. This, the first Korotkoff sound, correlates with systolic blood pressure as flow is just possible through the pressure applied by the compressive cuff. As the pressure is lowered further, subtle changes in pitch and volume occur; these are the second and third Korotkoff sounds and are not important clinically. With further lowering of the pressure in the cuff, the artery becomes less compressed, flow becomes less turbulent and the sounds over the brachial artery become muffled. This is the fourth Korotkoff sound. Shortly after this (usually 1–10 mmHg lower), the sounds die away completely as flow is unimpeded by the cuff; this, the fifth Korotkoff sound, correlates most accurately with diastolic blood pressure. Its identification is also less subjective than the fourth, but in some conditions (aortic regurgitation, arteriovenous fistula, pregnancy), the Korotkoff sounds remain audible despite complete deflation of the cuff. In such situations, phase 4 must be used for the diastolic measurement. Both systolic and diastolic values are recorded; the difference between these two values is called the pulse pressure. Certain conditions of the aortic valve may cause important abnormalities of pulse pressure. Supine and erect blood pressure measurements provide an assessment of baroreceptor function, a postural drop being defined by a fall in systolic blood pressure on standing. It is essential to work swiftly as well as accurately, as compression of a limb, by itself, will cause a rise in blood pressure. If several successive measurements are made, the air pressure in the cuff should be allowed to fall to zero between readings.

Jugular venous pulse

Fluctuations in right atrial pressure during the cardiac cycle generate a pulse that is transmitted backwards into the jugular veins. It is best examined in good light while the patient reclines at 45°. If the right atrial pressure is very low, however, visualization of the jugular venous pulse may require a smaller reclining angle. Alternatively, manual pressure over the upper right side of the abdomen may be used to produce a transient increase in venous return to the heart, which elevates the jugular venous pulse (hepatojugular reflux).

Jugular venous pressure

The jugular venous pressure (JVP) should be assessed from the waveform of the internal jugular vein, which lies adjacent to the medial border of the sternocleidomastoid muscle. Distention of the external jugular vein is a useful clue to an elevated JVP but, strictly speaking, it should not be used because it can be compressed as it passes under the clavicle. The JVP is measured in centimetres vertically from the sternal angle to the top of the venous waveform. The normal upper limit is 4 cm. This is about 9 cm above the right atrium and corresponds to a pressure of 6 mmHg. Elevation of the JVP indicates a raised right atrial pressure unless the superior vena cava is obstructed, producing engorgement of the neck veins (Box 13.12). During inspiration, the pressure within the chest decreases and there is a fall in the JVP. In constrictive pericarditis, and less commonly in tamponade, inspiration produces a paradoxical rise in the JVP (Kussmaul's sign) because the increased venous return that occurs during inspiration cannot be accommodated within the constrained right side of the heart (Fig. 13.5).

Waveform of jugular venous pulses

In sinus rhythm, the jugular venous pulse has a double waveform attributable to the 'a' and 'v'

Box 13.12	Causes of elevated jugular venous pressure

- Congestive heart failure
- Cor pulmonale
- Pulmonary embolism
- Right ventricular infarction
- Tricuspid valve disease
- Tamponade
- Constrictive pericarditis
- Hypertrophic/restrictive cardiomyopathy
- Superior vena cava obstruction
- Iatrogenic fluid overload, particularly in surgical and renal patients

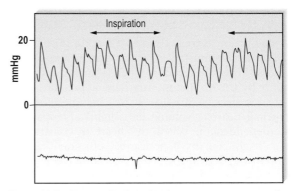

Figure 13.5 Kussmaul's sign. Jugular venous pressure recording in a patient with tamponade. The venous pressure is raised and there is a particularly prominent systolic 'x' descent, giving the waveform of the JVP an unusually dynamic appearance. Note the inspiratory rise in atrial pressure (Kussmaul's sign) reflecting the inability of the tamponaded right heart to accommodate the inspiratory increase in venous return.

waves separated by the 'x' and 'y' descents. The 'a' wave is produced by atrial systole. It is followed by the 'x' descent (marking descent of the tricuspid valve ring), which is interrupted by the diminutive 'c' wave caused by tricuspid valve closure. Atrial pressure then rises again, producing the 'v' wave as the atrium fills passively during ventricular systole. The decline in atrial pressure as the tricuspid valve opens to allow ventricular filling produces the 'y' descent. Important abnormalities of the pattern of deflections are shown in Figure 13.6.

In atrial fibrillation, there is no atrial contraction. Consequently, there is no 'a' wave and the jugular venous pulse loses its double waveform. It is not always easy to differentiate venous from arterial pulsations in the neck, but several features help to distinguish the jugular venous pulse from the carotid arterial pulse (Box 13.13).

Palpation of the chest wall

The apex beat is defined as the lowest and most lateral point at which the cardiac impulse can be palpated. Inferior or lateral displacement from its normal

Box 13.13	Characteristics of the jugular venous pulse

- Double waveform (in sinus rhythm)
- Varies with respiration
- Varies with posture
- Impalpable
- Obliterated by pressure at base of waveform
- Transient increase in volume and height with hepatojugular reflux

location in the fifth intercostal space in the mid-clavicular line usually indicates cardiac enlargement. Chronic volume loading of the left ventricle (mitral regurgitation, aortic regurgitation) causes left ventricular dilatation which can be appreciated clinically. In contrast, isolated pressure loading of the left ventricle (hypertension, aortic stenosis) causes left ventricular hypertrophy which does not

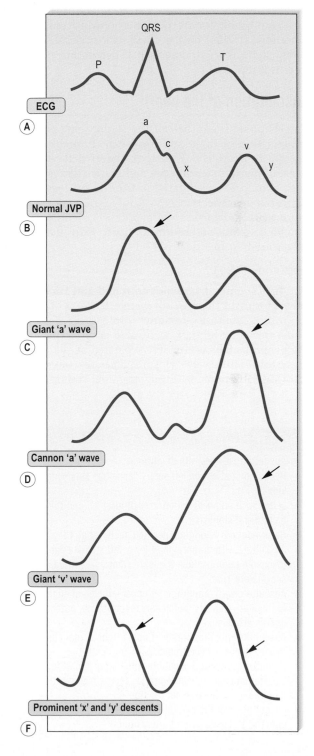

Figure 13.6 Waveform of the jugular venous pulse. **(A)** The ECG is portrayed at the top of the illustration. Note how electrical events precede mechanical events in the cardiac cycle. Thus, the P wave (atrial depolarization) and the QRS complex (ventricular depolarization) precede the 'a' and 'v' waves, respectively, of the JVP. **(B)** Normal JVP. The 'a' wave produced by atrial systole is the most prominent deflection. It is followed by the 'x' descent, interrupted by the small 'c' wave marking tricuspid valve closure. Atrial pressure then rises again ('v' wave) as the atrium fills passively during ventricular systole. The decline in atrial pressure as the tricuspid valve opens produces the 'y' descent. **(C)** Giant 'a' wave. Forceful atrial contraction against a stenosed tricuspid valve or a non-compliant hypertrophied right ventricle produces an unusually prominent 'a' wave. **(D)** Cannon 'a' wave. This is caused by atrial systole against a closed tricuspid valve. It occurs when atrial and ventricular rhythms are dissociated (complete heart block, ventricular tachycardia) and marks coincident atrial and ventricular systole. **(E)** Giant 'v' wave. This is an important sign of tricuspid regurgitation. The regurgitant jet produces pulsatile systolic waves in the JVP. **(F)** Prominent 'x' and 'y' descents. These occur in constrictive pericarditis and give the JVP an unusually dynamic appearance. In tamponade, only the 'x' descent is usually exaggerated.

cause displacement of the apex beat. Palpable third and fourth heart sounds give the apical impulse a double thrust. In the past, considerable importance was attached to the character of the apical impulse ('thrusting' in aortic valve disease, 'tapping' in mitral stenosis), but this is of very limited practical value in the modern era.

Left ventricular aneurysms can sometimes be palpated medial to the cardiac apex. Right ventricular enlargement produces a systolic thrust (heave) in the left parasternal area. The turbulent flow responsible for murmurs may produce palpable vibrations (thrills) on the chest wall, particularly in aortic stenosis, ventricular septal defect and patent ductus arteriosus.

Auscultation of the heart

The diaphragm and bell of the stethoscope permit appreciation of high- and low-pitched auscultatory events, respectively. The apex, lower left sternal edge, upper left sternal edge and upper right sternal edge should be auscultated in turn. These locations correspond respectively to the mitral, tricuspid, pulmonary and aortic areas, and loosely identify sites at which sounds and murmurs arising from the four valves are best heard (Box 13.14).

First sound (S1)

The first sound corresponds to mitral and tricuspid valve closure at the onset of systole. It is accentuated in mitral stenosis because prolonged diastolic filling through the narrowed valve ensures that the thickened leaflets are widely separated at the onset of systole. Thus, valve closure generates unusually vigorous vibrations. In advanced mitral stenosis, the

---

Box 13.14 Routine for auscultation of the heart

- Auscultate at apex with diaphragm
- Reposition patient on left side: 'Please turn onto your left side'
- Listen with diaphragm (mitral regurgitation) and then bell (mitral stenosis)
- Return patient to original position, reclining at 45°
- Auscultate with diaphragm at lower left sternal edge (tricuspid regurgitation, tricuspid stenosis, ventricular septal defect)
- Auscultate with diaphragm at upper left sternal edge (pulmonary stenosis, pulmonary regurgitation, patent ductus arteriosus)
- Auscultate with diaphragm at upper right sternal edge (aortic stenosis, hypertrophic cardiomyopathy)
- Sit patient forward. Auscultate with diaphragm at lower left sternal edge in held expiration (aortic regurgitation): 'breathe in … breathe out … stop'
- Auscultate over the carotid arteries (radiation of murmur of aortic stenosis, carotid artery bruits)

---

valve is rigid and immobile and S1 becomes soft again.

Second sound (S2)

The second sound corresponds to aortic and pulmonary valve closure following ventricular ejection. S2 is single during expiration. Inspiration, however, causes physiological splitting into aortic followed by pulmonary components because increased venous return to the right side of the heart delays pulmonary valve closure. Important abnormalities of S2 are illustrated in Figure 13.7.

Third and fourth sounds (S3, S4)

The third and fourth sounds are low-frequency sounds that occur early and late in diastole, respectively. When present, they give a characteristic 'gallop' to the cardiac rhythm. Both sounds are best heard with the bell of the stethoscope at the cardiac apex. They are caused by abrupt tensing of the ventricular walls following rapid diastolic filling. Rapid filling occurs early in diastole (S3) following atrioventricular valve opening, and again late in diastole (S4) owing to atrial contraction. S3 is physiological in children and young adults, but usually disappears after the age of 40. It also occurs in high-output states caused by anaemia, fever, pregnancy and thyrotoxicosis. After the age of 40, S3 is nearly always pathological, usually

Figure 13.7 Splitting of the second heart sound. The first sound, representing mitral and tricuspid closure, is usually single, but the aortic and pulmonary components of the second sound normally split during inspiration as increased venous return delays right ventricular emptying. Abnormal splitting of the second heart sound is an important sign of heart disease.

indicating left ventricular failure or, less commonly, mitral regurgitation or constrictive pericarditis. In the elderly, S4 is sometimes physiological. More commonly, however, it is pathological, and occurs when vigorous atrial contraction late in diastole is required to augment filling of a hypertrophied, non-compliant ventricle (e.g. hypertension, aortic stenosis, hypertrophic cardiomyopathy).

Systolic clicks and opening snaps

Valve opening, unlike valve closure, is normally silent. In aortic stenosis, however, valve opening produces a click in early systole that precedes the ejection murmur. The click is only audible if the valve cusps are pliant and non-calcified, and is particularly prominent in the congenitally bicuspid valve. A click later in systole suggests mitral valve prolapse, particularly when followed by a murmur. In mitral stenosis, elevated left atrial pressure causes forceful opening of the thickened valve leaflets. This generates a snap early in diastole that precedes the mid-diastolic murmur.

Heart murmurs

Heart murmurs are caused by turbulent flow within the heart and great vessels (Fig. 13.8). Occasionally the turbulence is caused by increased flow through a normal valve, usually aortic or pulmonary, producing an 'innocent' murmur. However, murmurs may also indicate valve disease or abnormal communications between the left and right sides of the heart (e.g. septal defects).

Rheumatic heart disease has become much less common in developed countries, although it remains common elsewhere, and is the cause of many of the classic heart murmurs (Box 13.15). Degenerative valve disease (calcific aortic stenosis, mitral regurgitation owing to chordal rupture) is increasingly common. Heart murmurs are defined by four characteristics: loudness, quality, location and timing.

The loudness of a murmur reflects the degree of turbulence. This relates to the volume and velocity of flow and not the severity of the cardiac lesion. Loudness is graded on a scale of 1 (barely audible) to 6 (audible even without application of the stethoscope to the chest wall). The quality of a murmur relates to its frequency and is best described as low-, medium- or high-pitched. The location of a murmur on the chest wall depends on its site of origin and has led to the description of four valve areas (see above). Some murmurs radiate, depending on the velocity and direction of the blood flow. The sound of the high-velocity systolic flow in aortic stenosis and mitral regurgitation, for example, is directed towards the neck and the axilla, respectively; that of the high-velocity diastolic flow in aortic regurgitation is directed towards the left sternal edge. Murmurs are timed according to the phase of systole or diastole during which they are audible. It is inadequate to describe the timing of a murmur as systolic or diastolic without more specific reference to the length of the murmur and the phase of systole or diastole during which it is heard: systolic

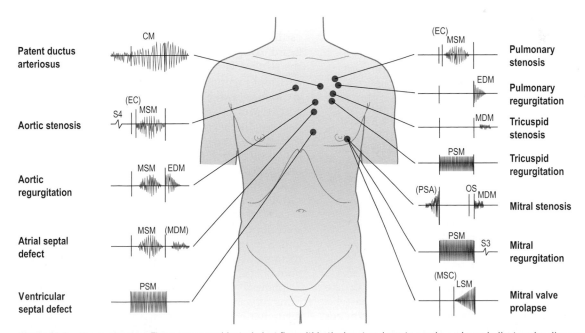

Figure 13.8 Heart murmurs. These are caused by turbulent flow within the heart and great vessels, and may indicate valve disease. Heart murmurs may be depicted graphically as shown in this illustration. CM, continuous murmur; EC, ejection click; EDM, early diastolic murmur; LSM, late systolic murmur; MDM, mid-diastolic murmur; MSC, mid-systolic click; MSM, mid-systolic murmur; OS, opening snap; PSA, presystolic accentuation of murmur; PSM, pansystolic murmur; S3, third heart sound; S4, fourth heart sound. Parentheses indicate those auscultatory findings that are not constant.

Box 13.15　Rheumatic heart disease

Typical patient

- Middle-aged woman, less commonly man, with a history of childhood rheumatic fever (often not recognized or dismissed as trivial feverish illness). The mitral valve is almost invariably affected, commonly with associated aortic valve involvement. Right-sided valves less commonly affected. Presentation is usually with exertional dyspnoea, less commonly with unexplained atrial fibrillation or unheralded stroke.
- Pregnant woman presenting abruptly with atrial fibrillation and pulmonary oedema

Major symptoms

- Mitral valve disease: dyspnoea or symptoms of frank congestive failure
- Aortic valve disease: dyspnoea, sometimes angina or syncope

Major signs

- Mitral stenosis: atrial fibrillation, signs of fluid retention (raised JVP ± peripheral oedema and basal crackles in lung fields), loud S1, opening snap in early diastole followed by low-pitched mid-diastolic murmur best heard at cardiac apex. With increasing calcification, the valve gets more rigid and the loud S1 and opening snap disappear.
- Mitral regurgitation: atrial fibrillation, signs of fluid retention, pansystolic murmur best heard at cardiac apex, often with third heart sound
- Aortic stenosis: slow-rising carotid pulse, ejection systolic murmur best heard at base of heart
- Aortic regurgitation: fast-rising carotid pulse, ejection systolic murmur with early diastolic murmur best heard at left sternal edge

Diagnosis

- Echocardiogram: diagnostic of rheumatic heart disease, Doppler studies providing additional information about the severity of valvular stenosis or regurgitation

Treatment

- Diuretics for fluid retention and vasodilators to increase forward flow through regurgitant left-sided valves. Digoxin or β-blockers for rate control in atrial fibrillation plus warfarin to protect against embolism. Symptomatic mitral valve disease that fails to respond to treatment requires valve surgery (repair or replacement) or, in selected cases of mitral stenosis, percutaneous valvuloplasty. Symptomatic aortic valve disease always requires consideration for valve replacement.

murmurs are either mid-systolic, pansystolic or late systolic; diastolic murmurs are either early diastolic, mid-diastolic or presystolic in timing. Continuous murmurs are audible in both phases of the cardiac cycle.

A mid-systolic ('ejection') murmur is caused by turbulence in the left or right ventricular outflow tract during ejection. It starts following opening of the aortic or pulmonary valve, reaches a crescendo in mid-systole and disappears before the second heart sound. The murmur is loudest in the aortic area (with radiation to the neck) when it arises from the left ventricular outflow tract, and in the pulmonary area when it arises from the right ventricular outflow tract. It is best heard with the diaphragm of the stethoscope while the patient sits forward. Important causes of aortic ejection murmurs are aortic stenosis and hypertrophic cardiomyopathy.

Aortic regurgitation also produces an ejection murmur owing to increased stroke volume and velocity of ejection. Pulmonary ejection murmurs may be caused by pulmonary stenosis or infundibular stenosis (as in Fallot's tetralogy).

In atrial septal defect, the pulmonary ejection murmur results from right ventricular volume loading and consequent increased blood flow through the pulmonary valve and does not indicate organic valvular disease. 'Innocent' murmurs unrelated to heart disease are always mid-systolic in timing and are caused by turbulent flow in the left (sometimes right) ventricular outflow tract. In most cases, there is no clear cause, but they may reflect a hyperkinetic circulation in conditions such as anaemia, pregnancy, thyrotoxicosis or fever. They are rarely louder than grade 3, often vary with posture, may disappear on exertion and are not associated with other signs of heart disease.

Pansystolic murmurs are audible throughout systole from the first to the second heart sounds. They are caused by regurgitation through incompetent atrioventricular valves and by ventricular septal defects. The pansystolic murmur of mitral regurgitation, which is loudest at the cardiac apex, radiates into the left axilla. It is best heard using the diaphragm of the stethoscope with the patient lying on the left side. The murmurs of tricuspid regurgitation and ventricular septal defect are loudest at the lower left sternal edge. Inspiration accentuates the murmur of tricuspid regurgitation because the increased venous return to the right side of the heart increases the regurgitant volume. Mitral valve prolapse may also produce a pansystolic murmur but, more commonly, prolapse occurs in mid-systole, producing a click followed by a late-systolic murmur.

Early diastolic murmurs, which are high-pitched, start immediately after the second heart sound, fading away in mid-diastole. They are caused by regurgitation through incompetent aortic and pulmonary valves and are best heard using the diaphragm of the stethoscope while the patient leans forward. The early diastolic murmur of aortic regurgitation radiates from the aortic area to the left sternal edge, where it is usually easier to hear, in maintained expiration with the patient leaning forward. Pulmonary regurgitation is loudest at the pulmonary area. Mid-diastolic murmurs are caused by turbulent flow through the atrioventricular valves.

They start after valve opening, relatively late after the second sound, and continue for a variable period during mid-diastole. Mitral stenosis is the principal cause of a mid-diastolic murmur which is best heard at the cardiac apex using the bell of the stethoscope while the patient lies on the left side. Increased flow across a non-stenotic mitral valve occurs in ventricular septal defect and mitral regurgitation and may produce a mid-diastolic murmur. In severe aortic regurgitation, pre-closure of the anterior leaflet of the mitral valve by the regurgitant jet may produce mitral turbulence associated with a mid-diastolic murmur (Austin Flint murmur). A mid-diastolic murmur at the lower left sternal edge, accentuated by inspiration, is caused by tricuspid stenosis and also by conditions that increase tricuspid flow (e.g. atrial septal defect, tricuspid regurgitation).

In mitral or tricuspid stenosis, atrial systole produces a presystolic murmur immediately before the first heart sound. The murmur is perceived as an accentuation of the mid-diastolic murmur associated with these conditions. Because presystolic murmurs are generated by atrial systole, they do not occur in patients with atrial fibrillation.

Continuous murmurs are heard during systole and diastole; they are uninterrupted by valve closure. The most common cardiac cause is patent ductus arteriosus, in which flow from the high-pressure aorta to the low-pressure pulmonary artery continues throughout the cardiac cycle, producing a murmur over the base of the heart which, though continuously audible, is loudest at end systole and diminishes during diastole. Ruptured sinus of Valsalva aneurysm also produces a continuous murmur.

Friction rubs and venous hums

A friction rub occurs in pericarditis. It is best heard in maintained expiration with the patient leaning forward as a high-pitched scratching noise audible during any part of the cardiac cycle and over any part of the left precordium. A continuous venous hum at the base of the heart reflects hyperkinetic jugular venous flow. It is particularly common in infants and usually disappears on lying flat.

Finishing the cardiovascular examination

The assessment of the cardiovascular system should be concluded with the examination of the abdomen for organomegaly (hepatomegaly in heart failure, splenomegaly in infective endocarditis and renal abnormalities in hypertension) and abdominal aortic aneurysm, auscultation of the chest bases for crackles related to impaired left ventricle (LV) function and urinalysis for proteinuria and haematuria.

The electrocardiogram

The electrocardiogram records the electrical activity of the heart at the skin surface. A good-quality 12-lead ECG is essential for the evaluation of almost all cardiac patients.

Electrophysiology

Generation of electrical activity

The stimulus for every normal ventricular contraction (sinus beat) begins with depolarization of an area of specialized conducting tissue high in the right atrium called the sinoatrial (SA) node. The depolarization spreads through the walls of the atria causing contraction of the atrial muscle before reaching another area of specialized conducting tissue in the lower part of the right atrium called the atrioventricular (AV) node. Conduction through the AV node is relatively slow, which allows atrial contraction to be completed and the ventricles to fill before depolarization travels down the bundle of His and then into the left and right bundle branches. The left bundle branch divides further into the left anterior fascicle and the left posterior fascicle. From here, the depolarization spreads through the Purkinje fibres in the ventricular muscle, which stimulates ventricular contraction. Once ventricular contraction has occurred, the muscle cells repolarize and the ventricles relax to allow ventricular filling to occur.

The wave of depolarization that spreads through the heart during each cardiac cycle has vector properties defined by its direction and magnitude. The net direction of the wave changes continuously during each cardiac cycle and the ECG deflections change accordingly, being positive as the wave approaches the recording electrode and negative as it moves away. Electrodes orientated along the axis of the wave record larger deflections than those orientated at right angles. Nevertheless, the size of the deflections is determined principally by the magnitude of the wave, which is a function of muscle mass. Thus, the ECG deflection produced by depolarization of the atria (P wave) is smaller than that produced by the depolarization of the more muscular ventricles (QRS complex). Ventricular repolarization produces the T wave.

Inscription of the QRS complex

The ventricular depolarization vector can be resolved into two components:
1. Septal depolarization: spreads from left to right across the septum.
2. Ventricular free wall depolarization: spreads from endocardium to epicardium.

Left ventricular depolarization dominates the second vector component, the resultant direction of which is from right to left. Thus, electrodes orientated to the left ventricle record a small negative deflection (Q wave) as the septal depolarization vector moves away, followed by a large positive deflection (R wave) as the ventricular depolarization vector approaches. The sequence of deflections for

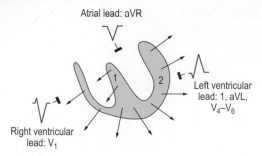

Atrial lead: aVR

Left ventricular
lead: 1, aVL,
V_4–V_6

Right ventricular
lead: V_1

Figure 13.9 Inscription of the QRS complex. The septal depolarization vector **(1)** produces the initial deflection of the QRS complex. The ventricular free-wall depolarization vector **(2)** produces the second deflection, which is usually more pronounced. Lead aVR is orientated towards the cavity of the left ventricle and records an entirely negative deflection.

electrodes orientated towards the right ventricle is in the opposite direction (Fig. 13.9).

Any positive deflection is termed an R wave. A negative deflection before the R wave is termed a Q wave (this must be the first deflection of the complex), whereas a negative deflection following the R wave is termed an S wave.

Electrical axis

Because the mean direction of the ventricular depolarization vector (the electrical axis) shows a wide range of normality, there is a corresponding variation in QRS patterns consistent with a normal ECG. Thus, correct interpretation of the ECG must take account of the electrical axis. The frontal plane axis is determined by identifying the limb lead in which the net QRS deflection (positive and negative) is least pronounced. This lead must be at right angles to the frontal plane electrical axis, which is defined using an arbitrary hexaxial reference system (Fig. 13.10).

Normal 12-lead ECG

A normal 12-lead ECG is illustrated in Figure 13.11. Leads I–III are the standard bipolar leads, which each measures the potential difference between two limbs:

- Lead I: left arm to right arm
- Lead II: left leg to right arm
- Lead III: left leg to left arm

The remaining leads are unipolar, connected to a limb (aVR to aVF) or to the chest wall (V_1–V_6). Because the orientation of each lead to the wave of depolarization is different, the direction and magnitude of ECG deflections is also different in each lead. Nevertheless, the sequence of deflections (P wave, QRS complex, T wave) is identical. In some patients, a small U wave can be seen following the T wave. Its orientation (positive or negative) is the same as the T wave, but its cause is unknown.

Analysis of the ECG

Heart rate

The ECG is usually recorded at a paper speed of 25 mm/s. Thus, each large square (5 mm) represents 0.20 s. The heart rate (bpm) is conveniently calculated by counting the number of large squares between consecutive R waves and dividing this into 300.

Rhythm

In normal sinus rhythm, P waves precede each QRS complex and the rhythm is regular. Absence of P waves and an irregular rhythm indicate atrial fibrillation.

Electrical axis

Evaluation of the frontal place QRS axis is described above.

P-wave morphology

The duration should not exceed 0.10 s, prolongation indicating left atrial enlargement, often the result of mitral valve disease or left ventricular failure. Tall-peaked 'pulmonary' P waves indicate right atrial enlargement, caused usually by pulmonary hypertension and right ventricular failure.

PR interval

The normal duration is 0.12–0.20 s measured from the onset of the P wave to the first deflection of the QRS complex. Prolongation indicates delayed atrioventricular conduction (first-degree heart block). Shortening indicates rapid conduction through an accessory pathway bypassing the atrioventricular node (Wolff-Parkinson-White (WPW) syndrome).

QRS morphology

The QRS duration should not exceed 0.12 s. Prolongation indicates slow ventricular depolarization caused by bundle branch block (Fig. 13.12), pre-excitation (WPW syndrome), ventricular tachycardia or hypokalaemia.

Exaggerated QRS deflections indicate ventricular hypertrophy (Fig. 13.13). The voltage criteria for left ventricular hypertrophy are fulfilled when the sum of the S and R wave deflections in leads V_1 and V_6 exceeds 35 mm (3.5 mV). Right ventricular hypertrophy causes tall R waves in the right ventricular leads (V_1 and V_2). A dominant R wave in lead V_1 can also be caused by right bundle branch block, posterior myocardial infarction, WPW syndrome and dextrocardia. Diminished QRS deflections occur in myxoedema and also when pericardial effusion or obesity electrically insulates the heart. The presence of pathological Q waves (duration >0.04 s) usually indicates previous myocardial infarction.

QT interval

The QT interval is measured from the onset of the QRS complex to the end of the T wave and represents

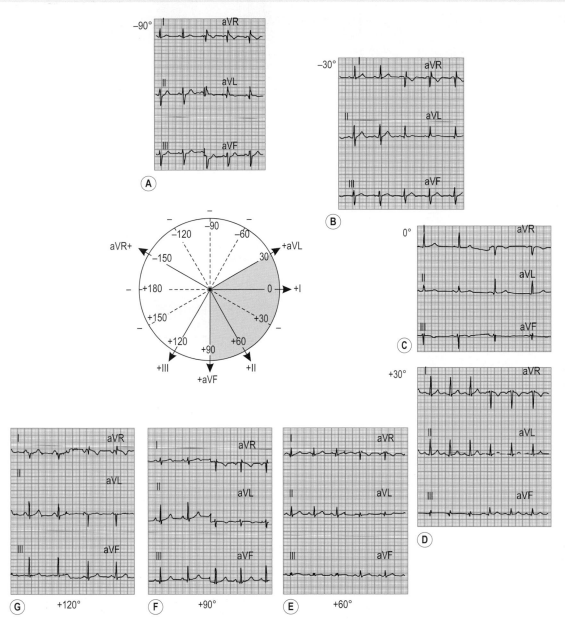

Figure 13.10 Mean frontal QRS axis. This is the mean direction of the left ventricular depolarization vector in those leads (I–aVF) that lie in the frontal plane of the heart. It lies at right angles to the lead in which the net QRS deflection is least pronounced. It is quantified using a hexaxial reference system. The QRS axis shows a wide range of normality from −30° to 90°. Thus, despite the different ECG patterns in this illustration, only recordings **(A)** and **(G)** are abnormal, owing to left and right axis deviation, respectively.

the duration of electrical systole (mechanical systole starts between the QRS complex and the T wave). The QT interval (0.35–0.45 s) is very rate sensitive, shortening as heart rate increases. A commonly used way to correct the QT interval (the so-called QTc) involves dividing the measured QT interval by the square root of the RR interval in seconds. As an example, at 60 bpm, the RR interval would be 1 second: the QTc would be equal to QT √1. Abnormal prolongation of the QT interval predisposes to ventricular arrhythmias and may be congenital or occur in response to hypokalaemia, rheumatic fever or drugs (e.g. quinidine, amiodarone,

tricyclic antidepressants). Shortening of the QT interval is caused by hyperkalaemia and digoxin therapy.

ST segment morphology

Minor ST elevation reflecting early repolarization may occur as a normal variant (Fig. 13.14), particularly in subjects of African or West Indian origin. Pathological elevation (>2.0 mm above the isoelectric line) occurs in acute myocardial infarction, variant angina and pericarditis. Horizontal ST depression indicates myocardial ischaemia. Other important causes of ST depression are digoxin therapy and hypokalaemia.

Figure 13.11 Standard 12-lead ECG. This is a normal recording. The QRS deflections are equiphasic in lead aVF. This is at right angles to lead I (see Fig. 13.10), which is dominantly positive. The frontal plane QRS axis is, therefore, 0°. The square wave calibration signal is 1 mV.

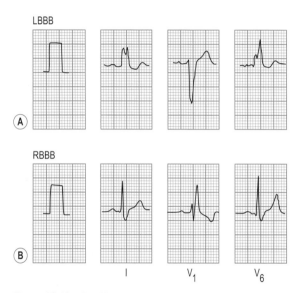

Figure 13.12 Bundle branch block. **(A)** Left bundle branch block (LBBB); the entire sequence of ventricular depolarization is abnormal, resulting in a broad QRS complex with large slurred or notched R waves in I and V_6. **(B)** Right bundle branch block (RBBB); right ventricular depolarization is delayed, resulting in a broad QRS complex with an 'rSR' pattern in V_1 and prominent S waves in I and V_6.

T-wave morphology

The orientation of the T wave should be directionally similar to the QRS complex. Thus T-wave inversion is normal in leads with dominantly negative QRS complexes (aVR, V_1 and sometimes lead III). Pathological T-wave inversion occurs as a non-specific response to various stimuli (e.g. viral infection, hypothermia). More important causes of T-wave inversion are ventricular hypertrophy, myocardial ischaemia and myocardial infarction. Exaggerated peaking of the T wave is the earliest ECG change in ST elevation myocardial infarction. It also occurs in hyperkalaemia.

Clinical applications of ECG

Diagnosis of coronary artery disease

The territories supplied by the three major coronary arteries, although variable, are highly circumscribed, the left anterior descending artery supplying the anterior wall, the circumflex artery the lateral wall and the right coronary artery the inferior wall of the left ventricle. The regional distribution of coronary flow has important implications for electrocardiography (and diagnostic imaging), patients with coronary artery disease showing regional electrocardiographic (or wall motion) abnormalities and patients with diffuse myocardial disease (e.g. cardiomyopathy) showing more widespread changes.

Stable angina

The ECG is often normal in patients with stable angina unless there is a history of myocardial infarction, when pathological Q waves or T-wave inversion may be present.

Exercise stress testing

The patient is usually exercised on a treadmill, the speed and slope of which can be adjusted to increase the workload gradually. In patients with coronary artery disease, exercise-induced increases in myocardial oxygen demand may outstrip oxygen delivery through the atheromatous arteries, resulting in regional ischaemia. This causes planar or downsloping ST segment depression, with reversal during recovery (Fig. 13.15). The ready availability of the exercise test means that it is one of the most widely used tests for evaluating the patient with chest pain, but its diagnostic accuracy is limited to about 70%, false-positive or false-negative results being common when the pre-test probability of coronary disease is very low (as in young women) or very high (as in elderly patients with typical symptoms), respectively. Non-invasive imaging modalities (see

Figure 13.13   Ventricular hypertrophy. **(A)** Left ventricular hypertrophy. The QRS voltage deflections are exaggerated such that the sum of S and R waves in V_1 and V_6, respectively, exceeds 35 mm. T-wave inversion in V_5 and V_6 indicates left ventricular 'strain'. **(B)** Right ventricular hypertrophy. Prominent R waves in V_1 and V_2 associated with T-wave inversion are shown.

later: magnetic resonance perfusion imaging, stress echocardiography, computed tomography (CT) coronary angiography) have higher rates of diagnostic accuracy and are now preferred in the assessment of patients with suspected coronary artery disease, where available. The exercise ECG also provides prognostic information in patients who are known to have coronary artery disease: an increased risk of myocardial infarction or sudden death is indicated by ST depression very early during exercise, by an exertional fall in blood pressure or by exercise-induced ventricular arrhythmias. In these cases, urgent coronary angiography should be considered.

Acute coronary syndromes

Acute myocardial infarction and unstable angina present similarly with unprovoked—often severe—ischaemic cardiac pain. Reliable differentiation between the acute coronary syndromes on clinical grounds cannot be made and requires measurement of cardiac biomarkers, in particular troponin I or T (see below), and observation of the 12-lead ECG. The combination of typical symptoms plus raised troponins is diagnostic of myocardial infarction, which is categorized as ST elevation myocardial infarction (STEMI) or non-ST elevation myocardial infarction (non-STEMI) by the ECG findings.

Figure 13.14 ST segment morphology: common causes of ST segment elevation and depression. Note that depression of the J point (junction between the QRS complex and ST segment) is physiological during exertion and does not signify myocardial ischaemia. Planar depression of the ST segment, on the other hand, is strongly suggestive of myocardial ischaemia.

Figure 13.15 Exercise ECG: ischaemic changes in inferior standard leads (II, III and aVF). At rest, the ST segments are isoelectric. Exercise causes tachycardia and provokes 3 mm of downsloping ST depression in leads II, III and aVF. The changes reverse during recovery. The findings suggest exertional ischaemia affecting the inferior wall of the heart. The probability of coronary artery disease is high.

Typical symptoms not associated with either troponin release or ST elevation are diagnosed as troponin-negative acute coronary syndrome or unstable angina. It therefore follows that acute myocardial infarction and unstable angina may be associated with a completely normal ECG or with ST depression (Fig. 13.16) or T-wave changes, the diagnosis depending on the presence or absence of raised troponins.

In STEMI, the evolution of ECG changes is characteristic, although it may be aborted by timely reperfusion therapy (thrombolysis or primary stenting). Peaking of the T wave followed by ST segment elevation occurs during the first hour of pain (Fig. 13.17). The changes are regional, and reciprocal ST depression may be seen in the opposite ECG leads. Usually a pathological Q wave develops during the following 24 hours and persists indefinitely. The ST segment returns to the isoelectric line within 2–3

days, and T-wave inversion may occur. The ECG is a useful indicator of infarct location. Changes in leads II, III and aVF indicate inferior infarction (Fig. 13.18), whereas changes in leads V_1–V_6 indicate anteroseptal (V_1–V_3) or anterolateral (V_1–V_6) infarction (Fig. 13.19). When the infarct is located posteriorly, ECG changes may be difficult to detect, but dominant R waves in leads V_1 and V_2 often develop (see Fig. 13.18).

Detection of cardiac arrhythmias

Electrocardiographic documentation of the arrhythmia should be obtained prior to instituting treatment. In patients with sustained arrhythmias, a 12-lead recording at rest is usually diagnostic, but a long continuous recording of the lead showing the clearest P wave (if present) should also be obtained. In patients with paroxysmal arrhythmias,

Figure 13.16   Unstable angina or non-ST elevation myocardial infarction (depending on troponin release): 12-lead ECG showing planar/downsloping ST depression in the inferolateral territory.

Hours after onset of chest pain

Figure 13.17   Acute myocardial infarction: evolution of ECG changes. Elevation of the ST segment occurs during the first hour of chest pain. The Q wave develops during the subsequent 24 hours, usually persisting indefinitely. Within a day of the attack, the ST segment usually returns to the isoelectric line and T-wave inversion may occur.

Figure 13.18   Acute inferolateral infarction. ECG 2 hours after the onset of chest pain. Typical ST elevation in leads II, III and aVF is diagnostic of inferior myocardial infarction. ST elevation in leads V_4–V_6 indicates lateral extension. There is reciprocal ST depression in lead aVL. Prominent R waves associated with ST depression in leads V_1 and V_2 indicate posterior wall infarction. This pattern may reflect occlusion of the right coronary artery or a dominant circumflex coronary artery.

Figure 13.19   Acute anterior infarction. ECG 1 hour after the onset of chest pain. Typical ST elevation in leads V_2–V_5 is diagnostic of anterior myocardial infarction. Additional ST elevation in standard leads I and aVL indicates lateral extension of the infarct. This pattern usually reflects proximal occlusion of the left anterior descending coronary artery.

the frequency and severity of symptoms determine which technique is used for electrocardiographic documentation.

In-hospital ECG monitoring

Patients who have had out-of-hospital cardiac arrest or severe, arrhythmia-induced heart failure should undergo continuous ECG monitoring in hospital under the surveillance of staff trained in the recognition and treatment of arrhythmia.

Patients with acute myocardial infarction should undergo ECG monitoring for 24 hours, after which time the risk of ventricular arrhythmia falls dramatically.

Ambulatory (Holter) ECG monitoring

Patients with frequent palpitation or dizzy attacks are commonly investigated by means of an ambulatory 24-hour ECG. The availability of portable recorders allows this to be performed as an outpatient. Analysis of the tape identifies any cardiac arrhythmias that occurred during the monitoring period (Fig. 13.20). A patient diary allows correlation between symptoms and heart rhythm.

Patient-activated ECG recording

For patients with infrequent symptoms, the detection rate with 24-hour ambulatory monitoring is low and patient-activated recorders are more useful. The patient can keep the recorder for several weeks and activate it when symptoms occur. Rhythm strips are stored for later analysis.

Implantable loop recording

Patients in whom there is clinical suspicion of serious arrhythmia but whose symptoms occur less than

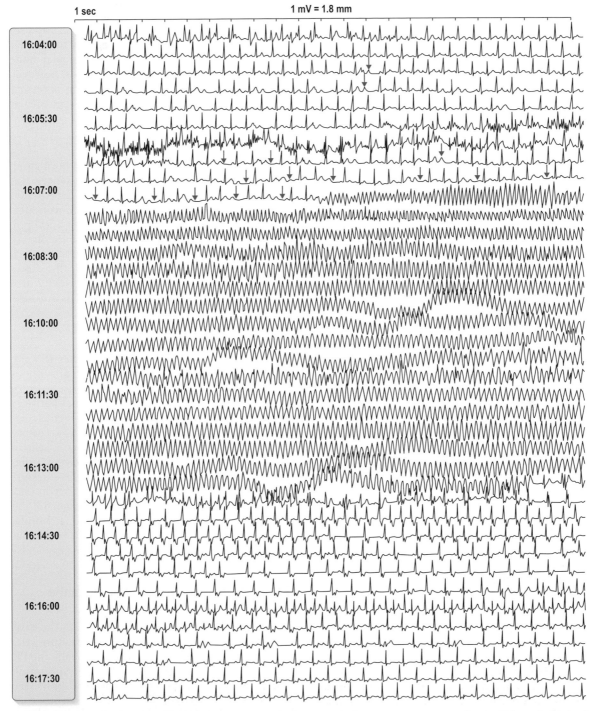

Figure 13.20 Ventricular tachycardia: Holter recording. When tachycardias are paroxysmal in nature, continuous ECG monitoring is often necessary to document the arrhythmia. Here a Holter recording illustrates a long burst of rapid VT lasting a total of 6 minutes. Preceding the VT there is second-degree heart block (*arrows*).

once a month pose particular diagnostic difficulty. In this group, a miniaturized recording device can be implanted subcutaneously using local anaesthetic and interrogated electronically through the skin in the event of symptoms.

Exercise testing

The ECG recorded during exercise may be helpful when there is a history of exertional palpitation. Arrhythmias provoked by ischaemia or increased sympathetic activity are more likely to be detected during exercise.

Tilt testing

When malignant vasovagal syndrome is suspected, ECG and blood pressure recordings during tilting from supine to erect posture can be helpful. Abnormal bradycardia or hypotension sufficient to produce presyncope or syncope indicates a 'vasodepressor response' or 'cardioinhibitory response', respectively, and either is strongly suggestive of the diagnosis.

Electrophysiological study

Electrophysiological study is a technique that requires cardiac catheterization with catheter-mounted electrodes. Premature stimuli are introduced into the atria or ventricles with a view to stimulating re-entry arrhythmias. In the normal heart, sustained arrhythmias are rarely provoked by premature stimuli. Thus, arrhythmia provocation is usually diagnostic, particularly when the arrhythmia reproduces symptoms. Electrophysiological study can identify accessory pathways and areas of focal atrial or ventricular ectopy as the prelude to radiofrequency ablation of the arrhythmia substrate.

Diagnosis of atrial arrhythmias

The ECG in atrial arrhythmias (Fig. 13.21) shows a narrow and morphologically normal QRS complex when ventricular depolarization occurs by normal His-Purkinje pathways. Rate-related or pre-existing bundle branch block, however, results in broad ventricular complexes that are difficult to distinguish from ventricular tachycardia.

Atrial ectopic beats

Atrial ectopic beasts rarely indicate heart disease. They often occur spontaneously, but may be provoked by toxic stimuli such as caffeine, alcohol and cigarette smoking. They are caused by the premature discharge of an atrial ectopic focus; an early and occasionally bizarre P wave is essential for the diagnosis. The premature impulse enters and depolarizes the sinus node such that a partially compensatory pause occurs before the next sinus beat during resetting of the sinus node.

Atrial fibrillation

Prevalence of atrial fibrillation increases with age and is common in hypertensive heart disease, mitral valve disease, thyrotoxicosis and left ventricular failure. It can be precipitated by pneumonia and major surgery and also by various toxic stimuli, particularly alcohol. Atrial activity is chaotic and mechanically ineffective. P waves are therefore absent and replaced by irregular fibrillatory waves (rate 400–600/min). The long refractory period of the atrioventricular node ensures that only some of the atrial impulses are conducted to produce an irregular ventricular rate of 130–200 bpm. If the atrioventricular node is diseased, the ventricular rate is slower; however, in the presence of a rapidly conducting accessory pathway in WPW syndrome, dangerous ventricular rates above 300 bpm may occur.

Atrial flutter

Atrial flutter is less common than atrial fibrillation, but it does occur under similar circumstances. Re-entry mechanisms produce an atrial rate close to 300 bpm. The normal atrioventricular node conducts with 2:1 block, giving a ventricular rate of 150 bpm. Higher degrees of block may reflect intrinsic disease of the atrioventricular node or the effects of nodal blocking drugs. The ECG characteristically shows sawtooth flutter waves, which are most clearly seen when the block is increased by carotid sinus pressure.

Diagnosis of nodal arrhythmias

Often called supraventricular tachycardias (SVTs), nodal arrhythmias are usually paroxysmal without obvious cardiac or extrinsic causes. They are re-entry arrhythmias caused either by an abnormal pathway between the atrium and the atrioventricular node (atrionodal pathway) or by an accessory atrioventricular pathway (bundle of Kent), as seen in WPW syndrome. Like atrial arrhythmias, ventricular depolarization usually occurs by normal His-Purkinje pathways, producing a narrow QRS complex which confirms the supraventricular origin of the arrhythmia. Rate-related or pre-existing bundle branch block, however, produces broad ventricular complexes difficult to distinguish from ventricular tachycardia.

Atrioventricular nodal re-entry tachycardia (AVNRT)

The abnormal atrionodal pathway provides the basis for a small re-entry circuit. In sinus rhythm, the ECG is usually normal, although occasionally the PR interval is short (Lown-Ganong-Levine syndrome). During tachycardia, the rate is 150–250 bpm (see Fig. 13.21). The arrhythmia is usually self-limiting. Sustained AVNRT will sometimes respond to carotid sinus pressure. If this fails, intravenous adenosine or verapamil usually are effective by blocking the re-entry circuit within the atrioventricular node. Antitachycardia pacing or direct current cardioversion may also be used. Many patients are now being treated by catheter ablation to destroy the abnormal atrionodal pathway and avoid the need for long-term drug therapy (see below).

Wolff-Parkinson-White syndrome

A congenital disorder that affects 0.12% of the population, Wolff-Parkinson-White syndrome, is caused by an accessory pathway (bundle of Kent) between the atria and the ventricles. During sinus rhythm, atrial impulses conduct more rapidly through the accessory pathway than the atrioventricular node, such that the initial phase of ventricular depolarization occurs early (pre-excitation) and spreads slowly through the ventricles by abnormal pathways. This produces a short PR interval and slurring of the initial QRS deflection (δ wave). The remainder of ventricular depolarization, however, is rapid because the delayed arrival of the impulse conducted through the atrioventricular node rapidly completes ventricular depolarization by normal His-Purkinje pathways (Fig. 13.22). Cardiac arrhythmias affect about 60% of patients with WPW syndrome and are usually re-entrant

Figure 13.21 Atrial arrhythmias. **(A)** Ectopic beats. After the fourth sinus beat there is a very early P wave which, finding the AV node refractory, is not conducted to the ventricle. This produces a pause before the next sinus beat, which itself is followed by a somewhat later atrial ectopic beat (*arrow*), which is conducted normally. This is followed by a sinus beat, following which the T wave is distorted by another early atrial ectopic (beat *arrowed*), which is also blocked. **(B)** Atrial fibrillation. Note the irregular fibrillatory waves and the irregular ventricular response. The ventricular rate is fairly slow because the patient was treated with a β-blocker. **(C)** A flutter. AV conduction with 2:1 block, giving a ventricular rate of about 150/min, which then gives way to 4:1 block. Sawtooth flutter waves at a rate of 300/min are clearly visible. **(D)** AV nodal re-entrant tachycardia (AVNRT). Often called supraventricular tachycardia (SVT), this arrhythmia causes a regular tachycardia, with a ventricular rate of about 180/min.

Figure 13.22 WPW syndrome: 12-lead ECG. Ventricular pre-excitation is reflected on the surface ECG by a short PR interval and a slurred upstroke to the QRS complex (δ wave). The remainder of the QRS complex is normal because delayed arrival of the impulse conducted through the AV node rapidly completes ventricular depolarization through normal His-Purkinje pathways.

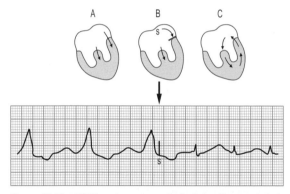

Figure 13.23 WPW syndrome: re-entry tachycardia recorded at fast paper speed. Just after the third pre-excited (broad) complex, a premature atrial pacing stimulus (S) initiates an impulse that is blocked in the bundle of Kent, but conducted normally through the AV node, producing ventricular depolarization without pre-excitation. Thus, the QRS complex is narrow and lacks a δ wave. The impulse is conducted retrogradely through the bundle of Kent, re-enters the proximal conducting system and completes the re-entry circuit, initiating a self-sustaining orthodromic re-entry tachycardia (last three complexes).

(rate 150–250 bpm) triggered by an atrial premature beat. In most patients, the re-entry arrhythmia is 'orthodromic', with anterograde conduction through the atrioventricular node and retrograde conduction through the accessory pathway (atrioventricular re-entry tachycardia (AVRT), Fig. 13.23). This results in a narrow complex tachycardia (without pre-excitation) that is indistinguishable from AVNRT. Occasionally, the re-entry circuit is in the opposite direction ('antidromic'), producing a very broad, pre-excited tachycardia.

Patients with WPW syndrome are more susceptible than the general population to atrial fibrillation. If the accessory pathway is able to conduct the fibrillatory impulses rapidly to the ventricles, it may result in ventricular fibrillation and sudden death. Digoxin (and to a lesser extent verapamil) should be avoided because it shortens the refractory period of the accessory pathway and can heighten the risk. Patients with dangerous accessory pathways of this type require catheter ablation of the pathway. Ablation therapy also cures AVNRT and is the treatment of choice in patients with frequent attacks.

Diagnosis of ventricular arrhythmias

Ventricular premature beats

Ventricular premature beats may occur in normal individuals, either spontaneously or in response to toxic stimuli such as caffeine or sympathomimetic drugs. They are caused by the premature discharge of a ventricular ectopic focus that produces an early and broad QRS complex (Fig. 13.24). The premature impulse may be conducted backwards into the atria, producing a retrograde P wave, but penetration of the sinus node is rare. Thus, resetting of the sinus node does not usually occur and there is a compensatory pause before the next sinus beat.

Ventricular tachycardia

Ventricular tachycardia is defined as three or more consecutive ventricular beats at a rate above 120 per minute. Ventricular depolarization inevitably occurs slowly by abnormal pathways, producing a broad QRS complex. This distinguishes it from most

Figure 13.24   Multifocal, ventricular ectopic beats. Frequent broad complex ectopic beats are seen early after the sinus beats. Note, however, that the ectopic beats have two different morphologies, indicating that they arise from different foci. Note also that the coupling interval (interval between QRS complex and ectopic beat) is identical for beats arising from any particular focus.

Figure 13.25   Paroxysmal AV nodal re-entrant tachycardia. This Holter recording shows sinus rhythm giving way to a broad complex tachycardia. However, this is clearly the result of temporary bundle branch block because it converts spontaneously to a narrow complex tachycardia, confirming that the arrhythmia is junctional, not ventricular, in origin.

Figure 13.26   Ventricular tachycardia: 12-lead ECG. The recording shows a broad complex tachycardia. The following features suggest or confirm the ventricular origin of the tachycardia: very broad QRS complex (>140 ms); extreme right axis deviation; atrioventricular dissociation: note the dissociated P waves in lead V_1; the 'rSR' complex in V_1.

atrial and junctional tachycardias that have a narrow QRS complex, although differential diagnosis may be more difficult for atrial or junctional tachycardias with a broad QRS complex caused by rate-related or pre-existing bundle branch block (Fig. 13.25). Nevertheless, ventricular tachycardia usually can be identified by careful scrutiny of the 12-lead ECG (Fig. 13.26). Support for the diagnosis is provided by a very broad QRS complex (>140 ms), extreme left or right axis deviation, concordance of the QRS deflections in V_1–V_6 (either all positive or all negative) and configurational features of the QRS complex, including an 'rSR' complex in V_1 and a QS complex in V_6. Confirmation of the diagnosis is provided by any evidence of AV dissociation: either P waves, at a slower rate than the QRS complexes, 'marching through' the tachycardia (Fig. 13.27A), or ventricular capture and/or fusion beats, in which the dissociated atrial rhythm penetrates the ventricle by conduction through the AV node

Figure 13.27   **(A)** Ventricular tachycardia: AV dissociation. P waves (*arrows*) can be seen 'marching through' the tachycardia, confirming its ventricular origin. The tachycardia is interrupted by a narrow capture beat. **(B)** Ventricular tachycardia (VT): fusion. In this example, VT is initiated by a very early ventricular ectopic beat (morphologically similar to the previous isolated ectopic beat) and is interrupted by a fusion beat (*arrow*), confirming the ventricular origin of the tachycardia.

Figure 13.28   Sinoatrial disease. **(A)** Sinus arrest with late junctional escape. After the second sinus beat there is a long pause, interrupted by a single junctional escape beat, before sinus rhythm is re-established. **(B)** Sinoatrial block. Pauses after the second and fourth complexes are the result of sinoatrial block, which has prevented sinus impulses from depolarizing the atrium. No P waves are seen but, because the sinus discharge continues uninterrupted, the pauses are each a precise multiple of the preceding PP interval. Sinoatrial block is probably rare. **(C)** Bradycardia-tachycardia syndrome. A slow junctional rhythm gives way to rapid atrial fibrillation.

and interrupts the tachycardia, producing a normal ventricular complex (capture, Fig. 13.27A) or, more commonly, a broad hybrid complex (fusion) that is part sinus and part ventricular in origin (Fig. 13.27B). *Torsades de pointes*, a broad complex tachycardia with changing wavefronts, also provides unequivocal evidence of ventricular tachycardia and is particularly characteristic of the arrhythmia that complicates long QT syndrome, often resulting in sudden death. The syndrome may be inherited as an autosomal-dominant (Romano-Ward syndrome) or as an autosomal-recessive (Lange-Nielsen syndrome) trait, when it is associated with congenital deafness. Another important cause of *Torsade de pointes* is the use of drugs (antiarrhythmics and others, such as anti-psychotic therapy) that cause prolongation of the QT interval.

Ventricular fibrillation

Ventricular fibrillation occurs most commonly in severe myocardial ischaemia, either with or without frank infarction. It is a completely disorganized arrhythmia characterized by irregular fibrillatory waves with no discernible QRS complexes. There is no effective cardiac output and death is inevitable unless resuscitation with direct current defibrillation is instituted rapidly.

Diagnosis of sinoatrial disease

Sinus node discharge is not itself visible on the surface ECG, but the atrial depolarization it triggers produces the P wave. The spontaneous discharge of the normal sinus node is influenced by a variety of neurohumoral factors, particularly vagal and sympathetic activity, which respectively slow and quicken the heart rate. In sinoatrial disease (Fig. 13.28 and Box 13.16), sinus node discharge may be abnormally slow, blocked (with failure to activate atrial depolarization) or absent altogether. Under these circumstances, the sinus rate may be very slow, the atrium may fibrillate, or pacemaker function may be assumed by foci lower in the atrium, the atrioventricular node or the His-Purkinje conducting tissue in the ventricles. The intrinsic rate of these 'escape' pacemaker foci is slower than the normal sinus rate.

Sinus bradycardia (<50 bpm)

Sinus bradycardia is physiological during sleep and in trained athletes, but in other circumstances

---

Box 13.16	Sinoatrial disease

Typical patient
- Elderly, often with no previous cardiac history

Causes
- Acute: myocardial infarction, coronary artery disease, drugs (e.g. β-blockers, digoxin), hypothermia, atrial surgery
- Chronic: idiopathic fibrotic disease, congenital heart disease, ischaemic heart disease, amyloid

Major symptoms
- Intermittent syncopal or presyncopal attacks
- Patients may also complain of exertional fatigue (chronotropic incompetence) or palpitations (tachycardia-bradycardia syndrome).

Major signs
- Often none
- Sometimes sinus bradycardia or slow atrial fibrillation

Diagnosis
- ECG: often normal. May show sinus bradycardia or slow atrial fibrillation
- Ambulatory ECG: 24-hour Holter recording may show pauses diagnostic of sinoatrial disease.

Comments
- Documentation of the sinus pauses (or very slow atrial fibrillation) during an attack of symptoms provides the most robust diagnostic information.

---

often reflects sinoatrial disease, particularly when the heart rate fails to increase normally with exercise.

Sinoatrial block

If the sinus impulse is blocked and fails to trigger atrial depolarization, a pause occurs in the ECG. No P wave is seen during the pause owing to the absence of atrial depolarization. The electrically 'silent' sinus discharge, however, continues uninterrupted. Thus, the pause is always a precise multiple of preceding PP intervals. Sinoatrial block that cannot be abolished by atropine-induced vagal inhibition usually indicates sinoatrial disease, particularly with pauses longer than 2 seconds.

Sinus arrest

Failure of sinus node discharge produces a pause on the ECG that bears no relation to the preceding PP interval. Pauses longer than 2 seconds are usually pathological. Prolonged pauses are often terminated by an escape beat from a 'junctional' focus in the bundle of His.

Bradycardia-tachycardia syndrome

In the bradycardia-tachycardia syndrome, atrial bradycardias are interspersed by paroxysmal tachyarrhythmias, usually atrial fibrillation. Nevertheless, it is the bradycardia that usually causes symptoms, particularly dizzy attacks and blackouts.

Diagnosis of atrioventricular block

In atrioventricular block (Fig. 13.29), conduction is delayed or completely interrupted, either in the atrioventricular node or in the bundle branches (Box 13.17). When conduction is merely delayed (e.g. first-degree atrioventricular block, bundle branch block), the heart rate is unaffected. When conduction is completely interrupted, however, the heart rate may slow sufficiently to produce symptoms. In second-degree atrioventricular block, failure of conduction, by definition, is intermittent; if sufficient sinus impulses are conducted to maintain an adequate ventricular rate, symptoms may be avoided. In third-degree atrioventricular block there is complete failure of conduction and continuing ventricular activity depends on the emergence of an escape rhythm. If the block is within the atrioventricular node, the escape rhythm usually arises from a focus just below the node in the bundle of His (junctional escape), and is often fast enough to prevent symptoms. If both bundle branches are blocked, however, the escape rhythm must arise from a focus lower in the ventricles. Ventricular escape rhythms of this type are nearly always associated with symptoms because they are not only very slow but also unreliable, and may stop altogether, producing prolonged asystole.

Figure 13.29 Atrioventricular conducting tissue disease. **(A)** 1° AV block. Delayed AV conduction causes a prolonged PR interval (>0.20 s). **(B)** 2° AV block, Wenckebach type. This, also called Mobitz type I block, occurs within the AV node. Three Wenckebach cycles are shown. Successive sinus beats find the AV node increasingly refractory until failure of conduction occurs. This delay permits recovery of nodal function and the process repeats itself. **(C)** 2° AV block at bundle branch level (Mobitz type II). This is standard lead I. Note that the PR interval of conducted beats is normal, but the QRS complex shows right bundle branch block. Intermittent block in the left bundle results in failure of conduction of alternate P waves. **(D)** 3° (complete) AV block at level of AV node. In this patient with acute inferior myocardial infarction there is complete failure of AV conduction, as reflected by the dissociated atrial and ventricular rhythms. Note the regular P waves and the regular slower QRS complexes occurring independently of one another. Because block is at the level of the AV node, a junctional escape rhythm has taken over with a narrow QRS complex. **(E)** 3° (complete) AV block at bundle branch level. The atrial and ventricular rhythms are dissociated because none of the atrial impulses is conducted. The ECG shows regular P waves and regular but slower QRS complexes. Because the escape rhythm is ventricular in origin, the QRS complexes are broad and the rate is slow.

Acute

- Myocardial infarction
- Drugs (e.g. β-blockers, verapamil, digoxin, adenosine)
- Surgical or catheter ablation of bundle of His
- Endocarditis complicated by aortic root abscess

Chronic

- Idiopathic fibrosis of both bundle branches
- Ischaemic heart disease
- Congenital heart disease
- Calcific aortic valve disease
- Chagas' disease
- Infiltrative disease (amyloid, haemochromatosis)
- Granulomatous disease (sarcoid, tuberculosis)

Figure 13.30 Normal chest X-ray: posteroanterior projection. Note the heart is not enlarged (cardiothoracic ratio <50%) and the lung fields are clear. AA, aortic arch; LV, left ventricle; PA, pulmonary artery; RA, right atrium; RV, right ventricle; SVC, superior vena cava.

First-degree atrioventricular block

Delayed atrioventricular conduction causes prolongation of the PR interval (>0.20 s). Ventricular depolarization occurs rapidly by normal His-Purkinje pathways and the QRS complex is usually narrow.

Second-degree atrioventricular block: Mobitz type I (Wenckebach)

Second-degree atrioventricular block (Mobitz type I) commonly occurs in inferior myocardial infarction. Successive sinus beats find the atrioventricular node increasingly refractory until failure of conduction occurs. The delay permits recovery of nodal function, and the process may then repeat itself. The ECG shows progressive prolongation of the PR interval, culminating in a dropped beat. Block is within the atrioventricular node itself and ventricular depolarization occurs rapidly by normal pathways. Thus, the QRS complex is usually narrow.

Second-degree atrioventricular block: Mobitz type II

Mobitz type II second-degree atrioventricular block indicates advanced conducting tissue disease affecting the bundle branches. The ECG typically shows a normal PR interval with bundle branch block in conducted beats, and intermittent block in the other bundle branch resulting in complete failure of atrioventricular conduction and dropped beats.

Third-degree (complete) atrioventricular block

The atrial and ventricular rhythms are 'dissociated' in third-degree atrioventricular block because none of the atrial impulses are conducted. Thus, the ECG shows regular P waves (unless the atrium is fibrillating) and regular but slower QRS complexes occurring independently of each other. When block is within the atrioventricular node (e.g. inferior myocardial infarction, congenital atrioventricular block), a junctional escape rhythm with a reliable rate (40–60 bpm) takes over (see Fig. 13.29).

Ventricular depolarization occurs rapidly by normal pathways, producing a narrow QRS complex. However, when the block is within the bundle branches (e.g. idiopathic fibrosis), there is always extensive conducting tissue disease. The ventricular escape rhythm is slow and unreliable, with a broad QRS complex (see Fig. 13.29).

Right bundle branch block

A right bundle branch block may be a congenital defect, but more commonly, it is the result of organic conducting tissue disease. Right ventricular depolarization is delayed, resulting in a broad QRS complex with an 'rSR' pattern in lead V_1 and prominent S waves in leads I and V_6.

Left bundle branch block

Left bundle branch block always indicates organic conducting tissue disease. The entire sequence of ventricular depolarization is abnormal, resulting in a broad QRS complex with large slurred or notched R waves in leads I and V_6.

The chest X-ray

Good-quality posteroanterior (PA) and lateral chest X-rays are always helpful in the assessment of the cardiac patient (Fig. 13.30).

Cardiac silhouette

Although the PA chest X-ray exhibits a wide range of normality, the maximum diameter of the heart should not be more than 50% of the widest diameter of the thorax. Cardiac enlargement is caused either

Figure 13.31   Pericardial effusion with tamponade: chest X-ray. There is a left hilar mass caused by carcinoma. Pericardial infiltration has produced effusion and tamponade, evidenced by the severely enlarged and globular cardiac silhouette. Malignant disease is now the most common cause of tamponade in most developed countries.

Figure 13.32   Left atrial dilatation. This is a penetrated PA chest X-ray in a patient with mitral stenosis. The dilated left atrium causes a bulge on the left heart border below the pulmonary artery which is also dilated, widening of the carina and the double-density sign at the right heart border.

by dilatation of the cardiac chambers or by pericardial effusion (Fig. 13.31). Myocardial hypertrophy only affects heart size if very severe.

Ventricular dilatation

The PA chest X-ray does not reliably distinguish left from right ventricular dilatation. For this, the lateral chest X-ray is more helpful. Dilatation of the posteriorly located left ventricle encroaches on the retrocardiac space, whereas dilatation of the anteriorly located right ventricle encroaches on the retrosternal space.

Atrial dilatation

Right atrial dilatation is usually caused by right ventricular failure, but it does occur as an isolated finding in tricuspid stenosis and Ebstein's anomaly. It produces cardiac enlargement without specific radiographic signs.

Left atrial dilatation occurs in left ventricular failure and mitral valve disease (Fig. 13.32). Radiographic signs are:

- Flattening and later bulging of the border on the left side of the heart below the main pulmonary artery
- Elevation of the left main bronchus, with widening of the carina
- Appearance of the medial border of the left atrium behind the right side of the heart (double-density sign)

Vascular dilatation

Aortic dilatation caused by an aneurysm or dissection may produce widening of the entire upper mediastinum. Localized dilatation of the proximal aorta, which occurs in aortic valve disease, produces a prominence in the right upper mediastinum (Fig. 13.33). Dilatation of the main pulmonary artery

Figure 13.33   Chest X-ray in a patient with Marfan's syndrome. Note the dilatation of the ascending aorta.

occurs in pulmonary hypertension and pulmonary stenosis and produces a prominence below the aortic knuckle (Fig. 13.34).

Intracardiac calcification

Because the radiodensity of cardiac tissue is similar to that of blood, intracardiac structures can rarely be identified unless they are calcified. Valvular, pericardial or myocardial calcification may occur, which usually indicates important disease of these structures. Calcification is best appreciated on the deeply penetrated lateral chest X-ray.

Figure 13.34 Atrial septal defect: chest X-ray. Note the prominent proximal pulmonary arteries and the pulmonary plethora reflecting increased pulmonary flow.

Lung fields

Common lung field abnormalities in cardiovascular disease are caused either by altered pulmonary flow or by increased left atrial pressure.

Altered pulmonary flow

Increments in pulmonary flow sufficient to cause radiographic abnormalities are caused by left-to-right intracardiac shunts (e.g. atrial septal defect; see Fig. 13.34, ventricular septal defect, patent ductus arteriosus). Prominence of the vascular markings gives the lung fields a plethoric appearance. Reductions in pulmonary flow, on the other hand, cause reduced vascular markings. This may be regional (e.g. pulmonary embolism) or global (e.g. severe pulmonary hypertension).

Increased left atrial pressure

Increased left atrial pressure, which occurs in mitral stenosis and left ventricular failure, produces corresponding rises in pulmonary venous and pulmonary capillary pressures. Prominence of the upper lobe veins is an early radiographic finding. As the left atrial and pulmonary capillary pressures rise above 18 mmHg, transudation into the lung produces interstitial pulmonary oedema, characterized by prominence of the interlobular septa, particularly at the lung bases (Kerley B lines). Further elevation of pressure leads to alveolar pulmonary oedema, characterized by perihilar 'bat's-wing' shadowing (Fig. 13.35).

Other lung field abnormalities

Pulmonary infarction

Localized and typically wedge-shaped areas of consolidation are occasionally seen in pulmonary

Figure 13.35 Chest X-ray in acute left ventricular failure: the patient had severe pulmonary oedema caused by acute myocardial infarction. The heart is not yet enlarged, but there is prominent alveolar pulmonary oedema in a perihilar ('bat's-wing') distribution. Note the bilateral pleural effusions.

embolic disease, although more often the bronchial circulation protects against ischaemic damage.

Pneumonic consolidation and abscess

In patients with right-sided endocarditis, infected pulmonary emboli commonly cause septic foci within the lung fields.

Interstitial lung disease

In longstanding pulmonary hypertension complicating rheumatic mitral valve disease, hemosiderosis (stippled shadowing throughout the lung fields) was once a common X-ray finding. It is now rarely seen.

Bony abnormalities

Bony abnormalities are unusual in cardiovascular disease, apart from coarctation of the aorta and thoracic outlet syndromes. In coarctation, dilated bronchial collateral vessels erode the inferior aspect of the ribs to produce notches, although they are rarely present before adolescence. Cervical ribs may compress the neurovascular bundle in the thoracic outlet, and special thoracic outlet views are necessary for radiographic diagnosis.

Echocardiography

Echocardiography is one of the most versatile non-invasive imaging techniques used in clinical cardiology. Because it does not use ionizing radiation, it is free of risk and can be employed safely throughout pregnancy. Transthoracic imaging with the transducer applied to the chest wall is usually satisfactory, but better quality information is obtained via the transoesophageal approach in which the transducer is mounted on a probe and positioned in the oesophagus, directly behind the heart. This provides higher resolution images because there are no intervening ribs or lung tissue and the probe is closely applied to the posterior aspect of the heart. It is particularly useful for imaging the left atrium, the aorta, the interatrial septum and prosthetic heart valves.

Principles

Physics

A transducer containing a piezoelectric element converts electrical energy into an ultrasound beam that is directed towards the heart. The beam is reflected when it strikes an interface between tissues of different densities. The reflected ultrasound, or echo, is converted back to electrical energy by the piezoelectric element, which permits the construction of an image using two basic units of information:

1. The intensity of the echoes, which defines the density difference at tissue interfaces within the heart.
2. The time taken for echoes to arrive back at the transducer, which defines the distance of the cardiac structures from the transducer.

Density differences within the heart are greatest between the blood-filled chambers and the myocardial and valvular tissues, all of which are clearly visible on the echocardiogram. Because the depth of the myocardial and valvular tissues with respect to the transducer changes constantly throughout the cardiac cycle, the time taken for echo reflection changes accordingly. Thus, real-time imaging throughout the cardiac cycle provides a dynamic record of cardiac function.

M-mode echocardiogram

The M-mode echocardiogram provides a unidimensional view through the heart. Continuous recording on photographic paper provides an additional time dimension, thereby permitting appreciation of the dynamic component of the cardiac image. By convention, cardiac structures closest to the transducer are displayed at the top of the record and more distant structures are displayed below. Thus, on the transthoracic M-mode echocardiogram, anteriorly located ('right-sided') structures lie above the posteriorly located ('left-sided') structures, but on the transoesophageal echocardiogram, the display is reversed. M-mode is particularly useful for measuring chamber dimensions and left ventricular wall thickness, and for timing events within the cardiac cycle (Fig. 13.36A).

Two-dimensional (2D) echocardiogram

A two-dimensional echocardiogram provides more detailed information about morphology than does the M-mode recording. By projecting a fan of echoes in an arc of up to 80°, a 2D 'slice' through the heart can be obtained, the precise view depending on the location and angulation of the transducer (Fig. 13.36B).

Clinical applications

Congenital heart disease

Echocardiography, particularly the 2D technique, has revolutionized the diagnosis of congenital heart disease, in most cases, obviating the need for invasive investigation by cardiac catheterization (Fig. 13.37). The relationships of the cardiac chambers and their connections with the great vessels are readily determined. Valvular abnormalities and septal defects can also be recognized. Recent technology has permitted in utero fetal imaging for the antenatal diagnosis of cardiac defects.

Myocardial disease

Echocardiography permits accurate assessment of cardiac dilatation, hypertrophy and contractile function. Dilated cardiomyopathy produces ventricular dilatation with global contractile impairment (Fig. 13.38). This must be distinguished from the regional contractile impairment that follows myocardial infarction in patients with coronary artery disease (Fig. 13.39). Hypertrophic cardiomyopathy is characterized by thickening (hypertrophy) of the left ventricular myocardium, usually with disproportionate involvement of the interventricular septum (asymmetric septal hypertrophy). In aortic and hypertensive heart disease, on the other hand, left ventricular hypertrophy is usually symmetrical (Fig. 13.40).

Valvular disease

Echocardiography is of particular value for identifying both structural and dynamic valvular abnormalities and any associated chamber dilatation or hypertrophy (Boxes 13.18–13.21). The severity of valvular involvement in congenital, rheumatic, degenerative and infective disease may thus be defined; the technique is diagnostic for bicuspid aortic valve and mitral valve prolapse, and readily identifies valve thickening and calcification in rheumatic and calcific disease (Figs 13.40 and 13.41). Vegetations in infective endocarditis usually can be visualized if they are large enough (>3 mm, Fig. 13.42). The transoesophageal approach is usually necessary for endocarditis involving prosthetic heart valves.

Pericardial disease

Although the echocardiogram is of little value in constrictive pericarditis, it is the most sensitive technique available for the diagnosis of pericardial effusion (Fig. 13.43). The effusion appears as an echo-free space distributed around the ventricles,

Figure 13.36 **(A)** M-mode echocardiography. The figure shows a sweep as the transducer is angulated from the left ventricle to the aortic root. **(B)** Transthoracic 2D echocardiography. Parasternal long-axis and apical four-chamber views are shown. The dots are a 1-cm scale. AV, aortic valve; CW, chest wall; IVS, interventricular septum; LA, left atrium; LV, left ventricle; MV, mitral valve; PW, posterior LV wall; RV, right ventricle.

Figure 13.37 Atrial septal defect: 2D echocardiogram (subcostal view). In this view, good views of the interatrial septum can usually be obtained without resorting to transoesophageal echocardiography. Note the atrial septal defect (*arrow*) and the dilatation of the right atrium (RA).

Figure 13.38 Dilated cardiomyopathy: echocardiogram. This M-mode study shows severe dilatation of the left ventricular cavity and severe global contractile impairment. The patient later underwent successful heart transplantation.

Figure 13.39 Heart failure: echocardiogram. This M-mode study shows considerable dilatation of the left ventricle. Note that the interventricular septum (IVS) is almost akinetic, but the posterior wall (PW) is contracting normally. Regional contractile impairment of this type indicates coronary heart disease. The phonocardiogram recorded simultaneously shows normal first and second heart sounds and also a third heart sound (*arrow*).

Figure 13.40 Aortic stenosis and left ventricular hypertrophy: 2D echocardiogram (long-axis view). The aortic valve (AV) is grossly thickened and calcified. Concentric left ventricular hypertrophy is present (*arrow*).

Box 13.18 Aortic stenosis

Typical patient

- Middle-aged (congenitally bicuspid valve) or elderly (degenerative calcific disease) man or woman

Major symptoms

- Exertional shortness of breath is usual presenting symptom.
- Angina may also occur and, in advanced cases, syncopal attacks or sudden death.

Major signs

- Carotid pulse: slow upstroke with plateau
- Auscultation: fourth heart sound at cardiac apex; ejection systolic murmur at base of heart, radiating to neck. The murmur may be preceded by an ejection click if the valve is mobile and not heavily calcified.

Diagnosis

- ECG: left ventricular hypertrophy
- Chest X-ray: dilatation of ascending aorta
- Echocardiogram: calcified immobile aortic valve with left ventricular hypertrophy. Doppler studies permit quantification of the severity of stenosis.

Additional investigations

- Cardiac catheterization is necessary to evaluate coronary arteries in patients being considered for aortic valve replacement surgery.

Comments

- Aortic stenosis is now the most commonly acquired valve lesion in developed countries.
- The use of percutaneous implanted aortic valves (TAVI) has significantly increased the number of patients with aortic stenosis who can now be treated.

Box 13.19 Aortic regurgitation

Typical patient

- Young men (Marfan's syndrome, etc.) or older patients (longstanding hypertension) with dilating disease of the aortic root

Major symptoms

- Exertional shortness of breath is usual presenting symptom.
- Angina may also occur.

Major signs

- Carotid pulse: sharp upstroke with early diastolic collapse
- Blood pressure: systolic hypertension with wide pulse pressure
- Auscultation: early diastolic murmur at left sternal edge. Third heart sound at cardiac apex in severe cases. Mid-diastolic murmur (Austin Flint) may be heard at apex owing to preclosure of mitral valve by regurgitant jet.

Diagnosis

- ECG: left ventricular hypertrophy
- Chest X-ray: cardiac enlargement with dilatation of ascending aorta
- Echocardiogram: often normal valve with dilated aortic root. Doppler studies confirm regurgitant jet.

Additional investigations

- Cardiac catheterization is necessary to evaluate coronary arteries in older patients (age >50) being considered for aortic valve replacement surgery.

Comments

- The timing of valve replacement surgery is difficult, but should anticipate irreversible left ventricular contractile failure.

Figure 13.41 Mitral stenosis: 2D echocardiogram (parasternal long-axis view). The mitral valve leaflets are densely thickened (*arrows*) and the left atrium is severely dilated.

Figure 13.42 Infective endocarditis: transoesophageal echocardiogram. A vegetation (*arrow*) is adherent to the aortic valve leaflet.

Box 13.20	Mitral stenosis

Typical patient

- Young to middle-aged woman with a history of rheumatic fever in childhood.

Major symptoms

- Exertional shortness of breath with orthopnoea in advanced cases.
- Palpitations commonly signal the development of atrial fibrillation, which puts the patient at serious risk of peripheral embolism and stroke.

Major signs

- Pulse: atrial fibrillation in many cases.
- Auscultation: loud S1 with early diastolic opening snap, followed by low-pitched mid-diastolic murmur best heard at cardiac apex. If the patient is in sinus rhythm, there is presystolic accentuation of the murmur.

Diagnosis

- ECG: atrial fibrillation usually.
- Chest X-ray: signs of left atrial enlargement (flat left heart border, widening of carinal angle and double-density sign at right heart border). Pulmonary congestion
- Echocardiogram: rheumatic mitral valve and left atrial dilatation. Doppler studies permit quantification of the severity of stenosis.

Additional investigations

- Cardiac catheterization is necessary to evaluate coronary arteries in patients aged >50 being considered for mitral valve replacement surgery.

Comments

- In patients with atrial fibrillation, anticoagulation with warfarin is mandatory to protect against stroke.

Figure 13.43 Pericardial effusion: 2D echocardiogram (parasternal long-axis view). Note the echo-free space (*arrows*) around the heart, but not behind the left atrium.

but usually avoiding the potential space behind the left atrium.

Other clinical applications

Intracardiac tumours, particularly myxomas (see Fig. 13.1) and thrombi (Fig. 13.44), are readily visualized by echocardiography. The transoesophageal technique is more sensitive for identifying thrombus in the left atrial appendage and is also helpful for diagnosing aortic disease, such as aneurysm and dissection, because it provides better views of the thoracic aorta than is possible with conventional 2D echocardiography (Fig. 13.45).

Stress echocardiography

Stress echocardiography is increasingly being used for the diagnosis of myocardial ischaemia in suspected coronary disease. Left ventricular imaging during increasing dobutamine infusion or exercise

Typical patient

- Mitral valve prolapse (floppy mitral valve) causes regurgitation of variable severity, and more commonly affects women at almost any age.
- Patients with subvalvular disease (papillary muscle dysfunction or chordal rupture) are usually elderly men or women.

Major symptoms

- Exertional shortness of breath with orthopnoea in advanced cases.
- Palpitations commonly signal the development of atrial fibrillation, which puts the patient at serious risk of peripheral embolism and stroke.

Major signs

- Pulse: often sinus rhythm, but may be atrial fibrillation
- Auscultation: pansystolic murmur at cardiac apex, radiating to axilla. Often associated with third heart sound.

Diagnosis

- ECG: atrial fibrillation, but may be normal.
- Chest X-ray: cardiac enlargement with variable signs of left atrial enlargement, though these are usually less marked than in mitral stenosis. Pulmonary congestion in severe cases.
- Echocardiogram: prolapsing (floppy) mitral valve may be seen; in subvalvular disease the valve often appears normal. Left ventricular and left atrial dilatation. Doppler studies confirm regurgitant jet.

Additional investigations

- Transoesophageal echo is sometimes necessary to clarify the severity and mechanism of regurgitation.
- Cardiac catheterization is necessary to evaluate coronary arteries in patients aged >50 being considered for mitral valve replacement surgery.

Comments

- In patients with atrial fibrillation, anticoagulation with warfarin is mandatory to protect against stroke.

permits assessment of regional wall motion in response to stress. Decreasing systolic wall motion or wall thickening indicates ischaemia and the need for further investigation. Stress echocardiography is also used to identify myocardial viability in patients with impaired cardiac function. Improvement in regional hypokinesia in response to dobutamine may indicate 'hibernating' (and hence potentially salvageable) myocardium likely to respond favourably to revascularization by angioplasty or bypass surgery.

Doppler echocardiography

Doppler echocardiography permits evaluation of the direction and velocity of blood flow within the heart and great vessels. It is widely used for measuring the severity of valvular stenosis and identifying valvular regurgitation and intracardiac shunts through septal defects.

Figure 13.44   Mitral stenosis: 2D echocardiogram (long-axis view). The left atrium is severely dilated and a large thrombus (*arrow*) is visible, emphasizing the importance of anticoagulation in patients with mitral valve disease and atrial fibrillation.

Figure 13.45   Aortic dissection: transoesophageal echocardiogram. Right panel: this long-axis transoesophageal echocardiogram reveals the dilated aortic root and an S-shaped flap (*arrow*) traversing the lumen. Left panel: same patient with colour Doppler superimposed to show flow in the true lumen.

Principles

Physics

According to the Doppler principle, when an ultrasound beam is directed towards the bloodstream, the frequency of the sound waves reflected from the blood cells is altered. The frequency shift or Doppler effect is related to the direction and velocity of flow. If continuous-wave Doppler is used, blood flow at any point along the path of the ultrasound beam is detected, such that a 'clean' Doppler signal from the area of interest may be difficult to obtain. Pulsed Doppler, however, has a range-gating facility that permits frequency sampling from any specific point within the heart, preselected on the echocardiogram. This lends greater precision to the technique. Nevertheless, pulsed Doppler is less able than continuous-wave Doppler to quantify very high-velocity jets, such as those that occur in aortic stenosis.

Colour-flow mapping

Colour-flow mapping has been a major technological advance. Instead of the unidirectional ultrasound beam used in continuous-wave and pulsed Doppler imaging, the beam is rotated through an arc. Frequency sampling throughout the arc permits the construction of a colour-coded map, red indicating flow towards and blue away from the transducer. Colour-flow data can be superimposed on the standard 2D echocardiogram to identify precisely the patterns of flow within the four chambers of the heart. This simplifies the interpretation of Doppler imaging and provides more useful qualitative data, although it is less useful for quantitative assessment of valve gradients, which requires the precision of conventional Doppler technique.

Clinical applications

In paediatric cardiology, the combination of 2D echocardiography and colour-flow Doppler mapping has made possible the 'non-invasive' diagnosis of a large majority of congenital defects, often without the need for cardiac catheterization. These techniques have also revolutionized the diagnosis of valvular disease in all age groups. In valvular regurgitation, the retrograde flow that occurs after valve closure is readily detected by Doppler echocardiography, although only an approximate estimate of its severity is possible (Fig. 13.46). In valvular stenosis, the peak velocity (as opposed to the volume) of flow across the valve is directly related to the degree of stenosis. Thus, measurement of Doppler flow velocity (ideally by continuous wave) permits quantification of the stenosis by the application of the Bernoulli equation:

$$\text{pressure gradient} = 4 \times \text{velocity}^2$$

Figure 13.46 Mitral regurgitation: colour-flow Doppler. This is an apical long-axis view of the heart showing a large jet of mitral regurgitation (*blue*) occupying most of the left atrial cavity (LA).

New developments

In recent years, real time three-dimensional imaging has emerged as a powerful technique—particularly in the assessment of valvular disease and in guiding percutaneous interventions such as minimally invasive transcatheter aortic valve implantation (TAVI).

Doppler imaging techniques can also be applied to the myocardium itself (tissue Doppler) to provide measures of myocardial strain. Abnormalities in strain often predate clinical symptoms and have been used to identify and treat patients at risk of developing cardiac disease.

Cardiovascular radionuclide imaging

Principles

All radionuclide techniques require the internal administration of a radioisotope; the distribution of radioactivity in the area of interest is then imaged with a gamma camera. Ideally, the isotope should be distributed homogeneously in that part of the cardiovascular system under investigation: thus, isotopes that remain in the intravascular space during imaging are used for radionuclide angiography. In myocardial perfusion scintigraphy, however, isotopes taken up by the myocardium are required. Because of their potential toxicity, isotopes with a short half-life are usually used.

Clinical applications

Radionuclide ventriculography

Radionuclide ventriculography is used for assessment of ventricular function. Red cells labelled with technetium-99m (^{99m}Tc) are allowed to equilibrate in the blood pool and the heart is then imaged under the gamma camera. The waxing and waning of radioactivity within the ventricular chambers during diastole and systole, respectively, permits the construction of a dynamic ventriculogram. Left ventricular contractile function can be evaluated quantitatively by calculating the ejection fraction, or qualitatively by observing wall movement. In clinical practice, this has now been replaced by other techniques, such as echocardiography and magnetic resonance imaging, for the assessment of left ventricular function.

Myocardial perfusion scintigraphy

Myocardial perfusion scintigraphy is used for the diagnosis and assessment of coronary artery disease (Fig. 13.47). The patient is 'stressed' in an

STRESS   REDISTRIBUTION

Figure 13.47   Isotope perfusion scan. These are tomographic slices across the short axis of the left ventricle. A posterior wall defect is seen during stress, but it largely disappears during rest as isotope 'redistributes' into the ischaemic area. A smaller fixed defect is seen in the anterior wall, indicating infarction in that territory.

attempt to provoke myocardial ischaemia, either by a standardized exercise test, an intravenous dobutamine infusion or an intravenous adenosine infusion. Isotope is injected intravenously at peak stress and the heart is imaged under a gamma camera. Thallium-201 (^{201}Tl) has now given way to ^{99m}Tc-labelled methoxy-isobutyl- isonitrile (MIBI) which provides better image quality. Isotope is distributed homogeneously in normally perfused myocardium, ischaemic or infarcted areas appearing as scintigraphic defects. If ^{201}Tl is used, repeat imaging after 2–4 hours' rest permits the reassessment of scintigraphic defects; those that disappear (reversible defects) indicate areas of stress-induced ischaemia, whereas those that persist (fixed defects) indicate infarcted myocardium. If ^{99m}Tc-labelled MIBI is used, resting images for assessment of reversibility require a separate injection of isotope 24 hours after (or before) the stress images.

Positron emission tomography

Positron emission tomography (PET) scanning is used to determine myocardial 'viability' in patients with heart failure (see stress echocardiography, above). Simultaneous assessment of myocardial perfusion using ^{13}N ammonia and glucose uptake using a glucose analogue permits the identification of viable but dysfunctional myocardium, in which perfusion is impaired but metabolic activity in terms of glucose uptake remains normal. This perfusion-metabolic 'mismatch' indicates viable muscle likely to respond favourably to revascularization by angioplasty or bypass surgery.

New PET tracers, such as rubidium, can be used to assess myocardial perfusion. A specialist cyclotron is not required for this tracer, reducing the costs involved.

Pulmonary scintigraphy (radioisotope imaging)

Pulmonary scintigraphy is used for the diagnosis of pulmonary embolism (Fig. 13.48). ^{99m}Tc-labelled microspheres injected intravenously become trapped within the pulmonary capillaries. The normal pulmonary perfusion scintigram shows a homogeneous distribution of radioactivity throughout both lung fields. Pulmonary embolism causes regional impairment of pulmonary flow, which results in a perfusion defect on the scintigram; however, the appearance is non-specific and occurs in many other pulmonary disorders, particularly chronic obstructive pulmonary disease. Specificity is enhanced by simultaneous ventilation scintigraphy (a ventilation/perfusion or V/Q scan). Inhaled xenon-133 (^{133}Xe) is distributed homogeneously throughout the normal lung, and in pulmonary embolism (unlike other pulmonary disorders), distribution remains homogeneous. Thus, a scintigraphic perfusion defect not 'matched' by a ventilation defect is highly specific for pulmonary embolism. CT pulmonary angiography is now the

Figure 13.48 Ventilation (right) and perfusion (left) lung scans in pulmonary embolism. Contrast the homogeneous distribution of isotope in the ventilation scan with the regional defects in the perfusion scan.

diagnostic test of choice for pulmonary embolism, but V/Q scanning is still valuable in patients with suspected pulmonary embolism who have severe renal impairment in whom X-ray contrast is contraindicated.

Computed tomography

Principles

Computed tomography measures the attenuation of X-rays after they have traversed body tissues. Attenuation is greatest for tissues such as bone, which are relatively radio-opaque, and least for tissues such as lung or fat, which are relatively radiolucent. From X-ray attenuation measurements, taken as a sensor rotates around the chest, cross-sectional images are constructed. Image resolution is excellent, and contrast injection into a peripheral vein opacifies the blood pool allowing assessment of the coronary arteries and intracardiac structures. In the past, the clinical application of cardiac CT was limited by image acquisition times of up to 5 seconds, during which the constant motion of the heart degraded the image, and by high radiation doses. The current generation of ultrafast CT scanners with image acquisition times of less than 1 second provides high-resolution cardiac images in both static and video mode, whereas radiation doses have reduced substantially.

Clinical applications

Computed tomography (with contrast enhancement) diagnoses pulmonary embolism and aortic dissection (Fig. 13.49) with a sensitivity of about 95%. It is also used for accurate assessment of pericardial thickness in constrictive disease (Fig. 13.50) and in the diagnosis of cardiac tumours. Recently, multislice CT has emerged as a useful investigative tool for the diagnosis of coronary artery disease. The quantification of coronary calcification has found application as a marker of coronary

Figure 13.49 Aortic dissection: CT scan (Marfan's syndrome). The ascending aorta is dilated and the intimal flap (*arrow*) clearly visible. This flap extends around the arch (not seen here) into the descending aorta, where again it is clearly visible.

Figure 13.50 Non-calcific pericardial constriction: CT scan. There is consolidation in the right lung and severe pericardial thickening. The patient had pulmonary tuberculosis with pericardial involvement and presented with fever and signs of constriction. Antituberculous therapy caused regression of all symptoms and signs, although the patient is at major risk of developing constriction later as the pericardium becomes fibrotic and calcified.

Figure 13.51 CT coronary angiogram: normal study in a 42-year-old man with atypical chest pain and a family history of premature coronary artery disease. **(A)** Multiplanar reformatted image of the left anterior descending artery (*arrow*). **(B)** Multiplanar reformatted image of the circumflex artery (*arrow*). **(C)** 3D volume rendered image of the right coronary artery (*large arrow*), its posterior descending branch (*upper small arrow*) and posterior left ventricular branch (*lower small arrow*).

risk in asymptomatic or low-risk individuals; a zero calcium score has a high accuracy rate for the exclusion of coronary artery disease. CT coronary angiography is able to diagnose normal coronary arteries or mild plaque disease extremely accurately (Fig. 13.51), but it cannot distinguish reliably between moderate and severe stenoses or determine the degree of stenosis in heavily calcified coronary segments. CT coronary angiography is therefore best used in the assessment of low- to medium-risk patients to 'rule out' significant obstructive coronary artery disease. Additional applications of CT include the evaluation of graft patency following coronary bypass surgery and analysis of ventricular wall motion.

Magnetic resonance imaging

Principles

Magnetic resonance imaging (MRI) utilizes the fact that certain nuclei with an intrinsic spin generate magnetic fields and behave like tiny bar magnets. Placed in a magnetic field, these nuclei align and adopt a resonant frequency that is unique to that nucleus and the strength of the magnetic field. If the nuclei are exposed to pulsed radiowaves of that frequency, they resonate and release energy, which allows their location to be determined.

For imaging purposes, the patient lies in a strong magnetic field that is artificially graded. The hydrogen protons of fat and water are imaged and, on exposure to pulsed radiowaves, they resonate at different frequencies in different parts of the imaging zone. Analysis of the emitted frequencies permits the construction of tomographic and 3D images of the heart. If data acquisition is gated to a specific part of the cardiac cycle, motion artefact is eliminated and excellent image resolution can be obtained. Different scanning parameters and patterns of gadolinium enhancement after its intravenous administration allow precise myocardial tissue characterization and detection of myocardial ischaemia.

Clinical applications

Cardiac MRI is now widely used for the assessment of cardiac structure and ventricular function. It can differentiate between myocardial infarction (Fig. 13.52), oedema, fibrosis and fat. MRI is well validated for the assessment of myocardial viability and ischaemia. Therefore, it is used in the diagnosis of coronary artery disease, myocarditis (Fig. 13.53) and cardiomyopathies. It is also used to guide therapy in patients with documented coronary artery disease, particularly those with chronic coronary occlusions or multivessel disease, the presence of viability or ischaemia, respectively, providing justification for revascularization. Cardiac MRI does not involve the use of ionizing radiation so it can be used safely for repeated follow up assessments. MRI provides an accurate assessment of valve regurgitant fraction and it is also highly sensitive for the diagnosis of aortic dissection (Fig. 13.54), intracardiac tumours and thrombi.

Cardiac catheterization

Catheters introduced into an artery or vein may be directed into the left or right sides of the heart,

respectively. Arterial access is gained percutaneously from the femoral or radial artery, or by surgical cutdown to the brachial artery. Venous access is usually from the femoral vein. Originally developed for diagnostic purposes, catheter techniques have now found widespread application in the interventional management of cardiovascular disease.

Cardiac angiography

Coronary angiography uses relatively small volumes of contrast (5–8 ml) injected manually, but other angiographic procedures require larger amounts (up to 40 ml), introduced by power injection. Digital subtraction techniques permit a reduction in contrast volume but at present have only a limited role in cardiovascular angiographic diagnosis (see below). The current generation of angiographic laboratories uses digital technology to provide high-quality dynamic images of ventricular wall movement, blood flow and intravascular anatomy.

Aortic root angiography

Injection of contrast into the aortic root demonstrates the vascular anatomy in suspected aneurysm or dissection, and also permits evaluation of aortic valve function (Fig. 13.55). The normal aortic valve prevents diastolic backflow of contrast, but in aortic regurgitation, variable opacification of the left ventricle occurs, depending on the severity of the valve lesion.

Left ventricular angiography

Contrast injection into the left ventricle defines ventricular anatomy and wall motion, and also permits evaluation of mitral valve function. Dilatation of the ventricle and contractile dysfunction occurs in left ventricular failure. An akinetic segment denotes previous myocardial infarction. Exaggerated contractile function with systolic obliteration of the cavity occurs in hypertrophic cardiomyopathy. Filling defects within the ventricular lumen may indicate thrombus or neoplasm. The normal mitral valve prevents systolic backflow of contrast into the left atrium, but in mitral regurgitation, variable atrial

Figure 13.52 Anteroapical myocardial infarction: MRI scan. Delayed gadolinium enhancement (*white arrows*) of the full thickness of the anteroapical left ventricular wall indicating infarcted, non-viable tissue.

Box 13.22	Indications for coronary angiography

- ST elevation myocardial infarction
- High-risk non-ST elevation acute coronary syndromes
- Severe angina unresponsive to medical treatment
- Angina or a positive exercise test following myocardial infarction
- Cardiac arrhythmias with clinical suspicion of underlying coronary artery disease
- Preoperatively in patients requiring valve surgery when advanced age (>50) or angina suggest a high probability of coronary artery disease

Figure 13.53 Myocarditis: MRI scan. **(A)** Still image from a cine loop of a two-chamber view of the left ventricle. Measurements of systolic function, chamber size and myocardial mass can be made from the cine loops. **(B)** Two-chamber view from the same patient with imaging for water content (T2 weighted) showing regions of myocardial oedema (*arrows*). **(C)** Late enhancement imaging following gadolinium infusion allows detection of areas of increased interstitial expansion from scar or oedema (*arrows*). The subepicardial pattern indicates myocarditis.

opacification occurs, depending on the severity of the valve lesion (Fig. 13.56).

Coronary angiography

Coronary angiography is the most reliable technique for diagnostic imaging of the coronary arteries and assessment of lesion severity. Indications are summarized in Box 13.22. The technique requires selective injection of contrast into the left and right coronary arteries to opacify the lumen (Fig. 13.57), and multiple views in different projections are necessary for a complete study. Intraluminal filling defects or occlusions indicate coronary artery disease, which is nearly always caused by atherosclerosis. In stable patients, coronary angiography often reveals a stenosis or stenoses of intermediate severity. Additional information regarding the functional significance and anatomic severity of the disease is required before treatment decisions can be made. This can be obtained either from non-invasive myocardial perfusion imaging that looks for ischaemia in the territory of the affected artery (see MRI perfusion imaging) or from catheter laboratory-based techniques.

Figure 13.54 Aortic dissection: MRI scan. The upper panel (coronal section) reveals an extensive aortic dissection extending from the aortic root through the arch and into the descending aorta. The lower panel reveals a transverse view through the heart and descending aorta. Note the thrombus in the false lumen surrounding the true lumen in the descending aorta (*arrow*).

Figure 13.55 Aortic root angiogram: normal study. Contrast injection provides an X-ray image of the ascending aorta. The coronary arteries arising from the sinuses of Valsalva are clearly seen.

Figure 13.56 Left ventricular angiogram showing mitral regurgitation. Contrast injection into the left ventricle has resulted in prompt opacification of the left atrium owing to backflow across the diseased mitral valve.

Pressure wire

Pressure wire, a relatively new catheter laboratory-based technology, is increasingly used to assess functional significance and guide management of coronary stenoses. The wire has a pressure sensor 3 cm from its distal tip. The pressure sensor is calibrated and then equalized to the pressure at the guide catheter tip in the left main stem, before being passed down the artery so that the pressure sensor is distal to the stenosis to be interrogated. Adenosine is administered by intravenous infusion to induce maximal hyperaemia in the myocardial capillary bed and simulate the physiological state during exercise. The fractional flow reserve (FFR) is calculated automatically by computer software from the pressure measured distal to the stenosis referenced against the pressure measured proximal to the stenosis at the guide catheter tip. An FFR <0.75 signifies a stenosis that is likely to cause myocardial ischaemia and the stenosis is deemed functionally significant. Clinical studies have shown that pressure wire-guided management is superior to angiographic-driven decision-making, predominantly through avoiding procedure-related myocardial infarction in patients who undergo revascularization.

Intravascular ultrasound

An ultrasound transducer mounted at the tip of a coronary catheter is used to provide cross-sectional images of the artery. The technique permits accurate measurement of the luminal area and provides information about plaque composition and structure that cannot be obtained from angiographic images (Fig. 13.58). Intravascular ultrasound has a clinical

Figure 13.57 Coronary angiograms. **(A)** Left anterior descending disease (*arrow*). This tight stenosis threatens the coronary supply to the anterior wall of the left ventricle. **(B)** Right coronary artery disease (*arrow*). Serial stenoses in this dominant right coronary artery threaten the supply to the inferior wall of the heart.

Figure 13.58 Intravascular ultrasound. **(A)** Non-obstructive, calcified plaque between the 5 and 7 o'clock position in a distal segment of the right coronary artery. The ultrasound's transducer is clearly visible at the intersection of the horizontal and vertical centimetre scales. **(B)** Coronary artery disease: a large semilunar, non-calcified coronary plaque that produced an intermediate severity stenosis on coronary angiography is shown extending from the 1 o'clock to the 7 o'clock position, severely reducing the vessel lumen.

role in quantifying the severity of intermediate stenoses identified on coronary angiography, optimizing stent deployment, assessing in-stent restenosis and stent thrombosis and in clarifying the cause of equivocal angiographic appearances owing to possible thrombus, dissection, calcium or plaque.

Pulmonary angiography

Injection of contrast medium into the main pulmonary artery opacifies the arterial branches throughout both lung fields. The normal flow distribution is homogeneous. Vascular occlusions with regional perfusion defects usually indicate pulmonary thromboembolism (particularly when intraluminal filling defects are present), but may also occur in advanced emphysema. The high diagnostic accuracy of CT pulmonary angiography means that invasive pulmonary angiography is now rarely performed.

Intracardiac pressure measurement

Cardiac catheterization for measurement of blood flow and pressure within the heart and great vessels is widely used both for diagnostic purposes and to guide treatment. The fluid-filled catheter is attached to a pressure transducer, which converts the pressure waves into electrical signals. For measurement of right-sided pressures, the catheter is directed by the venous route into the right atrium and then advanced through the right ventricle into the pulmonary artery. For measurement of left-sided pressures, the catheter is directed by the arterial route into the ascending aorta and advanced retrogradely through the aortic valve into the left ventricle. Because access to the left atrium is technically difficult, left atrial pressure is usually measured indirectly using the pulmonary artery wedge pressure.

The pulmonary artery wedge pressure is obtained during right-heart catheterization by advancing the catheter distally into the pulmonary arterial tree until the tip wedges in a small branch. Alternatively, a catheter with a preterminal balloon (Swan-Ganz catheter) may be used. Inflation of the balloon in the pulmonary artery causes the catheter tip to be carried with blood flow into a more distal branch, which becomes occluded by the balloon. Regardless of which method is used, the wedge pressure recorded at the catheter tip is a more or less accurate measure of the left atrial pressure transmitted retrogradely through the pulmonary veins and capillaries.

Haemodynamic evaluation of valvular stenosis

In the normal heart, there is no pressure gradient across an open valve. Such a gradient usually indicates valvular stenosis (Fig. 13.59) and, as stenosis worsens, the pressure gradient increases. This therefore provides a useful index of the severity of stenosis. However, it must be recognized that the pressure gradient is influenced by the flow through the valve. For example, if cardiac output is very low, the gradient may be small despite the presence of

Figure 13.59 Valvular stenosis: pressure signals. **(A)** Aortic stenosis: simultaneous left ventricular (LV) and aortic (AO) pressure signals. In the normal heart, the pressure signals essentially should be similar throughout systole. Here there is a peak systolic gradient of about 35 mmHg across the aortic valve. Note the prominent 'a' wave (*arrow*), reflecting the major contribution that atrial systole makes to filling of the hypertrophied, non-compliant ventricle. Note also the pulsus alternans indicating left ventricular failure. **(B)** Mitral stenosis: simultaneous recordings of the pulmonary artery wedge (PAW) and left ventricular (LV) pressure signals. In the normal heart, the pressure signals should be superimposed throughout diastole. Here there is a pressure gradient >10 mmHg, indicating severe mitral stenosis. Note that the patient is in atrial fibrillation and the pressure gradient varies inversely with the RR interval, tending to increase as the RR interval shortens.

severe stenosis. This applies particularly to the aortic valve because flow velocity is normally high. In patients with poor left ventricular function, the 2D appearances of the valve on echocardiography, the degree of calcification on CT and estimates of valve area should be considered before concluding that significant aortic stenosis is not present.

Haemodynamic evaluation of intracardiac shunts

Left-to-right intracardiac shunts through atrial or ventricular septal defects introduce 'arterialized' blood into the right side of the heart. This results in an abrupt increase or step-up in the oxygen saturation of venous blood at the level of the shunt, which can be detected by right heart catheterization. Thus, by drawing serial blood samples for oxygen saturation from the pulmonary artery, right ventricle, right atrium and vena cava, the shunt may be localized to the site at which the step-up in oxygen saturation occurs. The magnitude of the step-up is related to the size of the shunt, but precise quantification of the shunt requires measurement of pulmonary and systemic blood flow. The extent to which the pulmonary-systemic flow ratio exceeds 1 is a measure of the size of the shunt.

Haemodynamic evaluation of constriction and tamponade

In constrictive pericarditis and tamponade (Boxes 13.23 and 13.24), diastolic relaxation of the ventricles is impeded, preventing adequate filling. Compensatory increments in atrial pressures occur to help maintain ventricular filling, and because these disorders usually affect both ventricles equally, the filling pressures also equilibrate. Thus, simultaneous left- and right-sided recordings in constrictive pericarditis and tamponade show characteristic elevation and equalization of the filling pressures (atrial or ventricular end-diastolic), with loss of the normal differential (Fig. 13.60). Similar physiology characterizes restrictive cardiomyopathy, in which infiltrative disease (usually amyloid in the UK) impedes relaxation of the ventricles.

Measurement of cardiac output

Measurement of cardiac output usually is calculated by thermodilution using a Swan-Ganz catheter with a right atrial portal and a terminal thermistor positioned in the pulmonary artery. A known volume of cold saline (usually 10 ml) is injected into the right atrium and the temperature reduction in the pulmonary artery is recorded at the thermistor. The contour of the cooling curve is dependent on cardiac output, which is calculated by measuring the area under the curve using a bedside computer.

Cardiac output can also be measured by a variety of non-invasive methods, including oesophageal Doppler probe, pulse waveform analysis, bioimpedance and echocardiography. Stroke volume can be calculated using 2D echocardiography from

---

Box 13.23	Constriction

Typical patient
- Middle-aged or elderly patient with a long history of progressive debilitation

Major symptoms
- Dyspnoea and weight loss with abdominal discomfort

Major signs
- Fluid retention with raised JVP (prominent 'x' and 'y' descents), hepatomegaly and peripheral oedema; diastolic filling sound ('pericardial knock'); paradoxical rise in JVP with inspiration (Kussmaul's sign)

Diagnosis
- High level of clinical suspicion
- CT or MRI scan: increased pericardial thickness (±calcification)
- Cardiac catheterization: equalization of diastolic pressures in the four cardiac chambers

Additional investigations
- Chest X-ray: often normal, but occasionally shows pericardial calcification on lateral film

Comments
- Tuberculosis no longer most common cause in developed countries, where most cases are idiopathic

---

Box 13.24	Tamponade

Typical patient
- Either middle-aged or elderly patient with malignant disease (usually breast or lung), or patients of any age with tuberculosis

Major symptoms
- Dyspnoea and variable circulatory collapse

Major signs
- Low-output state (hypotension, oliguria, cold periphery); tachycardia; paradoxical pulse; raised JVP with rapid 'x' descent; paradoxical rise in JVP on inspiration (Kussmaul's sign)

Diagnosis
- This is a clinical diagnosis, confirmed by echocardiographic demonstration of pericardial effusion.

Additional investigations
- ECG: low-voltage QRS complexes with alternating electrical axis
- Tests for aetiological diagnosis: these might include serological tests for rheumatoid and systemic lupus erythematosus, and tests for malignant or tuberculous disease.

Comments
- Any cause of pericardial effusion may produce tamponade, malignant disease being the most common cause in developed countries. Pericardiocentesis relieves the tamponade. Pericardial fluid should always be sent for cytological and bacteriological analysis.

Figure 13.60   Pericardial constriction: left (LV) and right (RV) ventricular pressure signals. Like tamponade and restrictive cardiomyopathy, constriction usually affects both ventricles equally and the diastolic pressures must rise and equilibrate to maintain ventricular filling. Thus, in diastole, the pressure signals are superimposed with a typical 'dip and plateau' configuration ('square root' sign).

the estimated difference in left ventricular volumes at the end of systole and diastole. Alternatively, Doppler echocardiography can be used to measure stroke volume.

Cardiac output measurement is performed most commonly in intensive care units to characterize cardiovascular status and monitor responses to treatment. It is particularly valuable in the shocked patient whose intravascular volume status cannot be determined by clinical assessment.

Pathology laboratory support

Haematology laboratory

Anaemia exacerbates angina by adversely affecting the myocardial oxygen supply-demand relationship, and also exacerbates heart failure by increasing the cardiac work necessary to meet the oxygen demands of metabolizing tissues. Rarely, anaemia is a consequence of, rather than a contributor to, heart disease. In infective endocarditis, a normochromic normocytic anaemia is almost invariable, reflecting the adverse effects of chronic illness on erythropoiesis. Chronic haemolysis occasionally occurs in patients with mechanical prosthetic heart valves and is caused by traumatic erythrocyte damage. Anaemia is usually low grade; if severe, it may require removal of the prosthesis and substitution with a xenograft.

Biochemistry laboratory

Cardiac enzymes and other markers of myocardial injury

Following myocardial infarction, enzymes and structural proteins released into the circulation by the necrosing myocytes provide biochemical markers of injury. In the UK, for many years, creatine kinase (CK) was the most widely used marker, the CK-MB isoenzyme being the most specific for myocardial injury. However, newer serum markers of myocardial injury, particularly the highly specific troponins T and I, have replaced enzymatic markers. Indeed, these form the basis of the updated definition of myocardial infarction, which is diagnosed in any patient with raised circulating troponins who presents with cardiac chest pain, or who develops regional ST elevation on the 12-lead ECG. Implicit in this definition is the fact that myocardial infarction may be diagnosed in patients without ST elevation. In non-ST elevation myocardial infarction (non-STEMI), the increase in circulating troponin concentration is a useful measure of risk, troponin concentration correlating directly with rates of recurrent myocardial infarction and death; it is widely used to guide decisions about cardiac catheterization and coronary revascularization.

Increased ventricular wall stress (which occurs in heart failure, left ventricular hypertrophy, etc.) causes release of natriuretic peptides from the heart (brain natriuretic peptide—BNP and its precursor—N-terminal pro BNP), causing dilatation and natriuresis. High levels are associated with worsening symptoms and prognosis. They can be used to determine whether breathless patients need further cardiological investigations or need to be assessed for lung disease. Untreated patients with low levels of BNP are unlikely to have heart failure.

Renal function

Renal function should always be measured in the cardiac patient. Renal dysfunction is a major cause (and consequence) of hypertension whereas, in heart failure, progressive deterioration of renal function is almost inevitable as perfusion of the kidneys becomes threatened. Renal function may also deteriorate in response to treatment with diuretics and angiotensin converting enzyme (ACE) inhibitors, and careful monitoring is essential as these drugs are introduced. Cardiac drugs that are excreted through the kidneys (e.g. digoxin) should be used cautiously if renal function is impaired. In the patient with established renal failure, accelerated coronary artery disease and heart failure commonly occur, reflecting the combined effects of dyslipidaemia, hypertension, arterial endothelial dysfunction, anaemia and volume loading on the cardiovascular system. Cardiovascular disease is the major cause of death in patients with renal failure.

Electrolytes

Patients with hypokalaemia are at risk of lethal cardiac arrhythmias, whereas hyperkalaemia may cause bradyarrhythmias and heart block. Patients presenting with acute coronary syndromes commonly have hypokalaemia, owing to the effects of sympathoadrenal activation on membrane-bound sodium–potassium adenosine triphosphatase (ATPase), and this may require correction. In patients on thiazide or loop diuretics, potassium supplements (or potassium-sparing diuretics) are usually necessary to protect against hypokalaemia unless ACE inhibitors are also given. The combination of an ACE inhibitor and an aldosterone antagonist is used in patients with heart failure and can be complicated by hyperkalaemia. Serum potassium should always be measured in patients with hypertension, not only to provide a baseline before the introduction of diuretic therapy, but also as a simple screening test for primary aldosteronism. Hyponatraemia is common with chronic diuretic use.

Glucose and lipids

Blood glucose and lipid profiles (triglycerides, total cholesterol and high-density lipoprotein (HDL) and low-density lipoprotein (LDL) cholesterol) should be measured in all patients with suspected vascular disease. In high-risk individuals, particularly those with diabetes, and in all patients with established coronary artery disease, statin therapy is essential regardless of the baseline lipid profile; it reduces the cardiovascular event rate by about 25%. Statins lower LDL ('bad') cholesterol, but if HDL ('good') cholesterol is low, treatment with nicotinic acid or fibrates should be added. Treatment of diabetes protects against microvascular complications, and in hyperglycaemic patients with acute myocardial infarction, infusion of insulin and glucose is usually recommended.

Bacteriology laboratory

Blood culture

In suspected infective endocarditis (Box 13.25), treatment must not be delayed beyond the time necessary to obtain three to four blood samples for culture (Table 13.3). Aerobic, anaerobic and fungal cultures should be performed. Occasionally, bone marrow cultures are helpful for detection of *Candida* and *Brucella* endocarditis. *Coxiella* and *Chlamydia* can never be cultured from the blood and must be diagnosed by serological tests. Failure to detect bacteraemia may be owing to pretreatment with antibiotics, inadequate sampling (up to six

Box 13.25	Infective endocarditis

Typical patient

- Elderly man or woman with mitral or aortic valve disease (often not previously recognized)
- Younger patients with congenital heart defects (usually ventricular septal defect or patent ductus arteriosus)
- Patient of any age with prosthetic heart valve or history of intravenous drug abuse

Major symptoms

- Non-specific feverish ('flu-like') illness

Major signs

- Fever and heart murmur (usually aortic or mitral regurgitation)
- Splinter haemorrhages and vasculitic rash may occur
- Clubbing, Osler's nodes and Roth's spots are rare.

Diagnosis

- Blood culture: usually provides bacteriological diagnosis
- Echocardiogram: usually reveals valvular regurgitation ± vegetation

Additional investigations

- Haematology: leukocytosis; normochromic, normocytic anaemia
- Inflammatory markers: raised erythrocyte sedimentation rate and C-reactive protein
- Urinalysis: haematuria

Comments

- Formerly a disease of young adults, now seen more commonly in the elderly
- Diagnosis should always be considered in patients with fever and a heart murmur.

Table 13.3 Organisms implicated in endocarditis

Organism	Typical source of infection	First choice of antibiotics (pending sensitivity studies)
Streptococcus viridans	Upper respiratory tract	Benzylpenicillin: gentamicin
Streptococcus faecalis	Bowel and urogenital tract	Ampicillin: gentamicin
Anaerobic streptococcus	Bowel	Ampicillin: gentamicin
Staphylococcus epidermidis	Skin	Flucloxacillin: gentamicin
Fungi: *Candida*, histoplasmosis	Skin and mucous membranes	Amphotericin B*: 5-fluorocytosine*
Coxiella burnetii	Complication of Q fever	Chloramphenicol*: tetracycline*
Chlamydia psittaci	Contact with infected birds	Tetracycline* and erythromycin
Acute disease		
Staphylococcus aureus	Skin	Flucloxacillin: gentamicin
Streptococcus pneumoniae	Complication of pneumonia	Benzylpenicillin: gentamicin
Neisseria gonorrhoeae	Venereal	Benzylpenicillin: gentamicin

*These drugs are not bactericidal, and valve replacement is nearly always necessary to eradicate infection.

blood samples should be taken over 24 hours) or infection with unusual microorganisms.

Serology

If a recent streptococcal throat infection can be confirmed by demonstrating an elevated serum antistreptolysin O titre, Jones's criteria may be used for the diagnosis of rheumatic fever (Box 13.26). The presence of two major criteria, or one major and two minor criteria, indicates a high probability of rheumatic fever. In suspected viral pericarditis or myocarditis, the aetiological diagnosis depends on the demonstration of elevated viral antibody titres in acute serum samples, which decline during convalescence. Virus may sometimes be cultured from throat swabs and stools.

Box 13.26	Jones's criteria for the diagnosis of rheumatic fever

Major criteria

- Carditis
- Polyarthritis
- Erythema marginatum
- Chorea
- Subcutaneous nodules

Minor criteria

- Fever
- Arthralgia
- Previous rheumatic fever
- Elevated erythrocyte sedimentation rate
- Prolonged PR interval

Gastrointestinal system | 14

Sushma Saksena

General principles

A key requirement of being a good doctor is the ability to make a robust diagnosis. Making a diagnosis requires identifying departure from normal and involves answering two key questions:

1. Where is the problem (i.e. the anatomical site)?
2. What is the problem (i.e. nature of disease)?

A good history and a focused examination are the keys to making a diagnosis/differential diagnoses, and this is particularly true when patients present with diseases involving the gastrointestinal (GI) system. This chapter covers the key GI symptoms, how to take a focused history and the diseases likely to be associated with such symptoms. It then proceeds to cover examination technique for assessing the GI system, followed by a brief review of investigations required to confirm a diagnosis.

Anatomy of the GI tract

The human gastrointestinal tract can be seen as a system of serially connected tubular organs approximately 8 metres in length (Fig. 14.1) including mouth, oesophagus, stomach, duodenum, jejunum, ileum, colon, rectum and anus which, together with its connected secretory glands including the salivary glands, pancreas and biliary tree within the liver, controls the passage, processing, absorption and elimination of food. Symptoms of gastrointestinal (GI) disorders usually arise owing to an alteration in this transit, or an alteration in the function of this system, which includes absorption, processing and elimination of food.

The site of disease may lie in the lumen, its wall (including the mucosa, submucosa, muscle layer or serosa); involve the secretions that aid digestion (biliary and pancreatic diseases); and even lie outside the GI tract (extra luminal), affecting the GI system either through extrinsic compression or through neuroendocrine effects as seen in patients with diabetes or through electrolyte disturbances as in renal diseases. The liver, biliary system and pancreas, which are part of the GI system, are involved in aiding digestion. In addition, the liver is an important organ playing a key role in immunity as well as in metabolism of food and drugs, and also elimination of waste products such as bilirubin (a byproduct of haemoglobin breakdown) into bile.

Finally, from the standpoint of systematic history taking and examination, the kidneys, groin and genitalia are also considered in this chapter.

There are a large number of organs within GI tract, so to make it easier to diagnose the site of a problem, it may be helpful to consider the GI system composed broadly of three subsystems as follows:

1. Upper GI tract: This includes the oral cavity, oesophagus, stomach and proximal duodenum, traditionally as far as the ligament of Trietz: symptoms of diseases involving this section include dysphagia, odynophagia, reflux, heartburn, epigastric pain, and vomiting.
2. Lower GI tract: This includes small intestines, including distal duodenum, jejunum, ileum, colon, rectum and anus: common symptoms from diseases involving this section include change in bowel habit (this can range from constipation to diarrhoea, or a combination), bleeding per rectum, abdominal pain and distension.
3. Hepatopancreatico-biliary (HPB): This section includes liver, biliary tree including gall bladder and pancreas: diseases involving this section will present with symptoms that include jaundice and abdominal pain with biliary pain classically described as right upper quadrant abdominal pain radiating to the right shoulder. However, not all HPB diseases may be associated with jaundice and pure liver diseases rarely cause pain.

In addition to the above symptoms, GI diseases from all the three subsystems as above may present with diffuse or poorly localized abdominal pain, weight loss, loss of appetite and nausea. These symptoms, although of little localising value, may be useful in assessing the severity of underlying disease.

Diseases of the GI tract

A wide variety of diseases are associated with different sites of the GI tract. For simplicity, one way of classifying these is based on the underlying causes as shown in Box 14.1. However, in clinical medicine

Figure 14.1 Anatomy of the GI tract includes three sub-systems: upper gastrointestinal (UGI), includes all organs labelled in blue colour; hepatopancreaticobiliary (HPB), includes all organs labelled in orange colour; lower gastrointestinal (LGI), includes all organs labelled in green colour.

Box 14.1	The types of diseases seen in gastrointestinal system

- V-Vascular: Ischaemic bowel, hepatic infarction
- I-Inflammation/infection: Inflammatory bowel disease, viral hepatitis (A, B, C, D, E)
- N-Neoplasms: Cancers of oesophagus, stomach, small bowel, colon, liver, pancreas, biliary tree
- D-Drug (toxins)/degenerative/dysmotility: Drug-induced diarrhoea/hepatitis, irritable bowel syndrome
- I-Iatrogenic/idiopathic: Perforation of GI tract post endoscopy, bleed post liver biopsy/trauma
- C-Congenital/inherited/developmental: Pyloric stenosis, Hirschsprung's disease
- A-Autoimmune/allergy: Autoimmune hepatitis, coeliac disease
- T-Trauma
- E-Endocrine/metabolic/environmental: Diarrhoea caused by diabetic neuropathy

Table 14.1 Common GI diseases

Site	Diseases
Oesophagus	Oesophagitis, gastroesophageal reflux disease, hiatus hernia, oesophageal ulcer, benign oesophageal stricture, Barratt's oesophagus, oesophageal cancer, oesophageal varices
Stomach	Gastritis, gastric ulcer, gastric cancer, gastric varices
Small bowel	Duodenitis, duodenal ulcer, coeliac disease, Crohn's disease, lymphoma
Colorectal	Diverticulosis, ulcerative colitis, other colitis including infective, colonic/rectal polyps and cancers
Hepatic	Acute hepatitis, liver cirrhosis, liver abscess, liver cancers (primary/secondary)
Pancreatico-biliary	Gall bladder and CBD stones, cholangitis, cancer gall bladder and biliary tree, acute and chronic pancreatitis, cancer of the pancreas

it is important to be aware of the common diseases and to include these in the differential diagnosis before considering rare ones. Table 14.1 includes list of common GI diseases.

Symptoms of gastrointestinal disease

The common symptoms of GI and abdominal disease are listed in Box 14.2 and are discussed individually below.

An important aspect to remember while taking a history of GI symptoms is that certain symptoms and signs are associated with a higher likelihood of an underlying cancer, especially if recent in onset (i.e. less than 3 months in duration) and in an older patient (>55 years of age). These require urgent assessment, including referral to an appropriate specialist; to highlight this urgency such symptoms are referred to as red flags. The relevant red flags for GI diseases are shown in Box 14.3.

Box 14.2	Common symptoms of gastrointestinal and abdominal disease

- Dysphagia and odynophagia
- Heartburn and reflux
- Indigestion
- Flatulence
- Vomiting
- Anorexia
- Constipation
- Diarrhoea
- Alteration of bowel pattern
- Abdominal pain
- Abdominal distension
- Weight loss
- Haematemesis
- Rectal bleeding
- Melaena
- Jaundice
- Itching
- Urinary symptoms

Box 14.3	Gastrointestinal red flag symptoms

- Dysphagia
- Dyspepsia: new onset lasting for weeks
- Abdominal pain: new onset lasting for weeks
- Change in bowel habit: diarrhoea or constipation, sense of incomplete evacuation
- Rectal bleeding
- Weight loss
- Loss of appetite
- New onset iron deficiency anaemia in non-menstruating women or in men

Dysphagia (and odynophagia)

Dysphagia is defined as difficulty in swallowing. Patients may report an array of symptoms ranging from an awareness of something sticking in the throat or chest to an inability to swallow.

Dysphagia is a red flag symptom because it can be associated with oesophageal cancer or cancer of the gastric cardia or fundus. Other symptoms may accompany dysphagia and it is important to be familiar with the physiology of swallowing to understand the localizing value of these accompanying symptoms to help make an accurate diagnosis.

Swallowing is a complex movement composed of two phases: the initial oropharyngeal phase and the oesophageal phase (Fig. 14.2). The oropharyngeal phase involves multiple actions that happen synchronously, which are designed to allow safe passage of food bolus from the mouth into the oesophagus, without it going into the trachea (aspiration) or refluxing in the nasal cavity. As the food is moved to the back of the mouth by the tongue, the tongue closes the oral cavity, the soft palate closes the nasal cavity and the epiglottis closes the larynx, so the food is safely propelled into the proximal oesophagus. Diseases affecting the oropharyngeal phase of swallowing include local diseases of the throat, such as cancer of the throat, which may present with symptoms of dysphagia. More commonly neurological conditions, such as stroke, affect swallowing and patients may present with symptoms of choking, recurrent aspirations with frequent chest infections and, rarely, reflux of food through the nose.

The second phase of swallowing is the oesophageal phase, initiated on entry of food bolus into the proximal oesophagus; it involves movement of food down the oesophagus by peristalsis aided by gravity

Figure 14.2   Mechanism of swallowing. (From Hall JE, Hall ME, eds. Guyton and Hall Textbook of Medical Physiology, ed 14. Figure 64.1. 2021. Elsevier Inc.)

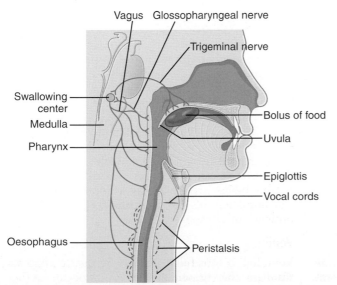

Box 14.4 Causes of dysphagia

Obstructive

- Intraluminal: Foreign body
- Within walls: Stricture, cancer
- Extraluminal: Goitre, thymoma, mediastinal lymphadenopathy, compression from enlarged aorta or heart

Non-obstructive

- Oesophageal: Achalasia cardia, eosinophilic oesophagitis, oesophageal dysmotility
- Systemic: Stroke, multiple sclerosis, myasthenia gravis

Box 14.5 Key features in history of dysphagia

- Onset: Sudden versus gradual
- Duration of symptoms: years or months or days
- Is it worse with solids than liquids?
- Difficulty in swallowing saliva
- Accompanied with reflux
- Loss of weight, loss of appetite, iron deficiency anaemia

---

and relaxation of the lower oesophageal sphincter (LOS) to allow passage of food into the stomach. Intact tone of the LOS is required to prevent reflux of gastric content into the oesophagus. Problems in the oesophageal phase can result in symptoms of dysphagia, reflux, heartburn and chest pain.

Box 14.4 shows the causes of dysphagia which can be broadly classified into obstructive and non-obstructive. Obstructive dysphagia may be caused by problems, firstly within the lumen such as foreign body, secondly within the wall, such as benign or malignant oesophageal strictures or thirdly extra-luminal compression of the lumen such as from goitre, thymoma, enlarged mediastinal lymph nodes or aortic aneurysm. Non-obstructive causes broadly refer to conditions that may affect oesophageal peristalsis, which can be caused by disorders within the oesophageal muscles—referred to as oesophageal dysmotility, the most prominent of these being localized to oesophagus such as achalasia of the cardia or eosinophilic oesophagitis or connective diseases such as systemic sclerosis. Dysmotility may also be owing to neurological disorders affecting the neuronal control of peristalsis, which include systemic diseases such as stroke, multiple sclerosis or myasthenia gravis.

Classifying dysphagia into obstructive and non-obstructive/dysmotility is relevant because these two types can be distinguished on the basis of an astute history, which should include questions in Box 14.5.

The presence of dysphagia worse to solids would suggest an obstructive dysphagia; if it is progressively worse over a short time and accompanied with weight loss, then oesophageal malignancy should be suspected. A benign stricture (or rarely an oesophageal pouch) may follow the same pattern, but much less

rapidly and only delayed weight loss. Neurogenic dysphagia may present with greater difficulty in swallowing with liquids than solids and, more importantly, may often be associated with aspiration or coughing and seen in patients with stroke, motor neuron disease and myotonic dystrophy.

In contrast, odynophagia is painful swallowing owing to inflammation in the oropharynx or proximal oesophagus, which may occur with or without dysphagia. Odynophagia indicates inflammation/infection of the oralpharyngeal or oesophageal mucosa, classically candida oesophagitis, which is commonly associated with recent therapy with steroids or antibiotics and the presence of diabetes. However, diffuse oesophageal candidiasis may be associated with immuno-compromised states, such as after chemotherapy or HIV infection.

Heartburn

Heartburn is a burning sensation perceived in the chest or neck. It is caused by acid reflux from the stomach into the oesophagus and seen in patients with gastro-oesophageal reflux disease (GORD). Occasionally it is difficult to distinguish from angina pectoris. It is reported as present particularly at night when the patient lies flat in bed or after bending or stooping when abdominal pressure is increased. Heartburn may be exacerbated by dietary intake (such as alcohol or very spicy or fatty foods, which lower tone of the lower oesophageal sphincter) and certain medications (such as bisphosphonates). However, not all patients with reflux will have symptoms of heartburn.

Reflux

Reflux or regurgitation is a symptom which refers to non-acidic fluid or bile regurgitation into the mouth, causing a bitter taste and a disagreeable sensation retrosternally. It is suggestive of underlying GORD, but not all patients with GORD have reflux symptoms.

Indigestion (dyspepsia)

Dyspepsia, a medical term for indigestion, includes a wide variety of symptoms, such as epigastric pain, heartburn, distension, nausea or 'an acid feeling' occurring after eating or drinking, bloating and belching. It may be associated with diseases of the upper GI tract such as *Helicobacter* infection of stomach or duodenum, peptic ulcer disease and GORD. Upper GI malignancy should be excluded in older patients who present with a new onset of dyspepsia. It can also be associated with diseases of the biliary tree, such as chronic cholecystitis (inflammation of the gall bladder), or just the presence of gallstones.

Vomiting

Vomiting is forceful expulsion of gastric contents through the mouth or nose. It occurs either consequent upon an obstruction in the transit of food through the GI tract or as a neurogenic response, in turn triggered either by chemoreceptors in the brainstem or as a reflex from irritation of the stomach. Vomiting consists of a phase of nausea, followed by hypersalivation, pallor, sweating and hyperventilation. Retching, an involuntary effort to vomit, then occurs, followed by expulsion of gastric contents through the mouth and sometimes through the nose. Most nausea and vomiting of GI origin are associated with local discomfort in the abdomen. Non-GI disease, such as raised intracranial pressure or metabolic disturbance, should be suspected if vomiting is not associated with food or any preceding abdominal discomfort.

It is important to take a history of the content of the vomit, its relationship with meals, frequency and association with other symptoms such as abdominal pain or constipation. The content of the vomit varies with the nature of the food ingested and it is important to note the absence or presence of bile or blood. In pyloric stenosis, the vomit is usually copious and sour-smelling. It frequently contains recognizable food eaten many hours before and exhibits froth on the surface after standing, but no bile. Faeculent vomit, characteristic of advanced intestinal obstruction, is brown in colour, and has a faecal odour. Vomit containing formed faeces is rare and may indicate a fistula between stomach and transverse colon, usually from an invading colonic carcinoma.

Haematemesis

Haematemesis, which is vomiting of blood, results from bleeding from lesions in the upper GI tract. Brisk haematemesis, such as from a large vessel in a gastric or duodenal ulcer, will cause the patient to vomit large volumes of pure blood. In addition this will often be accompanied with passage of black tarry stools, known as melaena (see below). Vomiting of dark-stained liquid is referred as coffee ground vomiting. It is owing to blood that lies in the acidic gastric juice for a period of time, during which it turns black and may be vomited looking like ground coffee. It is important to distinguish this from haemoptysis, which is coughing up blood and may be mixed with sputum.

Melaena

Melaena, the passage of black, tarry stool, is often described as the 5s': schwartz (black), sticky, smelly shiny, stool. The black colour is owing to blood as it gets denatured (digested), as it passes through the acidic milieu in stomach and long transit through the small bowel. It usually indicates bleeding in the upper GI tract. Less commonly, a small bowel bleed proximal to the ileo-caecal valve may produce melaena and, very occasionally, the bleeding source may be in the right colon, such as a large caecal polyp or cancer, with altered colour and partial digestion facilitated by slow transit.

Box 14.6	Characteristics of pain from frequent and important causes (see also Fig. 14.7)

- Peptic ulcer: Epigastric, burning or gnawing, radiates through to back, meal related, wakes the patient, relieved by antacid
- Gastric cancer: Epigastric, severe, partly meal related, not relieved by antacid
- Pancreatic: High epigastric, severe, felt front-to-back, immediately after eating, relieved by sitting forward
- Midgut: Periumbilical, colicky, some relation to meals
- Lower gut: Periumbilical or suprapubic, colicky, some relief from bowel action
- Biliary: Right upper quadrant, severe, colicky (but over a long period of time), radiates to right shoulder, accompanied by nausea
- Renal colic: Loin-to-groin, colicky, very severe, accompanied by nausea
- Functional: Anywhere in the abdomen, colicky, accompanied by bloating, relieved by bowel action

Abdominal pain

Abdominal pain is one of the most common GI symptoms and can be produced by a wide variety of underlying diseases. As with any pain, it is important to characterize it in terms of its **s**ite, **o**nset, **c**haracter, areas of **r**adiation, **t**iming including duration and frequency, **e**xacerbating and relieving factors and **a**ssociated features (the acronym SOCRATES is commonly used in practice as an aide-mémoire).

Acute abdominal pain is also discussed in Chapter 9 because it may be associated with serious life-threatening conditions and requires a distinct approach. The particular characteristics of pain from certain frequent and important causes are given in Box 14.6. Abdominal pain often radiates or spreads from one site to another. The pattern of radiation can indicate specific diseases. Pancreatic pain classically radiates through to the back and is relieved on bending forward, whereas pain from passage of ureteric stone radiates from loin to groin on the respective side.

It is important to be aware of referred pain in the abdomen when the pain is perceived away from the organ involved. The diaphragm is innervated by the phrenic nerve which derives from the C3, 4,5 nerve roots. Hence, pain may arise from diaphragmatic irritation owing to an inflamed gall bladder in cholecystitis or a liver abscess abutting the right diaphragm may be referred to the right shoulder, whereas pain from splenic pathology may be referred to the left shoulder. Pain from renal diseases is often referred to the lumbar area anteriorly or posteriorly.

Abdominal pain may also be owing to causes that are not specifically in the abdomen such as metabolic disorders including diabetic ketoacidosis, porphyria or lead poisoning.

Box 14.7 | Bristol stool chart

Bristol Stool Chart

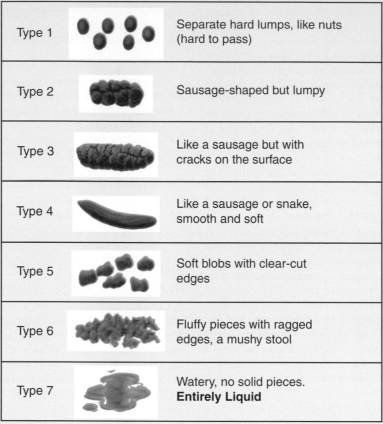

Type 1	Separate hard lumps, like nuts (hard to pass)
Type 2	Sausage-shaped but lumpy
Type 3	Like a sausage but with cracks on the surface
Type 4	Like a sausage or snake, smooth and soft
Type 5	Soft blobs with clear-cut edges
Type 6	Fluffy pieces with ragged edges, a mushy stool
Type 7	Watery, no solid pieces. **Entirely Liquid**

First published: Lewis SJ, Heaton KW. Stool form scale as a useful guide to intestinal transit time. *Scand J Gastroenterol*. 1997;32(9):920-924.

Source: https://www.nice.org.uk/guidance/cg99/resources/cg99-constipation-in-children-and-young-people-bristol-stool-chart-2

Abdominal distension

Abdominal distension is classically caused by one of the 'Five Fs': fluid (mainly ascites), fat (obesity), foetus (pregnancy), flatus and faeces. Consider whether the distension is symmetrical or asymmetrical. Common causes of symmetrical abdominal distension are obesity and ascites. Common causes of ascites include decompensated liver cirrhosis, congestive heart failure, nephrotic syndrome and abdominal malignancies.

Common causes of asymmetrical abdominal distension include marked enlargement of the major abdominal organs (hepatomegaly, splenomegaly) or the presence of a large mass lesion as seen in intra-abdominal cancers, lymphomas or peritoneal malignancies.

Change in bowel habit

Change in bowel habit is a broad term that includes diarrhoea, constipation, as well as a combination, where patients may report alternating diarrhoea and constipation. The frequency of 'normal' bowel action varies greatly from person to person and within different parts of the world. In high-income countries, with a greater ingestion of processed food, the statistical norm varies between three bowel actions per day to three per week. It is important to use a Bristol Stool chart (Box 14.7) to help objectively document the character of the stool, especially while monitoring response to an intervention or therapy.

Constipation

Constipation refers to a reduction in the volume or frequency of stool and/or an increase in the hardness of stool. In clinical practice, the passage of formed stool less frequently than three times per week is usually taken to indicate an abnormality of bowel frequency. If unresponsive to simple treatment, such as increasing fibre in diet, drinking more water or simple laxatives, or if associated with red flag symptoms, then investigation may be needed. Common causes for constipation are shown in Table 14.2 and it may be useful to consider these while taking the history to assess constipation. Any new onset constipation that persists for weeks in a middle-aged patient is a red flag and requires urgent assessment, although is less concerning than an alteration to looser bowels.

Patients may report being constipated when they sense that they have not adequately emptied their bowel by defaecation, and this is referred to as sense of incomplete evacuation. It is important to identify this symptom because it may be associated with rectal lesions, including rectal cancers, and will require urgent assessment, especially if of recent onset. Tenesmus is pain in the peri-anal area during defaecation or the sense of needing to pass stool when there is none there.

Diarrhoea

Diarrhoea is an increase in the frequency of bowel movements; however, because there is a wide variation in the norm, it is important to establish in the history what was normal for a patient. However, passage of more than three stools per day or the passage of a large amount of stool (>300 g/day) will be considered as diarrhoea. It is important to ask the following key questions while taking a history of diarrhoea to help ascertain the likelihood of underlying diseases:

1. Is it acute (present for days/weeks) or chronic (greater than 3 months to years)?
2. Does it contain blood? Does it contain mucus?
3. Does it wake the patient in the night?
4. Is it accompanied by weight loss?

Acute diarrhoea commonly results from viral or bacterial infection, whereas longer periods of diarrhoea (chronic diarrhoea) may have a variety of causes as shown in Table 14.3. The nature of the stool may give clues as to the underlying cause. In inflammatory bowel disease, the stool will be mixed with blood and mucus. The presence of blood in the stool excludes irritable bowel syndrome as the primary cause of any diarrhoea. In contrast, steatorrhoea is a distinct term that refers to the passage of pale, bulky stools containing excess fats that commonly float in water and are difficult to flush away. It is often described in patients with fat malabsorption owing to chronic pancreatitis with lipase deficiency or small bowel diseases with bile salt malabsorption. It is also important to distinguish diarrhoea from symptoms of incontinence or urgency as the underlying causes may be different.

Rectal bleeding

Bleeding from the rectum or anal canal typically causes bright red blood loss that is separate from the stool or just noticeable on the toilet paper: haemorrhoids are the most common cause. If darker red and mixed with the stool, this usually indicates a source above the rectum, of which carcinoma is the most important cause. Haemoatochezia is passage of large-volume red blood per rectum and, if not from the colon, may indicate a potentially exsanguinating bleed from an upper GI source.

Flatulence

Flatulence describes passage of excessive wind. It is associated with belching, abdominal distension and passage of flatus per rectum. It is often associated with excessively swallowed air. In some patients it is associated with ingestion of certain foods, such as legumes, beans, broccoli and cabbage. It is a socially embarrassing symptom yet infrequently associated with structural diseases of the GI tract.

Jaundice

Jaundice (or icterus) is a yellowish pigmentation of the skin and conjunctival membranes caused by high levels of bilirubin in the blood, which is a waste product from the breakdown of red blood cells. Its presence implies disease of the liver or the biliary tract, although it may also be the result of excessive haemolysis. Jaundice may be classified depending on its cause as pre-hepatic, owing to excess bilirubin from haemolysis; hepatic, owing to diseases of the liver; or post-hepatic, caused by obstruction in the flow of the bile within the biliary tree owing to

Table 14.2 Causes of constipation	
Types	**Causes**
Life style related	Low fibre, low fluid intake, drug related
Structural	Carcinoma, strictures, in colon or small bowel
Systemic	Metabolic (hypothyroid), neurological
Idiopathic/dysmotility	Irritable bowel syndrome

Table 14.3 Causes of diarrhoea		
	Causes	**Clues**
Inflammatory	Infections, ulcerative colitis, Crohn's disease	Blood in stools, abdominal pain, fever
Dysmotility	Irritable bowel syndrome	Abdominal pain Does not contain blood, not interrupt sleep
Malabsorption	Small bowel, pancreatic disease	Steatorrhoea, weight loss, anaemia
Secretory	Villous adenoma, ileal resection	Large volume No change with fasting

Table 14.4 Types of jaundice

	Pre-hepatic	Hepatic	Post-hepatic
History	No itch, Normal colour stools	May have itch Normal/pale stools	Itch Pale-coloured stool
Urine	Normal	Dark	Dark
Sclera	Lemon tinge	Dark	May fluctuate
Serum bilirubin	Often less than 70	Variable	Can go very high Plateaus at 500
Diseases	Gilbert's, drug-induced haemolysis	Hepatitis, cirrhosis, liver cancer	Stones in common bile duct Cancer head of pancreas, biliary tree

diseases of the biliary tree or pancreas. An important aspect of history taking is to be able to differentiate these three types of jaundice. The important questions to ask in the history are:

1. Presence of change in colour of urine
2. Presence of clay-coloured stools
3. Presence of itch

Haemolysis results in excess production of unconjugated bilirubin, which is water insoluble and does not get filtered in the urine. Hence, in jaundice caused by haemolysis, there is no change in colour of urine. In contrast, in hepatic and post-hepatic jaundice (also known as obstructive jaundice), the predominant type of bilirubin in the circulation is conjugated bilirubin which is water soluble and gets filtered out in the urine so the urine colour is darker or deeper yellow. In addition, post-hepatic jaundice is characterized by pale stools caused by a block in the passage of bile into the bowel and itch attributed to reflux of bile salts into the circulation. The differences between the three types of jaundice are shown in Table 14.4. In addition to the characteristic colour of the skin and conjunctiva, there may be other associated cutaneous and systemic features of liver disease, often with dark urine (see below).

Pruritus

Pruritus or itch is a symptom associated with liver disease or obstructive jaundice. It is most often seen in patients with liver diseases, such as primary biliary cholangitis, primary sclerosing cholangitis and cholestasis of pregnancy where it may be the only symptom and not accompanied by jaundice. In contrast, it often accompanies jaundice in patients with carcinoma of the head of the pancreas or a cholangiocarcinoma. Pruritus is attributed to the presence of elevated bile salts and diminishes more quickly than the jaundice when the biliary obstruction is relieved.

Anorexia

Anorexia, which refers to loss of appetite, may be associated with a wide variety of conditions, both GI and non-GI-related. It is important to recognize the symptom of anorexia as distinct from the psychiatric illness *anorexia nervosa*. Another symptom to look for is

Box 14.8	Peripheral stigmata (signs) of chronic liver disease

Skin, nails and hands

- Clubbing of the fingers
- Leuconychia: Expansion of the paler half-moon at the base of the nail
- Palmar erythema: Seen on the thenar and hypothenar eminence, often with blotchy appearance
- Bruising
- Dupuytren's contracture: Can occur in the absence of liver disease
- Hepatic flap: A sign of encephalopathy and advanced disease
- Scratch marks: Particularly in cholestatic liver disease

Face, neck, chest, groins

- Parotid swelling: Particularly in alcohol-related liver disease
- Spider naevi: Small telangiectatic superficial blood vessels with a central feeding vessel
- Hepatic foetor: Characteristic sweet-smelling breath
- Gynaecomastia
- Testicular atrophy: Loss of axillary and pubic hair

Feet

- Pedal oedema

early satiety where a patient may report feeling hungry but feels full after a few mouthfuls; this is indicative of decreased gastric capacity, either owing to extrinsic compression from an enlarged liver or spleen, an infiltrating type of gastric cancer called 'linitis plastica', which can reduce gastric capacity to distend, or more generally in patients with upper GI malignancy.

Weight loss

Weight loss may be owing to a decrease in food intake (as seen with anorexia, dysphagia or vomiting), malabsorption of nutrients or the effect of systemic diseases. Diseases that directly cause malabsorption include coeliac disease, pancreatic exocrine insufficiency and, occasionally, inflammatory bowel disease. Weight loss is also commonly associated with systemic conditions, such as cancer (within or outside the GI tract); chronic infections, such

Figure 14.3 A typical spider naevus, with a central arteriole and fine radiating vessels.

Figure 14.4 Palmar erythema in chronic liver disease (sparing the centre of the palms).

as tuberculosis (within or outside the GI tract); and endocrine conditions, such as thyrotoxicosis (despite an increased appetite) and Addison's disease.

Urinary symptoms

Urinary symptoms are discussed in Chapter 17.

Physical examination of the GI tract and abdomen

Physical examination involves a stepwise approach through the four steps of inspection, palpation, percussion and auscultation. In addition, for the GI tract, clusters of signs are linked with specific diseases and it is important to be aware of these as they provide clues to an underlying disease. Signs associated with chronic liver disease are shown in Box 14.8; of these, the most common and useful are spider naevi (Fig. 14.3) (the presence of up to five can be normal) and palmar erythema (Fig. 14.4) (the blotchy appearance often being more important than the overall redness). Inflammatory bowel disease may give rise to clubbing of the hands, arthritis, uveitis and skin changes, including erythema nodosum (tender raised red lumps on the extensor surface of the limbs) and the much rarer pyoderma gangrenosum. Anaemia accompanies many GI diseases, as does oedema, and lymphadenopathy can be secondary to GI malignancy.

It is helpful when examining the patient to record notes or communicate information to colleagues to remember the surface anatomy of the structures related to the GI tract and abdomen (Figs 14.5 and 14.6) and to think of the abdomen as divided into regions (Fig. 14.7). The two lateral vertical planes pass from the femoral artery below to cross the costal margin close to the tip of the ninth costal cartilage. The two horizontal planes, the subcostal and interiliac, pass

across the abdomen to connect the lowest points on the costal margin and the tubercles of the iliac crests, respectively.

Beginning the abdominal examination

1. Wash your hands and introduce yourself (if you examining as a student on a ward round; if you took the history, you will have already introduced yourself).
2. Confirm the patient's identity and explain the different steps of the abdominal examination in clear and easy to understand language, to seek patient agreement and consent for proceeding with the examination.
3. Position the patient appropriate for the examination: The patient should be lying supine with arms loosely at the sides, the head and neck supported by up to two pillows, sufficient for comfort. Make sure there is a good light, that the room is warm and that the hands are warm. A shivering patient cannot relax and vital signs, especially on palpation, may be missed.
4. Exposure of the abdomen: although it is important for the purpose of this examination that the area from 'nipples to knees' should be examined, it is not acceptable or appropriate to expose this area all at once. Instead, a stepwise approach is best, beginning with asking the patient to draw clothing up to just above the xiphisternum and a sheet folded down to the level of the symphysis pubis. The examination of the groins and genitalia must not be neglected and needs to be carried out with discretion, with full explanation as to the reasons, and leaving these areas exposed for a minimum amount of time. It is not unusual for a patient to present with intestinal obstruction owing to a strangulated femoral or inguinal hernia where the diagnosis has been missed initially owing to lack of proper inspection of the groins in an effort to save embarrassment.

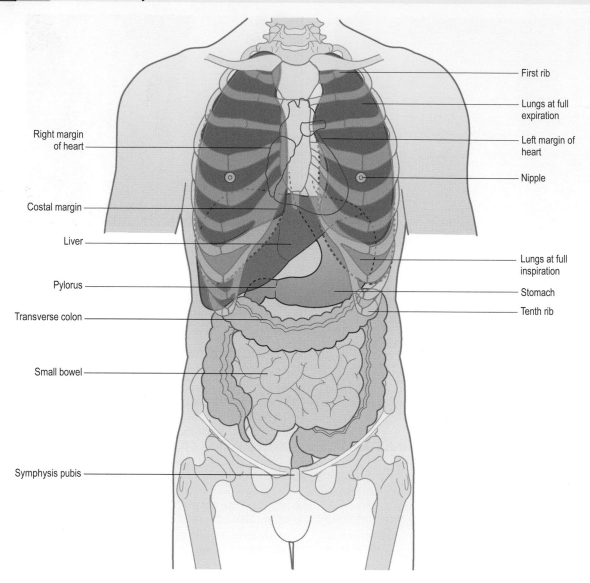

Figure 14.5 Anterior view of the external relationships of the abdominal and thoracic organs.

5. The last thing before beginning the examination is to ask if the patient is in pain and if he is comfortable to proceed.

Inspection

Inspection is an important and neglected part of abdominal examination. Initially, it is well worthwhile spending 30 seconds observing the abdomen from different positions to note the following features:

Shape

Is the abdomen of normal contour and fullness, or distended? Is it scaphoid (sunken)?

■ Generalized fullness or distension may be caused by fat, fluid, flatus, faeces or foetus.
■ Localized distension may be symmetrical and centred around the umbilicus as in the case of small bowel obstruction, or asymmetrical as in gross enlargement of the spleen, liver or ovary.

■ Make a mental note of the site of any such swelling or distension; think of the anatomical structures in that region and note if there is any movement of the swelling, either with, or independent of, respiration.
■ Remember that chronic urinary retention may cause palpable enlargement of the bladder felt in the lower abdomen.
■ A scaphoid abdomen is seen in advanced stages of starvation and malignant disease.

The umbilicus

Normally the umbilicus is slightly retracted and inverted. If it is everted, then an umbilical hernia may be present; this can be confirmed by feeling an expansile impulse on palpation of the swelling when the patient coughs. The hernial sac may contain omentum, bowel or fluid. A common finding in the umbilicus of elderly obese people is a concentration

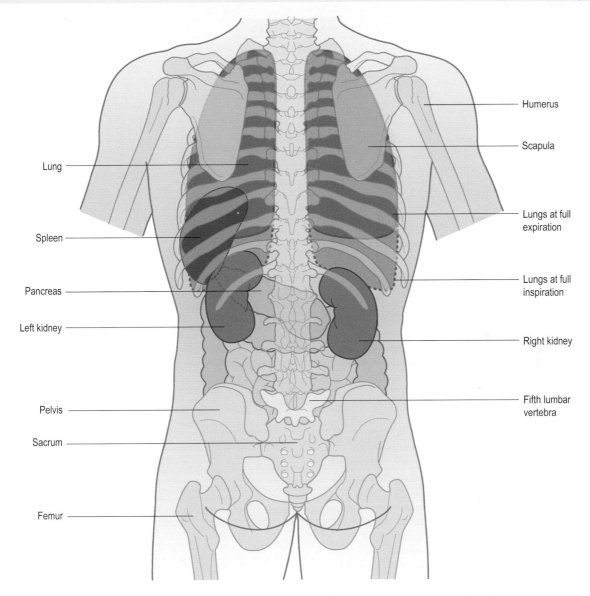

Figure 14.6   Posterior view of the external relationships of the abdominal and thoracic organs. The liver is not shown.

Labels: Humerus, Scapula, Lung, Lungs at full expiration, Spleen, Lungs at full inspiration, Pancreas, Left kidney, Right kidney, Pelvis, Fifth lumbar vertebra, Sacrum, Femur

of inspissated desquamated epithelium and other debris (omphalolith).

Skin and surface of the abdomen

On inspection of the surface of the abdomen, look for the following characteristics: scars, striae, superficial veins, stomas and pigmentation.

1. Scars: Note any scars present, their site, whether they are old (white) or recent (red or pink), linear or stretched (and therefore likely to be weak and contain an incisional hernia). Common examples of post-surgery scars are given in Figure 14.8.

2. Striae: Striae atrophica or gravidarum are white or pink wrinkled linear marks on the abdominal skin. Produced by gross stretching of the skin with rupture of the elastic fibres, they indicate a recent change in size of the abdomen, such as

is found in pregnancy, ascites, wasting diseases and severe dieting. Wide purple striae are characteristic of Cushing's syndrome.

3. Superficial veins: Look for prominent superficial veins, which may be apparent in three situations (Fig. 14.9: thin veins over the costal margin, usually of no significance; occlusion of the inferior vena cava; and venous anastomoses in portal hypertension). Obstruction of the inferior vena cava not only causes oedema of the limbs, buttocks and groins but, in time, distended veins on the abdominal wall and chest wall appear. These represent dilated anastomotic channels between the superficial epigastric and circumflex iliac veins below and the lateral thoracic veins above, conveying the diverted blood from the long saphenous vein to the axillary vein; the direction of flow is therefore upwards. If the

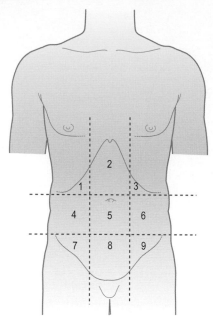

Figure 14.7 Regions of the abdomen. 1 and 3, right and left hypochondrium; 2, epigastrium; 4 and 6, right and left lumbar; 5, umbilical; 7 and 9, right and left iliac; 8, hypogastrium or suprapubic.

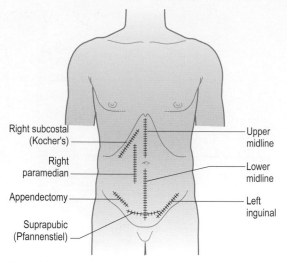

Figure 14.8 Some commonly used abdominal incisions. The midline and oblique incisions avoid damage to the innervation of the abdominal musculature and the later development of incisional hernia.

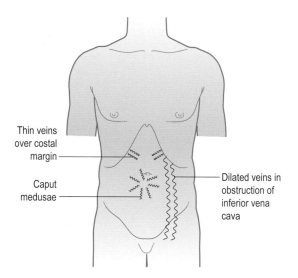

Figure 14.9 Prominent veins of the abdominal wall.

veins are sufficiently prominent, try to detect the direction in which the blood is flowing by occluding a vein, emptying it by massage and then looking for the direction of refill. Distended veins around the umbilicus (caput medusae) are uncommon, but signify portal hypertension, other signs of which may include splenomegaly, ascites and other cutaneous manifestations of chronic liver disease. These distended veins represent the opening up of anastomoses between portal and systemic veins and occur in other sites, such as oesophageal and rectal varices.

4. Stomas: Stomas are surgically created openings in the abdominal wall and are identified by the presence of a stoma bag overlying these. There are three different types of stoma: a colostomy, an ileostomy or a urosotomy (Fig. 14.10). The ileostomy, often on the right iliac fossa, is identified by an elevated spout. Colostomy stomas are often flat and can be either an end colostomy or a loop colostomy, in which case two lumens may be seen within the same stoma site. Urostomy is used to divert urine into a loop of bowel in the event of resection of urinary bladder.

5. Pigmentation: Pigmentation of the abdominal wall may be seen in the midline below the umbilicus, where it forms the *linea nigra* and is a sign of pregnancy. Erythema *ab igne* is a brown mottled pigmentation produced by constant application of heat, usually a hot water bottle or heat pad, on the skin of the abdominal wall or

back. It is a sign that the patient is experiencing severe persistent pain, such as from chronic pancreatitis.

Palpation

Palpation forms the most important part of the abdominal examination. Ask the patient to relax as much as possible, to breathe quietly and assure that you will be as gentle as possible. Enquire about the site of any pain and examine this region last. These points, together with unhurried palpation with a warm hand, will give the patient confidence and allow the maximum amount of information to be obtained.

When palpating, the wrist and forearm should be in the same horizontal plane where possible, even if this means bending down or kneeling by the patient's side. The best palpation technique involves moulding the relaxed right hand to the abdominal

The 3 Types of Ostomies

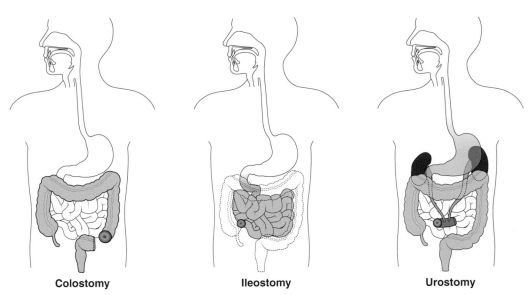

| Colostomy | Ileostomy | Urostomy |

Figure 14.10 Types of stomas on abdominal examination.

Figure 14.11 Correct method of palpation. The hand is held flat and relaxed and 'moulded' to the abdominal wall.

Figure 14.12 Incorrect method of palpation. The hand is held rigid and mostly not in contact with the abdominal wall.

Figure 14.13 Method of deep palpation in an obese, muscular or poorly relaxed patient.

wall, not to hold it rigid (Fig. 14.11). The best movement is gentle but with firm pressure, with the fingers held almost straight but with slight flexion at the metacarpophalangeal joints and avoiding sudden poking with the fingertips (Fig. 14.12).

Palpation of intra-abdominal structures is an imperfect process in which the great sensitivity of the sense of touch and pressure is heavily masked by the abdominal wall tissue. It is unusual for structures to be very easily palpable and so it is necessary to concentrate fully on the task and to try to visualize the normal anatomical structures and what might be palpable beneath the examining hand. It may be necessary to repeat the palpation more slowly and deeply. Putting the left hand on top of the right allows increased pressure to be exerted (Fig. 14.13), such as with an obese or very muscular patient.

A small proportion of patients find it impossible to relax their abdominal muscles when being examined. In such cases, it may help to ask them to breathe deeply, to bend their knees up or to distract their attention in other ways. No matter how experienced the examiner, little will be gained from palpation of a poorly relaxed abdomen. It is important to keep in mind the following three signs on palpation which can be markers of serious intra-abdominal pathology.

Guarding

Guarding is an involuntary reflex contraction of the muscles of the abdominal wall overlying an inflamed viscus and peritoneum, producing localized rigidity. It indicates localized peritonitis. What is felt on examination is spasm of the muscle, which prevents palpation of the underlying viscus. Guarding is seen classically in uncomplicated acute appendicitis. It is very important to distinguish this sign from the voluntary contraction of muscle.

Rigidity

Generalized or 'board-like' rigidity is an indication of diffuse peritonitis. It can be looked upon as an extension of guarding, with involuntary reflex rigidity of the muscles of the anterior abdominal wall. It is quite unmistakable on palpation; the whole abdominal wall feels hard and 'board-like', precluding palpation of any underlying viscus. The least downward pressure with a palpating hand in a patient with generalized rigidity produces severe pain. It may be differentiated from voluntary spasm by getting the patient to breathe: if there is voluntary spasm, the abdominal wall will be felt to relax during expiration.

Rebound tenderness

Rebound tenderness is present if, when palpating slowly and deeply over a viscus and then suddenly releasing the palpating hand, the patient experiences sudden pain. Rebound tenderness is not always a reliable sign and should be interpreted with caution, particularly in those patients with a low pain threshold, but is often a useful adjunct to detecting peritoneal inflammation.

To ensure comprehensive assessment of all intra-abdominal structures, it is helpful to have a logical sequence to follow and, if this is done as a matter of routine, then no important point will be omitted. Always consider the underlying anatomy when examining the abdomen. The following scheme is suggested, which may need to be varied according to the site of any pain, palpating the site of pain towards the end:

1. Light palpation: Start in the left lower quadrant of the abdomen, palpating lightly, and move in an anti-clockwise direction including all nine areas of the abdomen; adopting this routine reduces the risk of missing signs.

2. Deep palpation: Repeat using slightly deeper palpation examining each of the nine areas of the abdomen.
3. Focused palpation:
   a. Feel for the liver and gall bladder.
   b. Feel for the spleen.
   c. Feel for the left kidney.
   d. Feel for the right kidney.
   e. Feel for the urinary bladder.
   f. Feel for the aorta and para-aortic glands and common femoral vessels.
   g. Palpate both groins.
   h. Examine the external genitalia.
   i. If a swelling is palpable, spend time eliciting its features.

All of the organs in the upper abdomen (liver, spleen, kidneys, stomach, pancreas, gallbladder) move downwards with inspiration (with the spleen moving more downwards and medially). Thus, asking the patient to take a deep breath while examining makes detection of these organs easier. When the patient breathes in, the examining hand should be still so that the organ in question 'comes on to the examining hand' or 'slips by underneath it'.

Liver

Place the right hand below and parallel to the right subcostal margin. The liver edge will then be felt against the radial border of the index finger (Fig. 14.14). The liver is often palpable in normal patients without being enlarged. The lower edge of the liver can be clarified by percussion (see below), as can the upper border in order to determine overall size: a palpable liver edge can be owing to enlargement, or displacement downwards by lung pathology. Hepatomegaly conventionally is measured from the edge of the right costal margin in the mid-clavicular line. The degree of liver enlargement is often quoted in finger breadths, but

Figure 14.14 Palpation of the liver.

these are variable and it is better to use centimeters. One helpful tip is to place the left hand over the right costal margin and use the right hand to assess for hepatomegaly, starting from the right iliac fossa and moving the right hand gradually upwards with each inspiration.

Try to discern the character of the liver surface (i.e. whether it is soft, smooth and tender as in heart failure, very firm and regular as in obstructive jaundice and cirrhosis, or hard, irregular, painless and sometimes nodular as in advanced secondary carcinoma). In tricuspid regurgitation, the liver may be felt to pulsate. Occasionally a congenital variant of the right lobe, called Riedel's lobe, projects down lateral to the gallbladder as a tongue-shaped process. Although uncommon, it is important to be aware of this because it may be mistaken either for the gallbladder itself or for the right kidney.

Gallbladder

The gallbladder is palpated in the same way as the liver, although the normal gallbladder usually is not palpable. When it is distended, however, it forms an important sign and may be palpated as a firm, smooth or globular swelling with distinct borders, just lateral to the edge of the rectus abdominis near the tip of the ninth costal cartilage. It moves with respiration. Its upper border merges with the lower border of the right lobe of the liver or disappears beneath the costal margin and therefore can never be felt (Fig. 14.15). When the liver is enlarged or the gallbladder grossly distended, the latter may be felt not in the hypochondrium but in the right lumbar or even as low down as the right iliac region; hence, the importance of commencing palpation in the right iliac fossa and moving the examining hand upwards. An enlarged gallbladder may be easier to see moving on inspiration than to feel.

The ease of definition of the rounded borders of the gallbladder, its comparative mobility on respiration, the fact that it is not normally bimanually palpable and that it seems to lie just beneath the abdominal wall help to identify such a swelling as the gallbladder rather than as a palpable right kidney. A painless gallbladder usually can be palpated in the following clinical situations:

- In a jaundiced patient with carcinoma of the head of the pancreas or other malignant causes of obstruction of the common bile duct (below the entry of the cystic duct), the ducts above the obstruction become dilated, as does the gallbladder (see Courvoisier's law below).
- In mucocele of the gallbladder, a gallstone becomes impacted in the neck of an uninfected gallbladder and mucus continues to be secreted into its lumen (Fig. 14.16). Eventually, the uninfected gallbladder is so distended that it becomes palpable. In this case, the bile ducts are normal, and the patient is not jaundiced.
- In carcinoma of the gallbladder, the gallbladder may be felt as a stony, hard, irregular swelling, unlike the firm, regular swelling in the two above-mentioned conditions.

Murphy's sign

In acute inflammation of the gallbladder (acute cholecystitis), severe pain is present. Often an exquisitely tender but indefinite mass can be palpated; this represents the underlying acutely inflamed gallbladder walled off by greater omentum. Ask the patient to breathe in deeply and palpate for the gallbladder in the normal way; at the height of inspiration, the breathing stops with a gasp as the mass is felt. This represents Murphy's sign. The sign is not found in chronic cholecystitis or uncomplicated cases of gallstones.

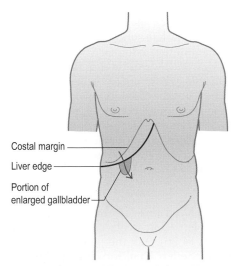

Costal margin
Liver edge
Portion of enlarged gallbladder

Figure 14.15   Palpation of an enlarged gallbladder, showing how it merges with the inferior border of the liver so that only the fundus of the gallbladder and part of its body can be palpated.

Figure 14.16   A mucocele of the gallbladder that is distended, pale and thin walled.

Courvoisier's law

Courvoisier's law states that in the presence of jaundice, a palpable gallbladder makes gallstone obstruction of the common bile duct an unlikely cause (because it is likely that the patient will have had gallbladder stones for some time and these will have rendered the wall of the gallbladder relatively fibrotic and therefore non-distensible). However, the converse is not true, because the gallbladder is not palpable in many patients who do turn out to have malignant bile duct obstruction.

Spleen

Like the left kidney, the spleen is not normally palpable. It has to be enlarged to two or three times its usual size before it becomes palpable and then is felt beneath the left subcostal margin. Enlargement takes place in a superior and posterior direction before it becomes palpable subcostally. Once the spleen has become palpable, the direction of further enlargement is downwards and towards the right iliac fossa (Fig. 14.17). Place the flat of the left hand over the lower-most rib cage posterolaterally and exert gentle traction, thus restricting the expansion of the left lower ribs on inspiration and concentrating more of the inspiratory movement into moving the spleen downwards. The right hand is placed beneath the costal margin more medially. Press in deeply with the fingers of the right hand beneath the costal margin, at the same time exerting considerable pressure medially and downwards with the left hand (Fig. 14.18), and then ask the patient to breathe in deeply. Repeat this manoeuvre with the right hand being moved more towards the left costal margin on each occasion (Fig. 14.19). If enlargement of the spleen is suspected from the history and it is still not palpable, turn the patient half on to the

Figure 14.18   Palpation of the spleen. Start well out to the left.

Figure 14.19   Palpation of the spleen more medially than in Figure 14.17.

right side, ask him to relax back on to your left hand, which is now supporting the lower ribs, and repeat the examination as above. Alternatively, the spleen may be very large and the lower edge may be much lower than at first suspected.

In minor degrees of enlargement, the spleen will be felt as a firm swelling with smooth, rounded borders. Where considerable splenomegaly is present, its typical characteristics include a firm swelling appearing beneath the left subcostal margin in the left upper quadrant of the abdomen, which is dull to percussion, moves downwards on inspiration, is not bimanually palpable, whose upper border cannot be felt (i.e. one cannot 'get above it') and in which a notch can often, though not invariably, be felt in the lower medial border. The last three features distinguish the enlarged spleen from an enlarged kidney; in addition, there is usually a band of colonic resonance anterior to an enlarged kidney (Table 14.5).

Left kidney

The right hand is placed anteriorly in the left lumbar region while the left hand is placed posteriorly in the left loin (Fig. 14.20). Ask the patient to inhale deeply and press the left hand forward and lift the right hand upward and inward. The left kidney is not usually palpable unless either low in position or enlarged. Its lower pole, when palpable, is felt

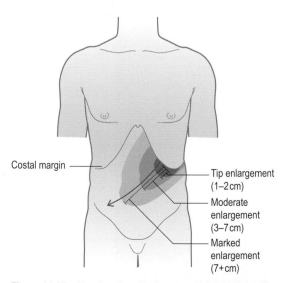

Costal margin

Tip enlargement (1–2 cm)

Moderate enlargement (3–7 cm)

Marked enlargement (7+ cm)

Figure 14.17   The direction of enlargement of the spleen. The spleen has a characteristic notched shape and the organ moves downwards during full inspiration.

Table 14.5 Features to differentiate kidney and spleen on examination

Spleen	Kidney
Dull to percussion	Band of colonic resonance anterior to an enlarged kidney
Moves diagonally downwards towards right iliac fossa on inspiration	Moves vertically downwards inspiration
Not bimanually palpable	Bimanually palpable
Upper border cannot be felt (i.e. one cannot 'get above it')	Can 'get above it'
Notch can often, though not invariably, be felt in the lower medial border	Is not notched

Figure 14.21 Palpation of the right kidney.

Figure 14.20 Palpation of the left kidney.

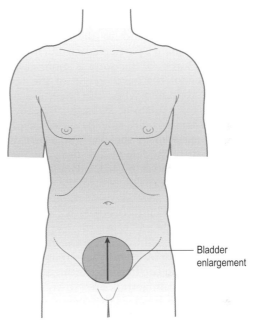

Bladder enlargement

Figure 14.22 Physical signs of urine retention: a smooth, firm and regular swelling arising out of the pelvis which one cannot 'get below' and which is dull to percussion.

as a rounded firm swelling between both right and left hands (i.e. bimanually palpable) and it can be pushed from one hand to the other, in an action which is called 'ballotting'.

Right kidney

Feel for the right kidney in much the same way as for the left. Place the right hand horizontally in the right lumbar region anteriorly with the left hand placed posteriorly in the right loin. Push forwards with the left hand, lift the right hand inward and upward (Fig. 14.21) and ask the patient to inhale deeply. The lower pole of the right kidney, unlike the left, is commonly palpable in thin patients; it is felt as a smooth, rounded swelling which descends on inspiration and is bimanually palpable and may be 'ballotted' (bounced back and forth between the two examining hands).

Urinary bladder

Normally the urinary bladder is not palpable. When it is full and the patient cannot empty it (retention of urine), a smooth, firm, regular oval-shaped swelling

will be palpated in the suprapubic region and its dome (upper border) may reach as far as the umbilicus. The lateral and upper borders can be readily identified, but it is not possible to feel its lower border (i.e. the swelling is 'arising out of the pelvis'). The fact that this swelling is symmetrically placed in the suprapubic region beneath the umbilicus, that it is dull to percussion and that pressure on it gives the patient a desire to micturate, together with the signs above, confirms such a swelling as the bladder (Fig. 14.22).

In women, however, a mass that is thought to be a palpable bladder has to be differentiated from a gravid uterus (firmer, mobile side to side), a fibroid uterus (may be bosselated and firmer) and an ovarian cyst (usually eccentrically placed to the left or right side).

The aorta and common femoral vessels

In most adults, the aorta is not readily felt; however, with practice, it usually can be detected by deep

Figure 14.23 Palpation of the abdominal aorta.

palpation a little above and to the left of the umbilicus. In thin patients, particularly women with a marked lumbar lordosis, the aorta is more easily palpable. Palpation of the aorta is one of the few occasions in the abdomen when the fingertips are used as a means of palpation. Press the extended fingers of both hands, held side by side, deeply into the abdominal wall in the position shown in Figure 14.23; identify the left wall of the aorta and note its pulsation. Remove both hands and repeat the manoeuvre a few centimetres to the right. In this way the pulsation and width of the aorta can be estimated. It is difficult to detect small aortic aneurysms; where a large one is present, its presence and width may be assessed by placing the extended fingertips on either side of it with the palms flat on the abdominal wall and the fingers pointing towards each other. When the fingertips are either side of an aneurysm, it should be clear that they are being separated by each pulsation and not just moved up and down (this latter manoeuvre can involve very deep palpation and the patient should be warned). In a patient with known aortic aneurysm or in those at high risk (elderly patients), caution must be exercised with deep palpation because examination can be very uncomfortable for patients and there is a risk of triggering rupture of the aneurysm.

Lymph nodes lying along the aorta (para-aortic nodes) are palpable only when considerably enlarged. They are felt as rounded, firm, often confluent fixed masses in the umbilical region and epigastrium along the left border of the aorta. Pulsations of the aorta are transmitted through the nodes which separates them from the expansile pulsations palpated in aneurysmal dilatation.

Causes of diagnostic difficulty on palpation

In many patients, especially those with a thin or lax abdominal wall, faeces in the colon may simulate an abdominal mass. The sigmoid colon is frequently palpable, particularly when loaded with hard faeces. It is felt as a firm, tubular structure about 12 cm in length, situated low down in the left iliac fossa, parallel to the inguinal ligament. The caecum is often palpable in the right iliac fossa as a soft, rounded swelling with indistinct borders. The transverse colon is sometimes palpable in the epigastrium. It feels somewhat like the sigmoid colon but rather larger and softer, with distinct upper and lower borders and a convex anterior surface. A faecal 'mass' usually will have disappeared or moved on repeat examination and may retain an indentation with pressure (not the case with a colonic malignancy).

In the epigastrium, the muscular bellies of rectus abdominis lying between its tendinous intersections can mimic an underlying mass and give rise to confusion. This usually can be resolved by asking the patient to tense the abdominal wall (by lifting the head off the pillow), when the 'mass' may be felt to contract.

What to do when an abdominal mass is palpable

An abdominal mass is an important finding and requires further characterization in order to establish the organ of origin and its pathological nature. The following are key parameters to include in the examination of a palpable abdominal mass.

Site

Note the region occupied by the swelling. Think of the organs that normally lie in or near this region and consider whether the swelling could arise from one of these organs. For instance, a swelling in the right upper quadrant most probably arises from the liver, right kidney, hepatic flexure of colon or gallbladder.

Feeling the swelling while the patient lifts his head and shoulders off the pillow to tense the anterior abdominal wall will differentiate between a mass in the abdominal wall and within the abdominal cavity. If the swelling is in the upper abdomen, try to determine if it is possible to 'get above it'; that is, to feel the upper border of the swelling as it disappears above the costal margin, and similarly, if it is in the lower abdomen, whether one can 'get below it'. If one cannot 'get above' an upper abdominal swelling, a hepatic, splenic, renal or gastric origin should be suspected. If one cannot 'get below' a lower abdominal mass, the swelling probably arises in the bladder, uterus, ovary or, occasionally, upper rectum.

Size and shape

It is important to characterize the outline of the lump and whether it is symmetrical or asymmetrical in nature. The larger a swelling arising from one of these structures, the more it tends to distort the outline of the organ of origin (e.g. a large renal mass can feel as if it is arising from intraperitoneal organs). Second, establish an approximate diameter of the lump, ideally using a tape measure.

Surface, edge and consistency

The pathological nature of a mass is suggested by a number of features. A swelling that is hard, irregular in outline and nodular is likely to be malignant, whereas a regular, round, smooth, tense swelling is likely to be cystic. A solid, ill-defined and tender mass suggests an inflammatory lesion such as may be seen in ileocaecal Crohn's disease.

Temperature and tenderness

Examine the overlying skin with the dorsum of the hand, comparing the temperature over the skin overlying the lump with that of the rest of abdomen. Inspect whether there are any overlying changes in the skin, such as erythema or tense skin overlying the lump. Elicit whether the lump is tender to palpation. Hot, tender lumps are likely to be inflammatory in origin or a site of infection.

Mobility and attachments

Swellings arising in the liver, spleen, kidneys, gallbladder and distal stomach all show downward movement during inspiration, owing to the normal downward diaphragmatic movement, and such structures cannot be moved with the examining hand. In contrast, tumours of the small bowel and transverse colon, cysts in the mesentery and large secondary deposits in the greater omentum are not usually influenced by respiratory movements, but may easily move on palpation.

When the swelling is completely fixed, it usually signifies one of three things:
1. A mass of retroperitoneal origin (e.g. pancreas)
2. Part of an advanced tumour with extensive spread to the anterior or posterior abdominal walls or abdominal organs
3. A swelling resulting from severe chronic inflammation involving other organs (e.g. diverticulitis of the sigmoid colon or a tuberculous ileocaecal mass)

In the lower abdomen, the side-to-side mobility of a fibroid or pregnant uterus rapidly establishes such a swelling as uterine in origin and as not arising from the urinary bladder.

Is it bimanually palpable or pulsatile?

Bimanually palpable swellings in the lumbar region are usually renal in origin. Occasionally, however, a posteriorly situated gallbladder or a mass in the postero-inferior part of the right lobe of the liver may give the impression of being bimanually palpable. Carefully note whether a swelling is pulsatile and decide if any pulsation comes from the mass or is transmitted through it.

Percussion

Details of how to percuss correctly are given in Chapter 12. The normal percussion note over most of the abdomen is resonant (tympanic) except over the liver, where the note is dull. A normal spleen is not large enough to render the percussion note dull. A resonant percussion notes over suspected enlargement of liver or spleen weighs against there being true enlargement.

In obese patients, tympanic areas of the abdomen may not give a truly resonant percussion note and palpation of organs such as a large liver is more difficult. If hepatomegaly is suspected, rhythmic percussion just above the suspected lower border of the liver, as the patient breathes in and out deeply, can elicit a note cyclically changing between dull to hollow, and eliciting this change may be more certain than the character of the fixed and unchanging note.

Defining the boundaries of abdominal organs and masses

Liver

The upper and lower borders of the right lobe of the liver can be mapped out accurately by percussion. Start anteriorly, at the fourth intercostal space, where the note will be resonant over the lungs, and work vertically downwards.

Over a normal liver, percussion will detect the upper border, which is found at about the fifth intercostal space (just below the right nipple in men). The dullness extends down to the lower border at or just below the right subcostal margin, giving a normal liver vertical height of 12–15 cm. The normal dullness over the upper part of the liver is reduced in severe emphysema, in the presence of a large right pneumothorax and after laparotomy or laparoscopy.

Spleen

Percussion over a substantially enlarged spleen provides rapid confirmation of the findings detected on palpation (see Fig. 14.18). Dullness extends from the left lower ribs into the left hypochondrium and left lumbar region.

Urinary bladder

The findings in a patient with retention of urine are usually unmistakable on palpation (see Fig. 14.22). The dullness on percussion and clear difference from the adjacent bowel provides reassurance that the swelling is cystic or solid and not gaseous.

Other masses

The boundaries of any localized swelling in the abdominal cavity or in the walls of the abdomen sometimes can be defined more accurately by percussion than palpation, as for the urinary bladder.

Detection of ascites and its differentiation from ovarian cyst and intestinal obstruction

There are three common causes of diffuse enlargement of the abdomen:
1. The presence of free fluid in the peritoneum (ascites)
2. A massive ovarian cyst
3. Obstruction of the large bowel, distal small bowel or both

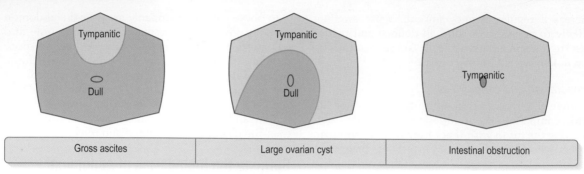

Figure 14.24   Three types of diffuse enlargement of the abdomen.

Box 14.9	Clinical features of marked abdominal swelling

Gross ascites

- Dull in flanks
- Umbilicus everted and/or hernia present
- Shifting dullness positive
- Fluid thrill positive

Large ovarian cyst

- Resonant in flank
- Umbilicus vertical and drawn up
- Large swelling felt arising out of pelvis which one cannot 'get below'

Intestinal obstruction

- Resonant throughout
- Colicky pain
- Vomiting
- Recent cessation of passage of stool and flatus
- Increased and/or 'tinkling' bowel sounds

Percussion rapidly distinguishes between these three causes, as can be seen in Figure 14.24. Other helpful symptoms or signs which are usually present are listed in Box 14.9.

The use of ultrasound to assess ascites has shown that at least 2 litres of ascites needs to be present to be detected clinically. It is unreliable to diagnose ascites unless sufficient free fluid is present to give generalized enlargement of the abdomen. The cardinal sign created by ascites is shifting dullness. A fluid thrill may also be present, but it would be unwise to diagnose ascites based on this sign without the presence of shifting dullness.

To demonstrate shifting dullness, ask the patient to lie supine. Place your fingers in the longitudinal axis on the midline near the umbilicus and begin percussion, moving your fingers laterally towards the right flank (Fig. 14.25). When dullness is first detected (in normal individuals, dullness is only over the lateral abdominal musculature), keep your fingers in that position and ask the patient to roll on to his left side. Wait a few seconds for any peritoneal fluid to redistribute and, if ascites is present, the percussion note will become resonant. This shift in the area of dullness can be confirmed by finding the left border of dullness with the patient still on

his left side and seeing if it shifts when the patient returns to the supine position or by repeating the original manoeuvre but towards the other side of the abdomen. It is important to have assessed for an enlarged liver or spleen before eliciting shifting dullness and, if present, ask the patient to roll over to the opposite side when eliciting shifting dullness.

To elicit a fluid thrill, the patient again lies supine. Place one hand flat over the lumbar region of one side, and get an assistant to put the side of his hand longitudinally and firmly in the midline of the abdomen. Then flick or tap the opposite lumbar region (Fig. 14.26). A fluid thrill or wave is felt as a definite and unmistakable impulse by the detecting hand held flat in the lumbar region. (The purpose of the assistant's hand is to dampen any impulse that may be transmitted through the fat of the abdominal wall.) As a rule, a fluid thrill is felt only when a large amount of ascites is present, which is under tension, and it is not a very reliable sign.

Auscultation

Auscultation of the abdomen is done to detect bowel sounds and vascular bruits.

Bowel sounds

The stethoscope should be placed on one site on the abdominal wall (just to the right of and below the umbilicus is best) and kept there until sounds are heard. It should not be moved from site to site. Normal bowel sounds are heard as intermittent low- or medium-pitched gurgles interspersed with an occasional high-pitched noise or tinkle.

In simple acute mechanical obstruction of the small bowel, the bowel sounds are excessive and exaggerated. Frequent, loud, low-pitched gurgles (borborygmi) are heard, often with a crescendo to high-pitched tinkles and occurring in a rhythmic pattern with peristaltic activity. The presence of such sounds occurring at the same time as the patient experiences bouts of colicky abdominal pain is highly suggestive of small bowel obstruction. In between the bouts of peristaltic activity and colicky pain, the bowel is quiet and no sounds are heard on auscultation.

Figure 14.25 Steps in eliciting shifting dullness to confirm presence of ascites on abdominal examination. **(A)** Patient in supine position: Percuss in midline to confirm percussion note is resonant due to gas-filled bowel loops in midline under the hand. Move the percussing hand in four steps to left flank. **(B)** Patient in supine position: Percussion note will change to a dull note due to presence of fluid under hand in left flank. Keep your hand fixed in left flank where you find the percussion note is dull and without moving hand position request patient to turn to right lateral position as in Figure C. **(C)** Patient in right lateral position (see Box): Maintain hand in left flank and percuss after 1 minute: percussion note will change from dull to resonant as fluid shifts from flank to midline and air-filled bowel move under the hand. **(D)** Patient in right lateral position: Move hand in four steps to midline: Percussion note will again change from resonant to dull as fluid is now in midline confirming dullness has shifted from left flank to midline.

If obstruction progresses leading to bowel necrosis, peristalsis ceases and sounds lessen in volume and frequency. In generalized peritonitis, bowel activity rapidly disappears and a state of paralytic ileus ensues, with gradually increasing abdominal distension. The abdomen is 'silent', but one must listen for several minutes before being certain that there are no sounds. Frequently, towards the end of this period, a short run of faint, very high-pitched tinkling sounds is heard. This represents fluid spilling over from one distended loop to another and is characteristic of ileus.

A succussion splash may be heard without a stethoscope and also on auscultation, when there is pyloric stenosis, in advanced intestinal obstruction with grossly distended loops of bowel and in paralytic ileus. This sign is particularly useful in paediatrics. It is generally less used in adults, but should be attempted in patients with chronic vomiting and weight loss, and not just after a meal. It is easiest to elicit without a stethoscope. After explanation, clasp the supine patient's lower ribs and, with your ear near his upper abdomen, give a sharp shake from side to side. A positive sign is when a splashing sound can be heard.

Figure 14.26 Eliciting a fluid thrill. (The hand in the middle of the abdomen is that of an assistant.)

Vascular bruits

Listen for bruits by light application of the stethoscope above and to the left of the umbilicus (aorta), the iliac fossae (iliac arteries), epigastrium (coeliac or superior mesenteric arteries), laterally in the mid-abdomen (renal arteries) or over the liver (increased blood flow in liver tumours—classically primary liver cancer). If an arterial bruit is heard, it is a significant finding that indicates turbulent flow in the underlying vessel, owing to stenosis, aneurysm or a malignant circulation.

Examination of the groin

The groin examination is carried out after examining the abdomen. Before beginning, explain what the examination involves, confirm patient consent, obtain a chaperone, wear gloves and make sure there is adequate light. Proceed to uncover and inspect both groins and the external genitalia. In male patients, inspect and examine the penis and scrotum for any swellings and to confirm that both testes are in their normal position. In the female patient, inspect and examine the external labial folds and the inguinal region for any obvious lumps, observing for general symmetry in structures.

Once the groins have been inspected, ask the patient to turn his head away from you to one side and cough. Look at both inguinal canals for any expansile impulse. If none is apparent, place the left hand in the left groin so that the fingers lie over and in line with the inguinal canal; place the right hand similarly in the right groin (Fig. 14.27). Now ask the patient to give a loud cough and feel for any expansile impulse with each hand. When a patient coughs, the muscles of the abdominal wall contract violently and this imparts a definite, though not expansile, impulse to the palpating hands which is a source of confusion to the inexperienced. Trying to differentiate this normal contraction from a small, fully reducible inguinal hernia is difficult, and the matter can usually be resolved only when the patient is standing up.

Figure 14.27 Palpating the groins to detect an expansile impulse on coughing.

Figure 14.28 Palpation of the femoral vessels.

The common femoral vessels are found just below the inguinal ligament at the mid-point between the anterior superior iliac spine and symphysis pubis. Place the pads of the right index, middle and ring fingers over this site in the right groin and palpate the wall of the vessel. Note the strength and character of its pulsation and then compare it with the opposite femoral pulse (Fig. 14.28). Now palpate along the femoral artery for enlarged inguinal nodes, feeling with the fingers of the right hand, and carry this palpation medially beneath the inguinal ligament towards the perineum. Then repeat this on the left side.

What to do if a patient complains of a lump in the groin

A patient who complains of a lump in the groin should be examined both lying down and standing up. A lump in the groin or scrotum is a common clinical problem in all age groups. Most lumps in the groin are caused either by herniae or enlarged inguinal nodes; inguinal herniae are considerably more common than femoral, with an incidence ratio of 4:1. In the scrotum, hydrocele of the tunica vaginalis or a cyst of the epididymis are common causes of painless swelling; acute epididymo-orchitis is the most frequent cause of a painful swelling. Generalized diseases, such as lymphoma, may present as a lump in the groin. Usually the diagnosis of a lump in the groin or scrotum can be made simply and accurately.

Ask the patient to stand in front of you, get him to point to the side and site of the swelling and note whether it extends into the scrotum. Ask him to turn his head away from you and give a loud cough; look for an expansile impulse and try to decide whether it is above or below the crease of the inguinal ligament. If an expansile impulse is present on inspection, it is likely to be a hernia, so move to whichever side of the patient the lump in the groin is on. Stand beside and slightly behind the patient. If the right groin is being examined, place the left hand over the right buttock to support the patient, the fingers of the right hand being placed obliquely over the inguinal canal. Now ask the patient to cough again. If an expansile impulse is felt, then the lump must be a hernia.

Next decide whether the hernia is inguinal or femoral. The best way to do this is to determine the relationship of the sac to the pubic tubercle. To locate this structure, push gently upwards from beneath the neck of the scrotum with the index finger (Fig. 14.29), but do not invaginate the neck of the scrotum because this would be painful. The tubercle will be felt as a small bony prominence 2 cm from the midline on the pubic crest. In thin patients, the tubercle is easily felt, but this is not so in the obese. If the tubercle is difficult to feel, follow up the tendon of adductor longus, which arises just below the tubercle.

If the hernial sac passes medial to and above the index finger placed on the pubic tubercle, then the hernia must be inguinal in site; if it is lateral to and below, then the hernia must be femoral in site.

If it has been decided that the hernia is inguinal, then one needs to know these further points:
- What are the contents of the sac? Bowel tends to gurgle and is soft and compressible, whereas the omentum feels firmer and is of a doughy consistency.
- Is the hernia fully reducible or not? It is best to have the patient lie down to decide this. Ask the patient if he is 'able to push the hernia back in' and, if so, ask him to do so and confirm yourself. (It is more painful if the examiner reduces it.)
- Is the hernia direct or indirect? Again, it is best to have the patient lie down to decide this. Inspection of the direction of the impulse is often diagnostic, especially in thin patients. A direct hernia tends to bulge straight out through the posterior wall of the inguinal canal, whereas in an indirect hernia the impulse can often be seen to travel obliquely down the inguinal canal. Another helpful point is to place one finger just above the mid-inguinal point over the deep inguinal ring (Fig. 14.30). If a hernia is fully controlled by this finger, it must be an indirect inguinal hernia.

Apart from a femoral hernia, the differential diagnosis of an inguinal hernia includes a large hydrocele of the tunica vaginalis, a large cyst of the epididymis (one should be able to 'get above' and feel the upper border of both of these in the scrotum), an undescended or ectopic testis (there will be an empty scrotum on the affected side), a lipoma of the cord and a hydrocele of the cord.

In considering the differential diagnosis of a femoral hernia, one must think not only of an inguinal hernia but of a lipoma in the femoral triangle, an aneurysm of the femoral artery (expansile pulsation will be present), a saphenovarix (the swelling disappears on lying down, has a bluish tinge to it, varicose veins are often present and there may be a venous hum), a psoas abscess (the mass is fluctuant and may be compressible beneath the inguinal ligament to appear above it in the iliac fossa) and an enlarged inguinal lymph node. Whenever the latter is found, the spine, the feet, legs, thighs, scrotum, perineum and the pudendal and perianal areas must be carefully scrutinized for a source of infection or primary tumour.

Figure 14.29 Locating the pubic tubercle. Note the position of the examiner, at the side of the patient, with one hand supporting the buttock.

Figure 14.30 Left hand: index finger occluding the deep inguinal ring. Right hand: index finger on the pubic tubercle.

The examination is completed by examining the opposite groin in a similar manner.

External genitalia

Examination of the genitalia is important in patients presenting with abnormalities in the groin and in patients with abdominal symptoms because disease of the genitalia may lead to abdominal symptoms, such as pain or swelling. This is an intimate examination and most patients will find this embarrassing and potentially distressing; it is vital to reassure the patient by ongoing explanation to the patient of what is involved throughout this part of the examination and to stop immediately in case you sense distress. A detailed description of the examination of the male genitalia is given in Chapter 17 and of the female genitalia in Chapter 5.

The anus and rectum

Although examination of the anus and rectum has been widely considered as important component of the examination of the gastrointestinal system, it is essential in patients with suspicion of incontinence, constipation, GI bleed or with peri-anal symptoms. As this is an intimate examination, it requires clear explanation of the steps of the examination in easy to understand language and clear patient agreement and consent, as well as clarifying if the patient is in pain, the need for a chaperone and if the patient is comfortable to proceed.

The left lateral position is best for routine examination of the rectum (Fig. 14.31). Make sure that the buttocks project over the side of the couch with the knees drawn well up and that a good light is available. Once patient consent is obtained, don disposable gloves and clinical apron, as well as having lubrication jelly and tissues close at hand. Stand behind the patient's back, facing the patient's feet. Reiterate briefly to the patient what you are about to do, that you will be as gentle as possible and that you will stop the examination, if requested, at any time.

Figure 14.31 Left lateral position for rectal examination.

Inspection

Separate the buttocks carefully and inspect the perianal area and anus. Note the presence of any abnormality of the perianal skin, such as inflammation or excoriation, which may vary in appearance from mild erythema to a raw, red, moist, weeping dermatitis or, in chronic cases, thickened white skin with exaggeration of the anal skin folds. The latter form anal skin tags, which may follow not only severe pruritus but also occur when prolapsing haemorrhoids have been present over a period of time. Tags should not be confused with anal warts (condylomata acuminata), which are sessile or pedunculated papillomata with a red base and a white surface. Anal warts may be so numerous as to surround the anal verge and even extend into the anal canal. Note any 'hole' or dimple near the anus with a telltale bead of pus or granulation tissue surrounding it, which represents the external opening of a fistula-in-ano. Usually it is easy to distinguish a fistula-in-ano from a pilonidal sinus, in which the opening lies in the midline of the natal cleft but well posterior to the anus.

A number of painful anorectal conditions usually can be diagnosed readily on inspection. An anal fissure usually lies directly posterior in the midline. The outward pathognomonic sign of a chronic fissure is a tag of skin at the base (sentinel haemorrhoid). If pain allows, the fissure can easily be demonstrated by gently drawing apart the anus to reveal the tear in the lining of the anal canal.

A perianal haematoma (thrombosed external haemorrhoid) occurs as a result of rupture of a vein of the external haemorrhoidal plexus. It is seen as a small (1 cm), tense, bluish swelling on one aspect of the anal margin and is exquisitely tender to the touch. In prolapsed strangulated haemorrhoids, there is gross swelling of the anal and perianal skin, which looks like oedematous lips, with a deep red or purple strangulated haemorrhoid appearing in between, and sometimes partly concealed by, the oedema of the swollen anus. In a perianal abscess, an acutely tender, red, fluctuant swelling is visible which deforms the outline of the anus. Usually it is easy to distinguish this from an ischiorectal abscess where the anal verge is not deformed, the signs of acute inflammation are often lacking and the point of maximum tenderness is located midway between the anus and ischial tuberosity.

Note the presence of any ulceration. Finally, if rectal prolapse is suspected, ask the patient to bear down (as if trying to pass stool) and note whether any pink rectal mucosa or bowel appears through the anus or whether the perineum itself bulges downwards. Downward bulging of the perineum during straining on bending down or in response to a sudden cough indicates weakness of the pelvic floor musculature, usually owing to denervation of these muscles. This sign is often found in women after childbirth, in women with faecal or urinary incontinence and in patients with severe chronic constipation.

Digital rectal examination (palpation)

Put a generous amount of lubricant (jelly) on the gloved index finger of the right hand, place the pad of the finger (not the tip) flat on the anus (Figs 14.32 and 14.33) and press firmly and slowly (flexing the finger) in a slightly backwards direction. After initial resistance, the anal sphincter relaxes and the finger can be passed into the anal canal. If severe pain is elicited when attempting this manoeuvre, then further examination should be abandoned because it is likely the patient has a fissure and the rest of the examination will be very painful and unhelpful.

Feel for any thickening or irregularity of the canal wall, making sure that the finger is carefully turned through a full circle (180° each way). Assess the tone of the anal musculature; it should normally grip the finger firmly. If there is any doubt, ask the patient to contract the anus on the examining finger by asking to 'squeeze as if trying to stop passage of urine or faeces'. A cough will induce a brisk contraction of the external anal sphincter which should be

Figure 14.32   Correct method for insertion of the index finger in rectal examination. The pad of the finger is placed flat against the anus.

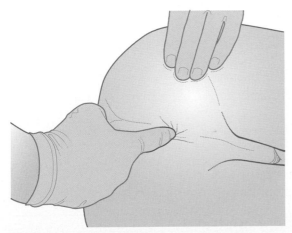

Figure 14.33   Incorrect method of introduction of the finger into the anal canal.

readily appreciated. In the old and infirm with anal incontinence or prolapse, almost no appreciable contraction will be felt. With experience it is usually possible to feel a shallow groove just inside the anal canal which marks the dividing line between the external and internal sphincter. The anorectal ring may be felt as a stout band of muscle surrounding the junction between the anal canal and rectum.

Now pass the finger into the rectum. The examiner's left hand should be placed on the patient's right hip and later it can be placed in the suprapubic position to exert downward pressure on the sigmoid colon. Try to visualize the anatomy of the rectum, particularly in relation to its anterior wall. The rectal wall should be assessed with sweeping movements of the finger through 360°, 2, 5 and 8 cm inwards or until the finger cannot be pushed any higher into the rectum. Repeat these movements as the finger is being withdrawn. In this way it is possible to detect malignant ulcers, proliferative and stenosing carcinomas, polyps and villous adenomas. The hollow of the sacrum and coccyx can be felt posteriorly. Laterally, on either side, it is usually possible to reach the side walls of the pelvis. In men, one should feel anteriorly for the rectovesical pouch, seminal vesicles (normally not palpable) and the prostate. In a patient with a pelvic abscess, however, pus gravitates to this pouch, which is then palpable as a boggy, tender swelling lying above the prostate. Malignant deposits will feel hard and, in infection of the seminal vesicles, these structures become palpable as firm, almost tubular swellings deviating slightly from the midline just above the level of the prostate.

Assessment of the prostate gland is important. It forms a rubbery, firm swelling about the size of a large walnut. Run the finger over each lateral lobe, which should be smooth and regular. Between the two lobes lies the median sulcus, which is palpable as a faint depression running vertically between each lateral lobe. Although it is possible to say on rectal examination that a prostate is enlarged, accurate assessment of its true size only comes with a lot of experience. In carcinoma of the prostate, the gland loses its rubbery consistency and becomes hard, whereas the lateral lobes tend to be irregular and nodular with distortion or loss of the median sulcus.

The cervix is felt as a firm, rounded mass projecting back into the anterior wall of the rectum. This is often a disconcerting finding for the inexperienced. The body of a retroverted uterus, fibroid mass, ovarian cyst, malignant nodule or a pelvic abscess may all be palpated in the pouch of Douglas (rectouterine pouch), which lies above the cervix. This aspect of the rectal examination forms an essential part of pelvic assessment in female patients.

On withdrawing the finger after rectal examination, look at it for evidence of mucus, pus and blood, either fresh or altered. If in doubt, wipe the finger on a white swab. Finally, make sure to wipe the patient clean before telling the patient that the examination is completed and also tell him to be careful as he rolls to the supine position as he will be very near the edge of the couch or bed.

Nutritional assessment

Nutritional assessment is important in all patients because most chronic and acute diseases affect nutrition and nutritional status has a key influence on prognosis of patients.

The following aspects constitute nutritional assessment:

1. Documenting a history of weight loss: The simplest nutritional assessment is to ask about weight loss and what the patient's weight was before the illness in all patients, including those who are obese. Patients at risk of weight loss and malnutrition may have GI disease preventing eating, reducing appetite or preventing absorption of nutrients or non-GI disease causing reduced appetite (especially malignancy). Increased energy consumption is also important in some patients with cancer and those with severe sepsis, thyrotoxicosis or burns.

2. Dietary history: Full medical clerking in a patient who has lost weight needs to include a simple assessment of the quantity and variety of foods eaten, as well as any restrictions on eating (e.g. poor dentition, social and financial circumstance) or special diets followed for medical reasons (e.g. a gluten-free diet in coeliac disease). If there are concerns then referral to a dietician for detailed diet history and a diet diary will be required.

3. Full examination including looking for signs of general and nutrient-specific malnutrition, see details in Table 14.6. Body weight and patient height are key parts of the general examination.

Table 14.6 Principal symptoms and signs caused by vitamin and mineral deficiencies

Nutrients	Deficiency syndrome	Principal symptoms/signs
Vitamin A, retinol (carotenoids)	Protein-energy malnutrition	Night blindness, Bitot spots, keratomalacia
Vitamin B$_1$, thiamine	Wernicke/Korsakoff, beri-beri	Nystagmus, sixth cranial nerve palsy, ataxia (Wernicke's encephalopathy) Symmetrical peripheral neuropathy (dry beri-beri), fulminant cardiac failure, lactic acidosis (Shoshin beri-beri), high output cardiac failure (wet beri-beri)
Vitamin B$_2$, riboflavin	Ariboflavinosis	Angular stomatitis, glossitis, magenta tongue
Vitamin B$_3$, niacin, nicotinic acid	Pellagra	Dermatitis of sun-exposed areas (including 'Casal's Necklace'), dementia, poor appetite, difficulty sleeping, diarrhoea
Vitamin B$_6$, pyridoxine	Deficiency associated with isoniazid use	Poor appetite, lassitude, oxaluria, seborrhea, neuropathy
Pantothenic acid		Nausea, abdominal pain, paraesthesiae, burning feet
Biotin		Dermatitis, depression, lassitude, muscle pains, electrocardiogram abnormalities, blepharitis
Folic acid	Deficiency associated with methotrexate use	Macrocytic anaemia, thrombocytopenia and megaloblastic bone marrow
Vitamin B$_{12}$	Pernicious anaemia	Subacute combined degeneration of the spine, macrocytic anaemia
Vitamin C, ascorbic acid	Scurvy	Poor wound healing, fatigue, limb pain, shortness of breath, difficulty sleeping, gingivitis, perifollicular purpura, hyperkeratosis
Vitamin D, ergo-/cholecalciferol	Rickets/osteomalacia	Bone pain, proximal myopathy, waddling gait, growth retardation
Vitamin E, tocopherol		Haemolysis, posterior column signs, ataxia, muscle wasting, retinitis pigmentosa-like changes, night blindness
Vitamin K, phylloquinone and other menaquinones	Chronic liver disease	Bruising, purpura, coagulopathy
Trace elements		
Iron		Koilonychia, smooth tongue, anaemia, ooesophageal web, impaired cognitive development
Zinc	Acrodermatitis enteropathica	Peristomal/perinasal/perineal erythema, thin hair, diarrhoea, apathy, anorexia, growth failure, hypoglycaemia
Copper		Microcytic hypochromic anaemia, neutropenia, scurvy-like bone lesions, osteoporosis
Chromium		Peripheral neuropathy, hyperglycaemia
Selenium		Cardiomyopathy
Iodine		Goitre

Table 14.7 World Health Organization classification of body weight

Category	BMI/Quetelet index
Underweight	<18.5
Healthy weight	18.5–24.9
Overweight	25–29.9
Moderately obese	30–34.9
Severely obese	35–39.9
Morbidly obese	>40

The two values are used to calculate the body mass index (BMI or Quetelet index). This is defined by body weight (in kilograms), divided by height (in metres) squared. The World Health Organization (WHO) classification of this index is given in Table 14.7. In the UK, the range 20–25 is often regarded as desirable, but the lower level of 18.5 is more applicable internationally. Patients with a BMI > 30 are at risk of a higher burden of health conditions and, therefore, are advised to undertake a structured weight loss program with full multidisciplinary team support in order to reduce their long-term health risks. These BMI values have been revised down for patients of South East Asian origin to reflect their higher risk of developing metabolic syndrome and cardiovascular complications at lower BMI. The state of nourishment can be assessed further by the more specialized measurements of mid-upper arm circumference (MUAC), skin-fold thickness, waist circumference and waist-to-hip ratio.

4. Malnutrition Universal Screening Tool (MUST): All UK hospital inpatients are now assessed for their risk of malnutrition. The most common assessment method used by health care staff is the MUST. This involves calculating the patient's BMI and then adding on a score for the percentage of unexpected weight loss and a score for the degree of acute illness. The final score is used to trigger a full dietary assessment and initiation of treatment in those who need it. Patients should be screened weekly whilst in hospital and at every outpatient attendance. It is important to be aware of the limitations of this tool, particularly in patients in whom there has been a lot of fluid retention which may have masked underlying weight loss.

Investigations: (see Box 14.10)

A large variety of investigations can be relevant to patients with GI diseases, including laboratory assessment of bloods, stool and ascitic fluid, endoscopic investigations and imaging as below (see Box 14.10). The choice and sequence of investigation is determined by the symptoms, suspected diagnosis and clinical presentation. A detailed description of each investigation is beyond the scope of this chapter, but it is important to be aware of the range available as a non-specialist as patients may refer to these while narrating their history.

Laboratory-based investigations (see Box 14.10)

Blood tests

Most patients seen in primary care and in hospital settings including within emergency departments have a 'routine' panel of blood tests that include full blood count, liver function tests, urea and electrolytes. Other blood tests may be added based on the diagnosis suspected as follows.

Blood tests for patients with liver disease

Liver function tests (LFTs) are usually included as part of a 'routine' panel of tests in most healthcare settings. If these are abnormal, a further panel of tests is usually required, often referred to as a liver screen. LFTs include serum bilirubin, alkaline phosphatase, serum alanine aminotransferase (ALT), serum aspartate aminotransferase (ALT), gamma glutamyl transferase (GGT) and serum albumin. In addition, prothrombin time is requested in any patient with abnormal LFTs, because it is a sensitive marker of the severity of acute and chronic liver injury.

Patients with abnormal LFTs and sometimes those with normal LFTs but with liver-related risk factors undergo a liver screen. This is a panel of tests that assesses the cause of liver disease and are requested in any patient suspected to have a liver problem, including those who may be asymptomatic and are found to have incidentally detected abnormal LFTs. The commonly used liver screen is shown in Box 14.11 as described below:

Viral hepatitis B and C are associated with chronic liver disease, whereas hepatitis A, B and E are associated with acute liver disease. Patients with chronic liver disease are screened for hepatitis B by testing for hepatitis B surface antigen (HBsAg); hepatitis C, D, E are screened for with antibody testing. If these tests are positive, then confirmatory tests include polymerase chain reaction (PCR) test for hepatitis B DNA, and hepatitis C, D and E RNA, respectively. Patients with acute liver injury are assessed by screening for IgM antibody (for hepatitis A, B, D and E), and confirmation by PCR testing. Hepatitis B assessment involves in addition detection of hepatitis e antigen and e antibody, which provide information about ongoing disease activity.

Box 14.10 Investigations in GI diseases including liver diseases

Laboratory-based investigations

1. Blood tests
2. Stool examination
   - Stool inspection
   - Stool microbiology, culture and sensitivities (MC&S)
   - Faecal occult blood
   - Faecal immunochemical testing (FIT)
   - Faecal calprotectin
   - Faecal elastase
   - Stool *H. pylori*
3. Ascitic fluid examination
   - Biochemistry: protein, albumin, amylase and SAAG (serum albumin ascites gradient)
   - Cell count
   - Malignant cytology
   - Culture

Endoscopic investigations

1. Upper GI endoscopy
2. Enteroscopy and wireless capsule endoscopy
3. Colonoscopy and sigmoidoscopy
4. Endoscopic retrograde cholangiopancreatography (ERCP)
5. Endoscopic ultrasound
6. Percutaneous transhepatic cholangiography

Imaging

1. Plain radiograph
2. Abdominal ultrasound
3. Transient liver elastography
4. Computed tomography (CT)
5. Positron emission tomography scanning (PET)
6. Magnetic resonance imaging (MRI and MRCP)
7. Barium studies
   - Barium swallow
   - Barium follow-through study
   - Small bowel enema
   - Barium enema

Other diagnostic and therapeutic investigations

1. Investigation for liver diseases
   - Liver biopsy
   - Hepatic venography, transjugular biopsy and transjugular intrahepatic porto-systemic shunt
2. Investigation for pancreatic diseases
   - Serum lipase
   - Faecal elastase
   - Pancreatic function test
3. Investigation for oesophageal diseases
   - Manometry
   - pH monitoring
4. Investigation for *H. pylori*
   - *H. pylori* antigen in stool
   - Endoscopic: Rapid urease test, culture
   - [14] Carbon labelled breath test
5. Investigation for complicated GI ulcer disease
   - Serum gastrin
6. Investigation for ongoing GI bleed
   - CT angiography of gastrointestinal arteries
   - Technetium tagged red cell scanning
7. Investigation to localize inflammation
   - Radioisotope scanning

Box 14.11 Liver screen: to determine cause of liver disease

Viral liver diseases

- *HAV:* IgM antibody to HAV
- *HBV:* Hepatitis B surface antigen (screening), HBV DNA, HBe antigen and HBe antibody for staging, isolated HB core antibody: marker of previous HBV exposure
- *HCV:* Hepatitis C antibody (screening), HCV RNA (diagnostic)
- *HDV:* Only in presence of HBV infection
- *HEV:* Hepatitis E antibody (screening), HEV RNA (diagnostic)

Immune liver diseases

- *Autoimmune hepatitis:* Elevated IgG and positive anti-nuclear antibody/anti-smooth muscle/anti-liver kidney microsomal antibody
- *Primary biliary cholangitis:* Elevated IgM and positive anti-mitochondrial antibody positive M2 subtype (diagnostic)
- *Primary sclerosing cholangitis:* Anti-neutrophil cytoplasmic antibody positive (ANCA)

Metabolic liver diseases

- *Alcohol-related liver disease*: History of alcohol excess, elevated mean corpuscular volume (MCV)
- *Non-alcoholic fatty liver disease*: Screen for presence of metabolic syndrome: T2DM, dyslipidaemia, central obesity and hypertension
- *Hereditary haemochromatosis*: Elevated serum ferritin and transferrin saturation (screening), HFE gene testing (diagnostic, so called because of H for high and Fe is the symbol for iron)
- *Wilson's disease*: Low serum caeruloplasmin (screening), elevated 24-hr urinary copper excretion (diagnostic)
- *Alpha 1 antitrypsin deficiency (A1AT):* Low levels (screening)

Tests to screen for autoimmune liver disease include antibodies to antinuclear antigen (ANA), smooth muscles (SMA) and liver kidney microsomes, which if present suggest autoimmune hepatitis. Anti-mitochondrial antibodies are found in the blood in primary biliary cholangitis in over 90% of cases.

A major cause for liver disease is alcohol. The most reliable screen for this remains an accurate history, documenting weekly consumption of alcohol in units (regular consumption of alcohol greater than 14 units per week is a risk for alcohol-related liver disease). Elevated mean corpuscular volume (MCV), elevated GGT and an ALT-to-AST ratio less than 1 are more often seen in patients with alcohol-related liver disease. It is also important to screen for the presence of alcohol dependence in patients with suspected alcohol-related liver disease using various validated tools (see Box 14.12).

CAGE: The CAGE uses four simple questions to assess alcohol use. Importantly, the questions should not be preceded by any questions about alcohol use; its sensitivity is increased by an open-ended introduction:

1. Have you ever felt the need to *C*ut down on your drinking?
2. Have people *A*nnoyed you by criticising your drinking?
3. Have you ever felt bad or *G*uilty about your drinking?
4. Have you ever had a drink first thing in the morning to steady your nerves or get over a hangover (*E*ye opener)?

A score of 2 or more is considered clinically significant

AUDIT: The alcohol use disorders identification (AUDIT) test is a longer screening tool recommended by the World Health Organisation.

Screen for other liver diseases include screening for liver disease owing to excess iron (hereditary haemochromatosis) or copper accumulation (Wilson's disease) and can be detected by measurements of elevated serum ferritin or low levels of serum caeruloplasmin, respectively. In primary haemochromatosis, genetic studies are used to confirm the diagnosis. Confirmation of Wilson's disease requires measurement of 24-hour urinary copper excretion and careful examination for copper deposition in the iris (Kayser-Fleischer ring) by slit-lamp examination.

Another common cause for chronic liver disease is non-alcoholic fatty liver disease (NAFLD), which is associated with the metabolic syndrome and screening for hypertension, dyslipidemia, central obesity and type 2 diabetes, and excluding other causes of liver disease, is a useful tool for diagnosing NAFLD.

Anaemia

Anaemia is a common finding in patients with GI and liver disease and an initial assessment will include measuring serum ferritin, vitamin B_{12} and folate levels and undertaking a coeliac screen (see below).

Coeliac screen

These include antibodies to tissue transglutaminase, endomysial and gliadin antigen. As these are IgA antibodies, it is important that IgA levels are checked at the same time to exclude IgA deficiency, which could lead to a false-negative result.

Weight loss screen

In addition to blood tests, as above, this includes thyroid function tests and erythrocyte sedimentation rate (ESR).

Patients with inflammatory bowel disease

In addition to routine blood tests, C-reactive protein (CRP) is used to assess the severity of inflammation and response to therapy.

Stool inspection used to be part of bedside assessment and is carried out less often owing to concerns regarding specimen handling and infection control issues. It may be possible to get a description of stools from the history. Watery stools are found in all cases of profuse diarrhoea and after administration of purgatives as well as antibiotic-associated diarrhoea in which case *Clostridium difficile* infection needs to be excluded. In cholera, the stools—known as rice-water stools—are colourless, almost devoid of odour, alkaline in reaction and contain a number of small flocculi consisting of shreds of epithelium and particles of mucus. Purulent or pus-containing stools are found in severe infectious dysentery or ulcerative colitis. Slimy stools are owing to the presence of an excess of mucus and point to a disorder of the large bowel. The mucus may envelop the faeces or may be intimately mixed with it. Presence of blood in stools varies in appearance according to the site of bleed within the GI tract and the volume of blood loss over time. If the bleeding takes place in the upper GI tract, the stools are black, shiny and foul smelling, called melaena. Red-currant jelly stools are classically described in children presenting with small bowel intussusception. Large bowel bleeding proximal to the rectum may produce darker red blood in stools, whereas bleeding within the rectum or anus is often brighter red and referred to as exit type per rectal (PR) bleed. There is blood streaking the side of faeces anal fissure and haemorrhoidal bleeding may be found mainly on the toilet paper or as drops of bright red blood in the pan. A brisk upper-GI bleed may lead to bright red rectal bleeding (haematochezia). The stools of bacillary dysentery initially consist of faecal material mixed with blood and pus, later of blood and pus without faecal material. Those of amoebic dysentery characteristically consist of fluid faecal material, mucus and small amounts of blood. The stools of steatorrhoea are very large, pale and putty- or porridge-like, sometimes frothy with a visible oily film, and often float. They are apt to stick to the sides of the toilet and are difficult to flush away.

Reliable microbiology, culture and sensitivity (MC&S) of the stool is vital for accurate diagnosis of acute and chronic diarrhoea. All stool samples for microbiological examination should be sent to the laboratory as fresh as possible; if amoebic or similar infection is suspected, then microscopy should be performed with the stool still as close to body temperature as possible (a 'hot' stool). Any microbiological finding must be correlated with the history, because many patients are healthy carriers of organisms that can be pathogenic in other situations. If *C. difficile* infection is suspected in a patient with diarrhoea following the use of antibiotics, the laboratory must be asked to look for the *Clostridium* toxin in preference to the organism.

The guaiac test (haemoccult) previously has been the most widely used method for testing for faecal occult blood. A filter paper impregnated with guaiac turns blue in the presence of haemoglobin when hydrogen peroxide is added. The test depends on the oxidation of guaiac in the presence of haemoglobin. Other substances with peroxidase activity, including dietary substances such as bananas, pineapple, broccoli and radishes, can produce a false-positive reaction, and ascorbic acid may cause false-negative results. Therefore, dietary preparation is necessary for accurate screening, for example, when screening a population in the early detection of colonic cancer. In ordinary clinical use, the test is sensitive to faecal blood losses of about 20 ml per day. This test can be used for patients on a normal diet, but it may not detect small amounts of GI bleeding. The test may be negative in the presence of lesions that bleed intermittently or slightly, particularly those situated in the upper GI tract.

Faecal immunofaecal (FIT) testing is increasingly used to check for the presence of occult blood in stool sample instead of above and is being rapidly adopted for use in primary care to screen patients with bowel symptoms or iron deficiency anaemia who may require referral to secondary care for further investigations including endoscopic assessment.

The faecal calprotectin test is used to assess for the presence of bowel inflammation and is most often used in primary care to differentiate inflammatory bowel disease from irritable bowel syndrome in younger patients. If elevated, it should prompt referral to secondary care for further investigations, including colonoscopy. It may also be elevated in patients taking nonsteroidal anti-inflammatory drugs.

Faecal elastase has largely replaced measurement of faecal fat in patients suspected to have diarrhoea owing to malabsorption from pancreatic diseases (steatorrhoea) and, if reduced, may indicate pancreatic exocrine insufficiency (although measurements can vary over time).

Helicobacter pylori is a common upper GI pathogen and it is associated with chronic gastritis, duodenitis and peptic ulcer disease. This stool test is used mainly in primary care to check for the presence of the infection, and often leads to treatment without needing endoscopy.

Ascitic fluid examination

Ascitic fluid sampling is carried out at the bedside taking a blood sample and is analysed for biochemistry, cell count, cytology and culture. It is indicated in all patients with new clinically apparent ascites to help ascertain its cause. All patients known to have ascites from liver cirrhosis who are admitted to hospital require an ascitic fluid examination to rule out the presence of spontaneous bacterial peritonitis which is potentially life-threatening. Ascitic fluid is sampled through the abdominal wall similarly to taking a blood sample.

Biochemical analysis includes measurement of total protein, albumin, amylase and a calcluation of the serum ascites albumin gradient (SAAG). Ascitic transudates, such as those that occur in heart failure, cirrhosis and nephrotic syndrome, normally have a protein content under 25 g/l (i.e. less than two-thirds the concentration of albumin in the plasma). Exudates occurring in tuberculous peritonitis or in the presence of secondary malignancy usually contain more than 25 g/l of protein. This method of distinction, however, is somewhat unreliable as it does not take into account the associated serum albumin levels. Therefore, it is now routine to measure serum albumin and ascitic fluid albumin to calculate the SAAG; a value of ≥11 g/l suggests that the ascites is secondary to portal hypertension (liver cirrhosis). If pancreatic ascites is suspected the amylase content of the fluid should be measured.

Lymphocytes in ascitic fluid are characteristic of chronic inflammation, the most common cause being tuberculous peritonitis, but acid-fast bacilli are often not seen on staining. In contrast, an elevated neutrophil count is seen in the presence of acute peritonitis. Very high neutrophil counts (>10,000 per mm³) in ascitic fluid are classically seen in patients with peritonitis secondary to perforation of the bowel. This needs to be differentiated from spontaneous bacterial peritonitis, a condition often seen in patients with liver cirrhosis who are suddenly less well. The neutrophil count is lower, but organisms may not be cultured: the diagnosis is primarily based on the finding of >250 or more neutrophils per mm³ fluid, results which should lead to the use of prompt and appropriate antibiotics.

In all new cases of ascites, the fluid should undergo careful examination for the presence of malignant cells, particularly if an underlying abdominal malignancy is suspected and/or ascitic aspiration reveals blood-stained fluid. (Fig. 14.34).

Figure 14.34   Ascites cytology. A group of tumour cells showing random orientation and large abnormal nucleoli indicating malignancy. Ascitic fluid from patient with ovarian carcinoma. May-Grünwald-Giemsa stain ×160.

Ascitic fluid cultures are positive in patients with peritonitis secondary to bowel perforation. However, in spontaneous bacterial peritonitis, the cultures are often negative and therefore in patients with ascites owing to cirrhosis, inoculating 10 ml of ascitic fluid sample into blood culture bottles may increase the yield.

Endoscopic investigations (see Box 14.10)

1. Upper GI endoscopy
2. Enteroscopy and wireless capsule endoscopy
3. Colonoscopy and sigmoidoscopy
4. ERCP
5. Endoscopic ultrasound
6. Percutaneous transhepatic cholangiography

Upper gastrointestinal endoscopy

In the last 50 years or so, the development of the fibreoptic endoscope and, more recently, of video-endoscopy, has revolutionized the assessment of the upper GI tract (Fig. 14.35). With these instruments it is possible to inspect directly as far as the proximal small bowel, with or without conscious sedation and local pharyngeal anaesthesia. Because of the ability to photograph and biopsy any suspicious lesions, this technique is the investigation of choice for demonstrating structural abnormalities in the upper gut. Therapeutic endoscopy is now the treatment of choice for bleeding varices, oesophageal obstruction and, in most cases, of bleeding peptic ulcer (Fig. 14.36). In inoperable cancer of the oesophagus, palliative prostheses (stents) can be inserted endoscopically. Enteral nutrition may be delivered via percutaneous endoscopic gastrostomy tubes.

Enteroscopy and wireless capsule endoscopy

Endoscopic examination of the small bowel, which requires the use of a longer small bowel endoscope,

is called enteroscopy. Samples of small intestine mucosa are valuable for histological diagnosis in various types of malabsorption. Direct biopsy of the lower duodenum at conventional upper GI endoscopy is usually sufficient for diagnosis of coeliac disease, but jejunal tissue can also be obtained from the first few small bowel loops using a push-type flexible enteroscopes. If coeliac disease is suspected, a coeliac blood screen is requested (as described), but a duodenal biopsy is essential to complete or fully exclude the diagnosis. The low-power view of the villi is as important as the detailed histology. Other malabsorption problems, such as Whipple's disease and chronic giardiasis, may also be seen on duodenal biopsy. Very occasionally, full-thickness jejunal biopsies are used for diagnosing neuromuscular gut disorders and can be obtained by laparoscopy. These tests are limited in view of the long length of the small bowel, but more recently virtual capsule endoscopy has evolved. Wireless capsule endoscopy provides excellent endoscopic images of the whole of the small bowel, without the need for intubation, but, as yet, biopsies are not possible by this method.

Colonoscopy and sigmoidoscopy

As in the upper gut, the use of flexible fibreoptic and video instruments has revolutionized the investigation of the colon. Sigmoidoscopy involves examination of the proximal sigmoid, rectum and anus, after a simple enema preparation, whereas colonoscopy allows examination up until the caecum and distal ileum and requires more extensive colon preparation. It is also an outpatient procedure, under conscious sedation. These techniques are invaluable for diagnosing and obtaining tissue for confirming inflammatory and neoplastic disease and for removal of all types of polyps (Figs 14.37 and 14.38). Dilation of strictures,

Figure 14.35 A patient undergoing endoscopy of the upper GI tract. The plastic guard between the teeth prevents the instrument from being bitten. The patient may have received pharyngeal local anaesthetic spray or light sedation with midazolam.

Figure 14.36 Endoscopic view of a duodenal ulcer that has recently bled with a visible blood vessel on its surface.

Figure 14.37 View of colonic epithelium at colonoscopy, showing severe ulcerative colitis with extensive ulceration and bleeding.

Figure 14.38 Colonoscopic view of a tubulovillous adenoma.

stenting or other thermal treatments of obstructing tumours can also be applied during endoscopy. A skilled colonoscopist should reach the caecum in more than 90% of examinations attempted and the terminal ileum in 50%. There is a small risk (1:1000) of colonic perforation associated with the colonoscopy. Sigmoidoscopy is particularly useful in the differential diagnosis of diarrhoea of colonic origin. Granularity, loss of vascular pattern and ulceration with bleeding may indicate the presence of ulcerative colitis; aphthous ulceration may suggest Crohn's disease; and multiple rounded white macules may be diagnostic of pseudomembranous colitis caused by *C. difficile* toxin, usually following antibiotic treatment. In suspected amoebic dysentery, the mucous membrane should be inspected and portions of mucus and scrapings from the ulcerated mucosa may be removed and examined microscopically for amoebic cysts.

The anal canal and lower rectum can be readily visualized with a rigid proctoscope. Place the patient in the position described for rectal examination and gently pass the lubricated instrument to its full depth. Remove the obturator and inspect the mucosa as the instrument is slowly withdrawn and air gently insufflated. Haemorrhoids are seen as reddish/blue swellings which bulge into the lumen of the instrument. Asking the patient to strain down as the proctoscope is withdrawn exaggerates any haemorrhoids. The internal opening of an anal fistula, an anal or low rectal polyp and a chronic anal fissure are other abnormalities that may be seen.

Endoscopic retrograde cholangiopancreatography (ERCP)

This technique is useful in the rapid diagnosis and localization of the different causes of jaundice owing to obstruction of the main bile ducts. Using a special side-viewing duodenoscope, the duodenal papilla is identified and a cannula passed through it into the common bile duct. Radiopaque contrast is then injected into the cannula and the whole of the biliary

system is visualized by X-ray imaging. Needle or forceps biopsy and brush cytology may give a specific diagnosis of strictures of the biliary tree. ERCP has an important therapeutic role in the treatment of jaundice because it allows the removal of bile duct stones or the placement of stents (tubes that facilitate the passage of bile into the duodenum past obstructing lesions, such as tumours of the pancreas or bile duct). More novel techniques allow direct visualization of the biliary system. Such therapies often involve performing a sphincterotomy during ERCP using a cutting diathermy wire passed into the bile duct via the ampulla. The sphincterotomy opens the ampulla and often allows the removal of stones in the bile duct. Rapid advances have been made in this field with dedicated mother and baby cholangioscopes, which provide greater accuracy and range of options to help in diagnosis, tissue biopsy and biliary interventions.

The entire pancreatic duct system can be visualized by ERCP. Therefore, the technique is valuable in the diagnosis of chronic pancreatitis. In patients with pancreatic carcinoma, a needle biopsy can be performed by ERCP, and brush cytology of the pancreatic duct may also provide histological confirmation of the diagnosis. ERCP carries a small mortality and may be complicated by pancreatitis, bleeding, perforation or infection. Prophylactic antibiotics should be used if there is biliary obstruction, and every procedure should be preceded by a large dose of nonsteroidal anti-inflammatory drugs (usually by suppository) to reduce the risk of pancreatitis afterwards. The advent of magnetic resonance imaging of the bile and pancreatic ducts now means that most ERCPs are therapeutic.

Endoscopic ultrasound

Endoscopic ultrasound is a relatively new tool that uses endoscopic access to carry out ultrasound assessment of luminal organs including the oesophagus, stomach, bowel and biliary tree. Endoscopic ultrasound is more sensitive in staging the mucosal depth of penetration of cancers in the oesophagus and stomach than computed tomography (CT) scanning; it is frequently better at lymph node detection, but is less effective at detecting distant metastases. It is also valuable in assessing biliary and pancreatic abnormalities. Endoscopic ultrasound

Figure 14.39 Plain X-ray of the chest showing gas under the right and left diaphragms after perforation of the duodenal ulcer. The patient was admitted in shock with abdominal pain and abdominal rigidity.

has the advantage of guiding fine needle aspiration cytology as well as other endoscopic interventions.

Percutaneous transhepatic cholangiography

Percutaneous transhepatic cholangiography complements the use of ERCP in patients with jaundice caused by obstruction of the main bile ducts, although it is usually only possible if the intrahepatic bile ducts are seen to be dilated on ultrasound. The site of the obstruction owing to tumours on the head of the pancreas or benign and malignant bile duct strictures can be localized and differentiated accurately. This technique is usually only used if ERCP fails. It also has a therapeutic function. Transhepatic drains can be placed to treat cholangitis and sepsis; stents can be placed to relieve obstruction; gallstones can be removed; and wires can be passed into the duodenum to facilitate stenting at ERCP.

Imaging (see Box 14.10)

Plain radiographs

Plain radiographs of the chest and abdomen with the patient supine and in the erect position are of great value in cases of suspected peritonitis owing to a perforated viscus, when gas may be seen under the diaphragm, usually on the right side (Fig. 14.39). A plain abdominal X-ray is useful in suspected intestinal obstruction or ileus when dilated bowel loops may be seen with fluid levels appearing on the erect X-ray (Fig. 14.40). It is important to use a plain abdominal X-ray to exclude toxic megacolon in fulminant colitis.

Abdominal ultrasound

In ultrasound scanning a probe emitting ultrasonic pulses is passed across the abdomen. Echoes

Figure 14.40   Plain X-ray of the abdomen. Obstruction of the large bowel owing to carcinoma of the sigmoid colon. Most of the colon is dilated with gas, indicating obstruction, but there appears to be no gas below the sigmoid region.

detected from within the patient are received with a transducer amplified and suitably displayed. Ultrasound examination of the liver, including Doppler assessment of the portal vein, remains the most useful and first-line imaging for all patients suspected to have a liver problem. It provides an assessment for the size and appearance of the liver, including the presence of focal liver lesions and for assessing the presence of liver cirrhosis. The ultrasound features that suggest liver cirrhosis include coarse echotexture with irregular liver outline, presence of splenomegaly, ascites and presence of reverse flow (flow away from liver-retrograde) on Doppler of portal vein. It is also useful for assessment of jaundice to assess the cause of jaundice as hepatic or obstructive from a pancreatic or biliary pathology. Patients with liver cirrhosis are at an increased risk of developing primary liver cancers known as hepatocellular carcinoma and require six-month surveillance using liver ultrasound. The main drawbacks with ultrasound are limitations of image quality owing to body shape, especially in those with obesity. It is also helpful in screening of focal liver lesions and is helpful in the diagnosis of fluid-filled lesions, such as cysts and abscesses. Liver biopsies and fine-needle aspiration of suspicious lesions can be undertaken under direct ultrasound guidance for cytology and for drainage of fluid, bile or pus. The gallbladder is most easily investigated by ultrasound. It appears as an echo-free structure. If stones are present, they are usually easily seen as mobile and echo-dense with a characteristic 'acoustic shadow' behind them. Ultrasound detects 95% of gallbladder stones, but only about 50% of stones in the bile ducts themselves. Ultrasound is particularly valuable in detecting dilation of the bile duct that may be owing to partial or complete obstruction by gallstones or tumour. Ultrasound has replaced oral cholecystography for imaging the gallbladder. Ultrasound is the usual initial technique for investigating the pancreas, is particularly useful in the diagnosis of true and pseudopancreatic cysts and is an essential tool for percutaneous needle biopsy. However, images may be obscured by overlying bowel gas and the tail of the pancreas is often poorly visualized. Ultrasound is used extensively for examining other intra-abdominal, pelvic and retroperitoneal organs and increasingly for imaging the bowel in inflammatory conditions such as in Crohn's disease. Blood flow patterns (such as in the portal vein) can be assessed by ultrasound using the Doppler principle.

Transient liver elastography

Transient liver elastography, an important tool for non-invasive assessment of liver fibrosis and quantification of liver steatosis (fat content), has reduced the need for liver biopsy. It measures liver stiffness by measuring speed of shear waves generated by ultrasound beams, with a higher score suggestive of an increase in liver stiffness and fibrosis (Fig. 14.41). Confounding factors, including obesity, concurrent significant liver inflammation, co-existent biliary dilatation and medical conditions such as heart failure and amyloidosis, may influence the accuracy. This tool is being used to screen patients who may have significant liver fibrosis/liver cirrhosis and require long-term follow-up with a liver specialist.

Computed tomography

Computed tomography is used to produce cross-sectional images of the liver and other intra-abdominal and retroperitoneal organs. It is particularly helpful in the accurate staging of all types of GI cancers, including cancers of the oesophagus, stomach, pancreas and colon (Fig. 14.42). Because it can be combined with injection of vascular contrast, it can be helpful in assessing intra-abdominal vascular abnormalities. It can facilitate guided biopsy of abnormalities and drainage of fluid and other collections. Also, increasingly it is being used to image the bowel, particularly if there is suspected obstruction, and is widely used in assessing patients with an acute abdomen. Clinicians should be aware of the radiation exposure associated with CT scanning and caution should be exercised for younger patients in particular. After scanning a patient with some gas put in the colon, the CT computer can be used to reconstruct a very accurate virtual image of the colon (CT virtual colonoscopy).

Positron emission tomography (PET) scanning

Radiolabelled isotopes that are taken up by cell metabolism are injected intravenously and the

Ribs

Pulse wave

Ultrasound wave

Probe/stroke transducer

Liver

Sample area for measuring liver stiffness by using ultrasound to measure the speed of compression wave by the pulse

Figure 14.41 **Transient liver elastography.** The probe delivers a pulse wave which spreads through the liver parenchyma. The speed of propagation of this pulse wave within the liver parenchyma is measured by the ultrasound, and in the absence of confounding factors is reflective of the degree of liver fibrosis. The measurements are expressed as kPa with <5 kPa indicating an absence of fibrosis, and >13 kPa suggesting established cirrhosis. The range from 5–13 kPa represents different fibrosis stages and can vary according to a number of variables including the underlying cause of liver disease, model of machine and other coexisting conditions such as heart failure, body habitus, liver inflammation, anti-viral therapy.

radiation that is detected is reconstructed into a cross-sectional image by the same techniques as for CT. It is a particularly sensitive technique for staging cancers, if baseline CT images are acquired at the same time

Magnetic resonance imaging (MRI and MRCP)

Magnetic resonance scanning is now replacing barium radiology for assessing the small and large bowel and perianal disease, especially when evaluating areas of stricturing and inflammation in patients with Crohn's disease and ulcerative colitis. Magnetic resonance cholangiopancreatography (MRCP) is used as a second-line imaging tool for patients with suspected biliary and pancreatic disease because it can provide high-quality images of the bile duct and pancreatic duct. The safety of this non-invasive technique has reduced the need for more invasive and hazardous examinations, such as endoscopic retrograde cholangiopancreatography (ERCP), which is reserved for patients requiring therapeutic intervention.

Magnetic resonance imaging, especially using contrast such as gadolinium, is a key tool to characterize focal liver lesions, including haemangiomas, adenomas, focal nodular hyperplasia and both primary and secondary liver cancers.

Barium studies

Barium study investigations involve administering radioopaque barium solution with direct observation of its passage using fluoroscopy through different parts of the GI tract. This study used to be first line; however, with the recent advances in the endoscopic tools, these investigations are being used less often as they involve radiation exposure and do not provide the opportunity of tissue diagnosis. Below is a brief summary of the different types.

Barium swallow
The direct observation of the passage of a radiopaque barium solution through the pharynx and oesophagus into the stomach remains an important investigation of dysphagia, especially in patients where no endoscopic diagnosis is evident, and especially where disorders of motility are suspected. Lack of progress of barium through an apparently normal lower oesophageal sphincter on swallowing in a patient with dysphagia usually indicates the presence of achalasia, a disorder of neuromuscular coordination of the oesophageal body and failure of the lower sphincter to relax.

Barium follow-through study
The small intestine may be studied by taking sequential X-rays of the abdomen after swallowing barium contrast. Abnormalities in the transit time to the colon and in small bowel pattern (e.g. dilation, narrowing, increase in transverse barring or flocculation) may be demonstrated in malabsorptive states. Areas of narrowing with proximal dilatation, fistulae and mucosal abnormalities may be produced by Crohn's disease. Small bowel diverticula or neoplasms may also be demonstrated. The amount and type of barium used for examination of the stomach/duodenum and of the small bowel is different, and so a barium follow-through should be requested as a specific examination and not as an add-on to a barium meal. However, this has been replaced largely by MRI assessment of the small bowel in view of the radiation exposure.

Small bowel enema
Small bowel enema is an alternative to the barium follow-through examination; it involves intubating the duodenum and passing small quantities of a non-flocculating barium suspension down the tube. This method is useful for detecting isolated focal lesions and strictures, but in most centres has been replaced by MR enterography and/or enteroscopy.

Barium enema
This contrast study was used to assess for colonic pathology and requires a full bowel preparation prior to barium enema (Figs 14.43 and 14.44).

Patients often find the preparation and procedure uncomfortable and there is a very small risk of perforating the colon. The inability to take diagnostic samples and the advent of CT virtual colonoscopy means that barium enemas are completely obsolete anywhere where CT scanning is available.

Other diagnostic and therapeutic investigations (see Box 14.10)

This section summarizes a battery of tests when a particular site of disease is suspected.

Investigation for liver diseases

Box 14.13 summarizes the key investigations for patients with liver disease. Most of these have

Figure 14.42   CT demonstrating liver metastases from colonic carcinoma. Large, lobulated, non-homogeneous masses (*arrows*) replace most of the left lobe of the liver.

Figure 14.43   Barium enema with air contrast. The right colon is outlined by barium sulphate and the rectum, left colon and part of the transverse colon are outlined by air, with a thin mucosal layer of barium sulphate. Note the normal haustral pattern in the colon and the smooth appearance of the rectum. The anal canal can also be seen.

Figure 14.44   Barium enema with air contrast. In this patient with ulcerative colitis, the normal mucosal pattern and the haustra themselves have been obliterated. The patient is lying on his right side so that there are clear fluid levels in the barium sulphate suspension in the bowel.

been covered in preceding sections. However, the following additional investigations may be required in some patients.

Liver biopsy

Liver biopsy is the gold standard for confirming the nature and assessing the severity of liver disease. Percutaneous needle biopsy is the standard technique for obtaining liver tissue for histological examination, under ultrasound guidance usually under local anaesthesia (sometimes with mild sedation). Although the method is safe and reliable, there is a small but definite mortality from the procedure owing to leakage of bile and/or blood into the peritoneal cavity from the puncture site. Therefore, the procedure should always be regarded as a potentially dangerous investigation for which there should be a clear beneficial indication for the patient and should be performed by an appropriately trained operator. Contraindications to percutaneous liver biopsy include patients with abnormal clotting times or thrombocytopaenia, obstructive jaundice or ascites. Patients with abnormal clotting and ascites can have liver biopsy via transjugular route under fluoroscopic guidance by a trained operator.

Box 14.13	Investigations for assessment of liver diseases

1. Liver function tests (LFTs)
2. Liver screen
3. Liver ultrasound and Doppler of portal vein
4. Transient liver elastography
5. MRI liver (gadolinium contrast)
6. Contrast-enhanced CT liver
7. Liver biopsy
8. Hepatic venography, transjugular biopsy and transjugular intrahepatic porto-systemic shunt

Hepatic venography, transjugular biopsy and transjugular intrahepatic porto-systemic shunt

This is a radiological intervention used for undertaking liver biopsies where the percutaneous route may be high risk owing to the presence of deranged coagulation or presence of ascites. It can also help confirm portal hypertension by enabling measurement of wedged hepatic vein pressures. It has a therapeutic role as it allows placement of transhepatic portosystemic shunts (TIPS; Fig. 14.45). This is used to treat patients with variceal bleed owing to liver cirrhosis and portal hypertension that have failed endoscopic therapy or control of ascites not responsive to routine management with

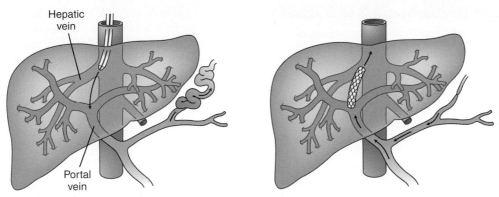

Figure 14.45 TIPS: Transjugular intrahepatic portosystemic shunt. (From Townsend C, Beauchamp RD, Evers BM, Mattox K, eds. Sabiston Textbook of Surgery: The Biological Basis of Modern Surgical Practice, ed 21. Fig. 54.21. 2022. Elsevier Inc.)

diuretics. It involves placing a stent within the hepatic parenchyma that links a branch of portal vein with hepatic vein thereby off-loading the elevated portal pressures into the systemic circulation. This helps to reduce the portal hypertension and its sequelae, including variceal bleed and ascites.

Investigation for pancreatic disease

The most specific blood test for acute pancreatitis is serum lipase, although it is not very helpful in chronic disease. The mainstay to diagnose pancreatic diseases is imaging, including abdominal ultrasound, contrast CT scan and MRCP.

Pancreatic function tests are now rarely used. In suspected pancreatic malabsorption, a therapeutic trial of pancreatic supplementation may be the easiest confirmatory test. If a definitive test is required, the pancreolauryl test can be used, a test which relies on the urine collection of a substance that can be absorbed only after GI breakdown by pancreatic enzymes. In chronic pancreatitis, faecal elastase may be reduced.

Investigation for oesophageal motility disorders

Oesophageal function studies are specialized tests indicated for patients suspected to have disorders of oesophageal motility. These include manometric studies and pH monitoring. Manometric studies of pressure changes during swallowing are used to localize functional abnormalities in the coordination of oesophageal peristalsis, for example, achalasia and oesophageal spasm. In patients with epigastric and retrosternal discomfort (heartburn) related to eating or to lying supine, reflux of acid from the stomach into the lower oesophagus should be suspected. Acid reflux can be detected best by monitoring the pH in the lower oesophagus during a 24-hour period. The pH measuring probe, passed via the nose, is placed in the lower oesophagus, 5 cm above the oesophagogastric junction, for 24 hours and the pH recorded continuously. The patient indicates when pain is experienced by pressing an electronic marker on the recorder to see if there is a correlation with the degree of acidity. This investigation has found a major clinical application in the differential diagnosis of acid reflux pain from atypical cardiac pain. A combined pH and impedance recording can also detect non-acid reflux.

Investigation for *Helicobacter pylori*

The role of infection by *H. pylori* in the pathogenesis of gastric and duodenal ulceration is well documented. *H. pylori* is a gram-negative spiral bacillus. The organism is found in the gastric antrum in about 60% of patients with gastritis or gastric ulceration and in almost all patients with duodenal ulceration. There are many asymptomatic carriers in the general population. Patients carrying *H. pylori* in the stomach will have IgG antibodies in the serum, but as these will remain present for a long period after successful treatment, serological testing is no longer recommended.

- Stool tests for *H. pylori* antigen, now the most widely used method in the community and before endoscopy, are indicated or performed.
- Endoscopic diagnosis of *H. pylori* involves carrying out a rapid urease test on a sample of gastric biopsy, referred to also as a CLO (campylobacter-like organism) test. As *H. pylori* is rich in urease, a gastric biopsy is placed in contact with a pellet or solution containing urea and a coloured pH indicator. The colour of the substrate changes when the pH is greater than 6, indicating the conversion of urea to ammonia by urease in *H. pylori*. Gastric biopsies may also be sent for culture and sensitivities testing and are indicated in those patients who do not respond to simple *H. pylori* eradication therapies.
- 13C-labelled urea breath testing, a variant of this method, utilizes 13C-labelled urea given to the patient by mouth. The patient's breath is monitored for labelled carbon dioxide, indicating breakdown of the ingested urea by urease-containing organisms in the upper GI tract. 13C-labelled urea breath testing should be used to confirm successful eradication. *H. pylori* can be rendered undetectable, but not eradicated by acid-suppression therapy, which should be stopped 2 weeks before any testing for reliable results (other than histology of gastric biopsies).

Investigation for complicated GI ulcer disease

The mainstay of investigation in such patients in endoscopy was covered in the preceding section. The following additional investigations may be required, in a sub-group of patients, depending on clinical presentations:

- Serum gastrin measurement is carried out in patients with complicated gastric and duodenal ulcer disease where a diagnosis of Zollinger-Ellison syndrome is suspected. Measurement of serum gastrin is made fasting, after a long period without acid-suppression therapy and collected into special preservative. In patients with Zollinger-Ellison syndrome the level of gastrin in the serum is increased above 100 ng/l. Serum gastrin levels are also increased in renal failure, pernicious anaemia, after vagotomy and during acid-suppression therapy.

Investigation for ongoing GI bleed

- Selective angiography of gastrointestinal arteries: This is carried out using CT-guided angiography by trained interventional radiologists in the investigations of patients presenting with ongoing haematemesis or melaena when gastroscopy and colonoscopy fail to identify the bleeding source. It is most useful if performed when the patient is actively bleeding, but may be of value if an aneurysm or abnormal tumour vasculature is present, and it can occasionally detect angiomas. It is an invasive technique that demands a great deal of skill on the part of the radiologist. It is possible to use therapeutic embolization to treat the side of bleed identified on angiography.
- Isotope scanning: Technetium-labelled red blood cells can be used to detect the location of sources of bleeding in the GI tract.

Investigation to localize inflammation

- Radioisotope studies: Technetium-labelled white cells can be used to localize inflamed bowel segments in inflammatory bowel disease; both the small and large bowel can be imaged with the same test. Isotopes taken up in the bile (hepatobiliary iminodiacetic acid, HIDA) can give images of the gallbladder and biliary tree and some information as to the functioning of these organs, such as in patients with typical biliary pain but a normal gallbladder on ultrasound examination.

Locomotor system | 15

Stephen Kelly

Introduction

Musculoskeletal symptoms are a major cause of pain and disability, accounting for a quarter of all general practitioner consultations in the United Kingdom (UK), with significant economic consequences. Common musculoskeletal conditions, such as back pain and osteoarthritis, are the dominant causes of chronic pain, disability and work loss in the UK and many other countries, consuming considerable health and social service resources. In addition, inflammatory arthritis and connective tissue disorders may present with musculoskeletal symptoms. As such, it is critical that clinicians are able to assess patients with such symptoms and initiate appropriate management or referral to a specialist centre. Early diagnosis and treatment of inflammatory arthritis, such as rheumatoid arthritis, has been consistently shown to improve patients' long-term outcome with the early initiation of disease-modifying therapy. The autoimmune rheumatic disorders, although much less common, cause significant morbidity with the potential for end-organ damage which may be fatal if not recognized and treated early.

The objectives of performing a musculoskeletal assessment are to:

- Make an accurate diagnosis
- Assess the severity and consequences of the condition
- Construct a clear management plan

Taking an effective structured history and making a simple, focused examination are likely to be more important than imaging and serology, which on their own may be falsely reassuring. Although modern musculoskeletal medicine uses complex imaging and immunological investigations, in most patients with locomotor disorders, diagnosis can be achieved at the bedside without complex investigations.

General assessment: the 'GALS' locomotor screen

This brief screening examination, which should take 1 to 2 minutes, has been devised for use in routine clinical assessment. This brief global assessment of the gait, arms, legs and spine (GALS) is typically used by both non-specialist and specialist alike (Box 15.1). The routine requires some practise to become proficient, but once achieved, it has been shown to be highly sensitive in detecting significant abnormalities of the musculoskeletal system. It involves inspecting carefully for joint swelling and abnormal posture, as well as assessing the joints for normal movement. Typically, the clinician will then focus on particular areas of interest with more dedicated and targeted examinations.

Screening history

If answers to the following four questions are negative, a musculoskeletal disorder is unlikely:

1. Do you have any pain or stiffness in your muscles, joints or back?
2. Have you ever had gout or arthritis?
3. Can you dress yourself completely without difficulty?
4. Can you walk up and down stairs without difficulty?

Positive answers imply the need for a more detailed assessment, as will be described in this chapter.

Screening examination

Gait

Watch the patient walking and turning back towards you. Normal: symmetry, smooth movement, arm swing, no pelvic tilt, normal stride length, ability to turn quickly.

With the patient standing in the anatomical position, observe from behind, from the side and from in front. Muscle symmetry should be noted along with limb alignment. Spine and limb alignment can be observed as well as abnormalities in the feet, such as pes planus or pes cavus.

Common gait abnormalities are listed in Table 15.1.

Spine

Inspect the standing patient. Normal on inspection: no scoliosis, symmetrical paraspinals, normal shoulder and gluteal muscle bulk and symmetry,

Table 15.1 Gait abnormalities

Type	Description	Causes
Antalgic	Avoiding weight bearing on affected side	Pain related to arthritis or tendonitis
Spastic	Leg swings outwardly from hip with extended knee	Hemiplegia related to stroke
Shuffling	Small shuffling steps, speeding up (festination), reduced arm swing and difficulty turning	Parkinson's disease
Ataxic	Wide-based gait, swaying torso	Cerebellar disease. Peripheral sensory ataxia (typically worsens with loss of visual input)
Waddling (Trendelenburg)	Exaggerated lateral movement of trunk and circumduction of hip to compensate for weak abductors	Bilateral gluteus medius tendinopathy
High stepping (foot drop)	Excessive hip and knee flexion to accommodate failure of ankle dorsiflexion	Peroneal neuropathy (multiple causes)

Box 15.1 GALS checklist

Gait

- Observe gait
- Observe patient in anatomical position

Arms

- Observe movement: hands behind head
- Observe backs of hands and wrists
- Observe palms
- Assess power grip and strength
- Assess fine precision pinch
- Squeeze metacarpophalangeal joints (MCPJs)

Legs

- Assess full flexion and extension
- Assess internal rotation of hips
- Perform patellar tap
- Inspect feet
- Squeeze metatarsophalangeal joints (MTPJs)

Spine

- Inspect spine
- Assess lateral flexion of neck
- Assess lumbar spine movement

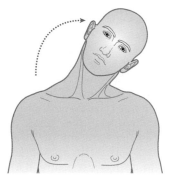

Figure 15.2 From the front, ask the patient: 'place your ear on your right then your left shoulder'.

Figure 15.3 Gently press the mid-point of each supraspinatus to elicit the hyperalgesia of fibromyalgia.

level iliac crests, normal cervical and lumbar lordosis. Movement: finger to floor distance less than 15 cm, lumbar expansion greater than 6 cm, ear touches acromion.

- From behind: look for abnormal spinal and paraspinal anatomy and look at the legs.
- From the side: look for abnormal spinal posture, then ask the patient to bend down and touch his toes (Fig. 15.1).

Figure 15.1 Inspect patient from behind and side, observing for normal spinal curves, then ask the patient: 'bend forwards to try to touch your toes'.

- From the front: ask the patient to 'put your ear on your left then right shoulder' and watch the neck movements (Fig. 15.2).
- Gently press the mid-point of each supraspinatus muscle to elicit tenderness (Fig. 15.3).

Arms

Ask the patient to follow instructions as in Table 15.2 (see Figs 15.4–15.9).

Table 15.2 Instructions for examining arms

Instruction	Normal outcome
'Raise arms out sideways and up above your head'.	180° elevation through abduction without wincing
'Touch the middle of your back'.	Touches above T10 with both hands
'Straighten your elbows right out'	Elbows extend to 180° or slightly beyond (females) symmetrically
'Place hands together as if to pray, with elbows right out'.	90° wrist extension and straight fingers
'The same with hands back to back'.	90° wrist flexion
'Place both hands out in front, palms down, fingers out straight'.	No wrist/finger swelling/ deformity, 90° pronation
Metacarpophalangeal (MCP) cross-compression	No tenderness
'Turn hands over'	90° supination No palmar swellings, wasting or erythema
'Make a fist and hide your nails'.	Can hide fingernails
'Pinch index, middle finger and thumb together'	Can do
Also look for swelling between the heads of the metacarpals and gently squeeze across the MCP joints to elicit tenderness.	Tenderness may be elicited

Figure 15.4 Ask the patient: 'Put your hands behind your head, elbows back'. Observe for pain or restricted movement.

Figure 15.5 Ask the patient: 'Put your hands out, palms down, and then turn your hands over'.

Figure 15.6 Ask the patient: 'Make a fist with both hands'.

Figure 15.7 Ask the patient: 'Place your hands together as if to pray, with elbows right out'.

Figure 15.8 Ask the patient: 'Do the same with your hands back to back'.

Figure 15.9 Look for swelling between the heads of the metacarpals and gently squeeze across the metacarpophalangeal joints to elicit tenderness.

Table 15.3 Instructions for examining legs

Instruction	Normal outcome
Flex hip and knee, holding knee	No bony crepitus, 140° knee flexion
Passively rotate hips	90° total pain-free rotation
Bulge test/patellar tap	No detectable fluid
Palpate popliteal fossa	No swelling
Inspect feet	No deformity, callosities or forefoot widening (daylight sign)
Test subtalar and ankle movement	Pain-free calcaneal mobility at subtalar joint, dorsiflexion beyond plantigrade and 30° plantarflexion

Legs

With the patient still standing:

- Examine the lower limbs for swelling, deformities or limb shortening. Normal: no knee deformity, anterior or popliteal swelling, no muscle wasting, no hindfoot swelling or deformity.
- Then, with the patient lying on a couch, continue the examination following the instructions in Table 15.3 (see Figs 15.10–15.14).

Figure 15.10 Gently flex the hips and knees, feeling for crepitus at the knee during movement, and look for pain and restriction of movement. Look for knee effusion.

(A)   Bulge test   (B)   Patellar tap

Figure 15.11 **(A)** Bulge test and **(B)** patellar tap.

This examination can be conducted in approximately 2 minutes, especially if the clinician performs the movements and asks the patient to follow them. The precise order of the examination is not important, and clinicians usually develop their own pattern of examination.

Children

Children should have their height and weight measured and plotted on centile charts to assess growth. When examining children, the assessment of the musculoskeletal system should be done with a parent present and include all the components of the adult version, with minor additions as follows:

Ask the child to walk on his tiptoes and then on the heels.

From the front, ask the child to put his hands together (as if praying) and also put his hands back to back and then have him reach his arms up towards the sky.

Additionally, when assessing the spine, ask the child to open his mouth and insert three of his own fingers into it.

Symmetry is key and any asymmetry should be assessed for pathology. It is normal for toddlers to be 'bow-legged,' 'knock-kneed' and 'flat-footed'. Various foot and toe appearances are also normal, including in-toeing, out-toeing and 'curly' toes. These appearances usually resolve as the child grows.

Recording the results

The incorporation of a brief musculoskeletal examination into the routine examination should lead to a more detailed assessment if any abnormalities are found (Table 15.4).

Figure 15.12   Palpate popliteal fossa.

Figure 15.14   Squeeze across metacarpophalangeal (MTP) joints and inspect the soles of the feet.

Figure 15.13   Test subtalar and ankle movement.

Table 15.4 How to record the locomotor screen routinely in the medical record

Screening issues:	Pain	0
	Gout or arthritis	0
	Dressing	✓
	Walking	✓
with positive answers being elaborated.		
Examination:		
A (Appearance)	M (Movement)	
G	✓	
A	✓	✓
L	✓	✓
S	✓	✓
with abnormal findings indicated, e.g. in rheumatoid arthritis:		
A (Appearance)	M (Movement)	
G	✗	
A	✗	✗
L	✗	✗
S	✓	✓
Slow painful gait.		
Synovitis of metacarpophalangeal (MCP), metatarsophalangeal (MTP), wrists and knee joints.		

Box 15.2 Common patterns of joint pain radiation

Pain may be referred or radiate from an affected joint, e.g.:
- Neck pain may radiate through the occiput to the vertex or to the shoulder and down the arm, with paraesthesiae if there is nerve-root impingement.
- Shoulder joint pain may radiate to the elbow and below.
- Thoracic spine nerve root pain may radiate around the chest and mimic cardiac pain.
- Lumbar spinal root pain may radiate through the buttock and leg to the knee and below, with paraesthesiae in the foot with a large disc prolapse; this is called 'sciatica'.
- Hip-joint pain may radiate to the knee and below.
- Knee pain may radiate above and below the joint.

Specific locomotor history

General demographic details, such as age, sex and occupation, should be recorded. Start the full musculoskeletal history with the presenting complaint and ask the patient to describe the sequence of symptoms, related features and events since the onset. Characteristic diagnostic points may emerge. Pain is a common presenting complaint and, as such, the clinician is expected to explore this fully. Using the WILDA (*Words, Intensity, Location, Duration, Aggravating/alleviating* factors) pain assessment approach may be helpful in drawing out key aspects of the patient's history and clarifying the nature of the complaint (see also Chapter 11).

Words

'I have pain' is not descriptive enough to inform a clinician about the character of the pain symptoms. Patients may have more than one type of pain and should be encouraged to describe their pain as much as possible. Neuropathic pain can be described as burning, shooting, tingling, radiating, lancinating or numbness. Somatic pain may be described as dull or throbbing and can usually be well localized. Somatic pain is most commonly described in the context of musculoskeletal pain afflicting joints and the spine.

Pain described as squeezing, pressure, cramping, distention, dull, deep and stretching is visceral in origin.

Intensity

It may be useful to use a simple visual analogue scale or ask the patient to rate his pain on a 0 to 10 scale. This may allow for monitoring and assessing progression of the underlying disorder.

Location

An accurate location of pain is often very helpful, although it must be remembered that joint pain may radiate. Patients should be asked, 'Where is your pain?' or 'Do you have pain in more than one area?'

Pain may be referred or radiate from an affected joint (Box 15.2).

Duration

The temporal description of pain is important in understanding the root cause. Pain may be constant, episodic or a combination of both. Is the patient ever pain free? Can he clearly identify the time of onset and is there a pattern of periodicity? For example, an osteoporotic vertebral fracture may be acute and self-limiting, which contrasts with the severe, constant and gnawing pain of a spinal metastatic deposit that prevents sleep.

Aggravating/alleviating factors

Aggravating and alleviating factors are often very helpful when trying to make a diagnosis. Back pain or stiffness that improves with exercise may point to an inflammatory cause, whereas pain that worsens after use is often described in the setting of degenerative arthritis.

Back pain is the most common musculoskeletal complaint; as such, it deserves further consideration. When taking a history of a patient's back symptoms

Table 15.5 Red flag symptoms associated with back pain with potential associated causes

Red flag	Potential cause
Elderly (>65 years) or young (<40 years) patient	Elderly patient: osteoporosis Young patient: inflammatory arthritis
Immunocompromised	Infection
Trauma	Fracture or displacement
History of cancer	Malignancy/metastasis
Nocturnal pain	Malignancy
Systemically unwell (temperature/weight loss/night sweats)	Infection
Thoracic pain	Inflammatory: ankylosing spondylitis Infection/malignancy Aortic dissection/pancreatitis
Saddle anaesthesia/bilateral sciatica/progressive neurological deficit	Cauda equina or cord compression
Bladder, bowel or sexual dysfunction	Cauda equina or cord compression

it is important to identify potential 'red flags,' which mandate further imaging or investigations, to exclude a potentially sinister underlying diagnosis. If red flag signs are present, then referral to a specialist for further evaluation is advised and a patient should be advised to rest and to avoid physical activity until then. Importantly, nerve root pain (unilateral sciatica) is not itself a cause for alarm, and conservative treatment should be effective. A list of red flag symptoms associated with back pain can be found in Table 15.5, with potential associated causes.

Pain may be referred or radiate from an affected joint (see Box 15.2). With these pain patterns in mind, the joints above and below the apparently affected area should be examined.

Chronic pain syndromes

Chronic pain syndromes need to be distinguished from other rheumatic disorders and a careful history is essential. A number of pain descriptors used by patients can indicate the influence of non-organic amplifying factors. For example, at least in the English language, words like 'searing,' 'torturing' and 'terrifying' can be used by patients with chronic widespread pain and fibromyalgia. Fibromyalgia falls under an umbrella term—Central Sensitization Syndromes (CSS) and so may present with overlapping symptoms with other conditions such as irritable bowel syndrome, chronic fatigue and temporo-mandibular joint (TMJ) disorders.

These debilitating disorders are often accompanied by poor sleep patterns, severe fatigue and depressed mood. The difficulty of cultural, religious and linguistic influences in interpreting pain should not be underestimated.

Joint disease

A combination of pain and stiffness, leading to loss of function, is a classic feature of joint disease. Usually one component predominates, as with stiffness in inflammation and pain in mechanical joint problems. Therefore, specific questions will establish whether symptoms are non-inflammatory (e.g. osteoarthritis) or inflammatory (e.g. rheumatoid arthritis). As with any condition, the good clinician will also draw out the consequences of the disorder in terms of the impact on the patient's day-to-day function and quality of life. The effect on relationships, work and social activities will help the clinician to gauge the severity of the problem and possibly elicit issues of stress and psychosocial pressure.

Non-inflammatory joint disease

Pain of a non-inflammatory origin is more directly related to function and use and usually is relieved with rest. This is in contrast to inflammatory joint pain, which is often present at rest as well as in use, and tends to vary from day to day and from week to week. Stiffness, particularly in the morning or after a period of inactivity, is often a feature in the history of inflammatory joint pain and typically lasts no more than 30 minutes. However, in severe cases the duration may be much longer. Subjective joint swelling may be described and indeed patients with knee osteoarthritis may present with a significant effusion. Joint swelling in this context tends to be more intermittent than the persistent joint swelling and warmth seen in inflammatory conditions.

Locking of a joint may occur. In the knee, this means that the knee becomes locked in such a way that it will not extend fully, although it may flex. In other joints, locking is less well defined and simply means that at some point through its range of motion the joint becomes stuck, usually associated with pain and often followed by swelling. Locking is caused by material within the joint interfering with movement at the articular surfaces. In the knee, this is usually part of one of the menisci or a cartilaginous loose body.

Inflammatory joint disease
Early morning stiffness

Early morning joint stiffness that persists for more than 30 minutes is an important symptom of active inflammatory joint disease. Ask about redness (rubor),

Figure 15.15 Gouty tophus on the ear. Other sites include the elbows, fingers and toes.

warmth (calor), tenderness/pain (dolor) and swelling (tumour), the classic features of inflammation.

Distribution of joint disease

The pattern of joint involvement is important. Common patterns are monoarticular (single joint), pauciarticular (up to four joints), polyarticular (many joints) and axial (spinal involvement). The pattern of joint involvement often aids in making a list of likely differential diagnoses. For example, rheumatoid arthritis is typically a symmetrical inflammatory arthritis of the small and large joints, often presenting with metacarpophalangeal (MCP), wrist and metatarsophalangeal (MTP) joint involvement. There are only a few causes of an exactly symmetrical arthropathy (Box 15.3). An asymmetrical inflammatory arthritis presentation is often seen in spondyloarthropathies, such as reactive arthritis. An inflammatory monoarthritis presentation must arouse a suspicion of infection alongside other potential conditions, such as gout or psoriatic arthritis. A history of fever or sweating may be helpful and, if possible, synovial fluid should be aspirated from the joint to look for an infection. Monoarthritis will certainly raise the suspicion of an infected joint, but may also be seen in the context of crystal arthropathies and spondyloarthropathies, particularly psoriatic arthritis in which the knee or elbow is often singularly affected. Other conditions have such a classic history that it is almost diagnostic. For example, acute inflammation in the first metatarsophalangeal joint (hallux) suggests a diagnosis of gout (Box 15.4). The pain and stiffness of the shoulder and hip girdles in polymyalgia rheumatica is also typical (Box 15.5). The pattern of the spondyloarthropathies can also be diagnostic with inflammatory sacroiliac and spinal pain and stiffness, lower limb arthritis, Achilles tendinitis and plantar fasciitis.

Recurrent attacks of joint pain

Ask if the same joint is always involved. If not, define the patterns of involvement, the severity and

Figure 15.16 Extensive rash in sun-exposed areas in a woman with systemic lupus crythematosus and anti-Ro antibodies.

Figure 15.17 Schirmer's test. A sterile strip of filter paper is hooked over the lower eyelid. Less than 5 mm of wetness after 5 minutes is abnormal and is associated with autoimmune rheumatic disease.

duration of the episodes and any associated clinical symptoms. Crystal arthropathies tend to affect the same joints recurrently with the first MTP joint most common followed by ankle and knee.

Episodic joint pain

Ask if attacks of joint pain are acute and associated with redness around the joint, with the attacks lasting about 48 hours (occasionally up to 1 week) and migrating to other joints. This is typical of palindromic rheumatism, which may progress to rheumatoid arthritis. Recurrent painful swelling of the same joint may be indicative of a crystal arthropathy, such as gout or calcium pyrophosphate disease.

Flitting or migratory joint pains

The term 'flitting' or migratory joint pains is used to describe inflammation beginning in one joint and then involving others, usually one at a time for about 3 days each. Gonococcal arthritis should be considered; this is characterized by typical fleeting skin lesions and urethritis, in addition to joint pain. In rheumatic fever, there is associated cardiac involvement, and erythema marginatum and subcutaneous nodules may occur.

The other features in the history that should be brought out are best considered under the differential diagnosis of polyarthritis (Box 15.6). Many arthropathies may have a monoarticular presentation.

Inflammatory connective tissue diseases

The autoimmune rheumatic disorders, such as systemic lupus erythematosus (SLE), Sjögren's syndrome, inflammatory myopathies, systemic sclerosis and the vasculitides, are multisystem disorders. It is critical that a full systems enquiry and physical examination are performed when inflammatory connective tissue is suspected. Associated features of these conditions include systemic symptoms, such as weight loss, malaise or fevers and rash, especially if the latter is photosensitive or vasculitic (Fig. 15.16). Alopecia, oral and genital ulceration, Raynaud's phenomenon and symptoms of neurological, cardiac, pulmonary and gastrointestinal involvement may occur. Dry eyes and dry mouth (sicca symptoms) are common and can be documented with Schirmer's test (Fig. 15.17). Renal disease is a serious complication of the autoimmune rheumatic disorders, especially in SLE and the systemic vasculitides. Clinical assessment should always include measuring blood pressure and dip-testing the urine for blood and protein and microscopy of the urine sediment for casts or dysmorphic red cells if this is positive. Ear, nose and throat involvement with sinusitis, facial pain and deafness are common in Wegener's granulomatosis and Churg–Strauss syndrome. A history of arterial and venous thromboses or miscarriages, especially in the context of livedo reticularis, should raise the suspicion of the antiphospholipid syndrome.

Soft tissue symptoms

Soft tissue problems, which are common, usually consist of pain, a dull ache, tenderness or swelling. In the elderly these symptoms often appear spontaneously, but in younger people there is

<table>
<tr><td>

Box 15.7 Localization of the site of articular and extra-articular features

Joint

- Diffuse pain and tenderness
- Generalized joint swelling
- Restriction of movement, usually in all directions of movement (specific to each joint)

Tendon

- Localized pain/tenderness at attachment (enthesis) or in the tendon substance
- Swelling, tendon sheath or paratendon
- Pain on resisted movement
- Sometimes pain on stretch (e.g. Achilles)

Ligament

- Localized pain/tenderness at attachment or in ligament substance
- Pain on stretch
- Instability, if major tear

Bursa

- Localized tenderness
- Pain on stretching adjacent structures

Muscle

- Localized or diffuse pain and tenderness
- Pain on resisted action
- Pain on stretch (e.g. hamstring)

</td></tr>
</table>

Figure 15.18 Thenar wasting owing to carpal tunnel syndrome. This is often associated with osteoarthritis. Note nodal change on the terminal interphalangeal joints of the index fingers.

Box 15.8 Examination of the musculoskeletal system

General observations

- Gait
- Posture
- Mobility
- Deformity
- Independence: use of wheelchair or walking aids
- Muscle wasting
- Long bones

Fractures

- Joints
- Tendons
- Skin

bursitis or enthesitis (inflammation at the attachment of a ligament or tendon to bone) accurately. A careful examination may reveal that the complaint and symptoms do not arise from joint pathology, but from soft tissue tendon or ligament structure next to the joint. This often changes the differential diagnosis. Movement of the joint region often elicits pain or discomfort in a particular direction, which can direct the clinician to the affected structure. Subacromial bursitis typically produces pain when the shoulder is abducted to 80° and resolves at 130° to 140°, described as a painful arc, whereas anterior and posterior movements are maintained.

The bones

Bone pain is characteristically deep seated and localized, but referred pain may confuse the clinical picture. In the case of fractures, unless pathological, almost always there will be a history of injury. In athletes, however, a fracture may be owing to chronic overuse, as in stress fractures of the tibia or metatarsals in runners. The spontaneous onset of pain may suggest Paget's disease (with bony enlargement, e.g. skull or tibia) or metastatic deposits. Infection must also be considered, particularly in younger patients or in immunodeficiency states. Consider also congenital or familial disorders as predisposing factors, for example multiple osteochondromata or brittle bone disease (osteogenesis imperfecta).

Examination

General Principles

Observe the patient entering the room (Box 15.8). Abnormalities of gait and posture may provide clues that can be pursued in history taking. Observation of any difficulty in undressing and getting onto the

usually a history of injury or overuse, through either occupation (e.g. tenosynovitis of the long flexor tendons of the hand) or sport (e.g. Achilles tendinitis in runners, shoulder rotator cuff tendinopathy in swimmers or throwers). It is important to define the exact site of the symptoms and the factors that either make them worse or induce relief. The mechanism of injury is also important and can help guide a focused examination. The localization of symptoms to specific soft tissue structures can be confirmed by careful examination (Box 15.7). The possible structures involved are joint, tendon, ligament, bursa and muscle. Local palpation may be enough to locate examination couch will further help in assessment. The patient must always be asked to stand and walk, even when it is obvious that this may be difficult. Note how much help the patient requires from others or from sticks, crutches, etc. The musculoskeletal system includes the muscles, bones, joints and soft-tissue structures, such as tendons and ligaments.

Remember that although muscle wasting may be caused by primary muscle disease (e.g. polymyositis), it is more commonly secondary to disuse, perhaps because of a painful joint, or to neuropathy owing to nerve root compression or peripheral neuropathy (Fig. 15.18). Examination of the muscles is discussed further in Chapter 16.

Figure 15.19 Paget's disease of the right tibia. Note tibial bowing and bony enlargement **(A)** and bony enlargement sclerosis with some patchy porosis in the X-ray of the upper tibia **(B)**.

Figure 15.20 Paget's disease, causing deformity of the skull **(A)**. Note the thickened skull vault with remodelled bone **(B)**.

The bones

The examination of the bones should always be directed by information obtained from the history.

Inspection

Look for any alterations in shape or outline and measure any shortening. In Paget's disease (osteitis deformans), bowing of the long bones, particularly the tibia (Fig. 15.19) and femur, is associated with bony enlargement and, usually, increased local temperature. The skull is also commonly involved, but this may not be apparent until the disease is advanced. Early involvement of the skull bones can be detected on X-rays (Fig. 15.20). Alterations in the shape of bones also occur in rickets as a result of epiphyseal enlargement. Deformity of the chest in rickets is caused by osteochondral enlargement (rickety rosary).

Localized swellings of long bones may be caused by infections, cysts or tumours. Spontaneous fractures may occasionally be the presenting symptom in the diagnosis of secondary carcinoma, multiple myeloma or generalized osteitis fibrosa cystica (hyperparathyroidism) or osteogenesis imperfecta.

Palpation

On palpation, bone tenderness occurs in local lesions when there is destruction, elevation or irritation of the periosteum, as in generalized osteitis fibrosa cystica, myelomatosis, bone infections, occasionally in carcinomatosis of bones and, rarely, in leukaemia. Injury is the most common cause.

Fractures

Fractures are common and may involve any bone. They are painful, distressing for the patient and expensive for the community (Box 15.9). Fractures in healthy bones commonly involve the long bones and are usually caused by trauma. Fractures of the wrists, hips and vertebrae are more frequently complications of bone disease, such as osteoporosis. Multiple rib fractures, caused by falls, may be found in heavy alcohol users but may only be seen as healed lesions on chest X-ray. Fractures occur without apparent trauma when a bone is weakened by disease, especially with metastatic malignant deposits in bone (pathological fractures). Traumatic fractures invariably present with local pain, swelling and loss of function, but pathological fractures may be relatively silent. The history will reveal the circumstances of the trauma, whether accidental or owing to physical abuse, and should be carefully documented, if necessary, with diagrams or digital photographs of the clinical findings. If clinical photographs are taken, prior written consent is needed.

Box 15.9	Fractures: clinical features

Type
- Closed
- Compound (open)

Complications
- Accompanying soft-tissue injury (indirect)

Features
- Haemorrhage
- Deformity
- Pain
- Crepitus
- Restricted movement

Cause
- Traumatic
- Spontaneous (osteoporosis or metabolic)
- Pathological

Examination of suspected fracture

Fractures may be open (compound) or closed. In closed fractures, the surrounding soft tissues are intact. In open fractures, the bone communicates with the surface of the skin, either because the primary injury has broken the overlying skin or because deformation at the fracture site has caused the bone ends to penetrate the skin. A major risk of infection exists when the fracture site communicates with the open air.

Deformity is an obvious feature in the majority of fractures, although in some patients this may be difficult to appreciate owing to a large body habitus. Comparison with the contralateral limb is often helpful. Deformity may be clinically characteristic, as in Colles' fracture, in which there is a fracture of the distal end of the radius characterized by dorsal displacement and angulation, shortening of the wrist and rotation of the fragment, well summarized in the description 'dinner-fork deformity'. Certain fractures may show little deformity; for example, a fracture of the femoral shaft may be accompanied by only slight deformity, because there is often little separation of the bones at the fracture site and other features are disguised by the thick overlying muscle. A fractured neck of the femur causes deformity through external rotation of the foot and shortening of the leg.

Most fractures are characterized by local tenderness and swelling, unless the overlying muscle mass is large, such as at the hip. Bony crepitus, owing to abnormal motion at the fracture site, is a feature of fractures, but this should not be elicited unless absolutely necessary for diagnosis because it is very painful. However, if it is perceived or has been recognized by the patient, it is diagnostic.

A fracture of the bone may damage the neighbouring soft tissues directly or, alternatively, a

Figure 15.21 Symmetrical joint involvement caused by rheumatoid arthritis.

Figure 15.22 Gouty tophus of the index finger.

Figure 15.23 Acute synovitis of the interphalangeal joint in reactive arthritis of the left hallux. Differential diagnosis includes gout.

fracture may be a marker of severe injury in which direct damage to the soft tissues, such as the nerves and vessels, may have taken place. A neuromuscular assessment distal to the fracture site is imperative. The presence or absence of pulses and cutaneous sensation and the colour and perfusion of the limb must always be recorded and any changes over time reported. Limb ischaemia distal to a fracture is a surgical emergency. Voluntary movement at joints distal to a fractured long bone, such as ankle movement in a fractured femur, should be noted. If this is absent, nerve injury must be suspected.

Figure 15.24 Nodal osteoarthritis (Heberden's nodes).

The joints

Examination of the joints can be summarized simply as 'look, feel and move' (i.e. inspection, palpation and range of movement). With practice, the clinician can develop a systematic review of the joints; for example, the jaw, cervical spine, shoulder girdle and upper limb, thoracic and lumbar spine, pelvis and lower limb, so that inconspicuous but important joints, such as the temporomandibular, sternoclavicular and sacroiliac joints, will not be overlooked. Compare the corresponding joints on the two sides of the body and always take care to avoid causing undue discomfort.

Inspection

The detection of joint inflammation is a crucial clinical skill. Inflammation is often associated with redness of the joint and with tenderness and warmth. Look also for swelling or deformity of the joint. The overall pattern of joint involvement should be recorded. Examine the contralateral joint where possible and note whether the distribution is symmetrical, as is usual in rheumatoid arthritis (Fig. 15.21), or asymmetrical, as in psoriatic arthropathy or gout (Fig. 15.22). The seronegative spondyloarthropathies (Fig. 15.23) tend to involve predominantly the joints of the lower limb.

Palpation

On palpation of a joint, check first for tenderness. Then determine whether the swelling is owing to bony enlargement or osteophytes (e.g. Heberden's nodes, Fig. 15.24), thickening of synovial tissues, such as occurs in inflammatory arthritis, or effusion into the joint space. Joint effusions usually have a characteristically smooth outline and fluctuation is usually easily demonstrable. Palpation of the whole joint is important because this may reveal localized enthesitis (e.g. lateral epicondylitis at the elbow) or reveal localized effusions (e.g. Baker's cyst in the posterior aspect of the knee joint). Tenderness and

Box 15.10	Assessment of joint tenderness

- Grade 1: The patient says the joint is tender.
- Grade 2: The patient winces.
- Grade 3: The patient winces and withdraws the affected part.
- Grade 4: The patient will not allow the joint to be touched.

Box 15.11	Extra-articular features of joint disease

- Cutaneous nodules
- Cutaneous vasculitic lesions
- Lymphadenopathy
- Oedema
- Tendon sheath effusions
- Enlarged bursae
- Ocular inflammation
- Diarrhoea
- Urethritis
- Orogenital ulceration
- Alopecia

Box 15.12	Types of subcutaneous nodules

- Gouty tophi caused by urate deposition
- Rheumatoid nodules
- Vasculitic nodules in systemic lupus erythematosus (SLE) and systemic vasculitis
- Xanthomatous deposits (hypercholesterolaemia)

Figure 15.25 Rheumatoid nodule overlying the olecranon of the right arm.

enlargement of the ends of long bones, particularly the radius, ulna and tibia, can occur in hypertrophic pulmonary osteoarthropathy; a chest X-ray is essential. Gross disorganization of a joint—nearly always the foot and ankle joints—associated with an absence of deep pain and position sense occurs in neuropathic (Charcot) joints. Charcot joints probably arise from recurrent painless injury and overstretching and are a feature of severe chronic sensorimotor neuropathy.

Joint tenderness may be graded depending on the patient's reaction to firm pressure of the joint between finger and thumb (Box 15.10). Grade 4 tenderness occurs only in septic arthritis, crystal arthritis and rheumatic fever.

If tenderness is present, localize it as accurately as possible and determine whether it arises in the joint or in neighbouring structures, for example in the supraspinatus or bicipital tendon rather than the shoulder joint. Other rheumatic conditions produce different types of pain. For example, in conditions such as complex regional pain syndrome (CRPS) type I (previously known as reflex sympathetic dystrophy), hyperalgesia (abnormal and excessive pain to mildly painful stimuli) and allodynia (a sensation of pain to stimuli not normally painful, e.g. light touch) may often be seen, together with altered sweating and discolouration. In fibromyalgia, there is widespread diffuse muscle and joint tenderness but no inflammation. A number of characteristic trigger points may be tender around the neck, trunk and upper and lower limbs.

Tendon sheath crepitus

Tendon sheath crepitus is a grating or creaking sensation defined by palpating the tendon while the patient is asked to contract the muscle tendon complex involved. It is particularly common in the hand and is seen in rheumatoid arthritis and systemic sclerosis. In tenosynovitis of the long flexor tendons in the palm, tendon sheath crepitus may be associated with the trigger phenomenon, in which the finger becomes caught in flexion and has to be pulled back into extension. Tendon sheath effusions can be distinguished from joint swelling by their anatomical location in association with tendons; where there is doubt, an ultrasonographic assessment will provide clarity.

Joint crepitus

Joint crepitus can be detected by feeling the joint with one hand while moving it passively with the other. This may indicate osteoarthritis or loose bodies (cartilaginous fragments) in the joint space, but should be differentiated from non-specific clicking of joints.

Range of movement

When examining joints for range of movement, it is usually sufficient to estimate the degree of limitation based on comparison with the normal side or on the examiner's previous experience. For an accurate description, the actual range of movement should be measured with a protractor (goniometer). Both active and passive movement should be assessed. Active movement, however, may give a poor estimation of the true range of movement because of muscle spasm owing to pain. If pain is very severe on attempting active movement and other findings suggest a fracture, take an X-ray before attempting any further examination. In testing the range of passive movement, always be gentle, particularly when the joints are painful. The direction of joint movement, particularly in ball and socket joints, may provide additional information as to the underlying lesion.

Limitation of movement in a joint may be owing to pain, muscle spasm, contracture, inflammation,

increased thickness of the capsular or periarticular structures, effusion into the joint space, bony overgrowths, bony ankylosis, mechanical factors such as a torn meniscus or to painful conditions quite unconnected with the joint.

Extra-articular features of joint disease

Some of the extra-articular features of joint disease are listed in Box 15.11.

Subcutaneous nodules

Subcutaneous nodules are associated with several conditions (Box 15.12). If gout is suspected, inspect the helix of the ear for tophi caused by the subcutaneous deposition of urate, which may also be found overlying joints or in the finger pads (see Figs 15.15 and 15.22). Subcutaneous nodules in rheumatoid arthritis are firm and non-tender; they may be detected by running the examining thumb from the point of the elbow down the proximal portion of the ulna (Fig. 15.25). They can also be found at other pressure and frictional sites, such as bony prominences, including the sacrum and in the hands. If an olecranon bursa swelling is found, feel also in its wall, as rheumatoid nodules, tophi or occasionally xanthomata may be found within the swelling. Subcutaneous nodules are not specific to rheumatoid arthritis and may occur in patients with SLE, systemic sclerosis and rheumatic fever. Ultrasonographic appearance may be helpful in distinguishing subcutaneous nodules and may facilitate a guide aspiration if necessary.

Cutaneous vasculitic lesions

Cutaneous vasculitic lesions may be seen in rheumatoid arthritis, SLE, Sjögren's syndrome and the systemic vasculitides. They may be small, punched-out necrotic lesions, palpable purpura or vasculitic ulcers, especially on the lower limbs. Small vessel involvement is typically seen at the nail fold (cutaneous infarct; Fig. 15.26), but it also occurs at pressure sites. Splinter haemorrhages, the classic feature of bacterial endocarditis, may also be a feature of vasculitis and the antiphospholipid syndrome.

Skin

Several rheumatological conditions occur with skin manifestations. Vasculitic skin lesions have already been mentioned earlier, but there may be other clues to possible underlying rheumatic conditions which should be actively sought during examination.

Skin psoriasis is a useful indication of possible psoriatic arthritis, particularly if there is associated nail pitting (Fig.15.27). Psoriasis is often noted on

Figure 15.26 Nail-fold vasculitis (**A**) A patient with dermatomyositis demonstrating nailfold infarcts at the cuticle and evidence of Gottrons papules on the dorsum of the MCP joints. (**B**) Nailfold infarcts seen in a patient with SLE.

Figure 15.27 Psoriartic arthritis. The patient has swelling of the distal interphalangeal joint (DIP) on the overlying right hand and third DIP joint of the left hand. Nail dystrophy with pitting is seen.

Figure 15.28 Patient with dermatomyositis presenting with a typical heliotrope rash around the eyes.

the extensor parts of the elbows and knees, but may be seen in the hairline, at the umbilicus, behind the ears as well as in the natal cleft.

Conditions, such as dermatomyositis, may present with the predominant dermatological manifestations such as peri-orbital oedema and purplish discolouration (Fig. 15.28). Gottrons papules are often noted on extensor surfaces at the level of the metacarpophalangeal joints (Fig.15.26).

Skin ulceration can also be seen in the context of vasculitis and typically are well-defined punched lesions, e.g. Felty's syndrome.

Lymphadenopathy

Lymphadenopathy may be found proximal to an inflamed joint, not only in septic arthritis but also in rheumatoid arthritis. Generalized lymphadenopathy, sometimes with splenomegaly, is common in active SLE.

Local oedema

Local oedema is sometimes seen over inflamed joints (Fig. 15.29), but other causes of oedema must be excluded. Pitting leg oedema may indicate cardiac failure, pericardial effusion or nephrotic syndrome, which can complicate rheumatoid arthritis and SLE.

Other soft-tissue swellings

Tendon sheath effusions are distinguished from joint swellings by their location in association with tendons. Enlarged subcutaneous bursae may be found over pressure areas, particularly at the olecranon surface of the elbow, owing to inflammatory joint disease or secondary to friction. Deeper bursae may be defined only by finding local tenderness or by stressing adjacent tissues (e.g. greater trochanter bursitis).

Figure 15.29 Pitting oedema, right hand.

Examination of individual joints

The range of movement of joints is described in the following pages. All motion should be measured in degrees from a neutral or zero position, which must be defined whenever possible and compared with the opposite side. Some special features seen at individual joints are set out in each section.

The spine

General examination of the vertebral column

Inspection

Examine the patient both in standing and in sitting in the erect posture. The normal thoracolumbar spine has an S-shaped curve. If there is an abnormality, note which vertebrae are involved and at what level any vertebral projection is most prominent. Note the presence of any local projections or angular deformity of the spine. Torticollis, if present, is usually obvious, resulting from muscle spasm of

Figure 15.30 Scoliosis of the lumbar spine owing to a prolapsed intervertebral disc.

Figure 15.31 Gibbus of the lumbar spine caused by tuberculosis.

Figure 15.32 X-ray of tuberculous discitis. This shows the underlying deformity shown in Figure 15.31. There is tuberculous infection of the intervertebral disc, causing the spinal deformity.

the sternocleidomastoid, trapezius and other neck muscles. This leads to the neck being in a tilted, rotated, partially flexed position.

Palpation

The major landmarks are the spinous processes of C7 (the vertebra prominens) and the last rib, which articulates with the 12th thoracic vertebra. In many patients, however, the last rib cannot be felt distinctly, which therefore makes this rather untrustworthy as a guide to this level.

The neutral position of the spine is an upright stance with the head erect and the chin drawn in. Note any curvature of the spinal column, whether as a whole or a part of it. Abnormal curvature may be in an anterior, posterior or lateral direction (Fig. 15.30). Anterior curvature (convex forward) is termed lordosis. There are natural lordotic curves in the cervical and lumbar regions. Posterior curvature (convex backward) is termed kyphosis. The thoracic spine usually exhibits a slight smooth kyphosis, which increases in the elderly and especially in osteoporosis. It must be distinguished from a localized angular deformity (gibbus, Fig. 15.31) caused by a fracture, by Pott's disease (spinal tuberculosis, Fig. 15.32) or by a metastatic malignant deposit.

Lateral curvature is termed scoliosis (see Fig. 15.30) and may be towards either side. It is always accompanied by rotation of the bodies of the vertebrae in such a way that the posterior spinous processes come to point towards the concavity of the curve. The curvature is always greater than appears from inspection of the posterior spinous processes. In scoliosis owing to muscle spasm (e.g. with lumbosacral disc protrusion syndromes), the spinal curvature and rotational deformity decrease in flexion. When scoliosis is caused by inequality of leg length, it disappears on sitting, because the buttocks then become level. Scoliosis secondary to skeletal anomalies shows in spinal flexion as a 'rib hump' owing to the rotation. Kyphosis and scoliosis are often combined, particularly when the cause is an idiopathic spinal curvature, beginning in adolescence.

The cervical spine

The following movements should be tested (Fig. 15.33):
- Rotation: ask the patient to look over one then the other shoulder.
- Flexion: ask the patient to touch chin to chest.
- Extension: ask the patient to look up to the ceiling.
- Lateral bending: ask the patient to bend the neck sideways and to try to touch the shoulder with the ear without raising the shoulder.

Note any pain or paraesthesiae in the arm reproduced by neck movement, especially on gentle sustained extension or lateral flexion, suggesting nerve-root involvement. If indicated, check for any associated neurological deficit, particularly of radicular or spinal cord type.

In rheumatoid arthritis, particular care is necessary when examining the neck, as atlantoaxial instability may lead to damage to the spinal cord when the neck is flexed. If there is any doubt about neck stability in a patient with rheumatoid arthritis, arrange for lateral X-rays of the cervical spine in flexion and extension, together with a view of the odontoid peg through the mouth, and defer clinical examination.

In patients with cervical injury, never try to elicit range of motion of the neck. Instead, splint the neck, take a history, look for abnormality of posture (usually in rotation) and check neurological function in the limbs, including both arms and both legs. Imaging the neck in the lateral (Fig. 15.34) and anteroposterior planes, *without* moving the neck, is essential and may be done with plain radiography or, in trauma patients, with computed tomography or magnetic resonance imaging (MRI) to assess injury to the cord. Only if imaging is normal should neck movements be examined.

The thoracic and lumbar spine

The main movement at the thoracic spine is rotation, whereas the lumbar spine can flex, extend and bend laterally. The following movements should be tested (Fig. 15.35):
- Flexion: ask the patient to try to touch his toes, without bending at the knees.
- Extension: ask the patient to bend backwards.
- Lateral bending: ask the patient to run the hand down the side of the thigh as far as possible.
- Thoracic rotation: ask the seated patient, with arms crossed, to twist round to the left and right as far as possible.

In flexion, the normal lumbar lordosis should be abolished. It is important to distinguish between flexion at the lumbar spine and compensated flexion

Figure 15.34 Lateral X-ray of cervical spine showing degenerative spondylosis with narrowing of the disc spaces and reversed cervical lordosis between C4 and C6.

Neutral   Rotation

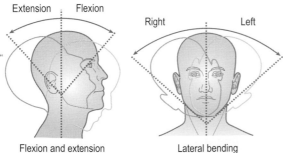

Flexion and extension   Lateral bending

Figure 15.33 Movements of the neck.

at the hips, which may deceive the examiner if only a cursory examination is carried out. A more objective assessment of lumbar spine flexion can be performed by marking a vertical 10-cm line on the skin overlying the lumbar spinous processes and the sacral dimples and measuring the increase in the line length on flexion (modified Schober's test); this should normally be 5 cm or more. Painful restriction of spinal movement is an important sign of cervical and lumbar spondylosis, but it may also be found in vertebral disc disease or other mechanical disorders of the back or neck in association with muscle spasm. A useful clinical aphorism is that a rigid lumbar spine should always be investigated for serious pathology, such as infection (e.g. staphylococcal or tuberculous discitis), malignancy or inflammation (e.g. ankylosing spondylitis). Spinal movements may be virtually absent in ankylosing spondylitis (Fig. 15.36), but in the early stages of this condition lateral flexion of the lumbar spine is typically affected first. In mechanical or osteoarthritic back problems, flexion and extension are reduced more than lateral movements. In prolapsed intervertebral disc lesions, sustained gentle lumbar extension may reproduce the low back pain and sciatic radiation.

Chest expansion is a measure of costovertebral movement and should be recorded using a tape measure with the patient's hands behind his head to reduce the possibility of muscular action in the shoulder girdle giving a false reading. The examiner stands behind the patient and the tape measure is placed around the chest at the level of the xiphisternal joint. The patient is asked to exhale and the tape is tightened before a maximum inhalation. An increase of 5 cm is expected in adults. Reduced chest expansion is a characteristic early feature in ankylosing spondylitis. Obviously, this may also be a feature of primary pulmonary disease, such as emphysema.

Examination of the back is completed by assessing straight leg raising (SLR) and strength, sensation and reflex activity in the legs. Pain and limitation on SLR are features of a prolapsed intervertebral disc when there is irritation or compression of one of the roots of the sciatic nerve. Tight hamstring muscles may cause a similar picture, but if there is severe pain, it is more considerate to lower the leg to just below the limit of SLR and then to see whether gentle passive dorsiflexion of the foot brings back the same pain. If in doubt, dorsiflex the foot once the limit of SLR has been reached. This further stretches the sciatic nerve (the pain increases) but does not affect the hamstrings (Lasègue's sign). The femoral stretch test is a useful confirmatory test. It is performed with the patient lying prone: if there is a prolapsed disc at that level, flexion at the knee will produce

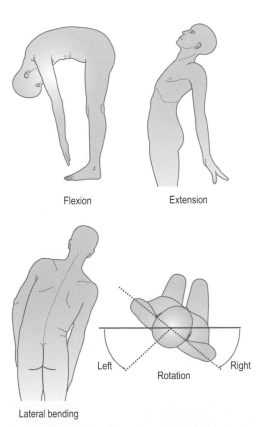

Flexion   Extension

Left   Rotation   Right

Lateral bending

Figure 15.35 Movements of the lumbar and dorsal spine.

Figure 15.36 Ankylosing spondylitis. Note dorsal kyphosis and protuberant abdomen owing to poor chest expansion with abdominal breathing.

Neutral (adduction)

Rotation in neutral adduction

Extension   Flexion

Flexion and extension

Abduction

Painful arc

External

Internal

(A)   Rotation in abduction

Elevation

(B)

Figure 15.37   **(A)** Movements of the shoulder. **(B)** Painful arc of supraspinatus tendinitis.

pain in the lower lumbar spine. Sacral sensory loss must always be carefully assessed because, if there is a large central lumbosacral disc protrusion, bilateral limitation of SLR may be associated with bladder or bowel dysfunction and sacral anaesthesia. This combination is an emergency and requires immediate investigation and treatment.

The sacroiliac joints

The surface markings of these joints are two dimples low in the lumbar region. Test for irritability in the following ways:

- Direct pressure over each sacroiliac joint
- Firm pressure with the side of the hand over the sacrum
- Inward pressure over both iliac bones with the patient lying on one side, in an attempt to distort the pelvis
- Flex the hip to 90° and exert firm pressure at the knee through the femoral shaft (this should only be done if the hip and knee are not painful).

In the last three, a positive test is only indicated by the patient localizing discomfort to the sacroiliac joint.

The shoulder

Shoulder examination involves the assessment of a number of other joints in addition to the glenohumeral articulation. Abduction of the shoulder particularly involves movement at the sternoclavicular, acromioclavicular, glenohumeral and scapulothoracic joints. Pain is also referred and the shoulder examination should be accompanied by an examination of the cervical spine, because radicular pain may be localized by the patient at the shoulder and vice versa.

Inspection of the shoulder should be from the posterior, lateral and anterior positions. Where possible, the contralateral shoulder should be exposed and comparisons made in muscle bulk.

Palpation of the shoulder should include the long head of the biceps tendon in the bicipital groove, acromioclavicular joint, clavicle, sternoclavicular joint and the acromion.

The neutral position is with the arm to the side, elbow flexed to 90° and forearm pointing forwards. Because the scapula is mobile, true shoulder (glenohumeral) movement can be assessed only when the examiner anchors the inferior angle of the scapula between finger and thumb on the posterior chest wall. The following movements should be tested (Fig. 15.37):

- Flexion
- Extension
- Abduction
- Rotation in abduction
- Rotation in neutral position
- Elevation (also involving scapular movement)

In practice, internal rotation can be compared best by recording the height reached by each thumb up the back, representing combined glenohumeral and scapular movement. Similarly, external rotation can be assessed by the ability to get the hand to the back of the neck. Limitation of external rotation is a good sign of true glenohumeral disease, which may occur in adhesive capsulitis (frozen shoulder) or erosive damage from inflammatory arthritis.

Note any pain during the range of movement. In supraspinatus tendinitis, a full passive range of movement is found, but there is a painful arc on abduction, with pain exacerbated on resisted abduction (see Fig. 15.37). Other tendon involvement should also be defined by pain on resisted action.

Subacromial impingement owing to a bursitis or rotator cuff abnormality may produce severe pain at the end of abduction, blocking full elevation. Acute bursitis, however, may be so painful that no abduction is allowed (grade 4 discomfort). Acromioclavicular joint pain is always very localized and is typically felt in the last 10° of elevation (170° to 180° arc).

Special tests, as follows, are used in shoulder examination.

Supraspinatus

The supraspinatus muscle can be tested using the 'empty can' test, which involves forward flexion of the arm to 90° and abduction to 30° with the thumb pointing upwards. The shoulder is then internally rotated so that the thumb is now facing downwards. The examiner places his hand on the arm and exerts downward pressure while the patient resists. Weakness or significant pain may indicate a muscle tear and further imaging is recommended (ultrasound (US) or MRI). It is recommended that both arms be used in this test for comparison purposes.

Subscapularis

The patient is asked to place his hand behind the back with the dorsum of the hand resting in the region of the mid-lumbar spine (mainly internal rotation at the glenohumeral joint). The ability actively to lift the dorsum of the hand off the back constitutes a normal test with no dysfunction or rupture of subscapularis.

Infraspinatus and teres minor

Hornblower's sign is an inability to rotate the elevated arm externally. This movement indicates severe infraspinatus and teres minor weakness.

Long head of biceps

Hueter sign may indicate a ruptured tendon. The patient is seated with the elbow extended and

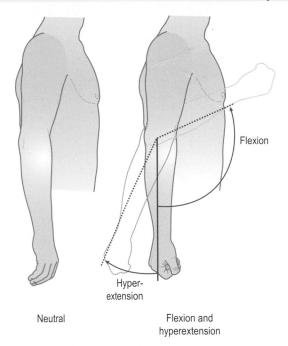

Figure 15.38 Movements of the elbow.

forearm supinated. The elbow is then flexed by the patient against resistance. If the tendon is ruptured, a biceps 'ball' develops.

Yergason's test indicates if there is bicipital tendinitis. The patient's elbow is flexed and the forearm pronated. The examiner holds the arm at the wrist while the patient actively supinates against resistance. If this resisted movement produces pain located to the bicipital groove area, then pathology within the long head of the biceps tendon sheath is likely.

The elbow

The neutral position is with the forearm in extension. The following movements should be tested (Fig. 15.38) as follows:
- Flexion
- Hyperextension

Medial (golfer's elbow) and lateral (tennis elbow) epicondylitis are the most common causes of elbow pain. They are characterized by pain on active use but, if severe, may be associated with night pain.

Examination must define localized epicondylar tenderness with pain on resisted movement. Wrist extension exacerbates lateral epicondylar tenderness and wrist flexion exacerbates medial epicondylar tenderness. An elbow effusion may be palpated in the posterior triangle formed by the epicondyles and the olecranon.

Placing the thumb and second and third fingers on the lateral, medial epicondyles and olecranon, respectively, with the joint in an extended position produces a straight alignment. In a flexed position

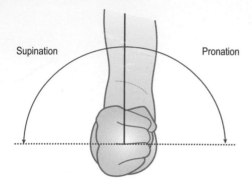

Supination and pronation

Figure 15.39   Movements of the forearm.

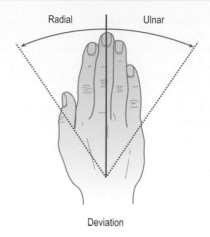

Deviation

these three points form a triangular shape. Disturbance of this geometric shift may indicate a supracondylar fracture.

The forearm

The neutral position is with the arm by the side, elbow flexed to 90° and thumb uppermost. The following movements should be tested (Fig. 15.39):
- Supination
- Pronation

The wrist

Inspection of the wrist may reveal clear evidence of joint swelling or localized tenosynovitis. The distal ulna is usually visible as a smooth, rounded protrusion. Loss of the normal anatomical landmarks may suggest joint or tendon inflammation.

Palpation of the wrist for warmth and swelling should be performed as well as specific palpation for tendon and bone discomfort. Palpation over the anatomical snuff box resulting in pain may indicate a scaphoid fracture if there is a history of trauma. Tenderness along the ulnar aspect of the wrist may suggest inflammation of the extensor carpi ulnas tendon, commonly involved in early rheumatoid arthritis. At the distal end of the anatomical snuff box the base of the thumb (first carpal-metacarpal joint) can be palpated, which is a commonly affected joint in generalized osteoarthritis in middle-aged and older patients.

The neutral position is with the hand in line with the forearm, and palm down. The following movements should be tested (Fig. 15.40):
- Dorsiflexion (extension)
- Palmar flexion
- Ulnar deviation
- Radial deviation

Even minor limitation of wrist flexion or extension can be detected by comparing movement in both

Neutral

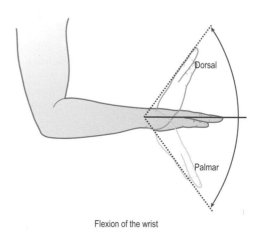

Flexion of the wrist

Figure 15.40   Movements of the wrist.

wrists (Fig. 15.41). Limitation of the wrist joints is usually caused by inflammatory arthritis. Primary osteoarthritis of the wrist is rare, but secondary degenerative change is common.

The fingers

When identifying fingers, use the names thumb, index, middle, ring and little. Numbering tends to lead to confusion. The neutral position is with the fingers in extension. Test flexion at the metacarpophalangeal

Figure 15.41 Minor limitation of left wrist extension compared with the right. Note the slightly different angulation of the left forearm.

Neutral

Flexion of MCP   Proximal IP   Distal IP joints

Figure 15.42 Movements of the fingers.

Neutral

Extension   Opposition

Figure 15.43 Movements of the thumb.

- Extension
- Flexion (measured as for the fingers)
- Opposition
- Abduction (not illustrated; movement at right angles to plane of palm)

The hand

Deformities in joint disease

Examination of the individual joints of the hand may be less informative than inspection of the hand as a whole (Fig. 15.44). The combination of Heberden's nodes and thumb carpometacarpal arthritis occurs in osteoarthritis (see Fig. 15.24). Pain and subluxation of the carpometacarpal joint is a typical feature of primary nodal osteoarthritis, leading to a 'square hand' appearance on making a fist.

A variety of patterns of deformity are characteristic of long-standing rheumatoid arthritis. For example, metacarpophalangeal joint subluxation, ulnar deviation of the fingers at the metacarpophalangeal joints, 'swan neck' (Fig. 15.45) and 'boutonnière' deformities (flexed proximal and hyperextended distal interphalangeal joints) of the fingers are typical in advanced disease. This is owing to the head of the phalanx sliding dorsally between the lateral slips of the extensor tendon, the middle slip having been damaged. In psoriatic arthritis, terminal interphalangeal joint swelling may occur, with psoriatic pitting and ridging of the nail (onychopathy) on that digit. Jaccoud's arthropathy

(MCP), proximal interphalangeal (PIP) and distal interphalangeal (DIP) joints (Fig. 15.42).

In fractures of the fingers, the most common deformity is rotational. If the finger will flex, make sure it points to the scaphoid tubercle (all the fingers will point individually in this direction). If it will not flex, look end-on at the nail and make sure it is parallel with its fellows.

The thumb (carpometacarpal joint)

The neutral position is with the thumb alongside the forefinger, and extended. The following movements should be tested (Fig. 15.43):

Figure 15.44 Functional ability. Severe joint deformity owing to psoriatic arthropathy, but retention of function and artistic ability.

Figure 15.45 Swan-neck deformity of the right hand. Note also wasting of the small muscles of the hand owing to disuse in this patient with rheumatoid arthritis.

produces a similar appearance to swan neck and boutonnière deformity alongside thumb subluxation and ulnar deviation. However, these deformities are reducible when the patient is asked to make a fist as a result of no underlying structural joint damage. This arthropathy may be seen in SLE and Sjögren's syndrome.

Deformities owing to neuropathy

The hand may adopt a posture typical of a nerve lesion (see Chapter 16). Slight hyperextension of the medial metacarpophalangeal joints with slight flexion of the interphalangeal joints is the 'ulnar claw hand' of an ulnar nerve lesion. There is wasting of the small muscles of the hypothenar eminence, with loss of sensation of the palmar and dorsal aspects of the little finger and of the ulnar half of the ring finger. In a median nerve lesion, the thenar eminence (abductor pollicis brevis) will be flattened (see Fig. 15.18) and sensory impairment will be found on the palmar surfaces of the thumb, index, middle and radial half of the ring fingers. Remember that carpal tunnel syndrome may be a presenting feature of wrist inflammation.

Box 15.13 Hip movements to be tested

- Flexion: measured with knee bent. Opposite thigh must remain in neutral position. Flex the knee as the hip flexes.
- Abduction: measured from a line that forms an angle of 90° with a line joining the anterior superior iliac spines.
- Adduction (measured in the same manner).
- Rotation in flexion.
- Rotation in extension.
- Extension: attempt to extend the hip with the patient lying in the lateral or prone position.

Assessment of hand function

Assessment of hand function (see Fig. 15.44) should include testing hand grip and pinch grip (between index and thumb). The latter may be decreased in lesions in the line of action of the thumb metacarpal, particularly scaphoid fractures.

The hip

The neutral position is with the hip in extension and the patella pointing forwards. Ensure the pelvis does not tilt by placing one hand over it while examining the hip with the other hand. Look for scars and wasting of the gluteal and thigh muscles. The hip joint is too deeply placed to be accessible to palpation. Hip movements to be tested are listed in Box 15.13 (Fig. 15.46).

Additional examination of the hip joint

- Test for flexion deformity. With one hand flat between the lumbar spine and the couch, flex the normal hip fully to the point of abolishing the lumbar lordosis. The spine will come down onto the hand, pressing it onto the couch. If there is a flexion deformity on the opposite side, the leg on that side will move into a flexed position (Thomas' test).
- Trendelenburg test. Observe the patient from behind and ask him to stand on one leg. In health, the pelvis tilts upwards on the side with the leg raised. When the weight-bearing hip is abnormal, owing to pain or subluxation, the pelvis sags downwards owing to weakness of the hip abductors on the affected side.
- Measurement of 'true' and 'apparent' shortening. The length of the legs is measured from the anterior superior iliac spine to the medial malleolus on the same side. Any difference is termed 'true' shortening and may result from disease of either the hip joint or the neck of the femur on the shorter side. 'Apparent' shortening is caused by tilting of the pelvis and can be measured by comparing the lengths of the two legs, measured from the umbilicus, provided there is no true shortening

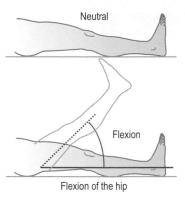

Neutral

Flexion

Flexion of the hip

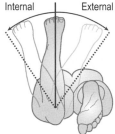

Internal External

Rotation in extension

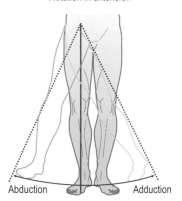

Abduction Adduction

Abduction and adduction

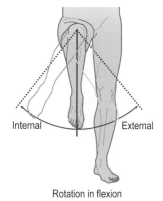

Internal External

Rotation in flexion

Figure 15.46 Movements of the hip.

of one leg. Apparent shortening is usually caused by an abduction deformity of the hip. Femoral or tibial shortening may be demonstrated with the patient lying on a couch and looking across both knees held equally flexed.

The knee

Magnetic resonance imaging scans of the normal knee are illustrated in Figure 15.47. The neutral position is complete extension. Observe any valgus (lateral angulation of the tibia) or varus (medial angulation) deformity on the couch and on standing. Look for muscle wasting. The quadriceps, especially the medial part near the knee, wastes rapidly in knee joint disease. Swelling may be obvious, particularly if it distends the suprapatellar pouch. Check the apparent height of the patella and watch to see if it deviates to one side in flexion or extension of the knee. Feel for tenderness at the joint margins, not forgetting the patellofemoral joint. Palpate the ligaments, remembering that the medial collateral ligament is attached 8 cm below the joint line. Measure the girth of the thigh muscles 10 cm above the upper pole of the patella.

Joint swelling

The presence of swelling in the knee joint may be confirmed by the patellar tap test or, for small effusions, by the bulge test, in which the medial parapatellar fossa is emptied by pressure of the flat of the hand sweeping proximally. The bulge is seen to refill as the suprapatellar area is emptied by pressure from the flat hand. Posterior knee joint (Baker's) cysts, particularly in rheumatoid arthritis, may be palpable in the popliteal fossa. They sometimes rupture, producing calf pain, and may then mimic a deep vein thrombosis. When intact, large posterior knee cysts can sometimes cause venous obstruction.

The movements of the knee are flexion and extension (Fig. 15.48). Loss of flexion can be documented by loss of the angle of flexion or loss of heel-to-buttock distance, either in the crouching position or on the couch. Loss of extension is detected by the inability to get the back of the knee onto the flat examining couch. Hyperextension must be sought by lifting the foot with the knee extended and comparing it with the normal side. Lack of full extension by comparison with the normal constitutes fixed flexion deformity. Loose bodies in the joint cause crepitus, interruption of movement (locking) and pain and effusion (Fig. 15.49).

Testing for stability

Cruciate ligaments

Anterior/posterior drawer test. The patient should be situated on the couch with the knee placed in 90° flexion. If there is a posterior sag on inspection, this may provide a false-positive anterior drawer sign. Place both hands around the upper part of the leg with both thumbs placed on the tibial tuberosity and fingers around the posterior aspect of the knee. With your forearm resting on the shin, firmly pull

Figure 15.47 Magnetic resonance imaging (MRI) scans of the normal knee (MRI, T1-weighted). **(A)** Scan to show the medial (5) and lateral (6) menisci, origin of the anterior cruciate ligament (4) and the articular cartilages (3) and synovial fluid (7). Other structures shown are (1) tibia, (2) articular surfaces of femur. **(B)** The anterior cruciate ligament (4). Other structures shown are (1) tibia, (2) femur, (3) patella. **(C)** The posterior cruciate ligament (4). Other structures shown are (1) tibia, (2) femur, (3) patella, (5) patellar tendon, (6) joint space.

the tibia anterior. A significant forward movement of the tibia plateau suggests an anterior cruciate tear. Pushing backwards with posterior movement of the tibial plateau may suggest a posterior cruciate pathology.

Collateral ligaments

The collateral ligaments are best assessed with the knee in 30° of flexion. Place your right hand on the lower limb (medial mid-calf) and left hand on the upper lateral thigh. Gradually apply opposing force to detect excessive medial movement of the lower limb. This tests the integrity of the medial collateral ligament. Reverse hand positions (left hand on lateral mid-calf and right hand on medial lower thigh) and repeat the movement to test the lateral collateral ligament. Pain on testing indicates possible

enthesitis or tear. Excessive movement can be seen in the context of joint hypermobility, which should be considered as part of the overall examination.

The ankle

The ankle is a hinge joint with movement only in the sagittal plane. The neutral position is with the outer border of the foot at an angle of 90° with the leg and midway between inversion and eversion. Observe the patient from behind in the standing position. With any long-standing ankle disorder, there will be a loss of calf muscle bulk.

Look at the position of the foot with the patient standing. The heel may tilt outwards (valgus deformity) in subtalar joint damage. Inward (varus

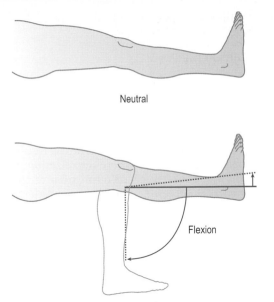

Neutral

Neutral

Flexion

Figure 15.48   Movements of the knee.

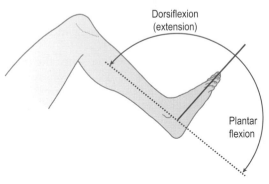

Dorsiflexion
(extension)

Plantar
flexion

Figure 15.50   Movements of the ankle.

Figure 15.49   Loose body in tunnel view X-ray of knee, showing the loose body in the intercondylar space.

Figure 15.51   Daylight sign owing to metatarsophalangeal joint synovitis in rheumatoid arthritis.

- Dorsiflexion: test with the knee in flexion and extension to exclude tight calf muscles.
- Plantarflexion: place a finger on the head of the talus to be sure that it is moving. A hypermobile subtalar joint can mimic movement in an arthrodesed ankle.

The foot

Remember that complaints apparently relating to the foot may be features of systemic disease, such as gout, or of referred vertebral problems, such as a prolapsed intervertebral disc. Look for abnormalities of posture.

Callosities are areas of hard skin under points of abnormal pressure. The most common site is beneath the metatarsal heads because loss of the normal soft tissue pad allows abnormal loading. There may be abnormal spread of two adjacent toes (daylight sign: Fig. 15.51) on weight-bearing if there

deformity) is much less common and usually not so painful. Flattening of the longitudinal arch of the foot (pes planus) also produces valgus at the heel, but the foot curves laterally as well because the change is in the mid-tarsal joints in addition to the subtalar joint.

The following movements should be tested (Fig. 15.50):

is synovitis between the metatarsal heads. Check for lateral deviation of the big toe (hallux valgus), usually associated with abnormal swelling at its base (a bunion). There may be deformities affecting any or all toes, with abnormal curvature (claw toes), fixed flexion of the terminal joint (hammer toes) or overriding.

The foot consists of three regions: hindfoot (subtalar joint), mid-foot (tarsal joints) and forefoot (MTP, PIP, DIP joints). The following movements should be tested (Fig. 15.52):

- Subtalar inversion and eversion: cup the heel in the hands and move it in relation to the tibia without any up and down movement; this eliminates movement at the ankle or mid-tarsal joints.
- Mid-tarsal inversion/eversion and adduction/abduction: hold the os calcis in the neutral position in one hand and grasp and rotate the forefoot in the other.
- Metatarsophalangeal and interphalangeal flexion/extension.

Also look for tenderness or swelling at the Achilles tendon insertion on the back of the calcaneum and for plantar tenderness at the site of the plantar fascial insertion. Inflammation of these attachments (enthesopathy) is common in ankylosing spondylitis and other spondyloarthropathies.

Achilles tendon rupture

Thompson test: This test requires the patient to be in the prone position with the feet hanging off the table. The clinician then squeezes the patient's calf muscle, which should shorten the Achilles tendon causing the ankle to plantar flex. It is important to note that false-negative results may occur in older injuries, where organization of a hematoma can cause some reconstitution of the tendon or with an incomplete partial tear. Patients may still be able to walk and actively plantar flex the ankle despite significant Achilles tendon tear. Achilles rupture is most often seen in the context of sport or with a clear history of trauma but may also occur in patients with spondyloarthropathies. When an index of suspicion of an Achilles tear or rupture arises, imaging with ultrasound or MRI is recommended.

The gait

It is best to study gait with the patient's legs and feet fully exposed and *without* socks, shoes or slippers. Ask the patient to walk away from you, to turn around at a given point and then to walk towards you.

Abnormalities of gait usually are caused either by joint problems in the legs or by a neurological disorder, although alcohol intoxication or malingering may occasionally cause difficulty. A full examination of the legs and feet should reveal any local cause, which may range from a painful corn to osteoarthritis of the hip. Abnormalities caused by neurological disorders are described in Chapter 16.

Eversion   Inversion

1

Forefoot adduction   Forefoot abduction   Flexion   Extension

2   3

Figure 15.52 Movements of the foot.

Figure 15.53 Hyperextensibility of the digits in Ehlers-Danlos syndrome.

Hypermobility

There is a wide variation in the range of normal joint movement, associated with age, sex and race. Excessive laxity or hypermobility of the joints (Fig. 15.53) can be defined in about 10% of healthy subjects and is frequently familial. It is also a feature of two inherited connective tissue disorders, Marfan syndrome and Ehlers-Danlos syndrome. Repeated trauma, haemarthrosis or dislocation may produce permanent joint damage. Hypermobility is often generalized but may occur at a single joint and must be considered if considerable joint laxity is demonstrated on examination. Hypermobility is often overlooked and should be considered in patients with joint pain with a lack of inflammatory or degenerative features on examination.

Work-related musculoskeletal disorders

Musculoskeletal pain arising as a result of a patient's occupation is an increasingly recognized cause of disability and economic loss. For example, spinal pain may be ascribed to poor seating in sedentary occupations. Likewise, an occupational history of repetitive movements may be relevant to upper limb pain. Assessment by an occupational health physician and an occupational therapist may be needed to consider workplace alterations.

Investigations in rheumatic diseases

When a full history and examination have been completed, investigations should be considered to support the working diagnosis or to distinguish between different possible diagnoses. They can be defined broadly as:
- Tests in support of inflammatory disease
- Diagnostic tests, including biopsies and imaging investigations

Tests in support of inflammatory disease

The acute-phase reactant tests that are used in the assessment of inflammatory disease activity and in the subsequent monitoring of the patient are listed in Box 15.14.

Diagnostic tests

Diagnostic tests differentiate between specific diseases and are relatively specific investigations.

Tests for rheumatoid factor

Rheumatoid factors are autoantibodies in the form of immunoglobulin (Ig) directed against other immunoglobulin G (IgG) molecules. IgM rheumatoid factor can be detected by its ability to clump particles coated with human IgG (latex test). This test is positive in about 80% of patients with rheumatoid arthritis. Results are reported as a titre, 1:80 or higher being a positive result. The original Rose-Waaler haemagglutination test used sheep erythrocytes coated with rabbit IgG to detect IgM (titres of 1:32 or more are positive); it has now been replaced by other tests. Enzyme-linked immunosorbent serum assay (ELISA) techniques are much more sensitive but produce positive results in many other conditions. Anti-citrullinated protein/peptide antibodies (ACPA) are a specific marker for rheumatoid arthritis and their presence indicates a poor prognosis, with patients at greater risk of joint damage, disability and loss of function.

These rheumatoid factor screening tests are useful where a diagnosis of rheumatoid arthritis is suspected, but they are not specific. Rheumatoid factor is frequently found in patients with other connective tissue diseases, for example SLE and Sjögren's syndrome, or other inflammatory disorders, such as subacute bacterial endocarditis and some viral infections.

Box 15.14	Common biochemical tests for inflammatory rheumatic conditions

Acute-phase reactant tests that are used in the assessment of inflammatory disease activity and in the subsequent monitoring of the patient:

- Erythrocyte sedimentation rate (ESR). This is a useful screening test, although it has poor specificity, being affected by the levels of haemoglobin, globulins and fibrinogen. Higher mean values are seen in healthy, elderly individuals.
- C-reactive protein (CRP). This is a more specific indicator of inflammation and is a good marker of the acute-phase response. A high ESR with a normal CRP is a useful pointer towards autoimmune rheumatic diseases, especially systemic lupus erythematosus (SLE).
- Plasma viscosity. This is a more specific measure of the acute-phase response than ESR, but may not be as widely available.
- Anaemia and thrombocytosis. Anaemia of chronic disease and a high platelet count often occur in inflammatory disease, but are non-specific. Other abnormalities on blood count, such as neutropenia, thrombocytopenia and lymphopenia, are common in SLE.
- Serum complement. Low levels of serum complement reflect activation owing to immune complex deposition; this may be a marker of disease activity in autoimmune diseases, such as SLE. Hereditary complement deficiencies are also associated with SLE.
- Muscle enzymes. Elevated creatine kinase levels occur in most patients with inflammatory myopathy.

Approximately 50% of patients with rheumatoid arthritis who present to a rheumatologist are positive for rheumatoid factor or anti-cyclic citrullinated peptide (CCP) antibodies when they initially present, rising to 70% to 80% at a later time point. Therefore, a negative serology test does not exclude rheumatoid arthritis as a diagnosis.

Antinuclear antibody tests

Antinuclear antibody (ANA), often referred to as antinuclear factor (ANF), is a very useful screening test for SLE as it is positive in up to 95% of patients. It is, however, non-specific, being positive in many other autoimmune rheumatic disorders, including about 20% of patients with rheumatoid arthritis. A positive test in children with arthritis may be associated with chronic iridocyclitis, which is frequently asymptomatic. Slit-lamp examination of the eye is mandatory to confirm the diagnosis.

The ANA test detects antibodies to intracellular nuclear and cytoplasmic antigens and is carried out by incubating the patient's serum with cells such as Hep-2 cells. After washing, a fluorescent antiserum to human IgG is used to detect human antibody adhering to the intracellular and nuclear antigens. A titre of 1:80 or more is significant, and adequate standardization is important.

DNA-binding test

Different immunochemical techniques (Farr assay or ELISA) may be used to detect antibodies to native double-stranded DNA. Another method is indirect immunofluorescence using the protozoon *Crithidia luciliae*, where the kinetoplast at the tail containing DNA fluoresces. The test is usually reserved for patients with a positive ANA test and is specific for SLE but not as sensitive as ANA. Occasionally it is positive in patients in whom the clinical suspicion of SLE is very high, but the ANA test is negative.

Box 15.16 Other helpful immunology tests in rheumatic disease

- Antineutrophil cytoplasmic antibodies are a marker for vasculitic conditions. Two immunofluorescence staining patterns occur:
  1. Cytoplasmic or c-ANCA, with specificity for proteinase 3 (a neutrophil enzyme), is specific for Wegener's granulomatosis (see Fig. 15.54)
- 2. Perinuclear or p-ANCA, with specificity for myeloperoxidase (and some other neutrophil enzymes), occurs in microscopic polyangiitis and other vasculitic diseases (and inflammatory bowel disease).
- Antiphospholipid antibodies, which include anticardiolipin antibodies, β2 glycoprotein 1 antibodies and the lupus anticoagulant tests, are associated with the antiphospholipid syndrome, characterized by arterial and venous thromboses and, in women, recurrent pregnancy loss and pregnancy morbidity. A false-positive VDRL test (see Chapter 18) may also be found in these patients.
- Anti-Jo 1 (histidyl t-RNA synthetase) is a marker for idiopathic inflammatory myopathies, such as dermatomyositis and polymyositis, especially when complicated by interstitial lung disease.
- Cryoglobulins are detected by clotting whole blood at 37°C and cooling the serum to 4°C and looking for a precipitate which is usually an IgM rheumatoid factor. Cryoglobulins are associated with vasculitis, infections such as hepatitis C and myeloproliferative disorders.
- Human leukocyte antigen (HLA) typing: the association of tissue antigen HLA-B27 with ankylosing spondylitis remains the strongest association in medicine. Although about 95% of patients with ankylosing spondylitis in the UK possess the B27 antigen, it is also found in 8% of the normal population. Ankylosing spondylitis, therefore, remains a clinical diagnosis, supported by typical radiographic findings. However, in early disease, in children with peripheral arthritis or where the clinical findings are atypical, HLA-B27 typing may provide supportive diagnostic value.
- Antistreptolysin-O (ASO) test: the presence in the serum of this antibody in a titre greater than 1/200, rising on repeat testing after about 2 weeks, indicates a recent haemolytic streptococcal infection.
- Viral titres. Certain viruses, notably parvovirus and Coxsackie virus, may cause transient musculoskeletal symptoms that may be mistaken for systemic diseases. Rising viral titres may be useful in the differential diagnosis.

Box 15.15 Extractable nuclear antigen (ENA) tests

The following tests may be indicated by a speckled staining pattern in the antinuclear antibody (ANA) test. They can be summarized in terms of their clinical associations:

- Anti-Ro (SSA) and anti-La (SSB), typically in Sjögren's syndrome. Also seen in systemic lupus erythematosus (SLE), where they are associated with photosensitivity, and the neonatal lupus syndrome, which may result in congenital heart block and neonatal rashes.
- Anti-Sm in 5% to 10% of patients with SLE; a very specific marker if present.
- Anti-RNP (ribonucleoprotein) in some cases of SLE. Also picks out certain patients who have clinical features of other autoimmune rheumatic disorders and who are therefore often diagnosed as mixed connective-tissue disease (MCTD). The test can be considered a marker for the combination of clinical features, but the major clinical component of the condition will define management.
- Anticentromere antibody is found in limited cutaneous systemic sclerosis or 'CREST syndrome' (calcinosis, Raynaud's phenomenon, oesophageal symptoms, sclerodactyly and telangiectasiae).
- Anti-Scl 70 (DNA topoisomerase I) and anti-RNA polymerase are found in scleroderma and are associated with severe disease.

Antibody tests to extractable nuclear antigens (ENA)

Box 15.15 shows tests that may be indicated by a speckled staining pattern in the ANA test. They can be summarized in terms of their clinical associations. Other diagnostic antibody tests are shown in Box 15.16.

Uric acid

A consistently normal plasma uric acid level (<375 mmol/l in women, <425 mmol/l in men) usually excludes the diagnosis of untreated gout. Raised levels occur in many circumstances and do not in themselves establish the diagnosis of gout (see later). On a low-purine diet, the 24-hour urinary urate excretion should not exceed 600 mg. Higher levels indicate 'overproduction' of urate and a risk of renal stone formation.

Synovial fluid examination

Synovial fluid may be obtained for examination from any joint in which it is clinically detectable. The knee is the most convenient source: after infiltration with a local anaesthetic, a 21-gauge needle is inserted into the joint between the patella and the femoral condyle. For smaller, more inaccessible joints, such as the wrist or MCP, an ultrasound-guided aspiration should be considered. The aspirated fluid should be placed in a plain sterile container; if a cell count is required, some of the fluid should be mixed with ethylenediaminetetra-acetic acid (EDTA) anticoagulant.

An injured joint can also be aspirated (Box 15.17). The joint swollen after injury may reveal clear pink fluid, suggesting a meniscal lesion, or show frank blood. The latter is usually indicative of a torn anterior cruciate ligament. If blood is aspirated,

look at its surface for fat globules. This is derived from the marrow and confirms an intra-articular fracture. Synovial fluid examination is diagnostic in two conditions—bacterial infections and crystal synovitis—and every effort should be made to obtain fluid when either of these is suspected. Polarized light microscopy can differentiate between the crystals of urate in gout and those of calcium pyrophosphate dihydrate in pseudogout. Outside these conditions, synovial fluid examination is unlikely to be diagnostic. Frank blood may point to trauma, haemophilia or villonodular synovitis,

Box 15.17	Findings in synovial fluid after aspiration of the knee joint

- Cloudy fluid or pus: bacterial infection (see text)
- Urate or pyrophosphate crystals: gout or pseudogout
- Pink fluid: torn meniscus
- Blood: trauma, haemophilia, villonodular synovitis

Box 15.18	Biopsy procedures and tissue harvesting that may be useful in the differential diagnosis of rheumatic diseases

- Muscle biopsy should be considered in patients with inflammatory myopathies, such as dermatomyositis, polymyositis and inclusion body myositis. Electromyography may show typical features of myopathy and biopsy may be guided by magnetic resonance imaging (MRI) of muscles (see Fig. 15.55).
- Rectal biopsy can be useful in the diagnosis of amyloidosis secondary to chronic inflammatory disease, but renal biopsy may still be necessary if the cause of renal impairment is not clear.
- Renal biopsy is essential in the vasculitides or systemic lupus erythematosus (SLE) where active glomerulonephritis is suspected. Vasculitis may also be confirmed on renal biopsy but, in general, tissues found to be abnormal on clinical examination or by further investigation (e.g. skin, muscle, sural nerve or liver) should be considered first for diagnostic biopsy in undifferentiated systemic vasculitis.
- Biopsy of a lip minor salivary gland may be useful to confirm Sjögren's syndrome.
- Temporal artery biopsy is often diagnostic in patients with clinical features of temporal (giant cell) arteritis. This is the investigation of choice.
- Synovial biopsy is of little value in the differential diagnosis of inflammatory polyarthritis, but should be considered in any unusual monoarthritis to exclude infection, particularly tuberculous, or rare conditions such as sarcoid, amyloid arthropathy or villonodular synovitis. This may be performed by arthroscopy or using a semi-automated guillotine needle under ultrasound guidance.
- Bone biopsy. May be useful in the diagnosis of osteomalacia, malignancy, renal osteodystrophy and Paget's disease. The bone marrow can also be aspirated at the same time if necessary.

Figure 15.54 Antineutrophil cytoplasmic autoantibodies with cytoplasmic staining (c-ANCA). This pattern has a high predictive value for a diagnosis of Wegener's granulomatosis.

Figure 15.55   Magnetic resonance imaging (MRI) scan of thigh muscles showing high signal lesions of inflammatory myositis.

Figure 15.56   Healed fracture of posterior left and right ribs in a 6-month-old infant, classic non-accidental injury (NAI).

Box 15.19	General principles of musculoskeletal imaging

- Use a systematic approach (see Box 15.13).
- Age, sex and clinical information are essential in interpretation.
- Radiographs reveal bones and soft tissues.
- Always obtain two views, at right angles, in trauma patients.
- Radiographs may be normal even in the presence of disease.
- Diffuse abnormalities are difficult to detect.
- Bone-based and joint-based disease must be differentiated.
- Normal variants can be confused with pathology.

Figure 15.57   Benign bone tumour (adamantinoma). Note the solitary well-defined lucent lesion with a sclerotic margin and the absence of matrix calcification.

whereas inflammatory (as opposed to degenerative) arthritis is suggested by opaque fluid of low viscosity, with a total white cell count greater than 1000/ml, neutrophils more than 50%, protein content more than 35 g/l and the presence of a firm clot. Culture of this fluid may produce a bacterial growth, usually of staphylococci, but occasionally *Mycobacterium tuberculosis* or other organisms.

Biopsies useful in differential diagnosis

Box 15.18 shows tests that may be useful in the differential diagnosis of rheumatic diseases.

Radiological examination

Certain general principles are important, particularly as clinicians may be asked to give an opinion on

radiographs of limbs after a traumatic injury, whether minor or more serious (Box 15.19). Common problems are shown in Figures 15.56–15.59. A systematic approach is essential (Box 15.20).

Bone density (Table 15.6) may be normal, reduced (osteopenia) or increased (osteosclerosis). These changes are easy to detect if focal, but difficult if diffuse. When a focal bone lesion (Box 15.21) is noted, look at its position in the bone and at its margins, and note whether there is any focal matrix

Figure 15.58 **(A)** Early rheumatoid arthritis: local osteopenia, loss of joint spaces, soft-tissue swelling. **(B)** Late rheumatoid arthritis: erosion of periarticular surfaces and ulnar subluxation.

Figure 15.59 Renal osteodystrophy: generalized demineralization, terminal phalangeal and subperiosteal bone resorption and vascular calcification.

Box 15.20	Systematic approach to musculoskeletal imaging

- Bone density
- Soft tissues
- Joints
- Bone
- Periosteum

calcification, whether the cortex of the bone is intact and whether there is any periosteal reaction around it. Most solitary bone lesions in young people are benign and show no periosteal reaction or swelling around them, and no associated soft-tissue swelling. Aggressive (malignant) bone lesions are more common in the elderly. Certain bone metastases have a characteristic appearance (Box 15.22). Isotope imaging is useful in detecting multiple sites of bony involvement in generalized disease and in metastatic cancer. Computed tomography (CT) imaging is also sensitive in detecting and analysing bony lesions, because it provides good images of the bony margins of the lesions and of the associated soft tissues. MRI is used to assess the extent of the lesion and any local soft-tissue invasion.

The most common use of plain radiographs is to document joint pathology, such as osteoarthritis (joint space narrowing, periarticular sclerosis, subchondral cysts and osteophytes), or inflammatory conditions, such as rheumatoid arthritis (joint space narrowing, periarticular osteopenia, erosions and subsequent bony ankylosis). Imaging of the hands and feet is most commonly performed when investigating an inflammatory arthritis, as subclinical inflammation and joint description may occur in the absence of frank joint inflammation. Osteoarthritis requires a more focused approach to imaging of symptomatic joints. Although imaging changes characteristic of degenerative joint disease can be detected by plain radiographs, they do not correlate well with symptom severity.

Fractures

X-rays are often the first investigation in suspected fractures and in joint disease. In traumatic fractures, X-rays are diagnostic and are used to check alignment of the fracture and healing. X-rays of a fracture are also important in excluding a pathological fracture associated with metabolic bone disease, a focal benign bone lesion or neoplastic invasion by metastases. When there is clinical doubt after

Table 15.6 Abnormal bone density

Generalized osteopenia	Generalized osteosclerosis	Benign focal lucent lesions	Benign focal sclerotic lesions
Ageing osteoporosis	Osteopetrosis (marble bone disease)	Simple bone cyst, aneurysmal bone cyst	Bone island
	Metastatic bone disease, e.g. prostate and breast cancer	Fibrous cortical defect	Callus after fracture
Disuse, e.g. trauma and neurogenic paralysis, osteogenesis imperfecta	Dietary causes, e.g. hypervitaminosis A, fluorosis	Non-ossifying fibroma	Paget's disease of bone
Acquired metabolic bone disease, e.g. rickets, osteomalacia, hyperparathyroidism	Acquired metabolic bone disease, e.g. renal osteodystrophy	Enchondroma	Bone infarction Osteoid osteoma
Myeloma	Myelofibrosis, sickle cell disease	Fibrous dysplasia, giant cell tumour of bone	Fibrous dysplasia

---

Box 15.21   Benign and malignant bone lesions

Benign

- Young person
- Single lesion
- Well-defined margin
- Intact cortex
- No periosteal reaction
- No growth
- Asymptomatic

Malignant

- Older age
- Multiple lesions
- Poorly defined margin
- Destroyed cortex
- Periosteal reaction
- Soft-tissue extension of lesion
- Lesions painful

Box 15.22   Bone metastases

- Expansile: thyroid, kidney, breast, bronchus, melanoma and myeloma
- Sclerotic: prostate and breast
- Lytic: breast, bronchus, kidney, thyroid and melanoma
- Mixed: breast, bladder or previously treated (irradiated) bone lesions

---

a non-diagnostic X-ray, an MRI scan often reveals the underlying fracture and is the investigation of choice. Radiographs taken to confirm or exclude a fracture must be taken in two planes. It is essential that either the whole limb is turned or the imaging equipment rotated. The limb must not be twisted at the fracture site. When looking for a fracture, run a pen tip or its equivalent around the cortex of the bone as seen on the film (without leaving marks). Any break in continuity will reveal itself; do not confuse an epiphysis with a fracture. Note soft-tissue swelling and distension of joints. Always seek a radiology opinion if in doubt.

In joint disease, MRI is the imaging method of choice because it can visualize all the soft-tissue components of the joints. Osteopenia is a non-specific feature of disuse, but it also occurs in relation to affected joints in rheumatoid arthritis and Still's disease of children. Involvement of the distal interphalangeal joint is a feature of psoriatic arthropathy. In rheumatoid disease, the involvement of joints is usually symmetrical, and the wrist is particularly susceptible.

Only radiographs likely to yield specific information should be requested. However, in unilateral joint disease, it is useful to examine both sides for comparison (Fig. 15.60). In patients with inflammatory polyarthritis, three routine films are helpful in the diagnosis and assessment of progression, with both hands and wrists on one plate and both feet on another to compare bone density and to look for periosteal reaction or erosive change, and one of the full pelvis (Fig. 15.61) to show the sacroiliac and hip joints. In the absence of so-called 'red flag' signs, for example weight loss, night pain, fevers or neurological signs, most spinal radiographs are unnecessary.

Specialized radiology

The following imaging techniques can provide precise information about localized pathology, but they are dependent on the clinician making a clear diagnostic request with as much clinical information as possible:

- High-resolution ultrasound is of value in defining soft-tissue structures, including muscles and tendons; it provides an excellent means for

Figure 15.61 X-ray of lumbosacral spine and upper pelvis. There is fusion of several vertebrae, and of the sacroiliac joints *(arrows)* from ankylosing spondylitis. The renal papillae on the left are calcified, evidence of previous papillary necrosis from prolonged analgesic use.

Figure 15.60 Left and right knee joints. The X-rays show normal joint anatomy, but with chondrocalcinosis **(A)** and osteoarthritic change **(B)** on the opposite side. Note the increased bone density and narrowing of the joint space.

guiding aspiration of joint effusions and biopsy procedures. Ultrasound consistently has been demonstrated to be more sensitive than clinical examination in the context of joint inflammation and it provides considerable additional information in the diagnosis and management of inflammatory arthritis. Grey-scale synovial thickening and power Doppler signal reflect histologically defined synovitis and can be used to differentiate between true joint pathology and fibromyalgia and other pain syndromes (Fig. 15.62). In addition, this imaging modality has the unique capacity to be used in a dynamic fashion, allowing tendon, ligament and joint function to be observed in real time. Rotator cuff pathology at the shoulder is amenable to ultrasound imaging and is often the first imaging investigation of choice when assessing the integrity of the muscle and tendons of these structures. Ultrasound can detect erosions and joint damage at a very early stage of disease before X-ray changes are demonstrated.

- CT. The combination of superior tissue contrast and tomographic technique permits definition of soft-tissue structures obscured by overlapping structures, including intervertebral discs and other joints normally difficult to visualize, such as sacroiliac (Fig. 15.63), sternoclavicular and subtalar. Bone pathology is particularly well

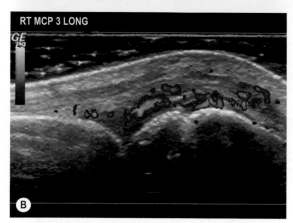

Figure 15.62 **(A)** Synovial thickening seen as hypoechoic *(darker grey)* material over the dorsal aspect of the metacarpal head and neck using ultrasound. **(B)** Power Doppler signal seen as *red/orange* signal located within the synovial thickening within the metacarpal-phalangeal joint.

Figure 15.63 Computed tomography (CT) scan of sacroiliac joints, showing a distinctive lesion on the left side with a sequestrum owing to tuberculosis.

Figure 15.64 A lumbar spine magnetic resonance imaging (MRI) scan. There is a disc protrusion at L4/5 with degeneration of the disc itself, shown by the less bright signal in the intervertebral disc at this level.

characterized on CT imaging (e.g. malignancy, erosive disease or fracture). MRI has unique advantages in evaluating the musculoskeletal system, but it is vital that the clinician defines the pathology suspected, as correct positioning and sequence selection (T-weighting) are vital in optimizing image quality. MRI is increasingly used to image the major joints in the limbs, especially the knee (see Fig. 15.47), hip, shoulder and elbow.

In the context of inflammatory arthritis, MRI has much to recommend it as an imaging modality. There is a clear relationship with bone marrow oedema on MRI and the subsequent development of erosive arthritis providing an early indicator of potentially poor prognosis. Erosive disease, when present, is detected earlier than with plain radiographs and changes in synovial inflammation can be readily detected after therapeutic intervention. A standardized, validated scoring system has been developed (RAMRIS: *R*heumatoid *A*rthritis *MRI* Scoring), which encompasses multiple elements of MRI-detected synovial inflammation and joint damage.

Enhancement by the use of intravenous paramagnetic contrast (e.g. gadolinium) has further improved definition in spinal imaging.

Magnetic resonance imaging is invaluable when assessing the degree of spinal involvement in spondyloarthropathies, such as ankylosing spondylitis, particularly in early disease where radiography ankylosis is absent. Both costovertebral

Figure 15.65 Magnetic resonance image (MRI) of cervical spine in a patient with transverse myelitis owing to systemic lupus erythematosus (SLE) **(A)** before and **(B)** after immunosuppression.

and sacroiliac joints are readily imaged with good sensitivity for inflammatory pathology.

It is of particular value in the non-invasive investigation of disc disease (Fig. 15.64), including spinal infection, and is a sensitive technique for the diagnosis of avascular necrosis. MRI scanning of the brain and spine is the single most important investigation in neuroimaging, as the neural tissues themselves, together with supporting tissues, are well visualized. Bone is less well seen with this technique. As a rule of thumb, most abnormalities appear dark on T1-weighted images and white on T2-weighted images. Some common problems are shown in Figures 15.55, 15.64 and 15.65.

- Isotopic scanning (scintigraphy) can be used in the diagnosis of acute (e.g. infection or stress fracture) or multiple (e.g. metastases) bone lesions by use of the first 2-minute (dynamic blood flow) phase,

second 10-minute (blood pool) phase and third 3-hour late phase (osteoblastic) (Fig. 15.66) following intravenous injection of diphosphonate compounds. Tomographic scintigraphy can further refine definition of the isotope uptake (e.g. in stress fracture of the pars interarticularis). Radionucleotide bone scans are more sensitive than plain radiographs for the diagnosis of Paget's disease and in polyostotic cases help to quantify the overall burden of disease. Scintigraphy has a high sensitivity to metabolically active lesions; however, it is relatively non-specific and is often used in conjunction with other imaging modalities.

- Dual-energy X-ray absorptiometry (DEXA) is widely used to assess bone mineral density in metabolic bone disease and osteoporosis. Scans recorded with long intervals (e.g. every 2 to 3 years) between them may be used to assess the

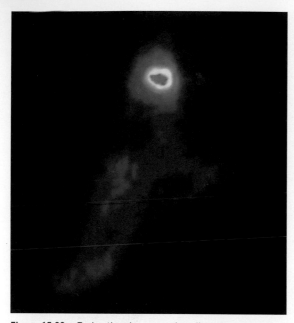

Figure 15.66 Technetium bone scan in a distance runner, showing focally increased uptake in the lower tibia owing to a stress fracture.

effects of therapy. Results are expressed in relation to a normal reference range.

- Positron emission tomography (PET) scanning is becoming more widely available, but remains expensive. This is a type of scintigraphic molecular imaging based mostly on the uptake of radiolabelled glucose by metabolically active structures. PET scans are mostly used in rheumatology investigations and have better signal-to-noise ratio than standard isotope bone scanning. The combined technology of CT and PET scanning allows the acquisition of structural information simultaneously with metabolic activity. It is extremely sensitive in detecting malignancy and is also proving useful in documenting large vessel inflammation in disorders such as Takayasu's arteritis and giant cell arteritis. The radiation exposure is considerable and, as such, this imaging modality should be used cautiously and appropriately.

Nervous system | 16

Rodney W.H. Walker and David A. Gallagher

Introduction

In recent years impressive advances have been made throughout the field of neurology—in delineating disease entities and understanding their aetiology and pathogenesis; in diagnostic methods, particularly imaging and genetic testing; and in treatment and management. However, despite advances in investigations, careful clinical assessment remains of central importance.

The fundamental importance of the clinical history and examination cannot be overemphasized. In the diagnosis of neurological disease, it is the history, rather than the examination, that is paramount, so it is even more important for this to be comprehensive. History taking has not changed significantly, but clinical neurological examination continues to evolve. Significant contributions have come from clinical assessment scales, some of which have been so successful as to have become internationally institutionalized, for example the Glasgow Coma Scale and the Mini-Mental State Examination (although the latter has recently been patented). On the other hand, clinical signs of limited sensitivity, specificity, reliability and localizing value can be dispensed with.

A thorough neurological examination does involve doing more than is the case for other systems. Some basic neuroanatomical knowledge is necessary, but most clinical neurology need not be daunting. In new patients presenting for diagnosis, a sensible formulation of the nature of the problem on the basis of the history and examination is critical in order to request appropriate investigations, should they be necessary. Modern imaging undoubtedly has been the biggest revolution in clinical neurology in recent years, but injudicious use of imaging frequently leads to confusion, delay in diagnosis and sometimes harm. Similar considerations apply to the other major investigational modalities.

This chapter will discuss some aspects of neurological history, concentrate on neurological examination and the formulation of the nature of the neurological diagnosis and include some remarks on neurological investigations. Coma, delirium and dementia are not covered in this chapter.

The neurological history

The essentials of history taking have been covered elsewhere, but some points are particularly salient to neurological conditions. The repertoire of neurological symptoms is actually quite limited, although perhaps larger than that of other specialties. Box 16.1 lists the usual ones that you should specifically ask about in taking a neurological history.

The time course of evolution and sometimes resolution of neurological symptoms very frequently indicate the nature of the problem, and so they need to be clarified as precisely as possible. Thus, sensory or motor symptoms, which start abruptly and are at their most marked at or very soon after their onset, strongly suggest a vascular causation (transient ischaemia or ischaemic or haemorrhagic stroke). In contrast, similar symptoms evolving over a few days, reaching a plateau in severity and then slowly receding typify inflammatory central nervous system (CNS) demyelination (a first episode or a relapse of multiple sclerosis). Subacute (developing over weeks to months), progressive symptoms can be caused by many kinds of pathology, but neoplasia is always a prime concern.

These statements are true enough to be clinically useful, although there are exceptions. For example, one of the reasons for requesting cranial imaging in all cases of stroke is to exclude a benign or malignant tumour or other pathology, which has caused a stroke-like presentation. Neurodegenerative conditions always develop insidiously with gradual progression, but occasionally patients present acutely. For example, motor neuron disease can present acutely with ventilatory failure. Alzheimer's disease commonly becomes evident after an episode of acute delirium caused by an intercurrent illness. Sometimes, gradually progressive neurological conditions seem to present suddenly, and only when they begin to interfere with the patient's daily functioning.

Two common neurological presentations require a history, not only from the patient but also, if at all possible, from others: attacks of loss of consciousness and memory impairment.

The three most common causes of attacks of reduced consciousness or awareness that lead to neurological consultations are neurocardiogenic syncope, epilepsy

Box 16.1	Neurological symptoms

- Cognitive symptoms, especially memory impairment
- Headache
- Loss of awareness
- Loss of consciousness
- Alteration of perception, including déjà vu
- Dizziness, vertigo
- Loss of balance
- Falls
- Loss of sense of smell
- Loss of taste
- Loss of vision
- 'Positive' visual symptoms, including components of migraine auras, unformed and formed hallucinations
- Double vision
- More than double vision (polyopia, palinopsia)
- Oscillopsia (a visual sensation of stationary objects swaying back and forth)
- Deafness
- Tinnitus
- Difficulty with speech
- Difficulty swallowing
- Weakness
- Abnormal movements of muscles (including cramp, fasciculations)
- Abnormal movements of parts of the body (including tremor, dystonia, myoclonus)
- Clumsiness
- Impairment of control of limbs
- Altered sensation
- Loss of sensation
- Pain
- Symptoms of postural hypotension
- Impairment of sexual function
- Impairment of bladder control
- Impairment of bowel control

and psychogenic non-epileptic attacks. It is far more informative to hear a description from a witness than to request potentially misleading and inappropriate investigations. Obtaining the witness's account may require a telephone call; this is time well invested. Table 16.1 summarizes some points, which help to distinguish syncope from seizures. In the case of recurrent attacks, asking patient's friends or relatives to record the episode, for example on a mobile phone camera, can be invaluable, particularly in psychogenic non-epileptic attacks.

Memory impairment is a common complaint. Distinguishing between the worried, but well, and those with real impairment is greatly facilitated by information provided by close family or other informants. In general, if a patient is brought to a doctor by a relative who complains that the patient has memory impairment, there is most often an organic disorder, usually dementia. In contrast, many but not all patients who come to a doctor alone with the same complaint have good cognitive function. Furthermore, it is the relative who can report on changes in personality, behaviour, self-care and capacity, which may be crucial to the diagnosis.

The most frequent symptom leading to neurological referral is headache. It is also a common reason for attending an emergency department. The vast majority of headaches are not caused by life-threatening disorders, such as aneurysmal subarachnoid haemorrhage, meningitis or brain tumour, but are caused by common primary headache syndromes, particularly migraine. Table 16.2 outlines some of the features, which may help to distinguish headaches of different sorts.

Vertigo (a hallucination of movement) is an important symptom that requires careful characterization. It indicates a disorder of one or both labyrinths, vestibular nerves, vestibular nuclei in the brainstem or, rarely, the

Table 16.1 Points that help to distinguish syncope from seizures involving loss of consciousness. Minor injury, incontinence and sleepiness after the event do not distinguish well.

Syncope	Seizure
In neurocardiogenic syncope, characteristic prodromal features include: tinnitus, muffled hearing, dimming of vision, loss of vision while still conscious, widespread altered sensation, dizziness (may be described as spinning), lightheadedness, feeling of impending faint, weakness	The symptoms of focal seizure activity which precede a secondarily generalized attack may or may not be remembered after the attack is over. For example, sensory hallucinations (olfactory, gustatory, visual, auditory or somatosensory) or perceptual distortions (appearance of change in shape or size); cognitive symptoms, such as loss of language or other cognitive domains or dysmnesia (altered memories), such as déjà vu or jamais vu; strong emotional symptoms (anxiety, elation, fear).
Marked pallor	Usually little or no pallor
Sweating (but not in those with autonomic failure)	Vocalization at onset of generalized convulsion (GC)
Any convulsion is brief (seconds)	Apnoea
Rapid recovery of lucidity and memory (registration and recall)	Cyanosis associated with GC
Patient comes round on the ground where he fell	Stertorous breathing
A second attack immediately on being sat up after the first attack is very suggestive of neurocardiogenic syncope	Tongue biting
Neurocardiogenic syncope is commonly set off by pain, squeamishness, gastrointestinal illness, public places indoors (clubs, restaurants, trains), prolonged standing	Postictal amnesia—paramedical staff present when patient 'comes round', or patient 'comes round' in hospital (although he walked to the ambulance)

Table 16.2 Headaches: points to consider in the history

Aspects of history	Feature	Diagnosis
Location of pain	Focal; retro-orbital or supra-orbital	Migraine
		Trigeminal autonomic cephalgias (cluster headache, paroxysmal hemicranias, SUNCT, hemicrania continua)
		Retro-orbital lesion
	Facial (lower two trigeminal divisions) or dental; severe and lancinating	Trigeminal neuralgia
	Occipital	Chiari malformation
		Intracranial hypotension
		Occipital neuralgia
		Cervical spondylosis
	Focal over frontal or maxillary sinuses; often with tenderness	Sinusitis
	Temporal; with scalp tenderness	Giant cell arteritis
Laterality	Unilateral	Migraine, trigeminal autonomic cephalgias
	Generalized	Migraine, tension-type headache
Onset and chronicity	New, explosive onset and severe	Subarachnoid haemorrhage
	New, acute or subacute onset	Meningitis, cerebral abscess, encephalitis
	Sporadic over years	Migraine
	Bouts lasting days or weeks	Migraine
		Cluster headache
		Trigeminal neuralgia
	Periodicity: diurnal (attacks at specific times or the day) or circannual (bouts at particular times of the year)	Cluster headache
Duration and frequency of attacks	Seconds (recurrent)	Trigeminal neuralgia
	5 to 300 seconds (multiple per day)	SUNCT
	2 to 30 minutes (usually 5 or more daily)	Paroxysmal hemicranias
	15 minutes to 3 hours (up to 8 per day)	Cluster headache
	Hours to days	Migraine
		Tension headache
Migrainous symptoms	Nausea or vomiting	Migraine
	Photophobia (sensitivity to light)	
	Phonophobia (sensitivity to noise)	
	Osmophobia (sensitivity to smell)	
	Motion sensitivity	
	Aura: visual, including photopsia (bright spots and flashes) or fortification (appearance of zigzag lines) or scotoma or other visual loss; sensory symptoms (usually positive) such as tingling or 'pins and needles'); and speech or language	
	Brainstem aura: such as dysarthria, vertigo, diplopia, ataxia or decreased conscious level.	
Cranial autonomic symptoms	Conjunctival injection ('bloodshot' eyes), lachrymation (tears), ptosis, nasal congestion, rhinorrhea (running nostril), eyelid oedema, facial sweating, miosis (small asymmetric pupil)	Can occur in migraine
		Unilateral autonomic symptoms are characteristic of trigeminal autonomic cephalgias (cluster headache, paroxysmal hemicranias, SUNCT or hemicrania continua)
Features of CSF dysregulation	High-pressure symptoms: orthostatic (worse on lying flat) or diurnal (worse at night or early morning) variation; exacerbation with Valsalva (coughing, sneezing, straining, etc.); transient visual obscurations; or pulsatile tinnitus	Craniocervical abnormality (such as Chiari malformation)
		Idiopathic intracranial hypertension (associated with papilloedema and typical body habitus)
		Intracranial lesion
	Low-pressure symptoms: orthostatic (worse on sitting or standing) or diurnal (deteriorate as day progresses)	Spontaneous CSF leak
		Post-lumbar puncture or epidural

Continued

Table 16.2 Headaches: points to consider in the history—cont'd

Aspects of history	Feature	Diagnosis
Situational headaches	Exertion	Benign exertional headache
		Exacerbates migraine
	Orgasm	Benign coital headache
		SAH should be excluded after single severe episode
	Sleep onset	Hypnic headache
		Migraine
		Cluster headache; so called 'alarm clock headache', wakes at same time every night.
Exacerbating or relieving factors	Provoked by alcohol	Migraine
		Cluster headache
	Menstrual association and other hormonal aspects (better or worse during pregnancy; after menopause)	Migraine
	Food precipitants	Migraine
	Facial touching or movement	Trigeminal neuralgia
General health	Systemic neoplasia	Metastases
	Body habitus (increased body mass index)	Idiopathic intracranial hypertension
		Obstructive sleep apnoea
Features of giant cell arteritis *Important to specifically consider in any patient over 60 years of age*	Amaurosis fugax (transient monocular visual loss) Jaw claudication (pain on chewing) Scalp tenderness Polymyalgia and weight loss	Giant cell arteritis

CSF, cerebrospinal fluid; SAH, subarachnoid hemorrhage; SUNCT, short-lasting, unilateral, neuralgiform headache attacks with conjunctival injection and tearing (a rare disorder).

cerebellum. A clear-cut description of a spinning feeling usually signifies true vertigo. Patients are more likely to complain of dizziness or giddiness than vertigo. Both dizziness and giddiness mean different things to different patients, including vertigo, oscillopsia (a visual sensation that stationary objects are swaying back and forth), lightheadedness, loss of balance or even sometimes headache. It is always important to establish whether a patient with vertigo has positional vertigo. Enquiring whether the patient's symptom is provoked by sitting from a lying position or standing from a sitting position will not distinguish vertigo from postural hypotension or ataxia, because all give rise to symptoms on rising. Symptoms brought on by lying down or turning over in bed or looking up at a high shelf or the sky more certainly signify real positional vertigo. It is not uncommon for patients with loss of balance to complain of dizziness; such patients will spontaneously comment that they feel secure sitting in a chair but dizzy as soon as they stand up and move around.

Focal weakness is self-explanatory. Many patients complain of feeling generally weak when they have no loss of muscle strength at all. Some patients become weak without realizing it. Thus, patients with unilateral or bilateral quadriceps weakness may present with falls rather than complain of weakness. Patients with bilateral ankle dorsiflexion weakness may complain of being off balance or of tripping rather than weakness. Exertional weakness or worsening of weakness is characteristic of neuromuscular junction disorders,

but it also occurs in cauda equina compression (spinal canal stenosis), spinal cord compression (cervical spondylotic myelopathy) and in multiple sclerosis and sometimes other disorders, so it is not specific but can be diagnostically helpful and so should be asked about.

Sensory symptoms may be negative (a reduction or absence of normal sensation) or positive (an abnormal sensation which is felt, e.g. buzzing, tingling, 'pins and needles', pain). In ordinary usage, the word numb would seem to be unambiguous, but some patients who are weak without sensory loss refer to numbness (particularly in Bell's palsy) and, conversely, patients with sensory migraine auras may be misdiagnosed as having hemiplegic migraine because of their impression of paralysis even though they can move the affected limbs. Patients who seem imprecise have some justification; the *Shorter Oxford Dictionary* defines numb as 'deprived of feeling, or of the power of movement' so it is important to clarify exactly what the patient is describing. As a rule, transient ischaemic attacks that involve the parietal cortex give rise to brief negative sensory symptoms. Conversely, focal sensory seizures are characterized by positive sensory symptoms.

Most organic neurological disorders that give rise to sensory symptoms involve structural or functional damage to nerves somewhere, whether it be in peripheral nerves, nerve roots, spinal cord or brain. Hypersensitivity (hyperaesthesia) to all modalities of sensation is therefore improbable or impossible. Patients who appear to have very sensitive skin as a

Table 16.3 Nomenclature of cutaneous sensory symptoms

Hypoaesthesia	Reduced cutaneous sensation of any modality
Paraesthesia	Spontaneous abnormal sensation including tingling, pins and needles and pain
Neuralgia	Pain in the distribution of a nerve or nerve root
Dysaesthesia	An abnormal perception of a sensory stimulus (e.g. touch causes tingling or pain)
Allodynia	Pain caused by a stimulus that does not normally cause pain
Hyperalgesia	An abnormally intense perception of a mildly painful stimulus
Hyperpathia	Perseveration, augmentation and, on occasion, spread of pain
	The pain threshold is normal or sometimes high
	The threshold for perceiving pain may be raised and there may be delay in perceiving a painful stimulus; once perceived, the pain is severe and prolonged and may spread
Hyperaesthesia	An ambiguous term, best avoided

result of a lesion (e.g. herpes zoster radiculitis) have combinations of paraesthesia, hypoaesthesia, dysaesthesia, allodynia, hyperalgesia and hyperpathia. Some of these terms are not without their ambiguities. Table 16.3 provides a definition for each.

Lhermitte's symptom (often called Lhermitte's sign) is a paroxysm of positive sensory symptoms—an electric shock feeling or a shower of paraesthesiae shooting down the spine and/or into the upper or lower limbs triggered by neck flexion. It is indicative of a cervical spinal cord lesion, commonly a multiple sclerosis plaque, although other cord lesions (e.g. spondylotic cord compression) and even cobalamin (vitamin B_{12}) deficiency may also produce this symptom.

Neurological examination is poor at identifying and characterizing disorders of the autonomic nervous system, making it particularly important that autonomic function (including bladder and bowel control and sexual function) is addressed in the history.

The neurological examination

Aspects of neurological examination can start from the moment the patient is first encountered, before and during the taking of the history, such as noting an abnormality of gait, difficulties with speech, parkinsonism or a hyperkinetic movement disorder. There is no such thing as a comprehensive neurological examination—it would take hours or days. However, too many patients without neurological symptoms have no neurological examination at all, which on occasions proves regrettable. Consider, for instance, the case of a man who develops areflexic weakness some days after

a hernia operation. How helpful would it be to know that the reflexes had been normal at the time of preoperative clinical clerking? A suggested minimal neurological examination for non-neurological patients would be assessments of the binocular visual fields, the eye movements, the biceps, triceps, knee and ankle reflexes, the plantar reflexes and fundoscopy. Most patients attending for a neurological consultation (with problems such as headache or epilepsy) have no neurological signs. A minimal routine neurological examination for such patients should include assessments of vision, the cranial nerves, motor and sensory examination and examination of gait. Bear in mind that many patients with early cognitive impairment are adept at concealing it, so that without probing it can be missed.

For most patients, it is best to be systematic with regard to neurological examination, adhering to a routine well rehearsed by the examiner and familiar to those with whom the examiner will communicate. Thus, even if the patient's problem is foot drop, it is entirely valid to start with examination of cranial nerves but sensible to explain to the patient that you are going to start at the top and work down. Certain situations require flexibility; patients with any degree of impairment of consciousness need assessment of their delirium or coma from the outset. In patients presenting with cognitive impairment, it is best to start the examination with cognitive assessment. It is important in all neurological patients to pay attention to and document mobility and, in patients presenting with a gait disorder, it is appropriate to examine the gait first. For most other patients, an appropriate order of examination is cranial nerves, speech if necessary, motor system, sensory system and gait, followed by cognitive testing if relevant.

Cranial nerve examination

Examination of the 12 cranial nerves actually involves an assessment of much more than just the nerves and nuclei, particularly with respect to the sensory visual system and eye movements. The naming and numbering of cranial nerves and their nuclei is in some measure idiosyncratic and confusing; for example, there is no olfactory nerve as such and the eighth cranial nerve is actually two nerves, as is the seventh. Within the brainstem, trigeminal sensory nuclei receive fibres not just from the fifth cranial nerve but also from the seventh, ninth and tenth nerves.

The olfactory (I) nerves

Olfactory receptor cells are bipolar sensory neurons situated under the nasal epithelium. Their central axons project in numerous bundles, not as a discrete nerve, up through the cribriform plate of the skull into the olfactory bulb on the inferior surface of the frontal lobe. These project via the olfactory tract to parts of the temporal lobe and frontal lobe.

Examination of the olfactory nerves

For ordinary clinical purposes, olfaction is tested using a small number of bottles containing either a fragrant or pungent smelling substance, such as lemon, clove or asafoetida. More detailed odour identification can be performed using specialist testing kits, such as the University of Pennsylvania Smell Identification Test (UPSIT), in which the patient scratches microencapsulated odorant in strips and identifies the smell. Each nostril should be tested separately. A necessary precondition is that a rhinological disorder does not preclude the test. Ideally, the patient should identify the smell rather than just report that it can be smelt. There is little value in routinely testing olfaction; it is uncommon to detect an abnormality and even less common for an abnormality to contribute to a diagnosis. A subfrontal tumour, such as a meningioma, may cause unilateral anosmia, but other features of the history and examination will mandate the imaging, which should establish that diagnosis. Subfrontal meningiomas can cause bilateral anosmia, so imaging is indicated in a patient presenting just with anosmia unless another cause is clearly evident. Olfactory nerve fibres passing through the cribriform plate are not uncommonly sheared as a result of head injury, frequently leading to permanent bilateral anosmia. Anosmia is commonly neurodegenerative, occurring particularly in Lewy body disease, so its presence in a patient with parkinsonism increases the likelihood that the patient has idiopathic (Lewy body) Parkinson's disease. Endocrinologists test olfaction when Kallman's syndrome is suspected.

The optic (II) nerves (see also Chapter 21)

The optic nerve runs from the back of the globe of the eye to the apex of the orbit and into the skull through the optic canal to the optic chiasm, where it is joined by the optic nerve from the other eye. Directly above the optic chiasm is the hypothalamus. Directly below is the pituitary gland. The pituitary stalk runs from the hypothalamus to the pituitary gland just behind the optic chiasm, between the optic tracts. Sensory afferents from all points of the retina run in the nerve-fibre layer on the inner surface of the retina to enter the optic nerve at the optic disc. Fibres from the temporal retina (nasal visual half-field) are placed laterally, whereas those from the nasal retina (temporal visual half-field) are medial. Fibres from the upper half of the retina run in the upper half of the optic nerve. At the optic chiasm, fibres from the nasal half of the retina (temporal visual half-field) cross (decussate) to the contralateral optic tract, whereas the fibres from the temporal half of the retina do not cross, but proceed posteriorly into the ipsilateral optic tract (Fig. 16.1). Starting within the chiasm and continuing further posteriorly within the optic tract, fibres which convey matching information

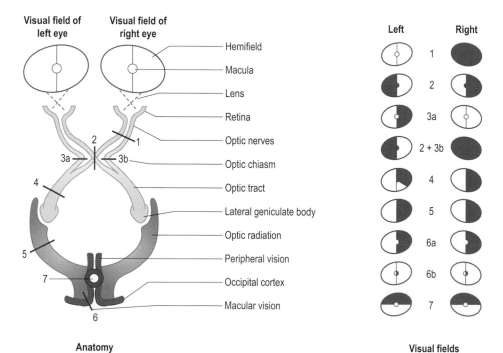

Anatomy

Visual fields

Figure 16.1 A diagram of the sensory visual pathways. Sites of lesions and the visual field defects they produce are shown. 1. Optic nerve lesion. 2. Optic chiasm lesion (bitemporal hemianopia). Lesions superior to the chiasm, for example craniopharyngioma, affecting upper chiasm fibres may cause bitemporal inferior quandrantanopia, whereas lesions inferior to the chiasm, for example the pituitary, may result in bitemporal superior quadrantanopia. 3a or 3b. Uniocular nasal hemianopia (rare). 3a plus 3b. Binasal hemianopia (very rare). 4. Optic tract lesion (incongruous homonymous hemianopia). 5. Visual radiation (homonymous quadrantanopia or hemianopia). Inferior optic radiation (temporal pathway or Meyer's loop) results in homonymous superior quadrantanopia, whereas superior optic radiation (parietal pathway) results in homonymous inferior quadrantanopia. 6a. Occipital cortex lesion sparing the occipital pole (homonymous hemianopia with macular sparing). 6b. Occipital pole lesion (homonymous paracentral hemiscotoma). 7. A bilateral occipital cortex lesion (homonymous altitudinal hemianopia).

from each eye (i.e. homonymous fibres, representing equivalent parts in the temporal retina for one eye, nasal retina for the other eye) become aligned with each other. Thus, each optic nerve conveys information from its respective eye, but every part of the sensory visual system behind the optic chiasm on each side deals with vision for the contralateral binocular visual half-field.

The majority of optic tract fibres pass, via the lateral geniculate nucleus, to the occipital cortex. The lower part of the visual radiation transmits visual information from the inferior temporal retina of the ipsilateral eye and inferior nasal retina of the other eye. A few optic tract fibres pass via the superior colliculus to the midbrain to mediate the afferent limb of the pupillary light reflex via connections to the Edinger–Westphal nuclei.

Visual acuity and colour vision

Visual acuity is of neurological as well as ophthalmological importance, because optic nerve disease may lead to any degree of loss of acuity. For ordinary clinical neurological purposes, the acuities measured using the Snellen chart are adequate. Severe loss of acuity (<6/60, the top letter on the Snellen chart) is documented as the ability to count fingers at 1 metre, ability to perceive hand movements, perception of light only and no perception of light.

Acquired unilateral loss of colour vision is a characteristic feature of optic neuropathy, and loss of colour vision can occur when visual acuity is well preserved. Thus, testing colour vision using Ishihara plates may be a sensitive bedside test for mild optic neuropathy.

Visual fields

Assessment of the visual fields is a key part of the neurological examination and need not take very long to perform. Field defects of importance are commonly missed because they have not been looked for adequately. Increasingly, opticians measure visual fields, but it cannot always be assumed that a recent ophthalmological assessment will have included the visual fields.

Visual field defects in one eye indicate a retinal or optic nerve disorder. They may affect any part of the field of the affected eye or nerve. Lesions at the optic chiasm or lesions behind the chiasm in the optic tracts, visual radiations or occipital cortex give rise to visual field defects affecting both eyes. Unilateral retrochiasmal lesions give rise to field defects affecting the contralateral binocular half-field, and the defects are homonymous (i.e. they affect equivalent parts of the temporal half-field of one eye and the nasal half-field of the other). Congruity refers to the extent to which the defects in the two half-fields match each other exactly. A congruous homonymous hemianopia indicates a lesion in the occipital cortex, whereas a non-congruous homonymous hemianopia is more likely to occur with an optic tract lesion.

When ophthalmologists do visual field testing, they tend to do Goldmann perimetry or to obtain automated Humphrey fields. The results of these tests are very useful, but in the clinic or on the ward, neurologists and general physicians test visual fields by simple confrontation field testing, comparing the patient's fields with their own, assuming their own to be normal.

Examination of the visual fields

It is best to start by testing the binocular visual fields (i.e. the patient and examiner both have both eyes open). Start by asking the patient to look at your face. Ensure that he avoids the common temptation to look to either side. Hold your hands up one on each side at face level, with your hands about 1 m apart and ask the patient whether he can see both hands. This simple test will detect a dense homonymous hemianopia. Next ask the patient to look into your eyes. Switch from hands held up to index fingers held up and move them up so that they are situated in the right and left superior quadrants of vision. Wiggle one of your fingers and instruct the patient to point to the finger he thinks is moving. Getting the patient to point is better than asking him to say whether it is the right or left finger that is moving; many patients will muddle left and right in this situation. First wiggle one finger, then the other, to check the integrity of the superior quadrants. Failure of the patient to see one of the fingers wiggling suggests a homonymous quadrantanopia. If that happens, carry on wiggling the finger that has not been registered by the patient and move it first across the midline to make sure that it becomes visible at the midline and then go back and do the same, this time moving the finger down into the inferior quadrant, where the finger will be visible if the patient has a quadrantanopia or remain unseen if the patient has a homonymous hemianopia. If the patient sees each finger wiggling consecutively in each of the upper quadrants, then wiggle both fingers simultaneously and ask the patient what is happening. If the patient only sees the wiggling of the finger on one side consistently, then he has visual inattention—an occipitotemporal or occipitoparietal disorder. Having tested the superior quadrants, move down to the inferior quadrants to test them in the same way. With a cooperative patient, all of this takes only a matter of seconds. The technique described will not detect a bitemporal hemianopia, optic nerve lesions or retinal disorders; these require testing of the field for each eye separately.

The best way to test the monocular visual fields at the bedside is to use a pin with a bright red pinhead of about 5–8 mm diameter. The patient needs to be positioned such that light is not shining from behind the examiner into the patient's eyes, so as to interfere with his ability to see the colour of the pinhead. The margin of the field is defined by the points at which perception of the colour of the pinhead changes from black to red. Ask the patient to cover one eye with the palm of his hand (or cover the eye with your own hand) and then ask him to look with his open eye straight into your own confronting eye (his left into your right and vice versa). First, put the pinhead into the middle of the visual field and check that the patient sees it as bright red. Swap to the other eye and compare the perceived brightness of red reported by the patient for his two eyes. Loss of perceived redness in one eye (red desaturation) raises the possibility of a mild optic neuropathy. A patient who is already known to have poor acuity in one eye may have a central scotoma, in which case the pinhead either will not be seen in the centre of the field or will be perceived black. A small central scotoma can be defined by moving the pinhead outwards in four different directions until the patient sees its redness. Next, put the pinhead into each of the four quadrants of vision close to the centre and check that the patient sees it as bright red. This may detect a paracentral scotoma and is also a good way of detecting temporal field defects caused by optic chiasm lesions such as pituitary tumours. Then finally, while ensuring that the patient maintains fixation into your eye, compare the periphery of his field with your own by moving the pin from outside the field in towards the centre at various points around the periphery, with the pin midway between you and the patient. The patient has to report not when he first sees the pin or your hand but when the pinhead colour changes from black to red.

The pupils

Examination of the pupils and their responses to light and accommodation provides information not only about specific neurological syndromes which affect the pupils, such as Adie's syndrome, but also information about the integrity of the anterior visual pathways (particularly the optic nerves), the brainstem and the efferent parasympathetic and sympathetic pathways to the pupillary sphincter and dilator muscles, respectively.

Pupil constriction is a parasympathetic function. Afferent optic pathways project to the pretectal nucleus, at the level of the superior colliculus, in the midbrain. The pretectal nucleus projects to both ipsilateral (uncrossed) and contralateral (crossed) Edinger–Westphal nuclei, adjacent to the oculomotor nucleus, in the midbrain, leading to direct and consensual pupillary responses, respectively. Pre-ganglionic parasympathetic axons travel in the oculomotor nerve to the ciliary ganglion in the orbit. Post-ganglionic axons innervate the pupillary sphincter. Lesions of the Edinger–Westphal nucleus or the pupilloconstrictor nerve fibres in the oculomotor (third) cranial nerve or in the orbit lead to dilatation of the pupil (mydriasis) unless there is simultaneously a lesion of the sympathetic innervation of the pupil. In either case, there is a failure of constriction of the pupil to light. In general, compression of the third cranial nerve (classically by a posterior communicating artery aneurysm) affects the pupilloconstrictor fibres (located on the dorsal surface of the oculomotor nerve and separately supplied by pial blood vessels), termed a 'surgical' oculomotor palsy. A microvascular ischaemic

lesion of the third nerve may spare the pupilloconstrictor fibres, giving rise to a pupil-sparing third nerve lesion, termed a 'medical' oculomotor palsy. Microvascular lesions of the oculomotor nucleus may spare the Edinger–Westphal nucleus with the same result. A mid-sized unreactive pupil caused by a lesion of both parasympathetic and sympathetic supplies is seen in aneurysms of the internal carotid artery within the cavernous sinus, along with other features of a cavernous sinus syndrome.

Pupil dilation is achieved by sympathetic innervation of pupillodilator muscle fibres. The first-order neurons are in the hypothalamus. They project down through the brainstem and cervical spinal cord to the ciliospinal centre in the lower cervical and upper thoracic spinal cord, from where second-order neurons project via the T1 nerve root and sympathetic chain to the superior cervical ganglion. Third-order axons run up the internal carotid artery as far as the cavernous sinus and from there through the orbit to the pupil. There is also sympathetic innervation of the superior tarsal muscle by the same route. A lesion of the sympathetic supply to the pupil at any point between the hypothalamus and the orbit will give rise to the two main features of Horner's syndrome: constriction (miosis) of the pupil (which will still react to light by further constricting) and partial ptosis (drooping of the upper eyelid but less marked that in a complete oculomotor (III) palsy).

Examination of the pupils

First, in normal illumination, establish whether the pupils are of equal size. If they are not, bear in mind that there are two possibilities: either one is smaller than it should be or the other is larger. Be careful not to jump to the wrong conclusion.

Ideally, the reactions of the pupils to light should be tested in moderately low illumination. Use a bright torch, not an ophthalmoscope. Shine the light into one eye and observe the response of the pupil (the direct response), the normal response being constriction of the pupil, which is sustained until the light is removed. Repeat the test, this time looking at the contralateral pupil, which will normally constrict (the consensual response). Then test the other eye. Next, test accommodation (constriction of the pupils when focusing on a near object). Ask the patient to look into the distance, then at your finger held at a distance and to keep looking as you advance your finger to a distance of about 20 cm from the patient's face. Advancing your finger in a wavy line allows you to check that the patient is looking at the finger. Observe the adduction of the eyes and the constriction of the pupils. Then ask the patient to look into the distance again.

Afferent pupillary defect

A patient with a severe lesion of the anterior visual system in one eye (an ophthalmological disorder or an optic nerve disorder, such as severe optic neuritis or an ischaemic optic neuropathy) will have an afferent pupillary defect (i.e. a failure of constriction of either pupil to light shone into the affected eye). If the visual system on the other side is unaffected, light shone into the normal eye will lead to a normal direct pupillary response and there will also be a consensual response in the visually impaired eye, assuming the efferent pathway is intact.

Relative afferent pupillary defect

A patient with a mild lesion of the anterior visual apparatus on one side will exhibit a direct pupillary response to light, but it will be less vigorous than the consensual response to light shone into the other eye. In this situation, the swinging torch test may reveal a relative afferent pupillary defect. If a patient has a mild optic nerve lesion in the left eye, then acuity and colour vision may be only mildly impaired and the field normal. Shine the torch into the affected left eye and note the seemingly normal response. After 2 seconds, move the torch briskly to shine into the normal right eye. The right pupil will already be constricted as a result of the consensual response. It will stay constricted and, if anything, will constrict a little further. After 2 seconds, move the torch briskly back to the left eye. Because of the subtle afferent defect, the signal strength of the input to the midbrain pupilloconstrictor (Edinger–Westphal) nuclei will be reduced, resulting in an apparently paradoxical dilation of the left pupil despite light being shone into it. If you keep swinging the torch back and forth from one eye to the other, the relative afferent pupillary defect will continue to be observed, although the defect is best seen within the first few attempts.

Afferent and relative afferent pupillary defects are important because they are objective. A person who gives the impression of having functional visual impairment in one eye, but who has an afferent pupillary defect, must have an organic problem. In contrast, a person who reports uniocular blindness and has normal pupillary responses to light will not be blind.

Efferent pupillary defect (part of a third cranial nerve lesion)

A lesion of the pupilloconstrictor nerve fibres in the oculomotor nerve will lead to dilation of the ipsilateral pupil (owing to the unrestrained effect of the intact sympathetic supply). Further, there will be failure of constriction of the pupil to light, although the consensual response in the other eye will be preserved. Light shone into the contralateral eye will elicit a normal direct response but no consensual response.

Other common pupillary abnormalities of neurological relevance

- Simple (physiological) anisocoria (inequality of pupil size): this is common. The pupillary inequality is not marked and the reactions to light and accommodation are normal.
- Tonic pupil: this is seen in Holmes Adie syndrome, a relatively benign polyneuropathy composed of a lesion of the ciliary ganglion and a degree of loss of

tendon reflexes. An acute Adie pupil is enlarged, does not react to light and there is a slow constriction to accommodation. Redilation of the pupil after accommodation is delayed such that, temporarily, the normal pupil may be larger than the affected one.
- Argyll Robertson pupils: these are small, irregular, unequal pupils, which do not react to light but do to accommodation. They were previously commonly seen in advanced syphilis. Without the irregularity but with the other features, diabetic small vessel disease is currently the most common cause.
- The pupils in coma: this is important but covered elsewhere (see Chapter 9).

Fundoscopy

Fundoscopy is described in Chapter 21. The neurological examination focuses on papilloedema, optic atrophy, pigmentary retinal degeneration and vascular disease.

The oculomotor (III), trochlear (IV) and abducens (VI) nerves—eye movements

Abnormalities of eye movements may result from disorders of the cerebral hemispheres; brainstem; cerebellum; cranial nerves III, IV and VI; the neuromuscular junctions between oculomotor nerves and eye muscles; the eye muscles themselves; and from lesions affecting the structure and contents of the orbits. Their importance in neurological and general physical examination is therefore obvious.

The nucleus for the third cranial nerve is in the midbrain (Fig. 16.2). The nerve emerges ventrally (anteriorly), medial to the cerebral peduncle, passing forward through the cavernous sinus to the superior orbital fissure. In the orbit, the superior ramus supplies superior

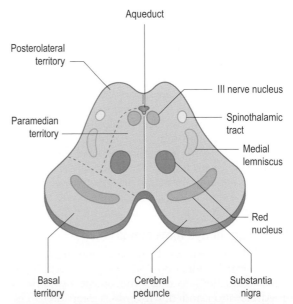

Figure 16.2 A diagram of the midbrain. Note the dorsally positioned third nerve nuclei. Vascular territories are shown on the left.

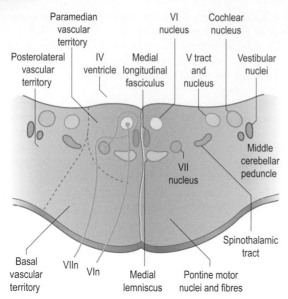

Figure 16.3 A diagram of the fifth, sixth and seventh nerve nuclei in the pons. Note how the nerve fibres of VII loop round the nucleus of VI.

Table 16.4 Actions of the eye muscles

Nerve	Muscle	With eye abducted	With eye adducted
Abducens; VI	Lateral rectus	Abduction	Abduction
Oculomotor; III	Inferior rectus	Depression	Depression; extorsion
Oculomotor; III	Inferior oblique	Extorsion; elevation	Elevation
Oculomotor; III	Medial rectus	Adduction	Adduction
Oculomotor; III	Superior rectus	Elevation	Elevation; intorsion
Trochlear; IV	Superior oblique	Intorsion; depression	Depression

The eye is offset laterally in relation to the apex of the orbit, which accounts for why the superior and inferior rectus muscles have only purely vertical actions when the eye is abducted. Adduction of the eye turns the superior and inferior oblique muscles into a pure depressor and elevator, respectively.

rectus and levator palpebrae superioris. The inferior ramus supplies inferior rectus, inferior oblique and medial rectus, and parasympathetic fibres from the inferior ramus pass to the ciliary ganglion and thence to the ciliary muscle and the pupil sphincter.

The fourth nerve nucleus lies just caudal to the third nerve nucleus in the brainstem. The nerve fibres of the fourth nerve decussate. The nerve starts on the dorsal aspect of the brainstem and passes around the brainstem through the cavernous sinus and superior orbital fissure to the superior oblique muscle. Consequent upon the decussation of fibres, the right trochlear nucleus innervates the left superior oblique and vice versa.

The sixth nerve nucleus is beneath the floor of the fourth ventricle in the pons (Fig. 16.3). Nerve fibres run forward (ventrally) through the pons emerging at its lower border, then up the skull base and forward through the cavernous sinus to the superior orbital fissure and into the orbit to supply the lateral rectus muscle. The nerve is long, thin and very susceptible to dysfunction, most notably in the setting of raised intracranial pressure of any aetiology, which may give rise to either unilateral or bilateral sixth nerve lesions. This is referred to as a 'false localizing sign', since a focal mass lesion causing raised intracranial pressure may be remote from the sixth nerves and their nuclei or there may be no focal cause of the raised pressure at all (e.g. idiopathic intracranial hypertension).

Table 16.4 and Figure 16.4 outline the actions of each eye muscle.

Terminology in eye movements

Horizontal movement of the eye outwards (laterally) is termed abduction and inwards (medially) is termed adduction. Vertical movement upwards is termed elevation and downwards is depression. The eye is also capable of diagonal movements (version) at

Figure 16.4 A diagram showing which muscles elevate and depress the abducted and adducted eye.

any intermediate angle. Rotary movements are those in which the eye twists on its anterior–posterior axis. Intorsion is rotation such that the upper part of the eye moves medially and the lower part of the eye moves laterally. Extorsion is the opposite. Convergence refers to adduction of both eyes to fixate on a near object. Lateral rotation of the head causes reflex movement of the eyes in the opposite direction (adduction of one eye, abduction of the other). A squint (the eyes point in different directions) is described as convergent or divergent strabismus, depending on whether the eyes point towards or away from each other. Saccades are abrupt, rapid, small movements of both eyes, such as those needed to shift fixation from one object to another. Nystagmus denotes rhythmic oscillations of one or (more usually) both eyes. In pendular nystagmus, the movement is slow in both directions. In jerk nystagmus, there is a slow phase in one direction and a fast phase in the opposite direction. By convention, the direction of nystagmus is the direction of the fast phase, but the defect is in fact the slow phase and is either an abnormal deviation of the eyes or a failure of the eyes to maintain position, and the fast phase is a compensatory saccade aimed at restoring the correct position of the eyes. Some types of nystagmus are outlined below.

Figure 16.5   A severe right third nerve lesion with complete ptosis **(A)**. With the paralysed eyelid raised, paresis of adduction is seen on attempted left gaze **(B)**. In this patient the pupil is spared, as is commonly seen in ischaemic lesions, but not in compressive lesions. The other features of a third nerve lesion are paresis of elevation of the eye and intorsion of the eye on attempting to look down, owing to the action of the superior oblique muscle on an eye that cannot be adducted. (Reproduced from Forbes and Jackson, Color Atlas and Text of Clinical Medicine, Mosby, 2002.)

Examination of eye movements

As with every other component of examination, the detail in which the eye movements are examined depends on whether there are relevant symptoms and whether abnormal signs are likely to be present. Ask the patient to keep his head still (assist him by putting your left hand on his head to steady it) and then to look at your right index finger held directly in front of his eyes at about half a metre distance. In the primary position of gaze, look for any visible abnormality of the alignment of the two eyes (an affected patient may or may not complain of double vision) and any pendular or vestibular nystagmus (see below). Now move your finger to the right, then left, and then up and down. The pursuit eye movements, which are elicited, should precisely follow your finger at the appropriate constant velocity. Eye movements, which are 'broken up' into a series of short saccades, indicate a brainstem or cerebellar lesion affecting eye movement control. Patients with diplopia usually will experience their diplopia at some point (or at all times) during this simple test. However, in patients with a complaint of diplopia it is important not just to test vertical eye movements from the primary position of gaze, but to test movements to the right and up and down and then to the left and up and down. During pursuit eye movement examination, gaze-evoked and vestibular nystagmus will be observable (see below). When looking for nystagmus, it is important not to get the patient to look too far in any direction because, at the extremes of gaze, nystagmus can be normal as the patient struggles to deviate his eyes beyond what is possible. Look for nystagmus at about 30° away from the primary position of gaze.

Diplopia testing

If a patient complains of double vision, first establish that it is true diplopia and not monocular diplopia. Monocular diplopia normally suggests a problem with the orbital globe, such as the cornea (e.g. kerato-conus, cone-shaped cornea; or astigmatism, abnormal curvature of the cornea), cataracts or lens disloca-tion (e.g. in Marfan's syndrome and homocystinuria). However, persistence of diplopia when one eye is covered, particularly in the absence of objective oph-thalmoparesis, may suggest a non-organic cause. In patients who have obvious, easily visible paresis of movement of one or both eyes, the reason for diplo-pia is self-evident.

Diplopia develops with even very subtle misalign-ment of the eyes, which cannot be seen on simple inspection. In this situation, if the ophthalmoparesis affects just one eye, it is possible to deduce which eye muscles are underactive by diplopia testing. The true image is the one generated by the eye with normal movements. The false image is the one generated by the eye with the paretic muscle or muscles. For exam-ple, if a patient develops double vision on looking to the right, with horizontal separation of the images, the false image will be the one further out to the right. This is true whether it is the right eye, which does not abduct adequately (right lateral rectus weakness) or if it is the left eye, which does not adduct adequately (left medial rectus weakness). If this does not seem immediately clear, consider the extreme case: one eye moves, the other does not. An image (an examiner's finger or a white pinhead) moves to the patient's right. The image remains in the middle of the field of the eye, which moves but moves progressively to the right of the field of the eye, which does not. The same rule applies in all directions of gaze. Diplopia is always maximal in the direction in which the weak muscle has its purest action (see Table 16.4).

The severity of the diplopia should be assessed in eight positions: looking to left and right, up and down, and obliquely up and down to the left and obliquely up and down to the right. To work out which muscle is underactive, where the diplopia is maximal, cover each eye in turn and get the patient to tell you which of the two images disappears. Inconsistent answers are common, however, and the assistance of an ophthal-mologist or optometrist is frequently desirable. The

Table 16.5 The effects of lesions of the oculomotor (III), trochlear (IV) and abducens (VI) nerves

Affected nerve	Signs	Comment
Oculomotor*	Paresis of adduction (medial rectus)	The eye becomes abducted because of unopposed action of lateral rectus, and slightly depressed because of action of superior oblique.
	Paresis of elevation (superior rectus and inferior oblique)	The pure depressor action of superior oblique cannot be tested because the eye cannot be adducted.
		Intorsion of the eye on attempted down gaze indicates intact trochlear nerve and superior oblique function.
	Paresis of depression (inferior rectus)	
	Ptosis owing to paresis of levator palpebrae superioris	With complete ptosis, of course, there is no diplopia.
	Dilated, unreactive pupil	This feature is not present in pupil-sparing lesions (microvascular lesions of nucleus or nerve).
Trochlear	Paresis of superior oblique	Extorsion of the eye owing to unopposed action of inferior oblique leads to diplopia such that a vertical line looks V-shaped.
		The patient compensates with a head tilt to the side opposite the lesion, intact intorsion on that side tending to correct the diplopia. This is the basis of the Bielschowsky head tilt test when double vision is improved by tilting the head away from the affected side and worsened by tilting the head towards the affected side.
Abducens	Paresis of lateral rectus	Horizontal diplopia to ipsilateral lateral gaze

*Figure 16.5 shows a patient with a severe oculomotor palsy.

features of lesions of the third, fourth and sixth cranial nerves are summarized in Table 16.5. It is important to assess for diplopia in sustained directional gaze, particularly if a neuromuscular transmission disorder (e.g. myasthenia) is considered, as otherwise fatigable ophthalmoparesis may be missed.

In assessing patients who have double vision, it is best first to establish which muscles appear to be weak and then try to decide what the nature of the problem is likely to be, taking into consideration all the physical signs. Thus, impairment of eye movements in one eye in combination with proptosis of that eye may occur because of mechanical restriction of eye movements by an intraorbital lesion. Weakness of muscles in both eyes with different patterns of involvement of the muscles in the two eyes is likely to be caused by a disorder of the muscles themselves (orbital myositis, thyroid eye disease) or by ocular or generalized myasthenia. The pupils will not be involved. Bilateral, asymmetrical combinations of cranial nerve lesions are relatively uncommon (neoplastic infiltration, cranial polyneuritis). Bilateral sixth cranial nerve lesions are common, usually but not exclusively as a feature of raised intracranial pressure. Multiple oculomotor neuropathies in one eye direct attention to the superior orbital fissure and the cavernous sinus (Box 16.2).

Horizontal gaze paresis; internuclear ophthalmoparesis

Neural control of voluntary lateral gaze to the right starts in the left cerebral hemisphere, such that a large left cerebral hemisphere lesion may be associated with failure of right gaze and a tendency for the eyes to deviate to the left (the side of the lesion). Output

Box 16.2 Cranial nerve involvement in lesions of the cavernous sinus and superior orbital fissure

1. Lesion of the cavernous sinus (e.g. internal carotid aneurysm, internal carotid artery dissection, meningioma):
   —potential involvement of cranial nerves III, IV, VI, V_1 (ophthalmic division), V_2 (maxillary division) and sympathetic pupillodilator nerve fibres
   —cavernous sinus thrombosis combines the above with proptosis, chemosis, papilloedema and visual failure
2. Lesion of the superior orbital fissure (e.g. Tolosa Hunt syndrome):
   —potential involvement of III, IV, VI and V_1 (ophthalmic division)
   —extension into the orbit may lead to involvement of the optic nerve

runs to the right paramedian pontine reticular formation (PPRF); hence, a right-sided pontine lesion may involve a right gaze paresis. Output from the right PPRF goes to the right sixth nerve nucleus, resulting in right eye abduction, and across, via the left medial longitudinal fasciculus (MLF), to the left third nerve nucleus, resulting in simultaneous left eye adduction. Attempted right gaze in the setting of a left MLF lesion results in abduction of the right eye, but failure of adduction of the left eye—an internuclear ophthalmoparesis (INO) (Fig. 16.6). Bilateral MLF lesions give rise to bilateral INO, in which case, with lateral gaze in either direction, only the abducting eye moves normally. Nystagmus is commonly seen in the abducting eye. The pathway for adducting both eyes for near vision is separate and sometimes in bilateral INO,

Figure 16.6 **(A)** A right internuclear ophthalmoparesis. **(B)** A diagram of the pathways for horizontal gaze. The command for left gaze originates in the right cerebral hemisphere. Descending nerve fibres decussate to reach the left pons. Lesion 1 produces a left horizontal gaze paresis. Lesion 2 produces a right internuclear ophthalmoparesis. Lesion 3 produces the 'one and a half' syndrome: a left gaze paresis and left internuclear ophthalmoparesis (failure of adduction of the left eye on right gaze)—only abduction of the right eye on right gaze remains. NPH, nucleus prepositus hypoglossi; MLF, medial longitudinal fasciculus; PPRF, paramedian pontine reticular formation.

preservation of adduction of the eyes for near vision (convergence) can be demonstrated, proving that the problem is not bilateral medial rectus weakness.

Vertical gaze paresis

The neural control of upgaze and downgaze is complex. Ultimately, output for upgaze is via components of the third nerve nucleus mainly to the superior rectus and inferior oblique muscles bilaterally. The output for downgaze is from the third and fourth nerve nuclei to the inferior rectus and superior oblique muscles, respectively. In general, defects of upgaze or downgaze localize rather poorly, but lesions, such as pineal tumours, which compress the midbrain and bilateral descending connections from the hemispheres, often cause upgaze paresis. For example, Parinaud's syndrome, from compression of the dorsal midbrain, owing to a pineal tumour, for example, causes restriction of upgaze, convergence-retraction nystagmus and pupillary light-near dissociation (pupils accommodate but respond poorly to light). Rare midbrain ischaemic strokes owing to occlusion

of a perforating vessel from the top of the basilar artery include downgaze paresis among the clinical manifestations.

Non-paralytic strabismus

Clinicians need to be able to recognize developmental non-paralytic strabismus. Decompensation of a long-standing squint may be a cause of acquired diplopia. The alternating cover test and unilateral cover test (cover–uncover test) are useful for detecting ocular deviation, when the misaligned eye will deviate inwards or outwards, on covering. This is particularly useful in detecting phorias (or latent strabismus), when ocular deviation is only evident when binocular vision is prevented, compared with tropias (exotropia or isotropia), when misalignment is evident during binocular vision, but often further exacerbated by the cover test.

Testing saccadic eye movements

Getting a patient to follow a moving finger tests pursuit eye movements. It takes very little time to test saccadic eye movements and useful signs may be detected. First, simply ask the patient to keep his head still and look to the left, to the right, up and down. Then hold your hands up in front of the patient, one in the primary position of gaze, the other to the side, with palms facing the patient, fists closed. Open the fist of the hand in front of the patient and ask him to look at it. Then close that fist and open the other and ask the patient to switch his gaze to the hand at the side. By alternating which hand is open you can get the patient to refixate briskly to and fro. Then check the other side. These manoeuvres test saccadic movements; in disease, saccades may be slowed or interrupted. A mild INO will be best seen during saccadic horizontal eye movements, with relative delay of adduction of eye on the affected side. Because detecting a mild INO requires observing a difference in the velocity of movement of the two eyes, it is difficult to appreciate if the examiner fixates on one or the other eye; perhaps, unintuitively, it is best to look at the bridge of the patient's nose to see the movement of the two eyes at the same time.

Supranuclear gaze pareses

Reflex eye movements related to head movements are generated and organized by vestibular, cerebellar and brainstem systems, whereas voluntary gaze is initiated in the cerebral hemispheres. A patient's gaze paresis is therefore supranuclear if reflex eye movements are intact. In a patient with selective paresis of downgaze, if brisk backward rotation of the head (extension of the neck) produced reflex depression of both eyes, a supranuclear lesion would be inferred. In practice, this is often not easily achieved because the relatively common disorder giving supranuclear downgaze paresis is progressive supranuclear palsy, a condition in which there is also axial rigidity affecting neck movements.

Peripheral vestibular nystagmus

Peripheral vestibular nystagmus occurs with lesions of the labyrinth or vestibular nerve. Normally there is tonic input to the brainstem vestibular nuclei from the periphery. Loss of this tonic input leads to deviation of the eyes towards the affected side (slow phase) with fast-phase nystagmus directed to the opposite side. In mild lesions, the nystagmus is only seen when the eyes look in the direction of the fast phase. In more severe lesions, the nystagmus is seen with the eyes in the primary position of gaze or even when looking away from the direction of the fast phase. Usually the nystagmus is of high frequency and relatively low amplitude.

Gaze paretic nystagmus

Gaze paretic nystagmus is a gaze-evoked nystagmus in which the eyes are not able to maintain a position away from their primary position, so the slow phase is a drift back to the primary position, whereas the fast phase is in the direction of gaze. In the primary position, the eyes are still. The nystagmus may be of large amplitude and low frequency. Drug-induced nystagmus (alcohol, benzodiazepines, antiepileptic medication) is of this sort and is seen in all directions of gaze. Structural brainstem or cerebellar lesions may cause asymmetric gaze paretic nystagmus. In cerebellar hemisphere lesions, the nystagmus may be unidirectional with the fast phase towards the side of the lesion.

Upbeat nystagmus (fast phase upwards) may occur with lesions at various locations in the brainstem and with cerebellar vermis lesions. Downbeat nystagmus is characteristic of cervicomedullary junction lesions, such as Chiari malformations, but may also be seen with cerebellar degenerations.

Congenital nystagmus

The rule here is that the nystagmus is horizontal, even when the patient looks up or down. On left gaze, it is left beating, and on right gaze, it is right beating. There may be a null point at which the nystagmus is least conspicuous, but it is not necessarily in the primary position, and the eyes may not be completely still. Congenital nystagmus is damped by convergence.

Pendular nystagmus

Pendular nystagmus may be seen as a complication of congenital or acquired very poor vision. It is also seen in pontine lesions (e.g. multiple sclerosis).

The trigeminal (V) nerve

The trigeminal nerve is a mixed motor and sensory nerve. The nerve trunk emerges from the pons as sensory and motor roots.

Sensory component of the trigeminal nerve

The primary sensory neurons are in the trigeminal ganglion, just behind the cavernous sinus at the apex of the petrous bone. Central projections run in the

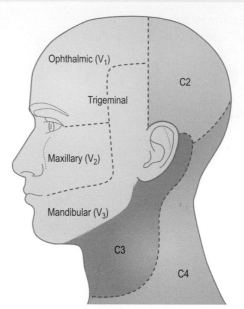

Figure 16.7   Areas of cutaneous innervation of the head and neck by the three divisions of the trigeminal nerve and the upper cervical nerve roots.

trigeminal nerve into the pons. Figure 16.7 shows the cutaneous distribution of the three divisions of the trigeminal nerve: ophthalmic (V_1), maxillary (V_2) and mandibular (V_3). These nerves also mediate general sensation inside the mouth and nose and proprioception. The ophthalmic nerve passes through the cavernous sinus and superior orbital fissure. The maxillary nerve also passes through the cavernous sinus, but leaves the inside of the skull through the foramen rotundum. The mandibular nerve passes through the foramen ovale.

Afferents mediating touch sensation pass to the principal sensory nucleus of the trigeminal nerve in the pons. Pain and temperature afferents go into the spinal tract and pass caudally into the medulla and into the spinal nucleus of the trigeminal nerve, which extends down from the medulla as low as the upper cervical spinal cord. Thus, lesions in the medulla can give rise to dissociated sensory loss in the trigeminal territory (loss of pinprick sensation with preserved light touch sensation). Afferents mediating masticatory muscle proprioception pass to the more rostral mesencephalic nucleus.

The afferent and efferent components of the jaw reflex are mediated by the sensory and motor components of the trigeminal nerve via the trigeminal mesencephalic nucleus.

Motor component of the trigeminal nerve

Motor nerve fibres from the motor nucleus in the pons run in the motor root of the trigeminal nerve, bypassing the trigeminal ganglion to enter the mandibular nerve. They supply the muscles of mastication: masseter, temporalis and the medial and lateral pterygoids.

Trigeminal territory sensory loss

Patients with impaired sensation on one side of the face may have a trigeminal nerve lesion, a trigeminal nucleus lesion or a lesion of central trigeminal sensory pathways. Not uncommonly, unilateral facial sensory symptoms remain unexplained, which does not necessarily make them 'non-organic'. Much is made of distinguishing between patients whose distribution of sensory loss is anatomical and those in whom it is not. Sensory loss, which ends at the jaw line and at the hairline, would be regarded as non-anatomical; however, too much dogma may be unwise—patients are often not very careful reporters of exactly where their sensory symptoms are located. Clearly defined symptoms of reduced sensation render examination almost redundant, but the area of hypoaesthesia can be delineated in the same way as sensory loss anywhere else using a pin and testing from a numb area outwards towards where sensation is normal.

The corneal reflex

A sensory stimulus applied to the cornea causes a reflex blink, which cannot be suppressed; its absence on one side establishes unequivocally the presence of a trigeminal lesion. Patients with an anaesthetic cornea are at risk of corneal injury, so it is important to identify affected individuals by testing patients who very clearly have symptoms and other signs of a trigeminal lesion. It is also an important test in coma. The test is uncomfortable and should not be part of a 'routine' neurological examination. The presence of a normal corneal reflex does not mean that there is no lesion of the trigeminal nerve or its connections.

Explain to the patient what is going to happen. Ask him to look in such a direction that the eyes are wide open. Using the corner of a clean tissue, touch the centre of the patient's cornea, approaching from the side. The normal response is a brisk blink. Some use cotton wool, but there is a risk of strands getting stuck in the eye because of the blink. In coma, a drop of saline applied to the cornea is a good stimulus. Remember that if there is ipsilateral facial paralysis (e.g. Bell's palsy), the reflex will be absent on the affected side, but will be readily seen on the other side.

Testing the motor component of the trigeminal nerve

Look for wasting of the temporalis and masseter muscles. Feel for contraction of the masseter muscles when the patient clenches his jaw. Ask the patient to open his mouth; the lateral pterygoid muscles on each side draw the mandible forward, such that a severe lesion of the trigeminal nerve will lead to deviation of the jaw towards the side of the lesion owing to weakness of the pterygoid muscles on the affected side. The pterygoid muscles may be further tested by asking the patient to push his open jaw sideways against your hand.

The facial (VII) nerve

The facial nerve is principally a motor nerve, supplying facial muscles on one side, but it also has small general somatic sensory and major gustatory sensory components, as well as important parasympathetic functions.

The facial nerve nucleus is in the caudal pons, lying ventrolateral to the sixth cranial nerve nucleus (see Fig. 16.3). It receives upper motor neuron input from both cerebral hemispheres. Lower motor neuron fibres from the facial nucleus first pass round the sixth nerve nucleus and then emerge from the pons to form the facial nerve. From here, it travels laterally, adjacent to the eighth cranial nerve, to the internal auditory meatus, thence to the facial canal, which has a relatively long and tortuous course through the skull, emerging at the stylomastoid foramen. The nerve then passes forward into the parotid gland and divides into branches, which supply all the facial muscles and the platysma muscle on one side. In the facial canal, a branch of the facial nerve supplies the stapedius muscle.

The nerve cell bodies of the sensory components of the facial nerve are in the geniculate ganglion in the facial canal. Gustatory sensory afferents from the anterior two-thirds of the tongue travel in the lingual nerve and then via the chorda tympani nerve to join the facial nerve in the facial canal. Central projections reach the medulla via the nervus intermedius between the facial and eighth cranial nerve.

The peripheral projections of the small general somatic sensory contribution innervate the tympanic membrane, external auditory meatus and tragus of the ear. This accounts for the herpetic vesicles seen in the ear in patients with the Ramsay Hunt syndrome of facial paralysis caused by herpes zoster affecting the facial nerve.

Secretomotor parasympathetic efferents leave the pontomedullary junction in the nervus intermedius, which joins the facial nerve in the internal auditory meatus. Some of the parasympathetic nerves leave the facial nerve at the geniculate ganglion in the greater petrosal nerve, and via the pterygopalantine ganglion, eventually mediating tear secretion from the lachrymal glands. Others leave via the chorda tympani nerve to reach submandibular and sublingual salivary glands, via the submandibular ganglion (note that the parotid salivary gland is innervated by the glossopharyngeal nerve via the greater auricular nerve).

These complexities are relevant to clinical neurology because a facial nerve lesion, depending on its location, may be associated with loss of taste, hyperacusis (if the stapedius is paralysed) and, in chronic lesions, gustatory lachrymation 'crocodile tears' (i.e. inappropriate tear production when salivary glands should be activated), attributed to aberrant reinnervation of salivary and lachrymal glands. Other aberrant reinnervation syndromes, relevant to recovering facial nerve palsies, include facial synkinesis (voluntary contraction of one facial muscle leads to contraction of an ipsilateral facial muscle—such as eye winking on smiling) or hemifacial spasm (spontaneous unilateral twitching, which usually responds to botulinum toxin treatment).

Facial weakness occurs because of muscle disorders (invariably bilateral weakness), myasthenia (invariably bilateral, but may be asymmetrical early on), polyneuropathies (e.g. Guillain-Barré syndrome or vasculitis, unilateral or bilateral), facial nerve or nuclear lesions (most commonly unilateral), motor neuronopathies (usually bilateral) or upper motor neuron disorders (usually unilateral, but occasionally bilateral).

A lower motor neuron lesion affecting the whole of the facial nerve nucleus or the whole of the facial nerve will cause weakness of all muscles of one side of the face. A unilateral upper motor neuron lesion, however, will cause weakness of the lower half of the face with sparing of the upper half of the face because there is bilateral representation of the upper half of the face in the motor cortex.

Testing the facial nerve

Look for asymmetry of the face. Ask the patient to raise his eyebrows (to look astonished), to blink and then to screw both eyes up, firmly closed. On a weak side, the eyelashes will be less buried by the eyelids. Attempt to raise the patient's eyebrows while his eyes are closed and screwed up; mild weakness may be detected. With severe lower motor neuron facial weakness, the patient will not be able to close the affected eye. Attempted eye closure will be accompanied by elevation of the eyes (Bell's phenomenon). Ask the patient to blow his cheeks out, to show his teeth (or gums) and then to grimace. Observe the patient's spontaneous smiles. (In some upper motor neuron disorders of facial muscle control, voluntary movement of the lower face is lost, but smiling is relatively preserved and vice versa 'emotional versus volitional'.) Ask the patient to purse his lips together and attempt to open them using your fingers. These tests usually suffice to pick up facial weakness and to distinguish between upper and lower motor neuron disorders.

The cochlear and vestibular (VIII) nerves

The cochlear and vestibular nerves convey afferents from the cochlea and the vestibular apparatus, respectively, via the internal auditory meatus to the pontomedullary junction in close proximity to the facial nerve, reaching cochlear and vestibular nuclei in the brainstem. Acute sensorineural deafness and acute vestibular neuritis reflect separate pathologies selectively affecting each of these nerves.

Testing the cochlear and vestibular nerves

The assessment of deafness is covered in detail elsewhere (see Chapter 22). At the bedside, a crude assessment of hearing can be achieved by rubbing your index finger and thumb together close to the patient's ear or by whispering numbers close to his ear, with the contralateral ear occluded. Rinne's test is good for distinguishing between conduction and sensorineural deafness, as long as you use the appropriate tuning fork (frequency 512 Hz—not the lower frequency tuning fork (128 Hz) used for testing vibration sense). Rinne's test is performed by placing the tuning fork on the mastoid, until the sound is no longer heard, and then placing the tuning fork a few centimetres from the auditory canal.

Conduction deafness is sometimes of neurological significance if an infective or neoplastic middle ear lesion has spread to affect the middle or posterior cranial fossa structures.

Unilateral sensorineural deafness is an important feature of 'cerebellopontine angle lesions', such as acoustic neuroma or meningioma, along with variable combinations of facial weakness (facial nerve), facial sensory symptoms (trigeminal nerve), nystagmus (brainstem and vestibular nerve), ataxia (brainstem and cerebellum) and ultimately long-tract signs (brainstem) and raised intracranial pressure.

Bilateral sensorineural deafness may be a feature of certain multisystem neurological disorders, particularly mitochondrial disorders.

Two important tests of vestibular function assess much of the vestibular system (the semicircular canals of the labyrinths, the vestibular nerves and the vestibular nuclei of the brainstem). These are the Dix-Hallpike test for positioning vertigo and nystagmus and the head thrust test. They should be performed in patients with vertigo.

The Dix-Hallpike test is described in Chapter 22. Far and away the most common cause of positioning vertigo is the condition benign paroxysmal positional vertigo, a labyrinthine disorder, and it is by far the most common cause of an abnormal Dix-Hallpike test. Vestibular neuritis is usually associated with nystagmus that does not require a change in head position to elicit it, but in this condition vertigo and nystagmus are usually exacerbated by positioning tests. Brainstem disorders may also be the cause of positioning vertigo and nystagmus. Typically, peripheral disorders are associated with a latent period between head movement and onset of vertigo and nystagmus, intense vertigo and a reduction of the vertigo and nystagmus with repeated testing, whereas central positioning nystagmus may be associated with rather mild vertigo, but with nystagmus that does not diminish with repeated testing.

The head thrust test (head impulse test) detects a failure of the afferent component of the vestibulo-ocular reflex. In a normal individual, fixating on an object straight ahead, an abrupt rotation of the head to one side or the other will not disrupt ocular fixation. In a patient with an acute unilateral peripheral vestibulopathy (vestibular neuritis), a head thrust rotating the front of the head towards the side of the lesion will result in the eyes turning with the head momentarily and a noticeable saccade to bring the eyes back to restore fixation. This test is useful in distinguishing acute vertigo caused by vestibular neuritis from vertigo caused by a brainstem stroke or transient ischaemic attack. With the patient's gaze fixed on the examiner's nose, the examiner then abruptly turns the patient's head successively about 30° to the right and left.

The glossopharyngeal (IX) nerve

Anatomical and functional relationships exist between the glossopharyngeal nerve, the vagus nerve and the cranial component of the accessory nerve. The nucleus ambiguus in the medulla (Fig. 16.8) contains the motor neurons, which innervate striated muscle of the palate, pharynx, larynx and upper oesophagus; fibres running partly in the glossopharyngeal nerve, mainly in the vagus nerve and partly in the cranial portion of the accessory nerve. Situated more dorsally in the medulla, the dorsal motor nucleus of the vagus and the inferior salivatory nucleus (whose fibres join the glossopharyngeal nerve) contain preganglionic parasympathetic neurons, which control glands and smooth muscle. Special visceral afferents (i.e. taste fibres from the intermediate nerve and the glossopharyngeal nerve) enter the solitary tract to end in the nucleus of the solitary tract in the medulla. General somatic sensory afferents in the glossopharyngeal and vagus nerves join trigeminal sensory nuclei.

The glossopharyngeal nerve rootlets emerge from the medulla just rostral to those of the vagus nerve. The glossopharyngeal nerve leaves the skull via the jugular foramen (together with the vagus and accessory nerves). It mediates somatic sensation of the palate and pharynx and gustatory sensation from the posterior third of the tongue; it has parasympathetic autonomic secretomotor fibres, which reach the parotid gland (via the otic ganglion); and supplies the stylopharyngeus muscle (which cannot be tested clinically).

Testing the glossopharyngeal nerve

The glossopharyngeal nerve is not tested in routine neurological examinations. With particular clinical indications to test it, such as a symptom of pharyngeal sensory impairment, pharyngeal neuropathic pain or a lesion of the vagus nerve, pharyngeal sensation can be tested using an orange stick to touch lightly the mucosa of the posterior pharyngeal wall. This requires tolerance and cooperation on the part of the patient. Some normal individuals will gag even at the approach of a tongue depressor or orange stick. In stuporous or comatose patients, testing the gag reflex may be useful. The afferent component of this reflex involves the glossopharyngeal nerves.

The vagus (X) nerve

The rootlets of the vagus nerve emerge from the medulla just below those of the glossopharyngeal nerve. Both nerves leave the base of the skull through the jugular foramen. The vagus nerve passes down the neck adjacent to the internal carotid artery and internal jugular vein. Motor efferent fibres supply pharyngeal muscles. The superior laryngeal nerve supplies the cricopharyngeus muscle of the larynx and conveys sensation from the larynx. Lower down in the thorax, the recurrent laryngeal nerve passes back up the neck to supply the laryngeal muscles other than the cricopharyngeus. The visceral afferent and efferent fibres of the vagus nerve downstream of the recurrent laryngeal nerves are not amenable to clinical neurological examination.

Testing the vagus nerve

A patient with a proximal unilateral lesion of the vagus nerve may complain of dysphagia and nasal regurgitation of swallowed fluids. There will be weakness of the muscles of the soft palate on the affected side. Attempted voluntary elevation of the soft palate (ask the patient to say 'Ahh', preferably fairly high pitched) reveals the weakness of elevation of the palate on the affected side, along with deviation of the uvula to the unaffected side, because of the unopposed action of the palatal muscles on that side. In addition, ipsilateral vocal cord paresis will lead to dysphonia. Bilateral lesions of the vagus nerves will invariably be associated with dysphagia. (Bilateral palatal weakness is not commonly caused by bilateral vagus lesions but rather by more diffuse disorders, such as polyneuropathy or myasthenia gravis.) The effects of bilateral lesions of innervation of the larynx vary depending on whether there is weakness mainly of vocal cord abduction or adduction or

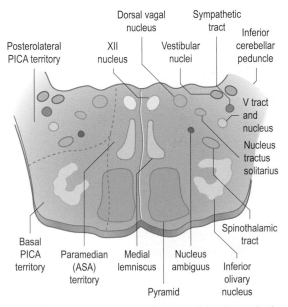

Figure 16.8 A diagram of cranial nerve nuclei and tracts in the medulla. Vascular territories are shown on the left. ASA, anterior spinal artery; PICA, posterior inferior cerebellar artery.

Labels in figure:
Dorsal vagal nucleus
Sympathetic tract
Inferior cerebellar peduncle
Posterolateral PICA territory
XII nucleus
Vestibular nuclei
V tract and nucleus
Nucleus tractus solitarius
Spinothalamic tract
Basal PICA territory
Paramedian (ASA) territory
Medial lemniscus
Nucleus ambiguus
Inferior olivary nucleus
Pyramid

both. Bilateral abductor weakness puts the patient at risk of stridor and respiratory obstruction. Bilateral adductor weakness leads to dysphonia and an inability to generate a normal explosive cough (the cough which the patient can manage is described as a 'bovine' cough).

The accessory (XI) nerve

The cranial accessory nerve is formed of nerve fibres from the nucleus ambiguus and they soon leave the accessory nerve to rejoin their equivalents in the vagus nerve. The spinal accessory nerve consists of motor nerve fibres from the cervical spinal cord (C2-6); instead of leaving the spinal cord in spinal roots, they pass rostrally up into the medulla and emerge as the accessory nerve which, along with the glossopharyngeal and vagus nerves, pass through the jugular foramen. The spinal accessory nerve supplies the sternocleidomastoid muscle and the upper part of the trapezius muscle.

Testing the accessory nerve

The left sternocleidomastoid muscle contributes to rotation of the head to the right and vice versa. Therefore, weakness of the left sternocleidomastoid is assessed by asking the patient to turn his head to the right with force, while the examiner opposes the rotation with the left hand, pushing carefully against the right side of the face. Failure of contraction of the muscle can be seen. Weakness of the upper part of trapezius is one of the causes of winging of the scapula, the other being weakness of serratus anterior owing to a lesion of the long thoracic nerve (see Table 16.6). Bilateral scapular winging can occur in primary muscle disorders, such as the genetic facioscapulohumeral muscular dystrophy. Scapular winging owing to trapezius weakness is most commonly caused by

a lesion of the accessory nerve in the posterior triangle of the neck, often iatrogenic related to surgical excision of a lymph node.

The hypoglossal (XII) nerve

The hypoglossal nucleus in the medulla contains motor neurons that innervate tongue muscles. The nerve leaves the lower medulla, passing through the hypoglossal canal to leave the base of the skull, then down and forward to reach the tongue.

Testing the hypoglossal nerve

A unilateral hypoglossal nerve lesion in the acute stage leads to weakness of tongue muscles on the affected side. Attempted protrusion of the tongue results in deviation of the tongue towards the weak side (Fig. 16.9). A chronic lesion will be associated with visible muscle atrophy of the affected side of the tongue. Bilateral wasting and weakness of the tongue with fasciculation are usually owing to the progressive bulbar atrophy of motor neuron disease.

Speech

Dysphonia is an abnormality of production of vocal sounds. Vocal cord paresis therefore causes dysphonia. Parkinson's disease may cause dysphonia and certainly hypophonia, a low-volume voice.

Dysarthria is an abnormality of articulation, for which neurological disease is an important cause. Those with a musical ear may be good at distinguishing spastic from cerebellar dysarthrias, but experienced neurologists sometimes get this wrong. The important thing is to detect mild dysarthria and look for other signs which will clarify its basis and to consider that a patient who has dysarthria may, more importantly, have dysphagia.

Figure 16.9 **(A)** The tongue of a patient with an acute left hypoglossal nerve lesion. She had noticed weight loss for 3 months and pain at the back of the neck on the left side for 1 month. She was afebrile and the only sign was the weak tongue. **(B)** A T2-weighted MRI scan at the base of the skull shows abnormal tissue (*thick arrow*) under the skull and infiltrating into the hypoglossal canal (*thin arrow*). The hypoglossal canal on the right side is normal (*dotted arrow*). MRI scans of the neck revealed lymphadenopathy (not shown). A fine needle aspirate from one of the nodes (hence, the adhesive dressing seen in the photograph) was not diagnostic. An open lymph node biopsy confirmed the diagnosis of tuberculosis.

Spastic dysarthria

An upper motor neuron disorder affects the tongue, pharynx and facial muscles. Tongue movements are slow, the jaw jerk (see below) is brisk and facial stretch reflexes may be present. If part of a pseudobulbar palsy is owing to diffuse small vessel cerebrovascular disease or motor neuron disease, there will be associated cognitive abnormalities and limb signs.

Cerebellar (ataxic) dysarthria

Look carefully for nystagmus and other eye movement disorders and for limb and gait ataxia.

Parkinsonism (hypokinetic dysarthria)

In parkinsonism, dysarthria and other disorders of speech and language, such as acquired stutter as well as dysphonia, may be seen.

Bulbar palsy (flaccid dysarthria)

Bulbar refers to the medulla oblongata, and bulbar palsy denotes any weakness of muscles supplied by the seventh to twelfth cranial nerves from the pons and medulla. Dysarthria and dysphagia are the main manifestations. Palatal weakness allows nasal escape of air during production of plosive sounds. Many causes are seen, ranging from muscle disorders, myasthenia gravis and polyneuropathies to lower motor neuronopathies. In myasthenia, fatigue may be evident, the dysarthria developing as the patient talks.

Severe upper motor neuron lesions, such as strokes, will produce dysarthria, which may also be a feature of certain dysphasias.

Motor system

For the purposes of clinical neurological examination and interpretation of neurological signs, the anatomical considerations can be kept simple. The motor neurons whose axons terminate at neuromuscular junctions and which activate voluntary striated muscle contraction are situated in the anterior horns of the spinal cord grey matter and in motor cranial nerve nuclei. These are the lower motor neurons. Upper motor neurons are those situated in the cerebral cortex whose axons leave the cortex to control, directly or indirectly, the lower motor neurons. Some of these are in the somatotopically organized primary motor cortex (Fig. 16.10) in the precentral gyrus at the back of the frontal lobe, but the distribution of upper motor neurons in the cortex is much wider than just the primary motor cortex and includes the supplementary motor area and premotor cortex in the frontal lobes. The cerebral control of posture and movement involves widely distributed cortical motor systems. Crucial also are circuits

involving the basal ganglia and cerebellum. Output from the cortex is either direct to motor neurons via corticospinal and corticobulbar tracts or indirect via projections to the brainstem which has major influences by various pathways.

The corticobulbar and corticospinal tracts pass via the internal capsule and cerebral peduncle to the ventral pons. The corticobulbar tract projects to motor nuclei of cranial nerves V, VII, IX, X and XII bilaterally. The corticospinal tract continues in the medullary pyramid. The majority of corticospinal tract fibres decussate in the lower ventral medulla, passing into the lateral corticospinal tract of the spinal cord to innervate contralateral spinal motor neurons. These fibres control movements of the limbs. A minority of corticospinal tract fibres do not decussate but proceed straight on into the spinal cord in the anterior corticospinal tract to project to motor neurons bilaterally. They control axial muscles involved in posture.

Lower motor neurons in the brainstem send their axons directly into cranial nerves. Lower motor neurons in the spinal cord send their axons via ventral nerve roots into spinal nerves. Spinal nerves divide into dorsal and ventral rami. Dorsal rami innervate paraspinal muscles of the back. Ventral rami innervate the other muscles. The anatomy of the thoracic spinal nerves is relatively simple, directly reflecting embryological segmentation. The ventral rami supply intercostal and abdominal trunk muscles. Cervical, first thoracic, lumbar and sacral spinal nerve ventral rami pass into plexuses (cervical, brachial and lumbosacral) from which are formed named peripheral nerves that mainly supply the limbs. The muscles supplied by a spinal nerve collectively constitute a 'myotome'. (The cutaneous area supplied by a spinal nerve is a dermatome.)

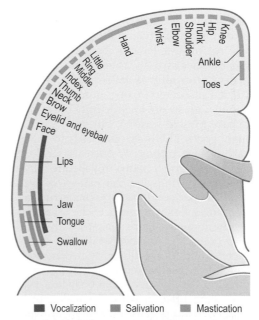

■ Vocalization   ■ Salivation   ■ Mastication

Figure 16.10 Somatotopic representation in the primary motor cortex.

The fundamental effect of a lower motor lesion is weakness (ultimately paralysis) of affected muscles with marked wasting. The effects of upper motor neuron lesions are more variable, depending on which descending pathways are affected. They are loss of dexterity, weakness and spasticity. An upper motor neuron lesion may cause mild weakness but, nevertheless, be incapacitating because of spasticity and impaired dexterity. On the other hand, a lesion restricted to cells in the primary motor cortex itself causes weakness without spasticity. With upper motor neuron lesions, muscle wasting is much less marked and it occurs late.

Motor system examination

The examination technique for formal assessment of the motor system depends very much on the circumstances. For instance, a follow-up outpatient assessment to gauge the response to treatment of a patient with myasthenia gravis, polymyositis or even chronic idiopathic demyelinating polyneuropathy may be effectively achieved in the consultation room without recourse to the examination couch. Here, it is assumed that the patient is presenting for a diagnosis; this requires complete exposure of limbs, shoulders, trunk and buttocks, and careful assessment of muscle power of a large number of muscles or muscle groups.

Inspection

Start by looking at the muscles of the limbs and trunk. Pathological hypertrophy of muscle is rare. Pseudohypertrophy is also uncommon. It is seen mainly in the calf muscles of individuals with certain muscular dystrophies. It is termed 'pseudohypertrophy' because it is associated with weakness; pathologically there is degeneration of muscle with replacement of muscle tissue by fat.

Wasting of muscle is a common sign of disease, but it does not always have a neurological basis. With disuse, muscles atrophy, sometimes quite fast. Generally, disuse atrophy is fairly mild. Power is preserved if it can be tested (e.g. quadriceps wasting in someone with severe knee arthritis). Cachexia involves diffuse muscle wasting, but usually power is surprisingly good. Thyrotoxicosis leads to diffuse muscle wasting and ultimately there is weakness (thyrotoxic myopathy). Many myopathic disorders give rise to wasting, and the pattern of wasting (proximal, distal, symmetrical, asymmetrical and selective, e.g. finger flexor muscles in the forearm in inclusion body myositis) helps diagnostically. Wasting is an important sign of peripheral nerve disease, which affects motor nerve fibres. It is denervated muscle, which wastes markedly, indicating motor nerve terminal or axon or nerve cell body loss. Focal motor nerve demyelination with conduction block, but without denervation, causes weakness, but there may be little or no wasting. In mononeuropathies, the wasting only affects muscles supplied by the affected nerve. Sometimes an ulnar neuropathy or median nerve lesion at the wrist or a common peroneal nerve lesion can be diagnosed correctly with reasonable confidence just by observing the pattern of wasting. In mononeuropathies, plexopathies and radiculopathies, wasted muscles will be weak. Motor and mixed motor and sensory polyneuropathies also cause wasting, most commonly distally and symmetrically. Disorders of motor nerve cell bodies lead to loss of associated axons and wasting. Thus, a range of pathologies of the spinal cord cause wasting, including processes which affect just motor nerve cell bodies, such as motor neuron disease, hereditary motor neuronopathies (spinal muscular atrophies) and poliomyelitis, and structural spinal cord disorders such as syringomyelia. Many elderly patients appear to have wasting of the small muscles of the hand, but if the strength is normal, there is probably actually no muscle wasting.

Fasciculations are spontaneous contractions of the muscle fibres of individual motor units within a muscle at rest, seen as twitches within a muscle. Although widespread fasciculations are rather characteristic of amyotrophic lateral sclerosis, they are not always seen in that condition, and they may be seen in peripheral neuropathies and radiculopathies and in normal individuals who are not fully at rest. They may also be an isolated, benign abnormality. Fasciculations restricted to the calf muscles are common in normal individuals.

Pes cavus (Fig. 16.11) with clawing of the toes may be idiopathic or an indication of long-standing imbalance of muscle power in the feet (mainly weakness of intrinsic foot muscles), caused commonly by

Figure 16.11 Pes cavus, with clawing of the toes in a patient with familial neuropathy. This patient had Refsum's disease and the peripheral nerves were slightly enlarged.

Charcot-Marie-Tooth disease, but also by other hereditary or congenital disorders of peripheral nerve or spinal cord. Contractures of joints can be a consequence of muscle disease, peripheral neuropathy or CNS disease. Scoliosis is common in neurofibromatosis, but it may be a complication of other neurological disorders, such as syringomyelia and Friedreich's ataxia.

Assessment of muscle tone

Some people can relax their muscles extremely well, whereas others tense up during an examination, sometimes making it difficult to assess tone. Generally, in adult neurological practice, apparent hypotonia is not very diagnostically useful. The two common and important forms of pathological increase in muscle tone are spasticity, reflecting an upper motor neuron disorder (imprecisely designated 'pyramidal' because the corticospinal tracts constitute the medullary pyramids) and the 'extrapyramidal' rigidity of parkinsonism.

Spasticity

Spastic hypertonia in the upper limbs affects flexor muscles more than extensor muscles. This may give rise to a characteristic posture of the limb, which is flexed at the elbow, wrist and fingers. There will be more resistance to passive extension of these joints than to passive flexion. The resistance increases in proportion to the speed of stretch of affected muscles until it suddenly reduces (so-called 'clasp-knife' rigidity). Accordingly, detecting spasticity is best achieved by fairly fast and vigorous movements of the patient's limb to stretch relevant muscles. Hold the patient's elbow and hand and extend the elbow briskly, from a fully flexed to a fully extended position. Similar considerations apply at the wrist and fingers. A spastic arm will also have increased tone in pronator muscles. Brisk passive supination of the forearm will elicit clasp-knife rigidity felt as a 'pronator catch'.

In the leg, spasticity typically affects adductors and extensors more than flexors. With spinal cord lesions, the spasticity is often bilateral (a spastic paraparesis). Mild bilateral adductor spasticity can be detected with the patient lying supine on a couch or a bed. Pick up one leg and abduct it. In doing so, adduction of the contralateral leg will be observed. Mild spasticity in quadriceps can be detected by asking the patient to relax. Then briskly flex his hip by lifting the leg behind the knee. In a normal limb, this will lead to flexion of the knee by gravity of the lower leg. The ankle will remain on the couch, being dragged proximally. If there is spasticity, however, the lower leg will be lifted off the bed briefly before falling back down. Spasticity at the ankle causes plantarflexion. Brisk passive dorsiflexion of the ankle, best done with the knee partially flexed, elicits the spasticity in the form of clonus—a succession of involuntary brief contractions of the calf muscles. Clonus may range from a few beats to sustained clonus in which there are repetitive calf muscle contractions until pressure on the sole of the foot is removed.

Parkinsonian extrapyramidal rigidity

Parkinsonian extrapyramidal rigidity takes two forms: either an increase in muscle tone affecting any movement of any muscle groups (so-called 'lead-pipe' rigidity) or rigidity, which is modified by tremor (so-called 'cogwheel rigidity', in which a high-frequency intermittency in the severity of the resistance to movement is felt owing to superimposed tremor on rigidity). Mild parkinsonian rigidity is sometimes absent when the patient is relaxed, but may be induced by getting the patient to use the arm contralateral to the arm being assessed (activated rigidity). Passive flexion and extension of the wrist or a rotatory movement of the hand at the wrist is a good manoeuvre to pick up parkinsonian rigidity. Test first with the contralateral arm at rest. Then, if appropriate, test again, this time for activated rigidity, with the patient moving his opposite arm up and down with the fist clenched. In early Parkinson's disease (PD), rigidity will be detected in a limb or the limbs of one side and, although the signs remain asymmetric throughout, in advanced PD rigidity will affect all the limbs and the neck and trunk. Extrapyramidal neck rigidity affects movements of the neck in all directions. This contrasts with the neck stiffness of meningitis (see Chapter 9) in which neck flexion is stiff, restricted and painful, whereas rotation is relatively supple.

Paratonia (Gegenhalten)

Paratonia is seen in patients with fairly advanced dementia. Whichever way you attempt to move the patient's limb, he puts up active resistance. In paratonia, the tone increases with continued movement and also with the speed of stretch of the affected muscle, similar to spasticity; however, spasticity differs in that there is the 'clasp knife' phenomenon and tone can often decrease after repeat manoeuvres.

Testing muscle power

Testing muscle power is a skill, which requires considerable practice in order to learn how to encourage patients to cooperate fully and demonstrate the full amount of power they have at their disposal and to be able to make correct judgements about the presence of weakness. With few exceptions, isometric contraction (in which a muscle exerts a force but does not change in length) is tested by the examiner opposing the action of the patient's muscle(s). Clearly the average healthy young doctor will be stronger than a child or a frail elderly person, but otherwise normal person, so judgement has to be applied. Conversely, some patients will be stronger than the examiner. It is important to be thinking about the patterns of muscle weakness which are likely to be found in different kinds of disease processes and to look for and register the evolving pattern of weakness as you go along.

A common problem is non-organic weakness. This may reflect malingering or a conversion disorder, but sometimes just indicates that the patient is keen to impress on you that there is something the matter. In non-organic weakness, intermittency of effort is apparent, with variability of power produced from second to second, often with a prominent tendency abruptly to give way or withhold effort. In contrast, the muscle of a patient with organic weakness exerting as much force as he can will give in a smooth, continuous way, not a jerky, fluctuating way. Non-organic paralysis is often quite easy to diagnose because of inconsistencies in the patient's capabilities. For instance, a patient may walk into the consulting room normally, mount the examination couch unaided but be unable to lift a leg into the air because of apparent paralysis of hip flexion. The non-organic nature of unilateral hip extension weakness may be established by Hoover's sign. A patient appears to have paralysis of hip extension. Keep a hand under the affected leg and ask the patient to flex the opposite hip against the resistance of your other arm. In doing so, the patient will unwittingly activate the previously paralysed hip extensors. Similarly, in non-organic hip flexion weakness, keep a hand under the unaffected leg. On attempted hip flexion, the absence of hip extension on the unaffected side suggests a lack of effort.

Clinical methods of recording the severity of muscle weakness have considerable shortcomings, but in neurological practice it is desirable to chart muscle strength in order to document progression or recovery and to gauge the effectiveness of therapeutic interventions. The Medical Research Council scale is widely used (Box 16.3), but a problem with this scale is that the vast majority of muscle weakness one will encounter is grade 4. It also performs badly for fingers and toes where gravity has scarcely any influence, so that grades 1, 2 and 3 are more or less identical. Many clinicians find a scale of normal power, mild, moderate and severe weakness and paralysis is practical for everyday use. Accurate quantitative myometry ought to be a way forward, but has hardly entered routine clinical practice.

There is not the space here to describe in detail the testing of all the important individual muscles and muscle groups. Tables 16.6 and 16.7 represent a summary of commonly tested muscles and their actions, but a number of specific points are important:

- There are two tests in which muscle strength is routinely tested isotonically (i.e. the muscle shortens while lifting a constant load) as opposed to isometrically. Abdominal trunk muscles are tested by asking the patient to sit up from lying flat with his arms folded on his chest. Standing up from a sitting position or rising from a crouched position is a good test of hip and knee extension and spine extension muscles and is useful in testing patients with myopathies. Normally these actions can be accomplished without use of the arms. Weak patients often have to resort to using their arms to push themselves up, either using surrounding furniture or, failing that, pushing themselves up with their arms on their own legs (Gowers' sign; Fig. 16.12).

Box 16.3	The Medical Research Council scale for grading muscle strength

- Grade 0: no contraction
- Grade 1: flicker or trace of contraction
- Grade 2: active movement with gravity eliminated
- Grade 3: active movement against gravity
- Grade 4: active movement against gravity and resistance
- Grade 5: normal power

Commonly Grade 4 is divided into 4−, 4 and 4+, denoting severe, moderate and mild weakness, and some use 5− to signify minimal weakness.

- Testing neck flexion and extension is important in myopathies, in myasthenia gravis and in motor neuron disease.
- Deltoids, spinati, the pectoralis major muscles, hip abductors and hip adductors can be tested bilaterally simultaneously, but all other muscles must be tested in each limb separately.
- People sometimes test ulnar nerve-supplied small hand muscles by squeezing together the abducted index and small fingers (first dorsal interosseous and abductor digiti minimi muscles). It is better to test these two muscles individually.
- Mild weakness of calf muscles (gastrocnemii and soleus) is difficult to detect on a couch. A good technique is to get the patient to walk around on 'tiptoes'. The ankle sags in a leg affected by mild plantarflexion weakness.
- Rather than thinking solely about the myotomes supplying the relevant muscles, it is better simultaneously to be thinking, 'Is this the pattern of weakness one sees in upper motor neuron disorders (monoparesis, hemiparesis, paraparesis, tetraparesis); is this the weakness of a polyneuropathy (usually distal symmetrical weakness except in demyelinating polyneuropathies which give substantial proximal weakness as well); is the weakness best explained by a nerve root lesion or lesions; is the weakness best explained by a lesion of an individual nerve or by a number of nerves or by a plexus lesion; is the pattern of weakness caused by a muscle disorder (often proximal symmetrical weakness)?'

Cerebellar system

The anatomy of the cerebellum is complex; it receives afferents of virtually every kind and its efferents connect to virtually every part of the brain and spinal cord. Important afferents include those from the motor cortex, visual cortex, vestibular nuclei and spinal cord. Vestibular afferents connect to the flocculonodular lobe. Lesions here cause dysequilibrium and gait ataxia. Spinocerebellar tracts go mainly to the vermis, in the midline of the cerebellum. Lesions here cause truncal and gait ataxia. Each cerebellar hemisphere receives a major input from the contralateral cerebral cortex via pontine

Table 16.6 Muscles of the upper limbs that are commonly examined (P is patient; E is examiner)

Action	Muscle	Nerve, nerve roots	Method	Comment
Shoulder				
Abduction	Supraspinatus	Suprascapular, C5, C6	P attempts to abduct arms from chest; E resists	
External rotation	Infraspinatus	Suprascapular, C5, C6	P holds upper arms down, forearms forward and attempts to externally rotate upper arms; E resists	
Abduction, extension	Deltoid	Axillary, C5, C6	Arms abducted; E pushes down	
Adduction of arms with shoulder flexed	Pectoralis major	Pectoral nerves, C5, C6, C7, C8	P arms stretched forward horizontal; P pushes fists together; E resists	
Lateral and forward movement and fixation of the scapula	Serratus anterior	Long thoracic, C5, C6, C7	P pushes arm forward against resistance	Serratus weakness causes winging of the scapula, noticed more with the arm forward. Trapezius weakness is the other major cause of scapula winging, noticed more with the arm abducted. Instability of the shoulder caused by either is disabling
Elbow				
Flexion	Biceps	Musculocutaneous, C5, C6	E holds P's distal forearm and shoulder; P pulls; E resists	
Flexion	Brachioradialis	Radial, C5, C6	P flexes elbow with forearm midway between pronation and supination; E resists	The muscle is not the major flexor, but can be seen and palpated. Weak, therefore less visible, with a radial nerve lesion. Weak and wasted in certain dystrophies
Extension	Triceps	Radial, C6, C7	E holds P's distal forearm and shoulder; P pushes; E resists	
Wrist				
Extension, abduction	Extensor carpi radialis longus (ECRL)	Radial, C6, C7	P makes a fist and extends wrist against resistance	
Extension, adduction	Extensor carpi ulnaris (ECU)	Posterior interosseous, C7, C8	P makes a fist and extends wrist against resistance	If ECU is weak and ECRL is not, on wrist extension there is radial deviation (abduction) of the wrist
Flexion, abduction	Flexor carpi radialis (FCR)	Median, C6, C7	P flexes supinated wrist up against resistance, fingers relaxed	Adduction (ulnar deviation) occurs if FCR is weak and FCU is not.
Flexion, adduction	Flexor carpi ulnaris (FCU)	Ulnar, C7, C8, T1	P flexes supinated wrist up against resistance, fingers relaxed	Abduction (radial deviation) occurs if FCU is weak and FCR is not.

Continued

Table 16.6 Muscles of the upper limbs that are commonly examined (P is patient; E is examiner)—cont'd

Action	Muscle	Nerve, nerve roots	Method	Comment
Fingers				
Extension	Extensor digitorum communis	Posterior interosseous, C7, C8	Hand prone, P extends fingers against resistance	
Flexion	Flexor digitorum profundus (FDP)	F2, F3: anterior interosseous, C7, C8, T1 F4, F5: ulnar, C7, C8, T1	P has back of hand on a flat surface; E holds middle phalanx down; P flexes distal phalanx against resistance	Finger flexion is achieved by FDP and flexor digitorum superficialis. The latter flexes the proximal interphalangeal (IP) joints and secondarily the metacarpophalangeal joints. FDP flexes the distal IP joints, and secondarily the other two. Testing grip (all flexors together) is useful, for instance in a patient with a hemiparesis. Testing each component of FDP individually is useful in anterior interosseous and ulnar nerve lesions.
Thumb abduction	Abductor pollicis brevis (APB)	Median, C8, T1	P has palm flat and sticks thumb up in the air and keeps it there while E attempts to push it towards the index finger.	APB can be seen and palpated and its strength can be tested (abductor pollicis longus has a different action, being more of an extensor, so action of APB can reliably be assessed more or less in isolation).
Abduction of the index finger	First dorsal interosseous muscle (1st DIO)	Ulnar, C8, T1	P spreads fingers; E attempts to adduct P's index finger; P resists	1st DIO can be seen and palpated and its strength tested. You can pit the strength of your 1st DIO against that of the patient.
Abduction of fifth finger	Abductor digiti minimi (ADM)	Ulnar, C8, T1	P spreads fingers; E attempts to adduct P's fifth finger; P resists	Usually not much added value over 1st DIO, except in a lesion of the deep palmar branch of ulnar nerve when ADM will be strong, but 1st DIO weak.

F2, index finger; F3, middle finger; F4, fourth finger; F5, fifth finger.

nuclei and the middle cerebellar peduncles. The major output from the cerebellum is via the superior cerebellar peduncles. Fibres from the cerebellar hemispheres cross to the contralateral red nucleus and thalamus, thence to spinal cord and basal ganglia and cerebral hemispheres. The red nucleus, thalamus and basal ganglia control the contralateral side of the body (e.g. rubrospinal tract crosses the midline after exiting the red nucleus); therefore, neural pathways originating in the cerebellum 'double cross'. Thus, whereas cerebral cortex lesions affect contralateral limbs, cerebellar hemisphere lesions cause incoordination of ipsilateral limbs.

Incoordination, ataxia and tremor are the main effects of cerebellar lesions. Given the widespread afferent and efferent connections of the cerebellum,

Table 16.7 Muscles of the lower limbs which are commonly examined (P is patient; E is examiner)

Action	Muscle	Nerve(s), nerve roots	Method	Comment
Hip				
Flexion	Iliopsoas	Lumbar plexus, femoral, L1, L2, L3	P flexes hip to 90° and flexes knee; E attempts to extend hip; P resists Can be done with P lying or sitting If sitting, stabilize P at shoulder	
Extension	Gluteus maximus	Inferior gluteal, L5, S1, S2	P lies on back; E attempts to lift the leg, lifting distal femur If P really tries, pelvis will lift off bed	Method described is quick, but to inspect or palpate the muscles, P needs to lie prone.
Adduction	Adductor magnus, longus and brevis	Obturator, L2, L3, L4	P squeezes legs together; E tries to prise them apart	
Abduction	Gluteus medius, gluteus minimus	Superior gluteal L4, L5, S1	P tries to separate legs; E pushes them together	
Knee				
Extension	Quadriceps femoris	Femoral, L2, L3, L4	P lying down, flexes knee to 90°; E puts left arm under knee; P extends knee (raises lower leg up into the air, not along the bed[a]); E resists with right hand Can also test knee extension with P sitting, legs dangling	P could extend knee pushing heel down bed or couch against resistance even with very weak quads by using hip extension.
Flexion	Hamstrings	Sciatic, L4, L5, S1, S2	P pulls heel towards bottom; E applies resistance, one hand behind ankle, the other at the front of the knee	If signs at the ankle and foot do not distinguish an L5 lesion from a common peroneal nerve lesion, look carefully for weakness here.
Ankle				
Dorsiflexion	Tibialis anterior (TA)	Deep peroneal, L4, L5	P dorsiflexes ankle fully; E attempts to plantarflex (extend) ankle	Another way of testing ankle dorsiflexion is to get P to walk around on his heels.
Inversion	Tibialis posterior (TP)	Tibial, L5, S1	P inverts foot against resistance Foot must be fully plantarflexed or otherwise TA contributes to inversion	Clear weakness of TP helps to distinguish an L5 radiculopathy from a common peroneal nerve lesion.
Eversion	Peroneus longus and brevis	Superficial peroneal, L5, S1	P everts foot against resistance	
Plantarflexion	Medial and lateral gastrocnemius; soleus	Tibial, L5, S1, S2	P uses E's hand as an accelerator or clutch pedal; E resists	Mild weakness is best appreciated by having P walk around on tiptoes. Muscle bulk on the two sides is best compared with P standing.
Toes				
Big toe extension	Extensor hallucis longus	Deep peroneal, L5, S1	P extends great toe against resistance	This may be the only weakness detectable in a mild L5 radiculopathy.

Continued

Table 16.7 Muscles of the lower limbs which are commonly examined (P is patient; E is examiner)—cont'd

Action	Muscle	Nerve(s), nerve roots	Method	Comment
Extension of the other toes	Extensor digitorum longus and brevis (EDL and EDB)	Deep peroneal, L5, S1	P extends toes against resistance	EDB wastes in individuals with weak feet owing to polyneuropathy but may remain bulky in those with myopathy.
Flexion	Flexor digitorum longus; flexor hallucis longus	Tibial, L5, S1	P flexes toes against resistance	The long toe flexors flex the distal interphalangeal joints primarily. Intrinsic foot muscles (plantar nerves) flex the toes at the metatarsophalangeal (MTP) joints. Weakness of them leads to extension of the toes at the MTP joints and flexion more distally, seen in association with pes cavus.*

*See Figure 16.11

Figure 16.12 Duchenne muscular dystrophy (Xp21 dystrophy). There is pseudohypertrophy of the weak muscles (e.g. the calves and deltoids). The child is 'climbing up himself' with legs widely placed as he gets up from the sitting position to the standing position. This is Gowers' sign.

it is clear that lesions outside the cerebellum itself may have clinical manifestations that closely resemble those of cerebellar disease, and this needs to be borne in mind when examining patients. Thus, gait ataxia may be seen with cerebral, brainstem or spinal cord disorders, and tremor and ataxia can be manifestations of brainstem lesions.

Examination of limb coordination

The finger-nose test

A mild cerebellar lesion gives rise to no limb signs at rest, but movements of affected limbs may be accompanied by action tremor. Actions are clumsy and inaccurate. Coordination of the arm is tested by the finger-nose test. Hold up an index finger in front of the patient. Ask him to touch it with the tip of his index finger, then with the same finger to touch his nose, and then ask him to carry on, touching alternately your finger and his nose. Some make the test a bit more difficult by moving the finger from place to place, but this adds little. More important is to make sure that the patient has to stretch a little to reach the finger, so that coordination is seen over the full range of movement of the arm. The observed action tremor is of fairly low tremor frequency, sometimes of quite large amplitude, and it becomes more marked in amplitude as the patient's finger approaches the target (his nose or your finger). This gives rise to the term 'intention tremor'.

In more severe cerebellar lesions, there will be postural as well as action tremor. In the extreme, the postural and action tremors are incapacitating. In such circumstances, the finger-nose test is inappropriate, being dangerous to the patient, whose finger might poke an eye or any other part of his face.

Dysdiadochokinesis

Ask the patient to tap his fingers rapidly on the back of his other hand. Then ask him to repeat the test, this time turning the tapping hand so that the tapping is alternately done with the palmar and the dorsal sides of the fingers. Each tap should be on the same spot, not adjacent parts of the back of the hand.

Irregularity and clumsiness indicate an ipsilateral cerebellar hemisphere disturbance. Dysdiadochokinesis is not very specific; impairment is also seen in pyramidal and extrapyramidal disorders as well.

The heel-shin test

The heel-shin test assesses lower limb coordination. The patient lies on a couch or bed. Ask him first to lift one leg into the air, then to put the heel of that leg on to the shin of the other leg just below the knee and run the heel down the front of the shin on to the dorsum of the foot. Cerebellar dysfunction is revealed as tremor when the patient attempts to place his heel at the top of the shin and as an inability accurately to run the heel down the shin.

In testing cerebellar function, make an allowance for any weakness, particularly spastic weakness, which by itself causes a certain amount of incoordination. Furthermore, it is essential to test proprioception, because proprioceptive loss can give rise to signs, which look just like cerebellar incoordination (sensory ataxia).

Reflexes

The jaw jerk, tendon reflexes, abdominal reflexes and plantar reflexes comprise the major commonly tested reflexes.

The jaw jerk and tendon reflexes

The jaw jerk and tendon reflexes are monosynaptic stretch reflexes. Sudden stretching of a muscle by striking its tendon sends an impulse from muscle spindle afferents, which synapse directly with motor neurons, leading to reflex contraction of that muscle. The reflexes provide information about both the motor system and the sensory system. Abnormally brisk reflexes contribute to the clinical picture of an upper motor neuron disorder. Absence of reflexes occurs in disorders of sensory afferents from muscle spindles in a wide range of sensory polyneuropathies, radiculopathies and mononeuropathies. Motor neuropathies and eventually myopathies may entail areflexia, but areflexia more commonly reflects a sensory rather than a motor system disorder. The other important cause of widespread areflexia, which can cause considerable confusion, is a spinal cord lesion, which is extensive up and down the cord. In this situation, interruption of afferents to motor neurons in the anterior horns or damage to the motor neurons themselves prevents the reflexes from occurring. Examples include syringomyelia, extensive myelitis, spinal cord infarction and extensive intramedullary spinal cord tumours.

Pathologically brisk reflexes below a particular myotome level raise the possibility of a spinal cord lesion between the lowest normal reflex level and the highest abnormal reflex level. Remember that a focal spinal cord lesion will interrupt the pathway of any reflex at that level. Thus, the combination of loss of a reflex at a particular level and abnormally brisk reflexes subserved by levels below points strongly to a focal spinal cord lesion. One of the limitations of these analyses is the restricted number of reflexes that can be examined. The biceps reflex is at C5 or C6 level and no reflex corresponds to C4 or higher, except for the jaw jerk. If all the reflexes are pathologically brisk but the jaw jerk is not, there may be a high cervical spinal cord lesion. Normal upper-limb power and reflexes and a spastic paraparesis with pathologically brisk lower-limb reflexes may indicate a thoracic spinal cord lesion, but there are no tendon reflexes between C8 (finger reflexes) and adductor reflexes (L2 or L3) to localize the lesion more precisely. A pathologically brisk jaw jerk in a patient with a spastic tetraparesis points to the site of the causative pathology being in the cerebral hemispheres (e.g. diffuse small vessel cerebrovascular disease, amyotrophic lateral sclerosis or hydrocephalus) rather than in the cervical spinal cord.

Testing the jaw jerk

Ask the patient to let his jaw hang down in a relaxed manner with the mouth slightly open. Place your index finger across his chin. Strike it lightly with a tendon hammer; reflex contraction of both masseters is the response. Sometimes an extremely brisk jaw jerk is accompanied by clonus. The jaw jerk tests trigeminal nerve function and localizes to the brainstem and therefore a brisk jaw jerk suggests an abnormality above the foramen magnum.

Testing the tendon reflexes

Eliciting tendon reflexes is not completely straightforward and requires practice. The aim is to ensure that the tendon of the relevant muscle being tested is briskly and effectively struck. Accordingly, sufficient force must be delivered. For the biceps reflex, place your own finger over the tendon and strike your finger. Similarly, the brachioradialis reflex can be elicited by applying the tendon hammer to your own fingers positioned just above the wrist on the lateral aspect of the radius bone. The other standard reflexes (triceps, knee (quadriceps) and ankle (gastrocnemii and soleus)) involve directly striking the tendon with the tendon hammer. The standard tendon reflexes examined are summarized in Table 16.8.

The range of briskness of normal reflexes is very variable both between and within individuals and often diminish with age, so it is important not to jump to conclusions about the presence of upper motor neuron lesions or polyneuropathies just on the basis of reflexes alone. For example, in young patients apparently brisk reflexes may be physiological, in the absence of other upper motor neuron signs. Normal individuals who have absent reflexes tested in the standard way usually will have reflexes if they are brought out by reinforcement. To reinforce lower limb reflexes, ask the patient to

Table 16.8 Frequently examined tendon reflexes

Reflex	Nerve	Nerve root(s)	Technique	Comment*
Biceps	Musculocutaneous	C5, C6	Elbow flexed 90°, arm relaxed Strike your finger or thumb located over the tendon.	Reduced or absent in radiculopathy or focal cord pathology at C5–C6 cord level
Brachioradialis	Radial	C5, C6	Elbow flexed 90°, arm relaxed Strike your finger over the distal radius.	Mainly of interest when it is inverted (see text)
Triceps	Radial	C6, C7	Elbow flexed 90°, arm relaxed Strike the tendon directly, just above the ulna at the back of the elbow.	Reduced or absent in high radial nerve lesion, radiculopathy or focal cord pathology at C6–C7 level
Finger	Median and ulnar	C8	Have the patient's hand supine on a flat surface. Put your index finger across the middle phalanges, which will be slightly flexed. Strike your finger so as to abruptly stretch the finger flexors.	Mainly of interest when abnormally brisk Hoffman's reflex is a variant.
Adductor	Obturator	L2, L3	Separate the legs. Apply fingers to medial thigh just above knee. Strike fingers.	Result is adduction of both legs when there is a spastic paraparesis (crossed adductor response). Retained adductor reflex with absent knee reflex suggests a femoral neuropathy rather than plexopathy or radiculopathy.
Knee	Femoral	L3, L4	Knee flexed 45–90°, supported and relaxed Strike the patellar tendon, just below the patella.	Reduced in radiculopathy, lumbar plexopathy or femoral neuropathy
Ankle	Tibial branch of sciatic	S1	Patient externally rotates hip and flexes knee. Hold the foot distally. Strike the Achilles tendon.	Absence may be the only sign other than restricted straight leg raising in S1 radiculopathy owing to L5/S1 disc prolapse.

*The remarks are made with reference to common abnormalities, not every possible one.

put his hands together with the fingers interlocked. Then get ready to elicit the reflex, ask the patient to squeeze with his hands and then directly test the reflex. Upper limb reflexes can also be reinforced. Ask the patient to squeeze firmly something held in the hand contralateral to the limb in which the reflexes are to be tested (e.g. the barrel of a standard ophthalmoscope).

Reflex spread, in which testing a reflex also causes muscle contraction at an adjacent spinal level, or reflex crossing, causing contraction of the corresponding contralateral muscle (e.g. crossed adductor reflexes) are useful upper motor signs.

Abdominal reflexes

The stimulus is a light stroke of the abdominal skin using an orange stick. The normal response is contraction of abdominal wall muscles in the region where the stimulus is delivered, noted as movement of the umbilicus towards the region where the response is positive. The reflex is absent in spinal lesions above the level at which the reflex is being tested, and the reflexes are sometimes absent at a very early stage in multiple sclerosis. With symptoms or signs of a sensory level on the abdomen, the reflexes may be absent below the sensory level and retained above.

Testing the abdominal reflexes

The patient should be supine, relaxed, with the abdomen fully exposed. Start the stroke of the orange stick right round in the flank, drawing it to the midline. Test all four quadrants of the abdomen.

The plantar reflex

Except in neonates and infants, the normal response to uncomfortable or painful cutaneous stimulation of the sole of the foot includes plantarflexion of the toes. In addition, there may be flexion withdrawal of the limb, composed of dorsiflexion of the ankle and flexion of the knee and hip, which can be suppressed voluntarily. A remarkably reliable feature of an upper motor neuron lesion (anywhere in the spinal cord above L5 cord level or in the brain) affecting the leg being tested is the extensor plantar response (the Babinski reflex). The minimum extensor response is extension of the great toe only and it is the key feature to look for. In addition, there may be fanning of the other toes and in the thigh contraction of tensor fascia lata. A marked response to plantar stimulation in a paralysed patient includes involuntary dorsiflexion of the ankle, flexion of the knee and flexion of the hip. If you are dealing with a patient who clearly has spasticity of the leg, a pyramidal distribution of weakness, pathologically brisk reflexes and ankle clonus, it hardly matters what the plantar response is. Occasionally, however, a patient has weakness without spasticity or hyperreflexia and the evidence that there is a CNS disorder hinges on the plantar reflex. Conversely, agitated individuals may have increased tone and very brisk reflexes, but the flexor plantar reflex responses reassure one that there is no neurological problem.

A patient with lower motor neuron paralysis of toe extension cannot have a conventional extensor response regardless of the severity of any upper motor neuron disorder he may also have. A small number of malingerers learn to produce extensor responses.

In dystonic syndromes and other extrapyramidal disorders, there may be apparent spontaneous extensor plantar reflex, in the absence of corticospinal tract dysfunction—the so called 'striatal toe'.

Testing the plantar reflex

The ideal instrument to use is an orange stick (Fig. 16.13). Hold the patient's foot. Apply the orange stick to the sole of the foot on the lateral border just in front of the heel. Draw it forward towards the base of the fifth toe. This may suffice. Some continue round across the ball of the foot. It is best to press fairly firmly, warning the patient that this is not a pleasant test. Try to do the test effectively once or twice, not a large number of times. If you remain in doubt as to whether a response is extensor or not, then later, when testing pinprick sensation, test the dorsum of the toe in question. Involuntary extension of the toe towards the pin is an extensor response.

Primitive reflexes

Certain reflexes found in neonates and infants can no longer be elicited once the cerebrum matures sufficiently, but in the setting of acquired disorders of one or both frontal lobes of the brain, they reappear and are useful as evidence of frontal lobe dysfunction.

The grasp reflex

Placement of the index and middle fingers into the palm of a normal adult will elicit no response, but a patient with a grasp reflex will, to a greater or lesser

Figure 16.13 The plantar response. A firm, stroking stimulus to the outer edge of the sole of the foot evokes dorsiflexion (extension) of the large toe and fanning of the other toes.

extent, grip the fingers. With a strong grasp reflex, it will be possible to pull the arm or indeed the whole patient forward without having given any instruction to the patient. A unilateral grasp reflex indicates a contralateral frontal lobe lesion, for instance a tumour or a stroke. Bilateral grasp reflexes are usually owing to diffuse disorders such as fronto-temporal lobar degenerations or advanced Alzheimer's disease, diffuse small vessel cerebrovascular disease or hydrocephalus. The sign is important when there is a paucity of other signs. An inert, mute individual could be depressed, but the presence of grasp reflexes would alert one to the likelihood of organic disease.

The pout reflex

A gentle tap on the lips of the patient causes reflex pouting of the lips. This also reflects bilateral frontal pathology. It can be elicited using the head of a tendon hammer held covered by a tissue for hygiene.

Movement disorders

This is a large field encompassing a whole range of abnormalities of posture, locomotor function and movement, with a spectrum from the very common to the distinctly rare. Both hypokinesia and hyperkinesia are abnormal, and the most common important disease in this sphere, Parkinson's disease, combines both, with akinesia, bradykinesia, dystonia, tremor and dyskinesia (the latter usually drug induced).

Tremor

Tremor by itself is a common reason for neurological referral. Tremor that has not hitherto been noticed by the patient or his doctors may contribute to a neurological diagnosis. Getting a tremor diagnosis wrong is rarely serious, but giving patients incorrect diagnoses or prognoses is unsatisfactory and may lead to futile and inappropriate treatments or deprive a patient of worthwhile treatment.

The common tremor disorders include enhanced physiological tremor, essential tremor, parkinsonian tremor, dystonic tremor, cerebellar ('intention') tremor, drug-induced tremor and psychogenic tremor (Table 16.9). Combinations of tremor and myoclonus are seen in encephalopathies, mainly in hospitalized patients.

The classic tremor of Parkinson's disease is called a rest tremor (a slight contradiction in terms), and it is not always easy to diagnose. The patient's limb shakes when it is relaxed and doing nothing. Getting a patient into a position that allows his arms completely to relax in a chair may be difficult; be aware you are not simply observing the postural tremor of a patient with essential tremor. Distracting the patient, by performing mental exercises (such as serial seven subtraction) or performing repetitive movements on the opposite side, can facilitate

true rest and also exacerbate the rest tremor on the affected side. In fact, you can quite often establish the presence of rest tremor as well from the history as from examination: 'When relaxed on a comfortable sofa watching television, does your arm start to shake?', 'Do any of your limbs shake when you are lying in bed?' Rest tremor may be observed in a relaxed patient sitting in a chair or lying on a couch. Furthermore, if a patient is walking and the fingers of one hand are shaking (and the arm is not swinging), it is likely to be the rest tremor of PD. PD tremor is seen most commonly in the fingers, wrist and forearm. It may also affect a foot. Classically, when a patient with Parkinson's disease with upper limb rest tremor holds his hands out in front of him, his tremor stops for 10–20 seconds, whereafter a postural tremor may become evident, called 're-emergence', whereas typical essential tremor is

Table 16.9 Common forms of tremor

Tremor variety	Comment
Physiological	Normal
Enhanced physiological	Normal in a stressful enough situation
	A constitutionally anxious person may have this and a psychogenic tremor.
Thyrotoxicosis	Perhaps a variant of enhanced physiological tremor
Drug induced	The mechanisms here are various: some drugs may also cause ataxia, some parkinsonism, some polyneuropathy.
Essential	Sporadic or familial
	Called benign, but severe cases are disabling
	Mainly upper limbs, but severe cases can affect legs too (see text)
	Postural or kinetic (on movement) tremor rather than resting tremor
	Immediate on posture and consistent throughout different positions
	Often reported improvement with alcohol
Parkinsonism	Mainly idiopathic Parkinson's disease (see text), but sometimes parkinsonian tremor is seen in other forms of parkinsonism
	Rest tremor more prominent than postural or kinetic tremor
	Latency of 10–20 seconds on posture ('re-emergence')
	Wilson's disease must be excluded in young people with tremor
	Drug-induced common, particularly neuroleptic use
Dystonic	More jerky and irregular than essential tremor, particularly with jerks occurring in one direction; often task-specific exacerbations (e.g. handwriting)
	Exacerbated in certain positions and often much less in other positions 'null point'
	Features of dystonia are also seen
	Often a neck tremor
Cerebellar	See text
Brainstem, thalamic or cerebellar outflow	Holmes tremor; previously referred to as 'rubral' tremor
	An irregular, low frequency and large amplitude tremor, predominantly proximal upper limb 'wing beating' and exacerbated by action
In association with polyneuropathy	Some patients with Charcot-Marie-Tooth disease
	Some patients with chronic idiopathic demyelinating polyneuropathy
Psychogenic	Typically exaggerated in clinic
	Variable amplitude, frequency, direction and laterality
	Settles when patient distracted from shaking
	Patient cannot maintain the same frequency of tremor when performing a repetitive task with the contralateral limb at a different frequency unless it is a harmonic 'entrainability'

immediate on posture, not re-emergent. Parkinson's disease tremor is almost invariably asymmetric, starting in one limb and remaining more marked on that side throughout.

Essential tremor is generally not present at rest. It is noted with maintained postures and during movement. It mainly affects upper limbs. It is usually not markedly asymmetric. The action tremor may be examined during the finger-nose test and may also be assessed by tasks such as drawing a spiral or a wavy line between two straight lines or while writing, and these can be documented in case records. Jaw and lip tremor can be seen in patients with Parkinson's disease and in those with essential tremor.

Even with all the other aspects of examination at one's disposal (rigidity, bradykinesia/akinesia, posture, gait), distinguishing Parkinson's disease and essential tremor is sometimes difficult. Where there is uncertainty, withholding judgement and reviewing after an interval is often helpful.

Dystonic tremors include task-specific tremors, for example handwriting tremor or 'writer's cramp' or focal limb or neck tremor, for example cervical dystonic tremor. These tremors are associated with dystonic posturing in the affected region or elsewhere, for example torticollis (lateral rotation) of the neck. Dystonic tremor tends to be focal and asymmetric; jerky and irregular; and exacerbated in certain positions and occasionally absent in other positions, 'null point'.

Parkinson's disease

The main motor features of Parkinson's disease are summarized in Box 16.4. Rigidity and tremor have been discussed above. Posture and gait are discussed below.

Impaired facial expression and generalized bradykinesia or akinesia are observations, but bradykinesia can also be tested formally; elements of the Unified Parkinson's Disease Rating Scale can be readily incorporated into routine clinical practice (Box 16.5). Postural stability is tested by the pull test, done after testing gait.

The pull test

The patient stands with his feet side by side. Stand behind the patient with one foot slightly behind the other. Explain that, without warning, you are going to pull the patient abruptly backwards by his shoulders.

The patient's task is not to fall over. He is allowed to step backwards in order to maintain his balance. Be prepared to catch the patient should he topple. A normal individual either remains upright even without moving his feet or does so by taking a single step backwards. 'Retropulsion' refers to the patient taking a number of small paces backwards, either succeeding or failing to reposition his centre of gravity; this is parkinsonian and abnormal. Some patients will simply fall backwards without taking any paces at all.

Other movement disorders (hyperkinetic movement disorders)

Generally hyperkinetic movement disorders are identified simply by history and by observation rather than any other component of examination. They are summarized in Table 16.10.

Sensation

The cell bodies of primary sensory neurons are in dorsal root ganglia and equivalent ganglia on cranial nerves (particularly the trigeminal ganglion). Their peripheral axons convey sensory information from sensory end organs in skin, muscle spindles and tendons and other tissues. Their central axons project into the spinal cord or brainstem. Large-diameter myelinated axons transmit proprioception, vibration and touch. Small diameter myelinated and unmyelinated axons transmit pain and temperature. The centrally projecting axons for proprioception and vibration

---

Box 16.4	Cardinal motor features of Parkinson's disease

- Tremor
- Akinesia, bradykinesia
- Rigidity
- Abnormalities of posture
- Impairment of postural control and balance
- Abnormalities of gait
- Dysphonia, dysarthria, stammer

Box 16.5	Tests for bradykinesia in Parkinson's disease

1. Finger tapping:
   - Ask the patient to tap repeatedly with his index finger on his thumb. The amplitude of each movement should be as large as possible and the speed should be as fast as possible. Test one side, then the other, not both together.
2. Hand movements:
   - Ask the patient repeatedly to fully open his fist and fully close it, again with maximum amplitude and speed. Test one side, then the other, not both together.

In these two tests, in PD there is slowness and progressive reduction of amplitude of the movement, sometimes such that the movement ceases altogether. Asymmetry is the rule.

3. Pronation-supination movements of the arms:
   - Ask the patient to hold both arms out, and repeatedly to pronate and supinate them, with maximum amplitude and speed. Test both arms together.

In this test, asymmetry with impaired amplitude on the more affected side is readily observed.

4. Leg agility:
   - Ask the patient to stamp his heel rapidly and repeatedly on the ground, lifting his whole leg at least 3 inches (8 cm) each time. Test each leg separately.

Table 16.10 Common kinds of movement disorders

Movement disorder	Characteristics
Parkinsonism	See text
Dystonia	Abnormal muscle contractions that may be sustained or repetitive, also involving co-contraction of antagonist muscles, leading to an abnormal posture, with or without jerks or tremor
	Associated pain and disability
	Can be focal, segmental, axial or generalized
	A wide range of causes
	In adults, idiopathic cervical dystonia is common.
Chorea and athetosis (choreoathetosis)	Chorea denotes irregular, brief, jerky, unrepetitive, unintentional movements, affecting differing parts randomly (unilateral in hemichorea).
	In mild cases, the patient just looks fidgety.
	Many causes, including metabolic, drug induced, autoimmune, neurodegenerative
	Athetosis denotes slower, more writhing movements than chorea.
	The two often coexist, particularly in levodopa-induced dyskinesia.
Ballism	Not very common
	Usually hemiballism owing to an ischaemic stroke affecting the subthalamic nucleus
	The movements are violent with flinging of the limbs.
Myoclonus	Sudden shock-like jerks of limbs or trunk
	Can reflect cortical, brainstem or rarely spinal cord pathology or an encephalopathy
	Epileptic myoclonus is fairly common.
Asterixis	Negative myoclonus. A sudden brief loss of tone. Particularly associated with hepatic encephalopathy
Tardive dyskinesia	A complication of dopamine antagonist neuroleptic medication
	Abnormal movements may affect any body part, but usually mainly affect the face, lips, jaw and tongue.
Tic	Usually fairly small twitchy movements made semivoluntarily by a patient
	Preceding urge to make the movement, and brief relief having done so
	Often affect the face (blinks, grimaces, twitches of the nose), neck, shoulders
	An individual may have one or several different tics.

sense enter the spinal cord and turn immediately to head rostrally in the posterior (dorsal) columns ipsilaterally, to synapse in the gracile and cuneate nuclei at the cervicomedullary junction. Axons from these nuclei cross in the medulla and proceed to the thalamus. In contrast, axons for pain and temperature, having entered the spinal cord, synapse in the dorsal horns. The axons of second-order sensory neurons cross over to the contralateral anteriorly (ventrally) situated spinothalamic tracts and run rostrally all the way to the thalamus. Touch sensation travels by both routes. Sensory pathways from the trigeminal sensory nuclei cross in the brainstem to project to the contralateral thalamus. From the thalamus, third-order neurons project via the posterior limb of the internal capsule to the primary sensory cortex in the parietal lobe, which is somatotopically organized (Fig. 16.14), akin to the primary motor cortex.

The anatomical separation of different modalities of sensation in the spinal cord accounts for dissociation of sensory loss in spinal cord lesions which affect one side of the spinal cord (Brown-Séquard syndrome) or which affect either the anterior (e.g. syringomyelia or spinal cord infarct-ischaemia) or posterior cord (subacute combined degeneration of the spinal cord, secondary to cobalamin deficiency) (see below).

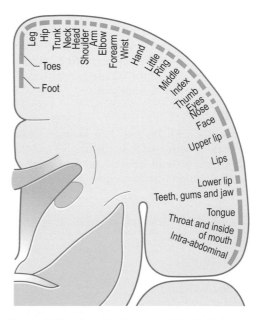

Figure 16.14 Somatotopic representation in the primary sensory cortex.

Similarly, anatomical separation in the brainstem can result in crossed patterns of sensory loss; for example, in a laterally medullary infarct, there is involvement of the lateral spinothalamic tract (contralateral pain and temperature in the body) and spinal trigeminal nucleus (ipsilateral pain and temperature sensation in the face).

With regard to the peripheral nervous system, cutaneous nerve fibres from dorsal root ganglia get to their end organs via spinal nerves, plexuses and peripheral nerves. A lesion of an individual peripheral nerve or a plexus lesion or a spinal nerve or nerve root lesion gives rise to loss of cutaneous sensation in a particular distribution which is diagnostically very helpful (Figs 16.15 and 16.16 and see Table 16.3). The cutaneous area supplied by a spinal nerve is called a dermatome. Loss of cutaneous sensation restricted to one dermatome indicates a spinal nerve or nerve root lesion. Loss of cutaneous sensation in all the dermatomes on both sides of the body below a particular level indicates a spinal cord lesion.

Cutaneous sensory examination

By the time sensation is examined, it may be apparent from the history and the clinical examination thus far what the diagnosis is and consequently what needs to be looked for during sensory testing. This is important because, in general, sensory testing needs to be goal directed; otherwise it tends to be fruitless or misleading. If a patient gives a very clear description of impaired sensation in the distribution of, for example, the ulnar nerve, diagnostically it makes little difference whether he can or cannot feel sharp pinpricks in the area of his symptoms. The symptoms still suggest an ulnar neuropathy either way. With very few exceptions (the corneal reflex would be one), all sensory tests are subjective; in other words, the examiner relies on what the patient reports. Patients with no sensory symptoms may have signs suggesting impaired cutaneous sensation; in that situation, the examiner has to exercise judgement as to whether they are of significance.

Disorganized sensory testing tends to confuse both the patient and the examiner. With cutaneous sensory testing, the goal is to see whether any hypoaesthesia conforms to a meaningful pattern (see Table 16.13 and Figs 16.15 and 16.16). Defining an area of hypoaesthesia is almost invariably better achieved by starting testing within the area of hypoaesthesia and moving the stimulus out into areas where sensation is normally perceived.

One of the less satisfactory modalities of sensation to test is light touch. It is often done by dabbing the skin lightly with a piece of cotton wool, but there may be differences between touching the skin and stroking it. Tickle is a different modality; moving hairs on hairy skin is different again. In the context of spinal cord pathology, an abnormality of light touch sensation will not differentiate a posterior column lesion from one affecting the spinothalamic tracts. When testing light touch sensation, it can be helpful to ask the patient to close his eyes and then to report when he perceives the touches because some patients with anaesthesia will report that they feel touches when they see them being applied. Touch/pressure can be somewhat more rigorously assessed using a 10-gram monofilament to apply a standard quantity of pressure, and this can be useful as a screening test in situations where a patient is at risk of development of sensory peripheral neuropathy (e.g. diabetes).

Pinprick testing, which is more informative diagnostically, is useful in mononeuropathies, polyneuropathies, radiculopathies and spinal cord lesions as well as brainstem and cerebral hemisphere lesions. It is, however, totally subjective. The patient reports whether the pinprick has a sharp, slightly painful quality or whether it is merely felt as a blunt touch. Testing can be done with the patient looking. In some clinical situations, it is worth testing pinprick sensation even when a patient has no sensory symptoms. A patient with a spastic monoparesis of one leg could have a brain or spinal cord lesion, but impaired pinprick sensation in the contralateral leg would strongly suggest a spinal cord lesion (Brown-Séquard lesion, see below). A patient with a slowly progressive spastic paraparesis or tetraparesis might have a neurodegenerative disorder, but the finding of a clear-cut sensory level on the trunk or neck would strongly suggest a structural spinal cord lesion.

Perception of heat and cold can be tested, but it adds little in routine clinical practice. A patient with impaired thermal sensation caused by a cerebral or spinal cord disorder will have impaired pinprick sensation in the same distribution. Impaired thermal sensation in patients with small fibre polyneuropathies is best assessed in a neurophysiology laboratory, but it does not contribute greatly to making the diagnosis.

Vibration sense

Patients do not complain of impaired vibration sense, but finding it on examination is a useful sign of either a polyneuropathy or a spinal cord lesion. Vibration sensation is conveyed in large-diameter sensory neurons, the central projections of which run in the posterior columns of the spinal cord.

Testing vibration sense

Set a low-frequency tuning fork vibrating noiselessly by striking it against the heel of your hand. Then apply the base of the tuning fork to bony parts of the limbs and ask the patient to report whether he feels the vibrations. Start distally and work proximally, if necessary. In the upper limb, start on a distal phalanx. If the patient has no vibration sense there, then test the wrist and, if necessary, the elbow. In the lower limb, test the distal phalanx of the big toe and then the medial malleolus and top of the

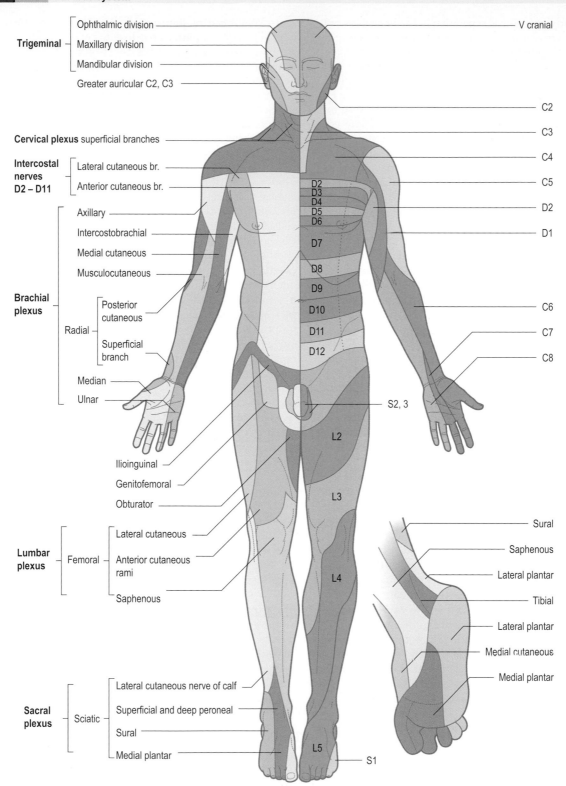

Trigeminal — Ophthalmic division ——————————————— V cranial
Maxillary division
Mandibular division
Greater auricular C2, C3

C2

C3

Cervical plexus superficial branches ——————— C4

Intercostal nerves D2 – D11 — Lateral cutaneous br. — C5
Anterior cutaneous br.
D2
D3
D4
D5
D6
D7 — D2

Brachial plexus — Axillary — D1
Intercostobrachial
Medial cutaneous
Musculocutaneous
D8
D9
Radial — Posterior cutaneous — D10 — C6
Superficial branch — D11 — C7
Median — D12 — C8
Ulnar

S2, 3

L2

Ilioinguinal
Genitofemoral
Obturator

L3

Lumbar plexus — Femoral — Lateral cutaneous
Anterior cutaneous rami
L4
Saphenous

Sural
Saphenous
Lateral plantar
Tibial
Lateral plantar
Medial cutaneous
Medial plantar

Sacral plexus — Sciatic — Lateral cutaneous nerve of calf
Superficial and deep peroneal
Sural
Medial plantar

L5
S1

Figure 16.15 Anterior view to show the segmental innervation of the skin, i.e. the dermatomes (left) and the peripheral nerve supply (right).

tibia, if necessary. If you suspect you are getting false-positive answers from the patient, ask him to close his eyes and then randomly apply the tuning fork, either vibrating or not vibrating to his limb; the patient reports whether it is or is not vibrating.

Proprioception

Impaired proprioception occurs in large-fibre sensory (or sensory and motor) polyneuropathies, spinal cord lesions affecting the posterior columns and in lesions

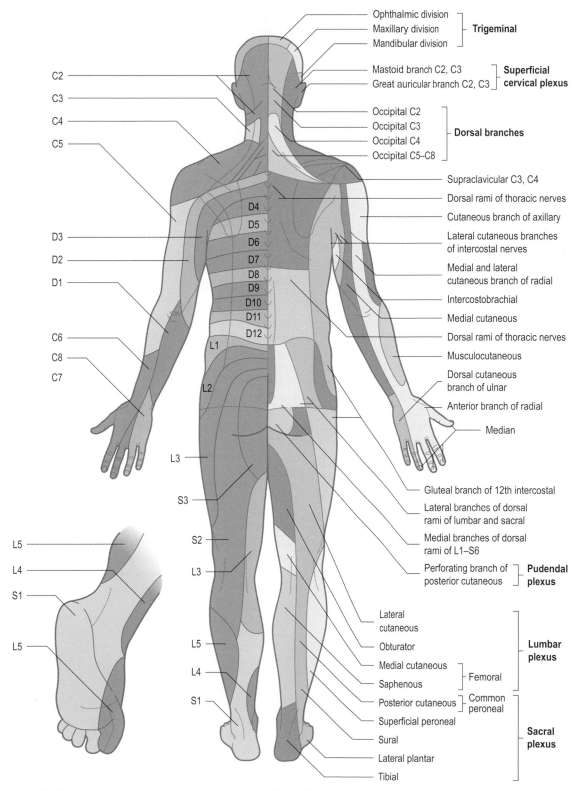

Figure 16.16 Posterior view to show the segmental innervation of the skin, i.e. the dermatomes (left) and the peripheral nerve supply (right).

at higher levels, including lesions of the sensory cortex. Proprioceptive loss is the basis of sensory ataxia. Patients with polyneuropathies which cause severe proprioceptive loss have gait and limb ataxia which looks very much like cerebellar ataxia. Several clinical tests or signs address proprioception: joint position sense (more strictly joint movement sense), pseudoathetosis and Romberg's test.

Testing joint position sense

Joint position testing does require the patient to look away or have his eyes closed. With the thumb and index finger of one hand, hold each side of the middle phalanx of the patient's middle finger. With your other hand, grasp the sides of the distal phalanx. Explain to the patient that he is to say which way his finger moves, that it will only go up or down and that the movements up or down will be random. Move the distal phalanx either up or down through a small angle; the patient should be able to perceive as small a movement as you will be able to make. Make sure each movement is random, not just up, down, up, down, etc. If the patient fails to understand the test or to concentrate, do it first with him looking at the joint being tested. If joint position sense is impaired at the distal interphalangeal joint, move more proximally to the metacarpophalangeal joint and, if necessary, to the wrist or elbow, employing bigger angles of movement. The same applies in the foot and leg: start with the interphalangeal joint of the big toe and, if necessary, the ankle or knee. The normal threshold for perception of joint movement in the toe is larger than in the finger.

Pseudoathetosis

Patients with impaired joint position sense in their fingers may exhibit so-called pseudoathetosis: outstretched fingers drift up or down or to the side when the patient has his eyes closed. This is because, proprioception having failed, vision is the only means by which the patient knows where his fingers are and can keep them in one place (Fig. 16.17).

Romberg's test

Ask the patient to stand with his feet together side by side. Having established that his balance is satisfactory with his eyes open, ask him to close his eyes, having reassured him that nothing untoward will happen. If he loses balance with his eyes closed, the test is positive. You need to be prepared to catch the patient if he shows signs of toppling. Sometimes this kind of proprioceptive loss is evident in the clinical history; the patient comments on loss of balance in the dark or when he closes his eyes to wash his face.

Cortical sensory loss

Cerebral hemisphere lesions may disrupt sensory afferents or the primary sensory cortex in such a way as to give rise to very straightforward sensory loss affecting the usually tested modalities. In the same way that

Figure 16.17 Paraneoplastic sensory neuropathy caused by small cell carcinoma of the lung. With the eyes closed, the patient's outstretched arms become flexed and abnormal postures develop in the fingers (pseudoathetosis).

occipital lesions may give rise either to visual loss or to disorders of visual interpretation, parietal lesions can cause sensory impairment without anaesthesia. One such disorder is sensory inattention, which is akin to visual inattention. A patient may feel sensory stimuli in limbs on the affected side, so does not have a hemianaesthesia, but sensory stimuli presented simultaneously on both sides are registered by the patient only on the normal side.

In tactile agnosia, a patient has no difficulty naming an item shown to him, but with his eyes closed and the item put into his hand, he is unable to work out by its size, consistency and texture what it is (astereognosis). Similarly, a patient may be unable to distinguish different very familiar coins by feel alone. Dysgraphaesthesia is another form of cortical sensory impairment. Use an orange stick or a pen with the cap on. Write numbers on the patient's palm, clarifying with him which way up they are going to be. With eyes open, the patient will cope with 2, 3, 6, 1, etc., but will not recognize the numbers with his eyes closed.

Clearly it is only valid to test these sorts of cortical sensory impairments in patients who do not have a hemianaesthesia.

Testing sensory inattention

Sensory inattention is tested with the patient's eyes closed. Randomly touch lightly his right or left hand (or foot) or both together, getting him to report each time whether he feels the touch on the right or left or on both sides. A patient who has right–left disorientation can still do this test, indicating which side or sides were touched by a finger movement. The lesion responsible for sensory inattention may be in the parietal cortex or in the subcortical white matter.

Stretch tests

In patients with pain radiating into a leg as a result of a painful compressive radiculopathy, usually caused by intervertebral disc prolapse, stretching the sciatic or femoral nerve may worsen the pain or bring it on. Straight leg raising with the patient lying on his back (see also Chapter 15) stretches the sciatic nerve and therefore the nerve roots which form it, and the test is most commonly positive in L4/L5 and L5/S1 disc protrusions causing L5 and S1 root lesions, respectively. The femoral nerve stretch test is performed with the patient lying on his front. The knee is flexed fully on to the back of the thigh and the thigh is raised, extending the hip. Pain provoked in the anterior thigh points to a L2/L3 or L3/L4 disc lesion (L3 or L4 root lesion, respectively). As with so many other tests, stretch tests are not specific. They can be positive in patients with painful inflammatory or infiltrative polyradiculopathies and false-positive results are not uncommon in patients with a lot of back pain but no neurological disorder.

Posture and gait

In the outpatient setting, a patient's gait will inevitably be observed, although it may well be desirable to inspect it in some detail, perhaps by taking him out into a corridor. In hospitalized patients, it is easy to neglect to test gait if the patient is encountered in his bed. Mobility is so fundamental that gait must be considered and assessed in every patient where it is appropriate to do so and it does not take long to do.

First, simply observe the patient standing. Look for abnormalities of posture. Established PD gives a kyphotic posture (Fig. 16.18). Neck extension weakness causes forward flexion of the neck; in extreme cases, a state of drop head is apparent. Axial dystonia may be observed. Muscular dystrophy may be associated with hyperlordosis. Check the patient's balance and perform the Romberg's test (see above). Then ask the patient to walk a short distance, turn around and walk back again. Mild gait ataxia can be brought out by getting the patient to walk heel to toe. If relevant, test for retropulsion (see section, the pull test).

Table 16.11 provides a summary of important kinds of neurological gait disorders. Sometimes it can be difficult to be certain that a patient with a frontal gait disorder does not also have PD. Patients with severe osteoarthritis of the hips sometimes have a gait disorder that looks deceptively like a myopathic gait. Finally, as in other domains, a functional gait disorder does not necessarily mean that there is no organic disease.

Patterns of motor and sensory signs

Formulating the nature of the neurological problem and its localization on the basis of the signs requires a combination of basic anatomical knowledge and pattern recognition. It is important to be able to recognize the limitations of information the physical signs convey in terms of localization. A patient with gait ataxia and extensor plantar reflexes and no other signs

Figure 16.18 Parkinson's disease, showing the typical rigid, flexed posture involving the trunk and limbs. The face is impassive.

could have a lesion in the thoracic or cervical spinal cord or in the cerebellum with early brainstem compression, or it could be a diffuse cerebral process, such as small vessel cerebrovascular disease or hydrocephalus. It may also be that two different lesions account for the two manifestations. Conversely, dysfunction affecting several different systems does not necessarily imply a multifocal disorder: diplopia, nystagmus, dysarthria, ataxia, upper motor neuron signs in the limbs, widespread sensory loss and impairment of bladder control might be caused by multiple sclerosis, but a single brainstem lesion could equally account for all of the symptoms and signs.

In the following section, patterns of motor signs and patterns of sensory signs are outlined separately. And, of course, the examiner encounters them sequentially, but for many syndromes it is the characteristic combination of motor and sensory features that allows accurate diagnosis.

Patterns of motor signs

Diagnosing lesions of individual motor or motor and sensory peripheral nerves requires knowledge of which muscles are supplied by which nerve; the same considerations apply to nerve root lesions.

Table 16.11 Common gait disorders

Gait	Characteristics
Myopathic (proximal, symmetrical myopathy)	Hyperlordosis (axial and pelvic muscle weakness) Waddling gait (weak gluteus medius muscles, among others, bilaterally)
High stepping or 'steppage'	A consequence of foot drop (unilateral or bilateral): common peroneal nerve lesion, motor polyneuropathy (e.g. Charcot-Marie-Tooth), distal myopathy The leg has to be lifted abnormally high to make a step. With mild ankle dorsiflexion weakness, the foot slaps onto the ground as weight is transferred on to the heel.
Ataxic	Midline cerebellar lesion (cerebellar vermis): wide-based unsteady gait with irregular sized paces and potential to topple in any direction; may be little or no limb incoordination Cerebellar hemisphere lesion: the patient veers towards the side of the lesion; there is ipsilateral limb incoordination. Sensory ataxia: there may be limb and gait incoordination with sensory signs (particularly joint position sensation) and positive Romberg's test.
Hemiparetic	The spastic arm is held adducted at the shoulder with the elbow flexed and the forearm in front of the chest with flexion at the wrist and fingers. Swinging of the affected arm is reduced. The spastic leg is stiff with impaired knee flexion and ankle dorsiflexion, with abduction of the leg to bring the plantarflexed foot round and forward when taking a step (circumduction).
Spastic (paraparesis; tetraparesis)	Bilateral spastic legs Bilateral circumduction, such that the leading leg may end up adducted in front of the trailing leg; hence, a 'scissor gait'
Parkinsonian	Kyphotic posture Start hesitation Initially small paces, which may get bigger Acceleration of rate of steps once walking initiated ('festinant gait') Reduced or absent arm swing unilaterally or bilaterally May suddenly get stuck (e.g. in a doorway) Increased number of paces to turn round Improvement of gait with visual cues on the ground
Frontal gait disorder This term has a number of mainly less satisfactory synonyms, including gait apraxia, lower body parkinsonism, atherosclerotic or vascular parkinsonism, marche à petits pas.	Gait ignition failure Start hesitation Small paces (but no acceleration) Unsteadiness Improvement of gait with visual cues on the ground Prominent swinging of the arms Ability to use the legs to make cycling movements on a bed or in a chair, yet inability to use legs to walk

Plexus lesions can be difficult, particularly if patchy and multifocal, but can sometimes be diagnosed confidently on clinical grounds simply from the anatomy. For example, a patient with a combination of what appears to be a radial nerve lesion and an axillary nerve lesion will have a lesion affecting the posterior cord of the brachial plexus.

Distal symmetrical weakness in the limbs would be typical for a generalized motor polyneuropathy. The same pattern can be seen in distal myopathies and some spinal muscular atrophies (hereditary motor neuronopathies), neither being common.

Demyelinating polyneuropathies (Guillain-Barré syndrome (GBS) being the most important) give rise to proximal as well as distal weakness, short nerves being as susceptible to conduction block as long ones. Hence, the presentation of GBS may be with exclusively 'proximal' and life-threatening weakness of muscles of swallowing and breathing.

Mainly proximal, symmetrical limb weakness should prompt consideration of myopathy, particularly polymyositis and dermatomyositis, and muscle disease secondary to metabolic or drug-induced disorders, such as steroid myopathy, thyrotoxic myopathy and osteomalacic myopathy. Ask your patient to get out of a chair or rise from a crouch. The different muscular dystrophies tend to have particular patterns of muscle involvement that may help diagnostically.

Table 16.12 Localization of upper motor neuron lesions

Pattern of weakness	Site of lesion
Spastic monoparesis	Cerebral hemisphere
	Arm (and face)—MCA territory
	Leg—ACA territory
	Brown-Séquard syndrome in thoracic cord gives a monoparesis of the ipsilateral leg
Spastic paraparesis	Thoracic spinal cord lesion (i.e. above lumbar cord, but below cervical cord)
	A parasagittal meningioma in the falx between the cerebral hemispheres affecting the motor cortex for the leg bilaterally is a much quoted but rare cause of a paraparesis.
Spastic hemiparesis	A large hemisphere lesion (e.g. MCA territory stroke, but the arm will be worse affected than the leg)
	A lesion of the internal capsule (pure motor hemiplegia is a lacunar syndrome)
	A brainstem lesion affecting the corticospinal tract on one side
	Brown-Séquard syndrome in the high cervical spinal cord
Spastic tetraparesis	High cervical spinal cord lesion (e.g. C3/C4 disc)
	Diffuse bilateral cerebral hemisphere disease affecting motor pathways bilaterally, e.g. small vessel cerebrovascular disease
	Hydrocephalus
	Brainstem disease affecting the corticospinal tracts bilaterally, e.g. basilar artery territory stroke (which causes locked-in syndrome)
'Cortical hand'	A small lesion in the primary motor cortex subserving the hand
	Weakness and difficulty using the hand, but little or no spasticity
'Cortical foot'	A small lesion in the primary motor cortex subserving the foot
	Weakness and difficulty using the foot, but little or no spasticity

ACA, anterior cerebral artery; MCA, middle cerebral artery.

Patients who have weakness and no sensory symptoms or signs and no upper motor neuron signs usually have muscle disorders or neuromuscular junction disorders (e.g. myasthenia gravis (MG), Lambert Eaton myasthenic syndrome or botulism). Typically, MG affects the eyelids, eye muscles, face, jaw, muscles of swallowing and breathing and axial and proximal limb muscles, but atypical cases do occur.

Upper motor neuron disorders affecting the leg

The lesion may be in the spinal cord or brain. Weakness affects the flexor muscles more than extensor muscles; hence, the abnormal findings are of weakness in hip flexion (iliopsoas), knee flexion (hamstrings) and ankle dorsiflexion (tibialis anterior). Spasticity usually predominates in the hip adductors and the extensor muscles of the leg and foot (gluteus maximus, quadriceps and calf muscles). These circumstances account for the characteristics of the hemiparetic and paraparetic gait (see Table 16.11).

Upper motor neuron disorders affecting the arm and hand

Here the typical pattern is almost the opposite of that in the leg: weakness mainly affects deltoid and the extensors of the arm and hand—elbow extension (triceps), wrist extensors and finger extensors. Spasticity is mainly in the flexors (biceps and brachialis, wrist flexors and finger flexors) and in forearm pronators. Thus, the typical posture of the arm in an ambulant patient with a hemiparesis is adduction at the shoulder, flexion at the elbow, pronation of the forearm and flexion of the wrist and fingers.

The distribution of weakness in upper motor neuron lesions of the limbs is often referred to as 'pyramidal', a useful but not completely accurate term. Table 16.12 summarizes where in the CNS lesions need to be to produce the various categories of upper motor neuron lesions.

Patterns of sensory loss (Table 16.13)

The diagnosis of lesions of individual sensory peripheral nerves or the sensory component of mixed nerves requires knowledge of anatomy, in this case the area of cutaneous sensation mediated by the nerve in question (see Table 16.13 and Figs 16.15 and 16.16). In lesions affecting mixed nerves, sensory symptoms with or without signs commonly precede motor symptoms and signs. Thus, a clear description by a patient of sensory loss in ulnar nerve distribution provides compelling evidence for an ulnar neuropathy even with no signs. The right combination of motor and sensory signs allows the diagnosis of a mononeuropathy to be made. Nerve conduction studies and electromyography may contribute to the assessment of the nature of the lesion (precise location, extent of conduction block, extent of axonal damage, subclinical involvement of other nerves, presence of an underlying subclinical polyneuropathy), but are not necessary for making the diagnosis if there are clear-cut signs.

Table 16.13 Patterns of sensory loss

Clinical sensory findings	Site of lesion
Hemianaesthesia (all modalities)	Parietal cortex or subcortical white matter (corona radiata)
Incomplete (e.g. face and arm)	Thalamus or internal capsule
Complete	Pure sensory stroke is a lacunar syndrome.
Crossed sensory deficit: loss of cutaneous sensation on one side of the face and loss of spinothalamic tract-mediated sensation on the other side of the body	Lateral medullary syndrome: lesion of spinal tract and nucleus of trigeminal ipsilateral to the facial sensory loss, and of crossed spinothalamic tract
Cape or half-cape distribution of dissociated suspended sensory loss (spinothalamic, with an upper and a lower level) with preserved proprioception and vibration sense	Central cord lesion: syringomyelia (and syringobulbia if there is no upper level but the sensory loss affects the face)
Loss of all modalities below a dermatomal level on legs (rare), trunk or neck	Transverse spinal cord lesion affecting posterior columns and spinothalamic tracts Cord compression by tumour, cord trauma, severe myelitis
As above, but with sacral sparing of cutaneous sensory loss	A severe intramedullary spinal cord lesion (e.g. tumour, bleed), but with sparing of the outermost spinothalamic fibres which come from sacral dermatomes
Brown-Séquard syndrome: loss of spinothalamic sensation on one side, with a sensory level, and loss of vibration and proprioception in affected limbs on the other side	Hemisection of the spinal cord: involvement of the posterior columns (uncrossed) and spinothalamic tract (crossed) on one side The lesion is on the side with the proprioceptive loss. Cord compression (tumour, disc), myelitis (e.g. multiple sclerosis), cord trauma
Anterior spinal artery syndrome	Infarction affecting the anterior (ventral) thoracic spinal cord Involvement of spinothalamic tracts bilaterally Posterior columns spared If the infarction extends down to the lumbar spinal cord, the lower limb reflexes are lost, otherwise, they become brisk because of the paraplegia caused by bilateral corticospinal tract involvement.
Radicular distribution of cutaneous sensory loss	Radiculopathy One of the clinical problems is that the distribution for nerve roots and individual peripheral nerves can be similar(e.g. C5 and axillary nerve, L4 and saphenous, L5 and common peroneal)
Extensive sensory loss in one limb, not accounted for by a nerve root or a peripheral nerve	Consider a plexopathy (brachial or lumbar) The motor features are likely to predominate.
Sensory loss in the distribution of individual sensory or sensory and motor nerves	Mononeuropathy Entrapment neuropathies of mixed nerves may present with sensory features only, or with motor and sensory features, which makes clinical diagnosis easier. For some nerves, you have to rely solely on clinical acumen: the nerve is not amenable to neurophysiological investigation (e.g. lateral cutaneous nerve of the thigh 'meralgia paraesthetica').
Distal sensory loss in limbs	Polyneuropathy: classically 'glove and stocking', but may be much less marked (toes only) or much more marked, only sparing the back close to the spine Multifocal polyneuropathies have features of a multiplicity of mononeuropathies.

Familiarity with the areas of cutaneous sensation mediated by nerve roots (dermatomes; see Figs 16.15 and 16.16) is important for two reasons. First, it enables lesions of individual nerve roots to be diagnosed. Second, the level of a spinal cord lesion can be ascertained to some extent (see below).

Distal cutaneous sensory loss (touch, pinprick) in all four limbs, often in a 'glove and stocking' distribution, usually indicates a sensory polyneuropathy. Vibration sense and joint position sense may also be affected, and loss of reflexes, particularly the ankle reflexes, provides strong clinical support for a diagnosis of sensory polyneuropathy. Cervical spinal cord lesions sometimes produce quite widespread sensory symptoms in both hands, which might make one think of peripheral nerve pathology, but the motor signs in the legs and possibly autonomic manifestations (sexual dysfunction, impaired bladder and bowel control) ought to clarify the situation. However, rarely, cervical spinal cord lesions can also give rise to distal lower limb sensory symptoms, which can be misleading.

Spinal cord and cauda equina lesions

The characteristic sensory disturbance associated with compression of the cauda equina or spinal cord is one of loss of all modalities of sensation below the level of the compression. If the compression is of the cauda equina (e.g. a big central posterior intervertebral disc prolapse), all nerve roots below and possibly at the level of the lesion will be affected, including the buttocks and perineum. A severe spinal cord lesion (often compression, but any process which functionally transects the cord at one site) will result in a sensory level on the trunk (abdomen and back, or chest, including the arms if the lesion is between C5 and T1 spinal cord level) or on the neck. Knowledge of the anatomy of the dermatomes allows the spinal cord level (not the same as the spinal column level) to be determined. In spinal cord lesions of mild to moderate severity, the sensory level (which is less dense than in severe lesions) is some distance below the spinal cord level of the lesion. As the lesion evolves, the patient develops progressively worse sensory symptoms, first perceived at a level well below that of the lesion, but which then extend up towards the level of the lesion. This process may not have been completed at the time the patient is evaluated and can sometimes lead to the wrong part of the spinal cord being imaged.

Brown-Séquard syndrome

Brown-Séquard syndrome refers to the signs resulting from a focal lesion affecting the right or left half of the spinal cord, such as an intramedullary inflammatory or an extramedullary compressive lesion. Disruption of the descending corticospinal tract on the affected side results in an ipsilateral upper motor neuron disorder below the level of the lesion (commonly in one leg but a high cervical lesion would affect the arm as well). Involvement of the posterior columns on the affected side results in ipsilateral loss of vibration sense and joint position sense in the leg or arm and leg below the lesion. The spinothalamic tracts on the side of the lesion are affected, but sensory input into the spinothalamic tracts comes from pain and temperature afferents on the opposite side that cross over on entering the spinal cord, so loss of pinprick and temperature sensation occurs below the level of the lesion on the opposite side (Fig. 16.19). Some patients with mild lesions comment that, although it is one leg that drags and feels weak and stiff, it is the other leg that has impaired sensation.

Central spinal cord lesion (especially syringomyelia)

A syrinx is a pathological tube-shaped cavity in the spinal cord, usually cervical and extending down into the thoracic area. It expands the spinal cord, but

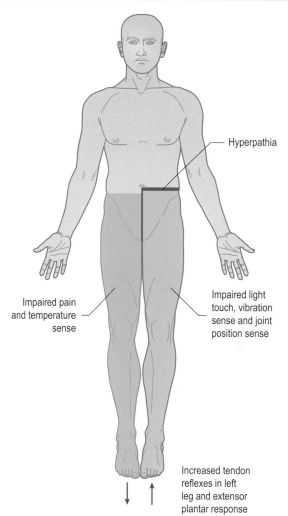

Figure 16.19   Brown-Séquard syndrome. Note the distribution of corticospinal, posterior column and lateral spinothalamic tract signs. The cord lesion is on the left side.

ascending and descending long tracts are unimpaired except in extreme cases. Anterior horn cells are damaged, leading to the motor manifestations of wasting and weakness of muscles in the arms and hands. Tendon reflex pathways are affected, which leads to upper limb reflex loss. There may be abnormalities of autonomic control of blood vessels and sweating in affected limbs. Most remarkable, however, are the patterns of sensory impairment. The classic findings are described by two adjectives: the sensory loss is *dissociated* and a sensory level is found that is *suspended*. Dissociated sensory loss denotes loss of pain and temperature sensation with preservation of vibration and proprioception. The central cord lesion interrupts the sensory afferents that cross the middle of the spinal cord from dorsal roots on one side to spinothalamic tracts on the other side. Sensory afferents proceeding directly from dorsal roots into posterior columns are unaffected. Spinothalamic afferents that have already crossed below the lower limit of the lesion are also unaffected. This dictates that the loss of pinprick sensation will have an upper level corresponding approximately to the top of the syrinx, but there will also be a lower level, usually on the trunk, so the sensory loss is suspended by comparison with the situation in lesions affecting the spinothalamic tracts themselves (such as complete transverse cord lesions, the Brown-Séquard lesion or anterior spinal artery territory spinal cord infarction).

Anterior spinal artery territory spinal cord infarction

A major component of the arterial supply to much of the cord, particularly the thoracic spinal cord, comes from the anterior spinal artery, which receives its main blood supply via the artery of Adamkiewicz from the thoracic aorta. Spinal cord infarction is uncommon; when it occurs, it is usually the thoracic cord that is affected. Occlusion of the artery of Adamkiewicz may be atherosclerotic, arteritic or consequent upon dissection of the aorta. The result is infarction of the anterior (ventral) half of the spinal cord over a variable length. The corticospinal tracts are involved bilaterally, resulting in abrupt-onset paraplegia. The major autonomic manifestations are loss of bladder and bowel control. The spinothalamic tracts are affected on both sides of the cord. Thus, there is dense loss of pinprick sensation with a sensory level on the trunk. The striking feature, in a numb paraplegic individual, is preservation of sensation mediated by the posterior columns—intact vibration and joint position sense in the toes and feet.

Patterns of sensory loss in lesions of the medulla

In the midbrain, pons and medulla, so many nuclei and nerve tracts are found in such restricted anatomical confines that inevitably the clinical manifestations resulting from small lesions in different parts vary substantially. Considering sensation in isolation, a lesion of the lateral medulla on one side may affect the spinothalamic tract on that side, conveying pain sensation from the contralateral side of the body and, at the same time, affect the spinal tract and nucleus of the trigeminal nerve, which mediates pain on the ipsilateral side of the face.

Hemianaesthesia

A lesion affecting the sensory afferent pathways rostral to the principal sensory nucleus of the trigeminal nerve in the pons (i.e. in the midbrain, diencephalon, thalamus or internal capsule) will result in a hemianaesthesia: loss of sensation on the whole of one side of the body, including the head and face. A large lesion, such as a middle cerebral artery territory ischaemic stroke affecting the whole of the primary sensory cortex, will have the same effect. Smaller lesions in the sensory cortex will affect sensation (all modalities) in only part of one side of the body.

Cognitive function

A risk exists in neurological examination that cognition may be neglected. It is a useful simplification to divide domains of cognition into those that are distributed and those that are localized. The anatomical substrates of distributed cognitive functions are bilateral and widespread in the brain. An implication is that a single focal neurological lesion will have little perceptible impact on that function. In contrast, a focal lesion in a particular place will have a major effect on a localized cognitive function.

The two major syndromes of cognitive impairment, which may be accompanied by no neurological signs, are dementia and delirium. They are covered in Chapter 7. In this section, emphasis is placed on cognitive deficits that, to some extent, have localizing value and that may be seen in patients with focal cerebral lesions as well as those with more generalized neurodegenerative disorders.

Amnesia

Memory is a distributed cognitive function. Dense amnesia requires bilateral hemisphere lesions, but those lesions may be very focal—bilateral thalamic infarction or damage to the mamillothalamic tracts in Wernicke's encephalopathy can cause devastating amnesia—and the anatomy of memory in each hemisphere is localized and well defined. Furthermore, unilateral lesions, such as a posterior cerebral artery occlusion causing temporal lobe infarction, do have discernible effects on memory. Normal episodic memory (memory of events which have been personally experienced) depends on integrity of the hippocampi and entorhinal cortex in the temporal lobes, the fornices, the thalami and the mamillary bodies. Anterior temporal lobes subserve semantic memory (memory for facts, learning and general knowledge). Verbal memory is dependent on the left temporal lobe, visual memory on the right temporal lobe. Some important causes of amnesia are listed in Table 16.14. Amnesia emerges mainly from the history taken from an informant rather than from the patient. Episodic memory may be assessed by testing recall of a name and address that the patient has registered and by testing the patient's recall of events from his past, both recent and distant.

Dysphasia

Dysphasia or aphasia is an acquired disorder of language function. The auditory processing of language involves the superior temporal gyri bilaterally. The meaning of words requires the dominant temporal lobe. The planning of speech production occurs in the dominant frontal lobe (including Broca's area in the inferior frontal lobe). The motor control of speech production depends on the sensorimotor cortex bilaterally. In routine practice, four major parameters of language can be used to assess dysphasia:

Table 16.14 Some causes of amnesia

Cause	Comment
Acute	
Transient global amnesia (TGA)	The name describes well what happens; the pathology remains obscure; imaging indicates a hippocampal process.
	Preserved autobiographical memory (self and family); prominent anterograde amnesia; alert and lucid with preservation of other cognitive domains; and resolves within 24 hours.
Transient epileptic amnesia	Here amnesia is the seizure; shorter than TGA (<1 hour); more likely to be recurrent; and associated aura or automatisms.
Epilepsy more generally	Temporal lobe seizures may involve amnesia and also other memory symptoms, particularly dysmnesia: deja vu (strong recollection of having an experience previously) and jamais vu (sensation of unfamiliarity); postictal amnesia follows any generalized convulsion
Closed head injury	Concussion involves retrograde and anterograde post-traumatic amnesia.
Drugs: benzodiazepines, alcohol	Amnesia can occur without significant impairment of alertness.
Chronic	
Hippocampal damage	
Herpes simplex encephalitis	Bilateral temporal lobe damage
Limbic encephalitis	Bilateral temporal lobe damage
Cerebral anoxia	
Temporal lobectomy with a lesion in the other temporal lobe	Should not happen in modern practice because of improvements in preoperative assessment
Bilateral posterior cerebral artery territory infarction	
Closed head injury	Bilateral temporal lobe damage is common.
Early Alzheimer's disease	Later there are other prominent cognitive deficits as well.
Diencephalic damage	
Korsakoff's syndrome	This is what results from untreated Wernicke's encephalopathy, owing to thiamine deficiency.
Third ventricular tumours and cysts	Potentially affecting the fornices and thalami bilaterally
Bilateral thalamic infarction	Either two separate events or, if the bilateral paramedian thalamosubthalamic arteries of Percheron branch from one common vessel (a not uncommon variant), one stroke
Subarachnoid haemorrhage from anterior communicating artery aneurysm	

The list on the left is adapted from John R. Hodges 1994 Cognitive Assessment for Clinicians, Oxford University Press.

fluency, comprehension, repetition and naming skills. Naming skills are affected in all forms of dysphasia. Dominant frontal lobe lesions are likely to give rise to a non-fluent dysphasia characterized by effortful speech, poverty of language and loss of grammatical structure (agrammatism), but with comprehension intact, whereas lesions in Wernicke's area (posterior superior dominant temporal lobe) result in impairment of comprehension, but with fluent speech that conveys rather little meaning. Single word or phrase repetition, in isolation, is impaired in conduction aphasia, localizing to the dominant peri-Sylvian region, for example the arcuate fasciculus which connects Broca's and Wernicke's areas. Global aphasia occurs as a result of large dominant hemisphere lesions of the frontal, temporal and parietal lobe. Dysphasia is often associated with dyslexia and dysgraphia. A severe comprehension deficit as a result of dysphasia makes it challenging to assess other aspects of cognition, although they may be intact. The most common cause of dysphasia is a dominant hemisphere stroke, but any appropriately placed focal lesion may cause dysphasia, and it is an important feature of neurodegenerative dementias.

Apraxia

Apraxia refers to an inability to do things in spite of having intact motor and sensory systems. Dressing apraxia, an inability to put on items of clothing, particularly jackets and gowns, is seen in patients with non-dominant parietal lesions. Visuospatial disabilities and neglect contribute to this form of apraxia. Constructional apraxia likewise reflects impaired visuospatial function. The main form of motor apraxia (ideomotor apraxia) manifests as difficulty using instruments and tools (toothbrush, scissors, etc.) in spite of knowing what the device in question is. Other manifestations of ideomotor apraxia include an inability to carry out actions, such as waving goodbye or saluting; an inability to mime actions (e.g. using a comb to comb one's hair, hammering a nail) and to copy finger and hand positions demonstrated by the examiner. This form of apraxia usually occurs in dominant parietal lesions. An apraxic individual may be unable to make a cup of tea, but agnosia (see below) might give rise to the same inability. Furthermore, a test for apraxia that requires a sequence of actions probes comprehension, memory and executive skills as well as praxis. Patients with dominant inferior frontal lobe lesions may have apraxia affecting the use of lips, tongue and mouth, often in association with a non-fluent dysphasia. Gait apraxia is covered in Table 16.11.

Agnosia

Agnosia is a failure of recognition by impaired cortical processing of sensory information. A simple classification is by the sensory modality affected: visual, auditory, tactile or olfactory. There is overlap between tactile agnosia and cortical sensory loss. Visual agnosia (potentially the most severely disabling agnosia) reflects visuoperceptual impairment owing to occipitoparietal and occipitotemporal lesions that are often bilateral and may be associated with a visual field defect, but basic visual function in the preserved field is intact. A patient with visual agnosia may not recognize a watch until it is put into his hand, but would answer correctly the question 'What do you wear on your wrist and use to tell the time?' Prosopagnosia is an inability to recognize familiar faces (though parts of the face are correctly identified, and the patient may be able to match correctly two different photographs of the face he cannot recognize). Bilateral occipitotemporal lesions underlie prosopagnosia, particularly the fusiform gyrus (face area).

Neglect phenomena

A lesion in either hemisphere may lead to a form of neglect affecting the opposite side, but neglect is much more commonly seen when the lesion is in the right cerebral hemisphere, affecting the left side. Usually the lesion is large, such as a stroke. Different forms of neglect may have different localizations. Parietal lobe involvement is often prominent. A patient with neglect of personal space may pay no attention to the affected side of the body, in the extreme even denying that the affected side belongs to him. Denial of a hemiplegia is anosognosia; unconcern about a hemiplegia is anosodiaphoria. Neglect of extrapersonal space leads to failure to eat the food off one side of a plate, failure to complete one side of a drawing, failure to read the left side of a text, even failure to write the first part of a word. Sensory and visual inattention are forms of neglect.

Localizing the neurological lesion

Having taken a history and undertaken a neurological and relevant general medical examination, it is important to decide where the likely lesion is and, ideally, its likely nature (e.g. vascular, inflammatory, degenerative, neoplastic). This can often seem bewildering for students and doctors in training. In addition to those points made above regarding the identification of muscle disorders, neuromuscular junction disorders, mononeuropathies, polyneuropathies, radiculopathies and spinal cord disorders, the following are some helpful principles regarding brainstem, cerebellar and cerebral hemisphere lesions.

If a patient has a hemiparesis and a hemianaesthesia on the same side, the lesion has to be above the decussation of the corticospinal tracts in the medulla. The lesion most likely is in the contralateral cerebral hemisphere, but could also be in the brainstem.

The range of possible manifestations of brainstem lesions is extensive, but a good general rule is that a cranial nerve lesion (III, V, VI, VII, VIII, X or XII) on one side and long-tract signs on the other side of the body indicate a brainstem lesion. The long-tract signs may be motor, sensory or both. A brainstem lesion has to be considered if there are bilateral long-tract signs and the lesion is above neck level. Nystagmus and long-tract signs indicate a brainstem lesion. Vertical gaze paresis of acute onset and internuclear ophthalmoparesis are indicators of midbrain and pontine lesions, respectively. Extensive brainstem lesions affecting the reticular formation will cause coma. A basilar artery thrombosis may spare the dorsal brainstem such that consciousness is preserved, but the devastating consequence is the locked-in syndrome.

Cerebellar lesions should be suspected with combinations of gait ataxia, limb ataxia, dysarthria and nystagmus. Ataxia by itself is rather non-localizing, being a feature of polyneuropathy and spinal cord, cerebellar, brainstem and cerebral hemisphere disease. Remember that anyone who is vertiginous will be ataxic until the vertigo settles, so ataxia in combination with vertigo may be caused by a peripheral vestibular rather than a neurological disorder. Cerebellar mass lesions readily compress the brainstem, which complicates the signs, and, moreover, brainstem compression readily causes hydrocephalus.

Common manifestations in large unilateral cerebral hemisphere lesions include contralateral hemianopia, horizontal gaze paresis, hemiparesis and hemianaesthesia together with cognitive impairment (dysphasia in dominant hemisphere lesions, neglect and visuospatial problems in non-dominant). A frontal lobe lesion affecting prefrontal structures may give rise to behavioural and cognitive deficits only. Anterior cerebral artery territory ischaemic strokes cause spastic paresis in the contralateral leg. Middle cerebral artery territory ischaemic strokes cause all of the features of large unilateral hemisphere lesions. The hemiparesis is maximal in the face and arm. Posterior cerebral artery territory ischaemic strokes cause hemianopia because of occipital lobe infarction and cause cognitive deficits owing to involvement of the temporal lobe.

The clinical manifestations of hydrocephalus depend on how acutely it develops. Acute hydrocephalus causes headache, papilloedema, drowsiness and coma. In the setting of established hydrocephalus, acute exacerbations cause hydrocephalic attacks, which may manifest with abrupt headache, paralysis, drop attacks and coma. In some cases, however, hydrocephalus occurs with hardly any raised pressure at all. In such cases, the manifestations are cognitive impairment, ataxia, urinary incontinence, upgaze paresis and extensor plantar reflexes. Hydrocephalus is a common cause of bilateral long-tract (corticospinal tract) signs of cerebral origin. The other is diffuse or multifocal bilateral white matter disease, which may be ischaemic or inflammatory. Large supratentorial mass lesions ultimately cause bilateral long-tract signs, pupillary changes and impending coma owing to brain herniation.

Investigations

It is crucial for investigations in neurological practice to be focused and directed on the basis of the clinical findings. Imaging, cerebrospinal fluid (CSF) examination and neurophysiological investigations may all play a role in diagnosis.

Imaging

Headache

A discussion about which patients with headache should be imaged is beyond the scope of this chapter, but a number of points are worth noting:

- Migraine, tension-type headaches, medication overuse headaches and post-traumatic headaches can be diagnosed with a high degree of accuracy without scans.
- Normal scans undoubtedly help reassure worried patients with headaches, but incidental abnormalities found on scans risk perpetuating worry.
- Normal scans do not cure headaches (though a proportion of patients who know their scan is normal do not attend their follow up appointment).
- Patients with serious intracranial disorders rarely just have headache.
- Occasionally migraine really is 'symptomatic' (i.e. caused by a structural intracranial disorder).

Computed tomography (CT) remains a good method to investigate for headache in the emergency setting, to image large tumours, particularly supratentorial tumours, abscesses, brain swelling, hydrocephalus and haemorrhage, particularly subarachnoid haemorrhage. However, the radiation dose is the equivalent of 200 chest X-rays so, if available, magnetic resonance imaging (MRI) is preferable, especially in an elective setting.

Epilepsy

The investigation of choice for late-onset epilepsy is an MRI head scan; the information required is whether there is an identifiable structural cause for the epilepsy. Electroencephalography (EEG) in this situation is less useful. In the paediatric/adolescent age group, imaging is usually normal, but the EEG may well be informative (see below).

Stroke

Imaging is central to the investigation of stroke and transient ischaemic attacks. The advent of thrombolysis and the possibility of other forms of emergency treatment of ischaemic stroke mandate extremely rapid, but accurate diagnosis of stroke and of stroke severity. CT, including CT angiography, and MRI both contribute.

Focal central nervous system lesions

All focal CNS lesions will require imaging. Usually MRI is preferable to CT, but the choice may depend on local resources. It is crucial, by means of the clinical methods outlined above, to decide where the focal lesion is, so as to image the appropriate part of the nervous system. This is particularly true of spinal imaging.

Multiple sclerosis

All patients presenting for the first time with manifestations of multiple sclerosis (often but not always the first attack) must have an MRI head scan, and imaging of the spinal cord may be necessary.

Cognitive impairment

As a rule, all patients with cognitive impairment should have structural imaging of the brain. Metabolic imaging contributes and molecular imaging (e.g. of amyloid) will soon become a clinical tool.

Peripheral nervous system

Magnetic resonance imaging is the technique used to investigate radiculopathies. MRI also has a role in the investigation of plexus lesions, but imaging of the brachial plexus remains problematic. The vast majority of compressive mononeuropathies are not imaged, but consideration should be given to imaging (MRI, ultrasound) in certain progressive and severe mononeuropathies to look for tumours and cysts.

Muscle diseases

Magnetic resonance imaging has a role in the investigation of muscle disorders, contributing to the assessment of some patients with dystrophies or inflammatory muscle disease, particularly in guiding the decision as to which muscle to biopsy.

Electroencephalography

Electrodes applied to the patient's scalp pick up small changes of electrical potential which, after amplification, are recorded on paper or displayed on a video monitor and recorded electronically. The main use of EEG is in diagnosing the nature of the epilepsy in young patients (particularly in distinguishing generalized from focal epilepsies), but it has significant limitations because, in the majority of cases, what is recorded is an interictal EEG which may or may not show diagnostically useful abnormalities. EEG is a poor test in individuals who have undiagnosed attacks of symptoms that might be epilepsy. Video telemetry is invaluable in clarifying whether attacks are epileptic or non-epileptic, the main limitation being that the attack frequency has to be high enough to make it likely that attacks will be recorded.

EEG may be a useful investigation in encephalopathic states where the clinical picture may be one of delirium. Here, EEG can identify non-convulsive status epilepticus or point to a diagnosis of encephalitis as opposed to a toxic or metabolic encephalopathy. It has a supportive role in diagnosing Creutzfeldt-Jakob disease.

Nerve conduction studies and electromyography

Sensory nerve conduction studies (NCS) are achieved by stimulating electrically a purely sensory nerve percutaneously and recording, usually by surface electrodes, the resulting sensory action potentials (SAP) in the relevant nerve, either more proximally or distally. The SAP amplitude and conduction velocity are measured. Motor NCS require stimulation of a motor or mixed nerve, recording the resulting motor action potentials from a muscle supplied by the nerve, again usually with surface electrodes. Stimulation of the nerve at two different sites allows calculation of the conduction velocity between the two sites. Electromyography (EMG) entails recording electrical activity generated by muscle fibres and motor units (groups of muscle fibres supplied by a single motor neuron) at rest and during contraction, using a needle electrode inserted into the muscle. Different abnormalities of EMG arise in denervation, disorders of neuromuscular transmission and disorders of muscle itself. NCS contributes to the diagnosis of many, but not all, entrapment neuropathies. It has to be anatomically possible to stimulate and record from the nerve proximal to the entrapment site. In patients with clear physical signs, NCSs are not needed to make the correct clinical diagnosis, but may help in the assessment of severity and prognosis. Every patient who is going to have surgical decompression of an entrapped peripheral nerve should have an NCS. NCS is invaluable in confirming the suspected diagnosis of nerve entrapment when there are no definite signs, a common circumstance in carpal tunnel syndrome.

NCS and EMG may contribute to the assessment of plexopathies and radiculopathies although, in the latter, the combination of careful clinical evaluation and imaging should suffice. NCS and EMG help to confirm a diagnosis of polyneuropathy and provide information about the nature of polyneuropathies (axonal, demyelinating, multifocal, small fibre). NCS and EMG are helpful in suspected disorders of neuromuscular junctions (e.g. amplitude decrement on repetitive stimulation and 'jitter'—an irregularity of neuromuscular transmission—on single fibre EMG). EMG helps in the diagnosis of myopathy and is an important test for patients with undiagnosed weakness.

Cerebrospinal fluid examination

Cerebrospinal fluid examination is usually obtained by lumbar puncture (LP), which is uncomfortable, invasive and attended by a number of potential complications, the most common one being post-lumbar puncture headache. There is a risk of death from brain herniation when LP is undertaken in a patient with raised intracranial pressure caused by a mass lesion or obstructive hydrocephalus. Papilloedema, any grade of impaired level of consciousness or any focal neurological signs mandate brain imaging before consideration of LP; it is contraindicated in patients with mass lesions and obstructive hydrocephalus. However, it is an essential investigation in patients with papilloedema owing to suspected raised intracranial pressure and in those who have a normal, good quality MRI, to pursue the possibility of idiopathic intracranial hypertension and to exclude low-grade chronic meningitis, as well as to treat the raised pressure. Pressure measurement, as well as CSF analysis, will be required.

Meningitis

The single circumstance in which LP is an emergency investigation is CNS infection, particularly meningitis. Controversy exists to whether CSF examination in meningitis is really necessary or at least whether the risk is worth taking. In adult neurology, the consensus remains that CSF should be obtained if possible but that, in cases of suspected pyogenic bacterial meningitis, there must be no delay in starting antibiotic treatment pending cranial imaging. Thus, if there is no contraindication to LP, it should be performed expeditiously immediately after clinical assessment and obtaining blood cultures, in order to provide a microbiological diagnosis. If cranial imaging is necessary, treatment should start directly after clinical assessment and blood cultures. CSF obtained after imaging has shown that LP is expected to be safe and may still be diagnostic even some hours after treatment has started.

CSF examination is important, sometimes critical, in the diagnosis of all forms of infective meningitis: bacterial, tuberculous, yeast, fungal and viral. The key parameters are the white cell count, the types of white cells (polymorphonuclear neutrophil white cells, lymphocytes), the CSF glucose concentration (low in bacterial meningitis), which must be compared with a simultaneous blood glucose concentration, microscopy for microorganisms (Gram stain, tuberculosis stain, India ink preparation for cryptococci), DNA analysis for viral and bacterial DNA (using polymerase chain reaction (PCR) techniques), other microbiological assays (cryptococcal antigen) and appropriate microbiological culture. The CSF protein concentration is of some importance and the CSF lactate concentration may be helpful.

CSF analysis is also urgent in encephalitis, which will be treated as herpes simplex encephalitis until CSF PCR tests for herpes simplex virus have proved negative. CSF examination in myelitis will follow imaging.

In all other situations, CSF examination is not so urgent, even if it is still essential. In low-grade meningitis, which is suspected to be owing to tuberculosis, to maximize the chance of identifying and culturing mycobacteria send up to three CSF samples on consecutive days before starting treatment.

Subarachnoid haemorrhage

In suspected subarachnoid haemorrhage with cranial imaging that does not show evidence of blood in the subarachnoid space, CSF must be examined. It is important to wait until 12 hours after the suspected bleed so that red blood cells will have lysed and haemoglobin will have undergone metabolism to oxyhaemoglobin and bilirubin, which can be detected by spectroscopy or seen with the naked eye as xanthochromia. Failure to allow time for xanthochromia to develop makes it impossible to distinguish a traumatic CSF tap from bloodstained CSF caused by a subarachnoid haemorrhage.

CNS inflammatory disorders

Cerebrospinal fluid lymphocytosis is usually a feature of conditions such as CNS vasculitis, neurosarcoidosis, Behçet's disease and sometimes systemic lupus erythematosus.

With regard to multiple sclerosis (MS), if the clinical features and MRI appearances are typical (particularly in a young patient), CSF examination may not be necessary. It remains important if scans do not fulfil diagnostic criteria or if there is ambiguity as to whether scan lesions are inflammatory or ischaemic, or reflect some other pathology. CSF protein electrophoresis to detect oligoclonal IgG immunoglobulins is the most sensitive test to provide evidence of chronic inflammatory CNS demyelination. Occasionally, in suspected MS, the results of CSF examination are incompatible with that diagnosis because of either a very high cell count or a very high protein concentration, mandating a revision of the diagnosis.

Guillain-Barré syndrome

A high CSF protein concentration without a high cell count is characteristic of Guillain-Barré syndrome, an acute inflammatory (usually demyelinating) neuropathy, but this takes time to develop so will not be found if the CSF is examined early in the course of the condition. Every patient with GBS should have CSF looked at in order to make sure that the patient does not have a rapidly progressive polyradiculopathy owing to diffuse neoplastic leptomeningeal infiltration. Accordingly, when the LP is done, take care to order cytology as well as a cell count, blood and CSF glucose concentration, protein concentration and, if appropriate, culture. High CSF protein, in the absence of other CSF abnormalities, is also a useful diagnostic marker of chronic inflammatory demyelinating neuropathies (CIDP).

Neoplastic leptomeningeal infiltration

Neoplastic leptomeningeal infiltration, either by a haematological malignancy (leukaemia, lymphoma) or metastatic carcinoma (lung, breast, others) may present as a cranial neuropathy or spinal polyradiculopathy or with headache, encephalopathy or hydrocephalus. High-protein and low-glucose concentrations in CSF are typical, but not diagnostic. The presence of malignant cells in the CSF is diagnostic, but they are not always seen. Sending serial samples on consecutive days (up to three) increases the chance of a positive result.

Neurodegenerative disorders

Cerebrospinal fluid neurodegenerative protein measurement may be used in the diagnosis of dementias, for example, raised CSF tau and reduced CSF amyloid-beta, with increased tau:amyloid-beta ratio, occurs in Alzheimer's disease. In prion disorders, there is raised CSF 14-3-3 protein and the real-time quaking-induced conversion (RT-QuIC) is a highly sensitive assay for prion protein.

Renal and urology system | 17

Sajeda Youssouf

Introduction

Many patients with renal disease have few or non-specific symptoms, whereas disease within the urinary tract usually does have symptoms, many of which are reasonably specific for the disease processes involved. As the kidney and urinary tract are clearly and closely linked, this chapter combines kidney and urinary tract problems in a coherent whole.

The diagnostic process in nephrology and urology

The clinical syndromes associated with kidney disease are more dependent than most on laboratory, histopathology and imaging techniques to complete the diagnostic process, but the basic principles of clinical assessment often lead towards an area of diagnosis and investigation. An understanding of the anatomy and physiology of the renal tract underpins the definition of nephrological 'syndromes' caused by groups of conditions with different types of pathological processes. These allow clinical investigation and assessment to be focused more clearly. Structural lesions tend to present in a more straightforward way with a constellation of symptoms and signs enabling a differential diagnosis that can be pursued in a more linear fashion. There is overlap between presentations and syndromes, particularly at different stages of a disease. This chapter describes symptoms and signs associated with renal and urological disease, as well as delineating some of the syndromes

The history

The history in nephro-urological disease can delineate specific structural abnormalities, intrinsic or systemic conditions causing renal disease, or the consequences of renal impairment, in particular salt and water overload and metabolic abnormalities. In addition, patients may be asymptomatic, with the presence of disease identified on screening, such as urinalysis or blood pressure monitoring. This can provide a way of dividing kidney disease into clinically meaningful syndromes, to aid diagnostic investigation.

Pain

Pain, which can occur throughout the urinary tract (Table 17.1), tends to be caused by infection, tumour or obstruction. Unilateral loin pain can be caused by pyelonephritis, renal stones causing obstruction, urinary retention and bleeding cysts. Pyelonephritis can be of abrupt or insidious onset, associated with fever, vomiting, lower urinary tract symptoms and urinary abnormalities. Laboratory analyses frequently show elevated markers of inflammation. Occasionally, pain may reflect tracking of pus upwards to the diaphragm, causing diaphragmatic pain, or in the retroperitoneal space to the psoas muscle, leading to pain when the muscle is stretched.

Renal stones cause pain in the presence of infection if they cause obstruction to urine flow. In ureteric tract obstruction, classically unilateral pain radiates from loin to groin, and may radiate to the testes or labia. A history of similar symptoms or family history of renal stone disease can be useful.

Kidney tumours classically cause a triad of pain, episodic macroscopic haematuria and a palpable mass, although this is rarely seen in practice. Attention should be paid to other systemic symptoms that may alert to the presence of metastases, such as weight loss, respiratory symptoms from lung metastases and back pain from tumour in the spine.

Polycystic kidney disease causes a spectrum from no symptoms at all, to recurrent or persistent loin pain caused by cyst infection, haemorrhage or local obstruction.

Bladder outflow obstruction (BOO) causes severe suprapubic pain when acute, and is most frequently owing to prostatic obstruction. BOO can also be caused by bladder or pelvic masses and prolapse in women. Acute urinary retention, which can also cause suprapubic pain, can be caused by medications and infection, and in post-operative patients.

Suprapubic and perineal pain most commonly arises from lower urinary tract infection owing to cystitis or urethritis. Such pain is frequently accompanied by dysuria, frequency or strangury (painful micturition). It is nearly always associated with urinary abnormalities on urine stick testing (protein, blood and leukocytes). In men prostatitis should be suspected in cases of severe perineal or rectal discomfort. In young children with urinary tract infection and cystitis the symptoms may be less obvious; cystitis should be suspected in any child who cries on micturating.

Bladder tumours infrequently cause pain; they are more commonly associated with painless haematuria and lower urinary tract symptoms.

Haematuria

Haematuria can be caused by bleeding anywhere in the genito-urinary tract. If visible to the naked eye it is termed macroscopic or visible haematuria; if seen only detectable using urine dipstick tests or microscopy it is termed non-visible, microscopic or dipstick haematuria. It can be continuous or intermittent, and painless or associated with pain and/or fever. Table 17.2 summarizes the causes of haematuria. Blood arising from renal parenchymal disease (glomerular bleeding) is usually, but not always painless, continuous and microscopic, but it can be macroscopic.. Haematuria from renal tumours is more frequently intermittent, macroscopic and associated with pain. Bleeding from bladder tumours is often intermittent, with associated local symptoms suggesting cystitis.

Infections in the urinary tract may also result in haematuria; the presence of microscopic haematuria should always be followed by urine microscopy and culture as part of the diagnostic process. It is important to decide whether haematuria originates from the kidneys or elsewhere in the urinary tract. This decision affects the order in which investigations should be conducted. Over the age of 40, bleeding should generally be assumed to be non-glomerular in the first instance, unless there is other compelling evidence for a glomerular lesion. Under the age of 40, the presence of associated proteinuria is likely to signify parenchymal renal disease, such as a glomerulonephritis.

Transient painless haematuria in the absence of any other urine abnormalities in women is most likely owing to contamination from menstrual blood. Other causes include exercise, intercourse and viral illnesses. Systemic conditions and medications can also cause haematuria; inquiry into a history of bleeding elsewhere may alert to this.

Discoloured urine with positive urine on dipstick can be owing to other causes. Myoglobin (released from muscle owing, for example, to rhabdomyolysis

Table 17.1 Site of pain in the renal tract and causes

Site	Cause
Loin pain	Renal stone causing obstruction
	Tumour
	Pyelonephritis; abscess
	Infected or bleeding renal cyst
Suprapubic pain	Acute bladder outflow obstruction
	Urinary retention
	Lower urinary tract infection (cystitis, urethritis, pyocystis)
	Bladder tumour
Strangury (painful micturition)	Urinary tract infection (UTI)
	Cystitis
Perineal pain	Prostatitis

Table 17.2 Causes of haematuria

Systemic	Glomerular	Non-glomerular
Sickle cell trait	IgA	Stones
Coagulation disorders	Thin basement membrane nephropathy (TBMN)	Tumours (kidney/ureter/bladder/prostate)
Anticoagulant medications	Alport's	Wilms' tumour (children)
	Post-infectious glomerulonephritis	UTI/pyelonephritis
	Membranous glomerulonephritis	Trauma
	Rapidly progressive glomerulonephritis (RPGN)	Infarction (e.g. renal cortical necrosis, papillary necrosis)
	Vasculitis (e.g. SBE, SLE)	Ureteric stricture/hydronephrosis
		Prostatitis/cystitis/urethritis
		Benign prostatic hypertrophy
		Post catheterization
		Rare infections (e.g. Schistosoma, bilharzia)
		Drugs (cyclophosphamide/radiation)
		Renal TB
		Cystic disorders: polycystic kidney disease, medullary sponge kidney
		Radiation cystitis
		Vascular: AV malformations

or trauma) and the presence of free haem both result in positive urine dipstick for blood in the absence of true blood in the urine. Various drugs and certain foods can also result in discoloured urine.

Oliguria/anuria

Oliguria is defined as the passage of less than 500 ml of urine per day, whilst anuria is the complete absence of urine flow. Progressive oliguria can be physiological, owing to inadequate intake, fluid loss such as in burns or blood loss, with preserved glomerular filtration rate (GFR). Here kidney function is not impaired; it is retaining sodium and water, resulting in concentrated urine; restoring adequate renal perfusion will restore normal urine output. However, if inadequate intake or excess loss leads to a significant reduction in the extracellular fluid compartment, the resulting decrease in renal blood flow leads to oliguria and a reduction in GFR. Oliguria owing to reduced renal blood flow is termed pre-renal; it can also occur in the context of cardiogenic or septic shock. Intrinsic renal disease causes loss of glomerular filtration in the absence of reduced blood flow to the kidneys; note that not all causes of intrinsic renal disease cause oliguria. Mechanical obstruction to urine flow, such as caused by stones, tumours or prostatic hypertrophy, is termed post-renal oliguria. When the lesion is at the level of the bladder, it may result in complete anuria.

Polyuria

Polyuria implies no more than a high urinary flow rate. It is caused by excessive intake, an osmotic diuresis, or renal tubular dysfunction (Table 17.3). Recovery from acute kidney injury, particularly following obstruction, can be accompanied by polyuria; the concentrating ability of the renal tubules recovers later than glomerular function. The description of polyuria should always be accompanied by a query about nocturia and polydipsia. The latter, in particular, is a presentation of diabetes. Medications, such as diuretics, can result in polyuria, whilst long-term lithium use is a common cause of nephrogenic

diabetes insipidus. A broader past medical history and systems inquiry assists in differentiating among causes.

Frequency of micturition

Increased frequency of micturition results from polyuria, a reduction in functional bladder capacity, or bladder/urethral irritation (Table 17.4). The most common cause is polyuria and excessive fluid intake, but it is also a feature of urinary tract infection (UTI). Incomplete bladder outlet obstruction, particularly when it is chronic, can result in frequency without accompanying polyuria. Some patients with neurological disease, in particular multiple sclerosis, have frequency of micturition. The detrusor muscle of the bladder contracts at an inappropriately low bladder volume, resulting in a low functional bladder capacity.

Nocturia

The term nocturia implies the need to empty the bladder during the hours of sleep. In the presence of a normal urinary tract and normal renal function, there is diurnal variation in the urinary flow rate: at night time there is a reduction in urine flow, and micturition is unnecessary. Polyuria can result in nocturia, along with a reduction in functional bladder capacity, which can happen with age. Polydipsia at night and the use of diuretics later in the day are also a cause. In chronic kidney disease, even in the early stages, the concentrating ability of the kidneys is reduced, and nocturia can be an early symptom of renal impairment. Sickle cell disease results in similar loss of concentrating ability.

Dysuria

Dysuria is discomfort arising from the urinary tract in which there is pain immediately before, during or after micturition. The urine is often described as 'burning' or 'scalding', and there is usually associated frequency and decreased functional bladder capacity. Infection or inflammation in the bladder or urethra are the most common causes. Malignancy in the lower urinary tract can also cause dysuria.

Table 17.3 Causes of polyuria

Cause	Example
Excessive water intake	Pathogenic polydipsia, beer drinking, caffeine
Osmotic diuresis	Glucose in diabetes mellitus Urea in chronic kidney disease (CKD) Sodium chloride in diuretic use
Renal tubular dysfunction	Cranial diabetes insipidus Nephrogenic diabetes insipidus Recovery following acute kidney injury (AKI)

Table 17.4 Causes of frequency of micturition

Polyuria	All causes
Reduced functional bladder capacity	Prostatic hypertrophy Bladder outlet obstruction Low capacity bladder Multiple sclerosis Post-stroke
Bladder/urethral irritation	Lower urinary tract infection Urethritis

An extreme form of dysuria, strangury, implies an unpleasant and painful desire to void when the bladder is empty or near empty.

Urgency of micturition, incontinence and enuresis

Urgency is the loss of the normal ability to postpone micturition beyond the time when the desire to pass urine is initially perceived. Incontinence is the involuntary passage of urine. Urgency may lead to urge incontinence. Stress incontinence is leakage of urine associated with straining or coughing, often owing to weakened pelvic floor muscles after vaginal childbirth. Enuresis is defined as involuntary micturition after the age at which bladder control begins, and usually refers to nocturnal enuresis. It can be primary, when in the vast majority of cases is a developmental delay, or secondary (nocturnal enuresis after a period of dryness). Occasionally, it can be a presentation of urinary tract infection or type 1 diabetes mellitus.

Slow stream, hesitancy and terminal dribbling

The triad of slow stream, hesitancy and terminal dribbling is most frequently seen in older men with prostatic hypertrophy. Here, the bladder outlet is partially obstructed by the enlarging prostate gland, and the maximum achievable urinary flow rate is reduced. There is often difficulty in initiating micturition (hesitancy) and in completing micturition (terminal dribbling). The symptoms are nearly always associated with frequency of micturition and nocturia. There is progressive bladder enlargement, with eventual overflow incontinence and continuous or intermittent dribbling of urine.

Urethral discharge

Urethral discharge is usually noticed only by men and always requires further investigation. There may be associated symptoms of urethral irritation and the underlying pathology is likely to be urethritis, which is often infective and sexually transmitted (see Chapter 18).

Past medical history

A history of urinary problems as a child may be suggestive of structural abnormalities such as posterior urethral valves. Previous urinary symptoms, specifically a history of UTI or recurrent dysuria, stones and prostate problems, should also be sought. Episodic macroscopic haematuria during upper respiratory tract infection is a classic presentation of IgA nephropathy. Haemoptysis is a feature of rare, but important, pulmonary renal syndromes, such as antineutrophil cytoplasmic autoantibody-associated vasculitis and antiglomerular basement membrane disease. Upper respiratory tract symptoms, such as epistaxis, may also be present. Systemic illnesses, in particular hypertension, diabetes and cardiovascular disease (ischaemic heart disease, stroke and peripheral vascular disease), are a risk factor for chronic kidney disease, which, particularly in the early stages, can present with few or no symptoms, and only be identified on screening.

Medication history

Many drugs can cause renal injury, or be nephrotoxic in the context of kidney disease. Table 17.5 summarizes some of the more common drugs of which to be aware.

Social history

Smoking increases the risk of cardiovascular disease and chronic kidney disease (CKD), and also the risk of many cancers, including urothelial cancer. Also enquire about risk factors for HIV and hepatitis B and C. Drug use, including ketamine, cocaine and cannabis, is important. Ketamine can cause 'ketamine bladder', a syndrome characterized by pain, microscopic haematuria and reduced functional bladder

Table 17.5 Common medications that can cause nephrotoxicity	
Medication	**Effect**
Diuretics	Polyuria, nocturia Pre-renal acute kidney injury (AKI)
Lithium	Polyuria, polydipsia, nocturia, chronic kidney disease (CKD)
Nonsteroidal anti-inflammatory drugs (NSAIDs)	Renal papillary necrosis Tubulo-interstitial nephritis Haemodynamically mediated injury
PPIs (chronic use)	Tubulo-interstitial nephritis
Angiotensin converting enzyme (ACE) inhibitors/ARB	Can exacerbate pre-renal AKI Hyperkalaemia
Metformin	Lactic acidosis at low glomerular filtration rate (GFR)
Spironolactone	Risk of hyperkalaemia in advanced CKD
Antibiotics (vancomycin, gentamicin, penicillins)	Acute tubular necrosis Tubulointerstitial nephritis
Chemotherapeutic agents	Thrombotic microangiopathy
Immunosuppressive agents (ciclosporin, tacrolimus)	Thrombotic microangiopathy Haemodynamically mediated injury
Antivirals	Crystal formation Acute tubular necrosis

capacity, whilst cocaine is associated with several patterns of renal injury. Occupation has been implicated in urothelial cancer (painters, dry cleaners, diesel fumes, metal-workers).

Family history

A family history of diabetes, hypertension, cardiovascular disease and CKD, including dialysis and transplantation, is important for assessing the risk of advanced kidney disease and identifying potential causes of CKD. Inherited kidney disease is relatively rare, the most common being autosomal-dominant polycystic kidney disease (ADPKD). Certain other rare genetic disorders may also have renal involvement, for example cysts and tumours in the kidney in von Hippel-Lindau syndrome.

Systems enquiry

Systems enquiry may point to a cause of kidney disease, or the consequences of CKD. Table 17.6 summarizes systemic conditions associated with CKD and associated signs on clinical examination.

Renal and urological syndromes

Renal and urological syndromes are listed in Table 17.7. Some are exclusively renal, others exclusively urological and some fall into both areas. Whilst there can be overlap between syndromes, they are a useful guide in delineating the level of a lesion, and a focus for further investigation.

Acute kidney injury

Acute kidney injury (AKI) is the onset of declining renal function occurring over a period of hours or days, usually but not always accompanied by oliguria.

There is a rapid decline in the GFR, leading to electrolyte dysregulation, and nitrogen retention. The outlook depends on the cause, which can be divided into pre-renal, intrinsic and post-renal (Table 17.8). The most common cause of intrinsic AKI is acute tubular necrosis (ATN)—loss of renal tubular epithelial cells, usually as a result of pre-renal ischaemia or nephrotoxins. A variety of classification systems for AKI use measurement of serum creatinine and urine output to stratify it into mild, moderate or severe. These are used as a guide to predict risk of mortality and outcome in hospitalized patients. It may reverse spontaneously (repair of ischaemic injury in tubular necrosis) or as a result of therapy (removal of stone or other cause of obstruction). Severe AKI can manifest with uraemic symptoms (see below). These are pre-terminal, but reversible with dialysis to remove the excess uraemic toxins. Failure to recover GFR partially or fully can result in progression to CKD.

Chronic kidney disease

Chronic kidney disease is defined by a persistent (>3 months) disorder of kidney function or structure. It can be caused by chronic renal ischaemia from renal parenchymal disease, failure of acute kidney injury to recover or unrelieved urinary obstruction. The most widely used classification for CKD divides it into stages based on GFR measurement and the presence or absence of albuminuria (Fig. 17.1), which, whilst imperfect, enables stratification of risk of progression to end stage kidney disease (ESKD).

If renal impairment is severe, there may be clinical manifestations of uraemia. These are usually evident when the GFR has fallen to <20 ml/min (CKD 4 or 5), and are most severe once GFR is <10 ml/min. Lethargy, poor concentration, irritability and failure of higher mental functions and ability to handle tasks are all commonly reported, as are nausea, anorexia and vomiting. In advanced renal insufficiency, there

Table 17.6 Systemic conditions associated with kidney disease		
System	**Association**	**Clinical signs**
Liver disease	Hepatorenal syndrome with cirrhosis Glomerulonephritis with hepatitis B or C	Jaundice, abdominal swelling (ascites), gastrointestinal (GI) bleeding (portal hypertension)
Auto-immune/inflammatory	Systemic lupus erythematosus (SLE) and other connective tissue disorders can cause glomerulonephritis or vasculitis Sarcoidosis causes an interstitial nephritis	Rash, joint pain or swelling, myalgia, mouth ulcers, Raynaud's, eye symptoms, dry eyes or mouth
Infection	Gastroenteritis (pre-renal acute kidney injury [AKI]) TB (granulomatous interstitial nephritis) HIV (HIV-associated kidney disease) Endocarditis (vasculitis)	Fever, sweats, weight loss, GI symptoms, shortness of breath
Malignancy	Secondary membranous nephropathy with malignancy Lymphoma Myeloma (cast nephropathy)	Weight loss, localizing symptoms, back pain, fractures (lytic lesions, bone metastases)
Haematological	Sickle nephropathy in sickle cell disease	Sickle pain, polyuria

Table 17.7 Renal and urological syndromes

Renal	Renal and urological	Urological
Chronic kidney disease	Acute kidney injury	Urinary tract infection
Acute nephritic syndrome	Asymptomatic urinary abnormality	Urinary tract obstruction
Nephrotic syndrome	Recurrent visible haematuria	Renal and urinary tract stone
Renal hypertension		
Tubular syndromes		

Table 17.8 Causes of acute kidney injury (AKI)

Pre-renal	Renal	Post-renal
Reduced renal blood flow	Acute tubular necrosis from any cause of renal ischaemia or nephrotoxic injury	Obstruction (tumour, stone, retroperitoneal fibrosis)
-hypovolaemia (e.g. blood loss, inadequate intake, fluid losses from burns)	Vascular—vasculitis, thrombotic microangiopathy, hypertensive emergency	Bladder outflow obstruction
Effective decreased blood flow:	Acute glomerulonephritis	Bilateral ureteric obstruction
-cardiac failure, vasodilation in sepsis	Acute tubule-interstitial nephritis	
-intrarenal vasomotor changes (drugs, such as nonsteroidal anti-inflammatory drugs [NSAIDs])		

Prognosis of CKD by GFR and Albuminuria Categories

				Albuminuria categories Description and range		
				A1	**A2**	**A3**
				Normal to mildly increased	Moderately increased	Severely increased
				<30 mg/g <3 mg/mmol	30–299 mg/g 3–29 mg/mmol	≥300 mg/g ≥30 mg/mmol
GFR categories (ml/min/1.73 m²) Description and range	**G1**	Normal or high	≥90			
	G2	Mildly decreased	60–90			
	G3a	Mildly to moderately decreased	45–59			
	G3b	Moderately to severely decreased	30–44			
	G4	Severely decreased	15–29			
	G5	Kidney failure	<15			

Green: low risk (if no other markers of kidney disease, no CKD); Yellow: moderately increased risk; Orange: high risk; Red, very high risk.
KDIGO 2012

Figure 17.1 Classification of chronic kidney disease. (Source: Kidney disease: Improving Global Outcomes (KDIGO) working group 2012. Available at: https://kdigo.org/guidelines/)

may be confusion, fits and stupor. The presence of these symptoms indicates the need for dialysis to remove uraemic toxins, or transplantation to restore GFR. Even in the absence of uraemic symptoms, renal replacement therapy (dialysis or transplantation) may be indicated once GFR falls to <15ml/min.

The nephritic syndrome

The nephritic syndrome is historically described as the constellation of oliguria, microscopic haematuria and hypertension, and is usually accompanied by mild proteinuria and impaired renal function. It usually has a fairly brisk onset (days, weeks or months). It is caused by injury to the glomerulus, which can be insidious or acute. Many of the causes of acute nephritis are associated with functional abnormalities of the immune system that may be detected by laboratory tests and which may also manifest with disease in other organs, for example the skin, joints or eyes, as in SLE, Henoch-Schönlein purpura (Fig. 17.2) and systemic vasculitis, post-infectious glomerulonephritis (GN), anti-GBM disease and membranoproliferative glomerulonephritis (MPGN).

The nephrotic syndrome

Nephrotic syndrome is defined as the presence of heavy proteinuria (usually >3 g/day, compared with normal of <150 mg/day), hypoalbuminaemia, hypercholesterolaemia and oedema. It is unusual for nephrotic syndrome to occur when the proteinuria is <2 g/day; conversely, some patients are able to maintain a normal or near-normal serum albumin concentration despite very heavy proteinuria in excess of 6 g/day.

Figure 17.2   Purpura in Henoch–Schönlein disease.

Proteinuria of this magnitude implies glomerular pathology and may coexist with a significant reduction in GFR. Thus, a number of the pathological entities capable of causing nephrotic syndrome may also present as acute nephritic syndrome, acute kidney injury or the syndrome of CKD.

Asymptomatic urinary abnormality

Asymptomatic urinary abnormality usually presents as part of a routine medical examination, often in the context of an employment or life insurance health check or at a screening visit to primary care. Urine testing leads to the finding of proteinuria, haematuria or pyuria in an otherwise healthy patient. Further assessment may reveal the coexistence of other renal syndromes. This syndrome may reflect disease of the kidneys, or be a manifestation of malignancy anywhere in the urinary tract, infection or stone.

An asymptomatic urinary abnormality can be the first sign of one of the other syndromes (nephritic, tubular, renal stones, malignancy) or can alert to renal disease in and of itself. Table 17.9 summarizes abnormalities seen. They should alert the clinician to take a more complete history, perform a clinical examination and check, as a minimum, blood pressure and renal function, with a view to further investigation.

Recurrent visible haematuria

Recurrent visible haematuria implies intermittent or in some cases continuous bleeding into the urinary tract. The source of the bleeding may be anywhere in the urinary tract, from the glomeruli to the urethra.

Urinary tract infection

Infection in the urinary tract leads to a range of symptoms and signs that reflect the location and severity of the infection. By far the most frequent site is the bladder, and local symptoms reflect bladder irritation. The presence of urinary tract infection is defined by the presence of a significant number of infecting organisms in the urine. A working definition of a proven urine infection would be the detection of more than 10^5 colony-forming units/millilitre urine in a mid-stream specimen of urine (MSU). In some infections, for example tuberculosis of the urinary tract, the number of organisms being excreted may be extremely low, and identification on the basis of urine culture is difficult. Sterile pyuria can be caused by a treated infection, parasites such as schistosomiasis, tuberculosis (TB), bladder stones, inflammation or a tumour.

Urinary tract obstruction

Urinary tract obstruction may be divided into lower and upper tract obstruction. Lower urinary tract obstruction is defined by residual urine in the bladder after micturition or an inability to empty

Table 17.9 Asymptomatic urinary abnormalities

Protein	Blood	Glucose	Leucocytes	Causes
±	+++	-	-	Nephritic syndrome, glomerulonephritis (GN), systemic lupus erythematosus (SLE), endocarditis, pulmonary renal syndromes, IgA nephropathy, renal stones
±	±	-	+++	Urinary tract infection (UTI)
+++	±	-	-	Nephrotic syndrome, DM, FSGS, amyloidosis, myeloma
±	-	+	-	Diabetes (with or without nephropathy) Rare tubular defects, pregnancy

the bladder at all. The most common causes relate to prostatic hypertrophy (benign hyperplasia or carcinoma), and signs include frequency, nocturia, poor stream, hesitancy and terminal dribbling.

The presence of an upper urinary tract obstruction is established in most cases by the demonstration of a dilated renal collecting system (renal pelvis and/or calyces), often seen to be proximal to a specific obstructing lesion. These features may be demonstrated by ultrasound and intravenous urography (IVU) as well as computerized tomography (CT) scanning. Upper and lower urinary tract obstruction may coexist, most frequently when the lower urinary tract obstruction is severe and/or long standing, and leading to progressive dilatation of the upper urinary tract with consequent renal parenchymal damage and loss of GFR. Unilateral renal obstruction should not result in a rise in the serum creatinine; if the creatinine is elevated, there is also dysfunction of the contralateral kidney.

An infected and obstructed urinary system is considered an emergency and is potentially life-threatening.

Renal and urinary tract stones

The operational definition of renal and urinary tract stones is largely observational, depending on the demonstration of stones in any part of the urinary tract. Resulting symptoms and signs depend on the location of the stone(s) and on their size. Small stones in the kidneys are frequently asymptomatic or lead to subtle urinary abnormalities, presenting initially with asymptomatic urinary abnormality. Larger stones in the kidneys can lead to renal pain; and stones in the ureter are particularly likely to cause acute obstruction and severe ureteric and renal pain. Remember that the pain of renal colic is one of the worst that a patient may experience. Bladder stones are usually associated with symptoms suggestive of cystitis, with frequency, haematuria and pain all common, and often associated with urinary tract infection.

Renal hypertension

The most common cause of sustained blood pressure elevation is essential hypertension. However, hypertension can be a cause and a consequence of renal disease. A minority of patients with raised blood pressure will have an underlying renal (or other) cause. Hypertension may be one of the presenting features of virtually any disease of the renal parenchyma, including GN, many forms of tubulo-interstitial disease, renal vascular disease, renal stone disease and obstruction. Thus, in any patient with newly identified hypertension, the possibility of underlying renal disease should be considered. Conversely, the exclusion of renal disease as a cause of hypertension is generally straightforward, composed of the absence of symptoms and signs of renal disease, the absence of urinary abnormalities on simple stick testing and the presence of a normal GFR and renal electrolytes.

Renal tubular syndromes

Most patients with parenchymal renal disease or obstructive renal damage manifest disordered tubular function. Much less common is the patient in whom the tubular defect dominates the clinical picture. These defects may be inherited or acquired. They usually require careful laboratory testing to characterize them fully. Proximal tubular abnormalities include renal phosphate wasting, aminoaciduria (of these, cystinuria with cystine stone formation is the most important) and renal tubular acidosis leading to chronic metabolic acidosis. Distal tubular defects are also associated with metabolic acidosis and with disturbances of potassium metabolism, sodium-losing nephropathy and nephrogenic diabetes insipidus, with resulting failure, respectively, of salt and water conservation.

Physical signs in renal and urological disease

These physical signs fall into four groups:
1. Local signs related to the specific pathology, such as an enlarged palpable tender kidney in renal

carcinoma or a palpably enlarged bladder in a patient with acute or chronic retention

2. Symptoms of disturbance of renal salt and water handling, with resulting clinical evidence of extracellular fluid volume expansion or contraction

3. Signs of failure of the kidney's normal excretory and metabolic functions

4. Signs caused by a systemic or underlying condition

In many renal patients, particularly those with advanced CDK and uraemia, signs from all of the above categories may be present. The effects of renal failure on other organ systems are summarized in Box 17.1.

General features

Patients with chronic renal failure (loss of the kidney's normal excretory and metabolic functions) look unwell. The skin is pallid, the complexion sallow and a slightly yellowish hue is often evident. The mucous membranes are pale, reflecting the associated normochromic, normocytic anaemia. There may be bruises, purpura and scratch marks owing to uraemic pruritus, and also an underlying disorder of platelet function and capillary fragility. The nails can appear pale and opaque (leukonychia) in the nephrotic syndrome and in chronic renal failure. Intercurrent episodes of severe illness in the past may have led to the appearance of Beau's lines, which appear as transverse ridges across the nails. Splinter haemorrhages in the nail beds point to underlying vasculitis, which may be the cause of the renal failure or be indicative of endocarditis; there may be an associated purpuric rash (see Fig. 17.2). When blood urea is very high, a uraemic frost may be seen on any part of the body and appears as a white powder; it is formed from crystalline urea deposited on the skin. It is rare and only usually seen in patients who have not been cared for and therefore not washed, as it may take days to develop. The onset of chronic renal failure in childhood is associated with impaired growth, causing short stature. Severe bony deformity (Fig. 17.3) may be evident in some cases, particularly in children, who may develop rickets. Advanced uraemia is also associated with metabolic flap, a coarse tremor which is best seen at the wrists when in the dorsiflexed position. The presence of metabolic acidosis leads to increased ventilation with an increased tidal volume, known as Kussmaul respiration.

The circulation in the renal patient

Correct assessment of the patient's fluid volume status is crucial. It is important to define whether the patient is euvolaemic, hypovolaemic or hypervolaemic. Objective assessment of volume status is made by assessing lying and standing

| Box 17.1 | Effects of renal failure on other organ systems |

Disturbances of water and electrolyte balance

- Breathlessness caused by salt and water overload
- Deep sighing breathing (Kussmaul respiration) owing to acidosis
- Weakness and postural fainting due to hypotension caused by salt and water depletion
- Lethargy and weakness from hypokalaemia

Disturbances of the haematological system

- Lethargy and breathlessness associated with anaemia owing to impaired production of erythropoietin by the kidneys
- Defective coagulation and excessive bruising (advanced renal failure)
- Haemorrhage from the gastrointestinal tract or lungs

Disturbances of the cardiovascular system

- Cardiac failure or angina associated with fluid overload, hypertension, anaemia and impaired ventricular function (uraemic cardiomyopathy)
- Precordial chest pain owing to pericarditis
- Cardiac arrhythmias associated with left ventricular hypertrophy and hyperkalaemia/hypokalaemia

Disturbances of the gastrointestinal system

- Nausea and vomiting, especially in the morning, owing to uraemia
- Anorexia

Disturbances of the respiratory system

- Breathlessness and haemoptysis from fluid overload
- Chest pain owing to pleurisy

Disturbances of the musculoskeletal system

- Muscular weakness and bone pain owing to impairment of vitamin D activation and to excessive parathyroid gland activity
- Acute pain caused by gout
- Muscle wasting

Disturbances of the nervous system

- Hypertensive stroke and encephalopathy
- Clouding of consciousness, fits and coma in advanced renal failure
- Impaired sensation or paraesthesia in the feet, caused by peripheral neuropathy in long-standing uraemia
- Impaired higher mental/intellectual function
- Entrapment neuropathies

Disturbances of the eyes

- Pain from conjunctivitis caused by local deposits of calcium
- Visual blurring from hypertensive retinal damage or retinal vascular disease

blood pressure, jugular venous pressure and pulse pressure. Subjective signs include skin turgor, mucous membranes and 'sunken eyes'. Patients who are hypervolaemic may be hypertensive, with evidence of excess extracellular fluid (oedema, ascites, basal crackles on lung auscultation). Oedema with expansion of the extracellular fluid is often accompanied by hypertension and, particularly if the cardiac reserve is poor, may progress to pulmonary oedema and other manifestations of heart failure. In patients with nephrotic syndrome (see below), oedema and salt and water retention are caused by reduced plasma oncotic pressure. The presence of oedema can coexist with intravascular volume depletion, especially in patients with nephrotic syndrome.

Abdominal palpation

The detection of the kidneys in the abdominal examination is described in Chapter 14. In slim people with relaxed abdominal muscles, it is sometimes possible to feel a normal right kidney (the right kidney is situated slightly lower than the left at the level of T12-L3). More often a palpable kidney can only be felt because it is enlarged, as in hydronephrosis, multiple cysts (polycystic kidney disease) or tumour (generally unilateral). A distended bladder is identified in the lower abdomen by a combination of palpation and percussion. Bimanual palpation of the bladder with rectal examination is a more reliable way of assessing bladder enlargement than is simple per abdominal examination. In men, rectal examination also allows evaluation of the prostate gland, both for benign enlargement and for the detection of malignant change suggested by hard irregularity of the gland and an absence of the central groove.

Auscultation

Uraemic pericarditis and pleurisy may be suggested by pericardial and pleural friction rubs, respectively. Their presence points to either advanced uraemia or a multisystem inflammatory disorder, such as systemic lupus erythematosus (SLE), which may have both renal and extra-renal manifestations. Added heart sounds (S3 and S4) suggest, respectively, volume expansion and incipient heart failure, and ventricular hypertrophy, often as a consequence of hypertension. The presence of vascular bruits and/or impairment of the major arterial pulses is an important finding, raising the possibility of renal vascular disease, which may underlie hypertension and/or renal failure if bilateral.

The eye in uraemia

Corneal calcification (limbic calcification) occurs in patients with long-standing hyperparathyroidism with elevation of blood calcium and phosphorus concentrations (see Chapter 19), seen medially and laterally or circumferentially. The presence of limbic calcification should not be confused with a corneal arcus (arcus senilis), which is a broader band at the edge of the superior and inferior cornea and

merges with the sclera. Retinal changes can be seen in patients with diabetes or hypertension. Diabetic nephropathy in type 1 diabetes is extremely rare in the absence of diabetic retinopathy. In type 2 diabetes, however, diabetic nephropathy is present in many patients without any diabetic eye changes. Patients with renal disease as part of systemic vasculitis may have manifestations of the latter in the retinae, with haemorrhages and exudates. Patients with CKD are at greatly increased risk of a range of vascular complications affecting both the macrovasculature and the microvasculature. In the retinae, thrombosis of the central retinal artery or its branches, or of the central retinal vein and its branches, is an important manifestation of this.

Laboratory assessment and imaging of the kidneys and urinary tract

The most important laboratory assessment in renal and urological disease is analysis of the urine, and measurement of renal GFR and electrolytes. Because of the kidneys' importance in other systems, including production of erythropoietin and regulation of bone metabolism, additional tests are frequently necessary if there is evidence of renal insufficiency.

The urine

Urine should be tested as part of every general medical examination and not just in patients with

Figure 17.3 X-ray of the hands of a patient with chronic renal failure and secondary hyperparathyroidism, showing renal osteodystrophy. There is a loss of density of the tips of the digits (acro-osteolysis) with loss of density on either side of the interphalangeal joints and subperiosteal bone resorption. The latter is best seen in the middle phalanges of the index and middle fingers.

known renal or urinary tract disease. The urine specimen should be passed into a clean container without additives, by placing a sterile container in the path of the urine stream once voiding has commenced (i.e. a mid-stream specimen). Normally, sample should be tested as soon as possible, or refrigerated (not frozen) and returned to room temperature before testing.

Quantity

Normal adults in temperate climates usually pass between 750 and 2500 ml of urine every 24 hours. The minimum daily urine output compatible with normal renal excretory function varies from person to person and also with other factors, such as diet.

Colour

The colour of urine is heavily influenced by the urinary flow rate, with high flow leading to dilute urine and hence a pale colour. Darkening occurs on standing as a result of oxidation of urobilinogen to coloured urobilin. Table 17.10 describes some common causes of discoloured urine.

Specific gravity and osmolality

Specific gravity and osmolality measurements are functions of the urinary concentrations of sodium, chloride and urea in the absence of significant glycosuria. The range of specific gravity is 1.001 to 1.035, which is equivalent to 50–1350 mOsmol/kg water (Fig. 17.4). In advanced renal disease, the osmolality becomes relatively fixed at about 300 mOsmol/kg water, close to that of the glomerular filtrate (Fig. 17.5). This is termed isosthenuria, and because the urine concentration cannot be varied, causes increased sensitivity to changes in sodium and water balance.

pH

The pH varies from 4 to 8 and can be measured using paper strips impregnated with an indicator.

If more accurate measurements are needed, as in suspected renal tubular acidosis, a pH electrode is used. Most people pass acid urine most of the time, exceptions being in some vegetarians, certain types of renal tubular acidosis, rapid water diuresis, metabolic alkalosis and urine infection with urea-splitting organisms.

Figure 17.4   Relationship between specific gravity and osmolality.

Figure 17.5   Relationship between renal concentration and diluting capacity, and serum creatinine concentration. The serum creatinine is plotted on a logarithmic scale. This therefore represents linear changes in glomerular filtration rate (GFR), such as might occur in progressive renal failure. End-stage renal failure is shown on the left, and normal renal function on the right. Curve (a) represents maximum concentrating capacity (e.g. in water deprivation, when the normal kidney can maintain the serum creatinine in the normal range by increasing urine osmolality). In renal failure, the urine cannot be concentrated and the serum creatinine rises. Curve (b) represents the maximum diluting capacity (e.g. after the ingestion of large volumes of water). The normal kidney excretes urine of low osmolality. In end-stage renal failure, urine osmolality cannot be reduced and the water load is not adequately handled. There is also isosthenuria (i.e. the urine tends towards an iso-osmolar state (specific gravity 1.010)).

Table 17.10	Causes of discoloured urine
Colour	**Cause**
Brown	Bile pigments
	Blood
	Myoglobin (brown/red)
	Nitrofurantoin
Red	Large volume of blood
	Intravascular haemolysis (free haemoglobin)
Cloudy	Leucocytes (infection)
	Large volume of red blood cells
	Phosphates
Orange	Rifampicin
	Senna
Grey	Methyldopa
Pale yellow	Dilution: polyuria/excess water intake

Glucose

Glucose oxidase-impregnated dipsticks provide a quick and semi-quantitative test for glucose in urine. By far the most common causes of glycosuria are diabetes and during pregnancy, in which glycosuria occurs with normal plasma glucose concentrations. Very rarely, tubular transport defects may be associated with glycosuria at normal plasma glucose concentrations, and more frequently, patients with CKD may exhibit glycosuria at normal plasma glucose concentrations.

Protein

The normal daily urine protein output is <150 mg and albumin <30 mg/day. Dipsticks reactive to urine albumin provide a simple semi-quantitative test and are sensitive to 200–300 mg protein/l. Albumin excretion in the range of 30 to 200 mg/day is termed microalbuminuria. Although this range is frequently too low to be detectable by stick testing, it is an important finding, particularly in people with diabetes in whom it predicts the later onset of overt diabetic nephropathy. The urinary protein excretion rate generally rises in the upright posture; with activity and, in some normal individuals, this may lead to apparently abnormal proteinuria (orthostatic proteinuria). Measurement of protein in an early-morning urine specimen, however, reveals no protein.

The albumin-to-creatinine (ACR) and protein-to-creatinine (PCR) ratios are useful surrogate markers for proteinuria. They are increasingly used instead of the 24-hour urine collection for quantification of protein excretion (Table 17.11). The diagnostic implications of proteinuria depend on its magnitude (Table 17.12). Heavy proteinuria (>1.5 g/day) is nearly always glomerular in origin, and albumin predominates over larger proteins, such as globulins. Other proteins, rarely measured, arise from the renal tubules; they include Tamm-Horsfall protein, retinol-binding protein and nephrocalcin, the latter helping to prevent the formation of urinary stones. It is worth noting that urine light chains (found in plasma cell dyscrasias, such as myeloma) may not be detected by some routine laboratory urine protein assays and have to be sought separately.

Microscopy

Microscopy (Figs 17.6–17.9) is performed after slow spinning of a fresh urine specimen for approximately 2 minutes. The pellet is resuspended in 0.5 ml of urine and examined unstained on a microscope slide under a coverslip. Important findings include leucocytes (suggestive of infection), red blood cells and tubular casts. The presence of tubular casts is indicative of parenchymal renal disease. They may be red cell casts or white cell casts in which Tamm-Horsfall protein matrix has solidified and is studded with red or white blood cells. Granular casts probably represent degenerate cellular casts and have a grainy appearance. Hyaline casts contain no elements or debris and may be seen in small numbers in normal urine. The presence of red cell casts should alert one to the possibility of an aggressive GN. Red cell morphology may be a useful indicator of the source of bleeding. Red cells with a normal outline usually, but not always, arise from the renal collecting system or from a point downstream of that, whereas red cells arising from the glomeruli are often distorted.

Table 17.11 Relationship between ACR, PCR and 24-hour urine protein excretion

	ACR (mg/mmol)	PCR (mg/mmol)	24-hour urine protein (g/day)
Microalbuminuria	3–30		
Proteinuria	>30	>50	>0.5

ACR, albumin-to-creatinine; PCR, protein-to-creatinine.

Table 17.12 Proteinuria

Mild (<500 mg/day)	Moderate (up to 3 g/day)	Heavy (>3 g/day)
Benign hypertensive nephrosclerosis	Chronic pyelonephritis	Acute glomerulonephritis
Obstructive nephropathy	Acute tubular necrosis	Chronic glomerulonephritis
Prerenal uraemia	Acute glomerulonephritis	Diabetic nephropathy
Renal tumour	Chronic glomerulonephritis	Pre-eclampsia
Fever	Obstructive nephropathy	Myeloma
Tubulointerstitial nephropathy	Accelerated phase hypertension	All causes of nephrotic syndrome
Chronic pyelonephritis	Orthostatic proteinuria	
Early diabetic nephropathy	Urinary tract infection	
Orthostatic proteinuria		
Urinary tract infection		

Figure 17.6 Erythrocytes in urinary sediment.

Figure 17.7 Leukocytes in urinary sediment.

Figure 17.8 Hyaline casts, leukocytes and bacteria in urinary sediment. (Reproduced with permission from Spencer ES, Petersen I 1971 Hand Atlas of Urinary Sediment. Munksgaard, Copenhagen.)

Microbiological examination of the urine

Mid-stream urine specimens are normally satisfactory, but they are always contaminated to a certain extent

Figure 17.9 Granular casts in urinary sediment.

during passage to the exterior. Extensive studies have shown that the finding of more than 10^5 bacteria per millilitre in a mid-stream specimen is usually associated with active urinary infection, especially when accompanied by leucocytes.

Measurement of the glomerular filtration rate

Accurate assessment of the GFR requires measurement in blood alone or blood and urine of a compound that is filtered freely at the glomerulus and neither reabsorbed nor secreted by the tubules. Inulin is the best agent but it is a laborious investigation that is generally confined to research and is not routinely available. A number of surrogates for the inulin clearance method exist and details of these are given in Table 17.13. The most frequently used surrogates, and also the crudest ones, are the plasma urea and plasma creatinine concentrations. Both compounds are produced endogenously (at an inconstant rate in the case of urea) and excreted by glomerular filtration. Neither is particularly accurate when used to establish the absolute level of glomerular filtration, although the plasma creatinine concentration is very useful when used to follow changes in an individual patient's renal function (Fig. 17.10). Creatinine clearance is more precise but it requires a 24-hour urine collection with measurements of plasma creatinine concentration and urine creatinine excretion. Only those compounds that are freely filtered at the glomerulus and neither secreted nor reabsorbed by the renal tubules are suitable for GFR measurement.

Several mathematical formulae are used to estimate GFR (Table 17.14), validated internationally and used by most laboratories. GFR estimation using some of these formulae has traditionally included a correction factor to account for differences in muscle mass in black patients; this is increasingly being phased out in recognition of the genetic diversity within black patients and lack of a scientific evidence to underpin clinical decision making based on race.

Table 17.13 Measurement of the glomerular filtration rate

Method	Comments
Plasma urea	Poor surrogate: – variable production rate – variable excretion rate – dependant on uptake
Plasma creatinine	Better than urea Poor discrimination at near-normal glomerular filtration rate (GFR)
Calculated GFR	Useful surrogate of creatinine clearance (MDRD or CKD-EPI formulae)
Creatinine clearance	Reasonable surrogate but depends on accurate timed urine collection (usually 24 hours) *UV/P* where *U* equals the urinary concentration of creatinine, *V* the urinary flow rate (usually expressed in ml/min) and *P* equals the plasma creatinine concentration.
^{51}Cr-EDTA	The best surrogate in clinical practice Expensive
Inulin clearance	Near-perfect measurement of GFR but: – needs continuous infusion – difficult urine and plasma assays – research studies only: not suited to clinical practice

Table 17.14 Estimation of GFR formulae

Cockcroft and Gault	Male GFR = [1.23 × weight (kg) × (140 − age)]/creatinine
	Female GFR = [1.03 × weight (kg) × (140 − age)]/creatinine
Modification of diet in renal disease	GFR = 186 × PCR − 1.154 × age − 0.203 × 1.212 (if black) × 0.742 (if female) PCR = plasma creatinine in mg/dl
CKD-EPI	CKD-EPI equation expressed as a single equation: **GFR = 141 × min (S_{cr} /κ, 1)$^\alpha$ × max(S_{cr} /κ, 1)$^{-1.209}$ × 0.993^{Age} × 1.018 [if female] × 1.159 [if black]** where: S_{cr} is serum creatinine in mg/dl, κ is 0.7 for females and 0.9 for males, α is −0.329 for females and −0.411 for males, min indicates the minimum of S_{cr} /κ or 1, and max indicates the maximum of S_{cr} /κ or 1

Figure 17.10 Relationship between creatinine clearance and plasma creatinine concentrations. The normal range of serum creatinine concentration can be maintained only when the renal creatinine clearance is greater than about 60 ml/min. The red area represents the normal range of creatinine concentration.

GFR peaks at 20 to 25 years of age and declines steadily thereafter at a rate of approximately 1 ml/min/year.

Other biochemical tests important in renal disease

The GFR is usually measured along with urea and electrolytes (sodium, potassium, chloride), expressed in mmol/l. Sodium balance can be an indicator of volume status, or may reflect an underlying tubular or endocrine disorder. An elevated potassium, owing to the failure of the K/H co-transporter in the distal tubule, is a common finding in renal insufficiency; high levels (>6 mmol/l) can result in arrhythmia and even sudden cardiac death, and require urgent assessment and treatment. A low potassium level can be an indicator of an underlying tubular disorder. Urea frequently rises in parallel with creatinine and is responsible for many of the symptoms associated with chronic kidney disease. Exceptions are in upper GI bleeding, when the passage of blood through the bowel results in reabsorption of urea into the circulation, and dehydration. In both these situations the urea can be elevated disproportionately to the rise in creatinine level.

In CKD 3 and above, measurement of bone parameters (calcium, phosphate, vitamin D, parathyroid hormone) should be undertaken to monitor the effects of CKD in bone mineralization. These tests are also useful when evaluating the patient with renal stones for underlying causes.

Anaemia is frequently seen in the patient with CKD, and in those with bleeding in the urinary tract from any cause. An elevated white cell count with associated neutrophilia may be seen in infection.

Immunological and serological tests for infection, viruses and auto-immune disease may be indicated in the investigation of renal syndromes, including nephrotic syndrome, nephritic syndrome, acute kidney injury and CKD.

Measurement of renal tubular function

The two tests most frequently utilized to measure renal tubular function are:

1. Tests of renal concentrating ability when investigating possible causes of polyuria
2. Tests of renal acidification in patients with metabolic acidosis and possible underlying renal tubular acidosis

Renal concentrating ability involves treating the patient in a way that should lead to the production of a concentrated urine. Water deprivation is the most common provocation: after 12 hours, the urine osmolality should be at least 750 mmol/kg (specific gravity 1.020). Failure to concentrate the urine indicates either impairment of vasopressin output (pituitary diabetes insipidus) or resistance of the renal tubules to the action of vasopressin (nephrogenic diabetes insipidus). These two possibilities may be distinguished by measuring the urine osmolality after an injection of vasopressin (or an analogue) when the urine osmolality should increase to at least 750 mmol/kg.

Renal tubular acidification can be assumed to be adequate if the pH of a random specimen of urine is below 5.5. Urine pH > 5.5 in the presence of metabolic acidosis usually indicates renal tubular acidosis. If the patient is only minimally acidotic and the urine pH is >5.5, a provocative test, in which ammonium chloride is given at a dose of 0.1 g/kg body weight to provide an acid load and an acute mild metabolic acidosis, can be performed. The pH should fall to <5.4 if acidification is normal.

Assessment of the urine in the stone-forming patient

Assessment of urine in a stone-forming patient involves measurement of the important constituents of stone whose outputs may be abnormally increased and also measurement of at least one of the natural inhibitors of stone formation, combined with analysis of the stone itself.

The identification of increased excretion rates of calcium, uric acid, oxalate or cystine indicates a strong predisposition to recurrent stone formation. Conversely, citrate is a natural inhibitor of stone formation, and a low urine citrate is associated with increased stone risk. All patients who make radiopaque stones should be screened for cystinuria using the nitroprusside test. If hypercalciuria or hypercalcaemia are noted, then the parathyroid and serum angiotensin-converting enzyme should also be measured.

Kidney biopsy

Kidney biopsy, in which one or two small cores of renal cortex are removed using a needle-biopsy, is performed in patients in whom renal parenchymal disease is suspected. However, not everyone with renal parenchymal disease requires a biopsy. The procedure is invasive and carries a small but definite risk of serious complications. It is therefore important to define the indications and contraindications carefully.

Kidney biopsy is often the only way to distinguish the various forms of GN, both from one another and from tubulo-interstitial diseases of the kidney.

Imaging of the urinary tract

Plain radiographs

In many people, one or both of the kidneys can be seen outlined by perirenal fat on plain abdominal films. The information gleaned is limited, although certain types of renal stone and renal calcification may be identified.

Ultrasound

Ultrasound provides good images of the renal parenchyma and collecting system, and gives a reliable estimate of renal size as well as identifying discrete lesions within the parenchyma, hydronephrosis and stones. Doppler studies often permit assessment of blood flow in the main renal arteries. The resistive index, measured by Doppler ultrasound, indicates the degree of chronic intrarenal ischaemic injury, but is very operator dependent. Although the upper ureter can be seen quite well in most patients, the lower ureter is not visualized adequately. Ultrasound allows calculation of the bladder capacity when full and after micturition (emptying should be virtually complete), as well as visualization of the bladder wall and lesions projecting into the bladder itself (e.g. tumours). It can be combined with a measurement of urinary flow rate along with post-micturition residual to assess the efficiency of micturition and bladder emptying in patients with lower urinary tract symptoms (LUTS) or incontinence. The volume of the prostate gland can be derived at an ultrasound examination, and can be compared with normal values.

Intravenous urography

Intravenous urography involves the intravenous injection of organic iodine compounds that are excreted and concentrated radiographically. It is an extremely good technique for examining the renal collecting system, the ureters and the bladder (Fig. 17.11). Imaging by IVU depends on renal function. This is useful in that it gives a crude measure of the symmetry, or otherwise, of excretory capacity, but it also means that the image quality is poor in patients with renal insufficiency in whom the GFR is low (Fig. 17.12).

Antegrade and retrograde urography

In antegrade and retrograde urography X-ray contrast material is instilled directly into the urinary tract

Figure 17.11 Normal excretion urogram. In this film, taken 15 minutes after intravenous injection of the iodine-based contrast medium, the calyces of both kidneys, the ureters and the bladder can be seen.

Figure 17.12 Excretion urogram. In this film, made 30 minutes after injection of contrast, the left kidney fails to excrete a detectable concentration of contrast (non-functioning left kidney) and the right kidney shows dilated, hydronephrotic calyces. The right ureter is partially obstructed at the level of the body of the fifth lumbar vertebra. The circular lucency in the bladder is the dilated balloon of a Foley catheter.

via a percutaneous needle (antegrade) or a ureteric catheter inserted via a cystoscope (retrograde). These tests are invasive and are most often used in the evaluation of patients with clear obstruction of the urinary tract.

Cystography

In cystography, the bladder is filled with contrast medium via a urethral catheter and X-rays are taken before, during and after micturition. The test assesses reflux and the completeness of bladder emptying. This also is an invasive test, the principal risk being the introduction of infection. Urodynamics (the measurement of pressure and urine flow) may be included in more detailed studies of bladder function.

Radionuclide studies

Diethylenetriamine penta-acetic acid (^{99}Tc-DTPA) is used to investigate the excretory function of each kidney selectively (Fig. 17.13). The test is very useful for the assessment of symmetry of function, delayed onset of excretion (as may happen in renal artery stenosis) and retention of excreted isotope (as seen in the presence of obstruction).^{99}Tc-DMSA (dimercaptosuccinic acid) is a similar technique used to show the gross renal morphology. An

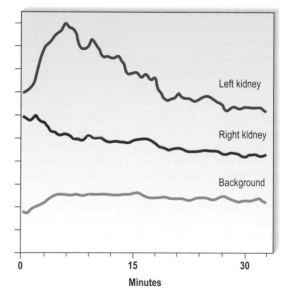

Figure 17.13 Radioisotope excretion (ordinate) during the 30 minutes after intravenous injection in a patient with right renal artery stenosis and hypertension. The left kidney achieves more rapid excretion of isotope. The malfunctioning right kidney caused the patient's hypertension.

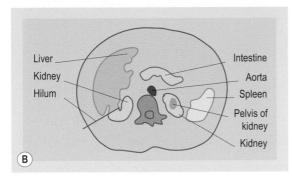

Figure 17.14 **(A)** CT scan with **(B)** drawing showing normal kidneys.

MAG3 (mercaptoacetyltriglycine) renogram can assess comparative function and demonstrate upper urinary tract obstruction.

Computed tomography and magnetic resonance imaging

Computed tomography scanning of the kidneys yields important information about the kidneys and surrounding structures in the retroperitoneum (Fig. 17.14). It is useful in patients with ureteric obstruction from, for example, retroperitoneal malignancy or retroperitoneal fibrosis. Triple-phase CT is used to discriminate malignant renal tumours from benign ones. Standard intravenous contrast used for CT scanning can result in an AKI if the baseline GFR is reduced. In some cases, more information is obtained using magnetic resonance imaging (MRI). Caution has to be exercised, however, if gadolinium is required, because its use has been associated with nephrogenic systemic fibrosis in patients with advanced renal disease. Current data suggest an increased risk of this condition in patients with a GFR below 30 ml/min.

Arteriography and venography

Arteriography and venography, which are both invasive, are used rarely in selected patients. The most common indication is the patient with hypertension and/or renal insufficiency in whom renal artery stenosis is suspected. In the context of renal insufficiency, contrast-induced deterioration of function can occasionally occur, mitigated by ensuring the patient is well hydrated. MRI can be used to generate images of the major renal vasculature and has the advantage of avoiding contrast nephropathy and of being non-invasive.

Sexually transmitted infections | 18

Laurence Dufaur and Liat Sarner

Introduction

The following chapter covers the history, examination and investigation of the patient who presents with genital symptoms and outlines the common sexually transmitted infections (STI) and non-infective conditions encountered in the sexual health clinic.

A fundamental principle in the treatment of the patient with genital symptoms is recognition of the stigma associated with the condition and the shame he may feel in presenting himself to you. To overcome these barriers and to facilitate an accurate assessment, carry out the consultation in total privacy with assurances of confidentially re-enforced. It is the responsibility of health services to ensure that protected characteristic groups (as defined by the Equality Act 2010) are free from discrimination. You should demonstrate a non-judgmental and relaxed approach by using both verbal and non-verbal cues and in doing so create a space where people feel able to discuss their sexual health issues without prejudice of their age, sexual orientation, gender/gender identity, race, disability, marital status or beliefs. Gay, bisexual and other men who have sex with men (MSM), trans people[a] and those from Black and Asian minority ethnic (BAME) groups are particularly vulnerable to systemic discrimination and are at higher risk of sexual ill health.

STI are frequently asymptomatic yet have significant long-term complications for patients and their sexual contacts. Routine sexual health screening and partner notification are therefore required to break the chain of infection, but also to provide an excellent opportunity to educate service users around 'safe-sex', STI prevention (including prophylaxis and vaccination) and effective contraception to prevent unplanned pregnancies.

Finally, many patients who present with genital symptoms will have no disease at all. It is your duty to reassure them and to explore the factors that have led them to question their sexual health, which may involve discussions around health anxiety.

Preparation

Following your own introduction, ask the patient how he would like to be addressed and what pronoun to use. Avoid making assumptions about any sexual orientation or level of understanding about sexual health. It is accepted practice to see all patients alone even if they request a friend or partner to be present in the consulting room. A partner who insists on being present can be a warning sign for intimate partner violence (IPV). IPV can be screened for in private by asking simple questions about fear and threats to the patient's safety and wellbeing. If a language barrier exists, always use a dedicated telephone translation service.

History

Begin with an open question that enables the patient ample time and space to state and describe in his own words the issue that has brought him into the clinic. Prompt the patient to expand but do not interrupt at this stage or you may inadvertently miss the most important features. This introductory phase allows the clinician to demonstrate interest and empathy and provides an opportunity to develop rapport before embarking on the more sensitive subject of the sexual history.

Presenting complaint

Urethral discharge

Urethral discharge is usually observed by the patient as an abnormal liquid draining from the penile urethra or as a stain on underwear. Clarify the colour and duration. Discharge may be associated with urethral irritation or itch, dysuria and, occasionally,

---

[a]Trans is an umbrella term used to describe people whose gender identity differs from the sex they were assigned at birth in contrast to cisgender whose gender identity is congruent with the sex they were assigned at birth.

urinary frequency (if the trigone of the bladder is involved).

A clear stringy secretion noticed following sexual arousal or on waking is likely to be physiological prostatic secretions and would not be associated with inflammatory symptoms. Men who have had little if any prior sexual education may not be aware that this is normal.

Vaginal discharge

Vaginal discharge is usually observed by the patient as a change in the appearance, smell or quantity of fluid that is normally produced by the vagina and cervix.

Clarify the duration, relationship to the menstrual cycle, colour, consistency, odour as well as associated soreness, itching and pain. A history of vaginal douching, pregnancy, diabetes mellitus as well as oral contraceptive, antibiotic and immunosuppressive drug use are important considerations.

Dysuria

The patient may present with dysuria in isolation, in association with a vaginal or urethral discharge, ulcers or with symptoms of a urinary tract infection.

Scrotal pain and swelling

Often a unilateral aching of the scrotal contents with or without enlargement may be a symptom of epididymo-orchitis.

Clarify the onset, duration and severity and make note of associated urethritis, lower urinary tract symptoms, lower abdominal and flank pain, fever and any history of trauma or surgery.

Abnormal vaginal bleeding

A change in the character of the menstrual period as being heavier (menorrhagia) or more painful (dysmenorrhea) is abnormal. Inter-menstrual bleeding (IMB) and post-coital bleeding (PCB) is typically spotting of blood between periods or in the hours or days following sexual intercourse. It may be a symptom of mucopurulent cervicitis and pelvic inflammatory disease (PID).

Clarify the relationship of the bleeding to the normal and last menstrual cycle (note the usual length and regularity), current and previous contraceptive use, obstetric and gynecological history, cervical smear tests history (including previous diagnoses, treatment and follow up) as well as human papilloma virus (HPV) vaccination history.

Abnormal vaginal bleeding requires exclusion of endometrial and cervical pathology and STI. In post-menopausal women, new onset vaginal bleeding requires urgent referral to exclude an endometrial malignancy.

Dyspareunia

Dyspareunia is pain experienced during sexual intercourse. Clarify first if it is superficial (felt in the vulvo-vagina on penetration) or deep (felt in the lower abdomen and pelvis).

If superficial dyspareunia is caused by vulvitis (e.g. owing to candida, herpes simplex or dermatitis), then it may be associated with an abnormal vaginal discharge or vulval skin changes.

Deep dyspareunia is often associated with lower abdominal pain (LAP) and is a symptom of PID. Clarify the site, onset, character, radiation, timing (including positional pain) severity and any associated abnormal vaginal discharge and bleeding, urinary symptoms, change in bowel habit and fever. Because deep dyspareunia and LAP can be caused by any abdominal or pelvic pathology (e.g. endometritis, ovarian cysts and adhesions), a detailed menstrual, obstetric, gynaecological and surgical history, including previous instrumentation, is relevant. Pregnancy risk should be assessed and an ectopic pregnancy must be excluded.

Anorectal symptoms

The patient may describe pain, soreness, itching, rectal discharge or bleeding or tenesmus, all of which are symptoms of proctitis.

Clarify the onset and duration and note a change in bowel habit. Non-infective proctitis may be an early presentation of Crohn's disease or ulcerative colitis so enquire about weight loss, fever and systemic complications.

Skin complaints

The patient may describe lumps or growths, a spot, a cut, a sore or a rash in the ano-genital area which can be painful, itchy or uncomfortable but otherwise may be symptom free. Generalized rashes are also seen and may be associated with ano-genital symptoms, fever and systemic illness.

Clarify the location, onset and duration, paying particular attention to the relationship with recent sexual intercourse, washing, the use of perfumed products and practices such as waxing and shaving pubic hair. The evolution of the symptoms over time is also important, including any previous similar episodes. Urethral and vaginal discharge, dysuria and anorectal symptoms may co-exist with skin complaints. Make note of a past history of genital herpes, syphilis and genital warts as well as dermatological conditions and atopy. A travel, medication and smoking history may be relevant. Document the HPV vaccination history (bivalent versus quadrivalent).

Sexual wellbeing

A difficulty in achieving or maintaining an erect penis may be associated with arteriopathy, polypharmacy or prostate surgery in older men. In younger men, along with premature and delayed ejaculation, it is mostly likely learned and psychogenic in nature. Vaginismus is the unconscious tightening of the vaginal walls following penetration. Vulvodynia is localized vulval tenderness or pain (not always associated with sexual intercourse) and is multifactorial in origin. Management of these conditions often involves input from the multidisciplinary team, including specialist psychology and physiotherapy.

The sexual history

It is important to sign-post this part of the history. 'I'm now going to ask you some important questions about your sexual relationships and the type of sex you have'. Enquire as to the most recent sexual encounter, when it occurred and the type of partner (e.g. steady established, new relationship, occasional, one-off or commercial sex). Ask 'what gender are they?' then clarify the type of sex (e.g. oral, vaginal or anal), whether they were insertive (active/top/giving) or receptive (passive/bottom/receiving) and if barrier protection was used. Work backwards sequentially, detailing previous sexual encounters and finally clarify the total number of different sexual partners in the preceding 3 months. If an index case is diagnosed with an STI, then it may be necessary to gather information on his sexual contacts to provide those at risk of infection with screening and epidemiological treatment. This process is known as partner notification (PN).

The sexual health screen (SHS) and STI history

Establish if the patient has ever had an SHS, when this occurred and the results. The last negative result for bacterial STI and blood borne viruses (BBV) will act as a baseline from which to assess sexual risk and provide PN. A past history of STI is a good predictor of risk. Include the date of diagnosis, treatment given and response (if applicable). This is also useful information when considering a presenting issue that is recurrent (e.g. in genital herpes) or when ordering serological tests (e.g. in syphilis and hepatitis).

Risk assessment for BBV

Human immunodeficiency virus (HIV), hepatitis B virus (HBV) and hepatitis C virus (HCV) are typically spread sexually or through intravenous drug use (IVDU), but may be passed from mother to child to varying degrees. Historically, infection through contaminated blood products, tattoos and piercings was an identifiable risk, but this has been ameliorated through widespread screening, single-use instruments and disinfection practices. The patient and their partner's country of birth is useful in assessing endemic risk (sub-Saharan African, South-East Asia and South America carrying the greatest risk for BBV acquisition). MSM, sex workers, intravenous drug users and prisoners are also all at increased risk.

Special groups

MSM

Men having sex with men are at increased risk of STI exposure owing to a high frequency of sexual partners built around dense geosocial sexual networking apps (e.g. Grindr, Scruff). Specific drugs, such as gamma hydroxybutyrate (GHB, G), crystal methamphetamine (tina) and mephedrone (meph), are taken to enhance the sexual experience (chem-sex) by increasing sexual appetite and reducing inhibitions. As the rectal mucosa is more fragile and susceptible to infection, condomless receptive anal intercourse, fisting and the use and sharing of sex toys significantly increase the risk of STI acquisition. A surge in IVDU amongst MSM has driven a rise in cases of HCV infection.

Sensitively enquire about group sex, toys and chem-sex, including the route of administration of any drugs taken.

Hepatitis A virus (HAV) is spread via the faeco-oral route and usually causes a self-limiting gastrointestinal illness but may, rarely, lead to fulminant hepatic failure. Sexually transmitted outbreaks in MSM occur periodically with oro-anal sex (rimming) being an important risk factor. Giardiasis, amoebiasis and bacterial dysentery (e.g. shigella and salmonella) are additional causes of diarrhoea in MSM, so examine stools for the presence of such organisms in addition to serological testing for acute HAV (IgM).

You should note previous infection and/or vaccination for HAV and HBV as all unexposed MSM should be vaccinated against these viruses. In addition, all MSM under the age of 45 should be offered vaccination with the quadrivalent HPV vaccine.

Trans people

There is a spectrum of trans identities, including but not limited to trans woman, trans man, transgender, genderqueer, non-binary and agender. Sensitivity and special care must be employed when assessing sexual health and wellbeing. If you inadvertently misgender someone, acknowledge and apologize for your error and move on. Clarify how patients refer to their body and genitals and echo this during your consultation. Particularly awkward pitfalls to avoid include taking a menstrual and obstetric history from a trans woman and forgetting to record the cervical smear test history in a trans man. Collect detailed information on hormonal treatment and surgery to date so that you are appropriately prepared for the examination and genital site sampling. Remember that a speculum examination may be more difficult for transgender people who have a vagina or a neovagina. Screen for IPV, general threats of violence and harassment, sex work, group sex, the use of sex toys as well as drug and alcohol misuse, including 'chem-sex'. Viral hepatitis screening and vaccination against HAV, HBV and HPV will be indicated based on the aforementioned risk behaviours.

Sex workers

Sex workers are at higher risk of STI and also for physical violence from clients as well as IPV, so screen for these specifically. Depending on their place of work (sauna, flat, street) they may also have issues with drug and alcohol dependence. Take a thorough history of services offered as it may dictate the anatomical sites to be screened. Vaccination against HAV and HBV is indicated as in MSM. Support to enable better negotiation around 'safe sex' should also be provided.

HIV prophylaxis

Strong evidence indicates that when taken correctly daily or on demand, pre-exposure prophylaxis (PrEP) is highly effective at reducing HIV transmission and is recommended for HIV prevention in those deemed at risk. This includes, but is not limited to, MSM, sex workers and other cis and trans people based on risk assessment. Post-exposure prophylaxis (PEP) is also available for those presenting within 72 hours of a high-risk HIV exposure, although the evidence base for efficacy is less robust.

Young and other vulnerable people

Bacterial STI and unplanned pregnancies are both more common in young people, so longer consultations are required in order to gather additional information and provide education and support on 'safe-sex' and initiating contraception. Recognizing child sexual exploitation (CSE) is of particular concern in the sexual health setting and an appropriate proforma (e.g. Spotting the Signs[1]) should be used to identify coercion, grooming, abuse and non-consensual sex in those under 18 years. Ensure the patient is aware that if serious concerns are raised these are likely to be discussed with the child safeguarding team. Vulnerable adults include those with mental health disorders and learning disabilities. Consultations will be longer and information gathering will be more challenging. Screen for signs of abuse as you would with young people.

Female genital mutilation (FGM)

Female genital mutilation is the deliberate cutting and altering of the female genitalia without medical need and is carried out on young females between infancy and age 15. It is illegal in the UK and should be screened for in consultations with people assigned female at birth. If FGM has occurred, record when and where it was performed, the patient's attitude towards FGM and if you have any safeguarding concerns for children in the family. FGM performed under the age of 18 is a matter for the police as well as the child safeguarding team.

Genital examination

Prior to performing the genital examination, it is essential that you take time to explain to the patient what will happen and in doing so you are also gaining consent to proceed. Familiarize yourself with your environment and equipment and develop a reliable routine. A fluent and systematic approach will instil confidence in you and the patient. A chaperone should be offered for every examination and gloves should be worn throughout. In cases of sexual assault and child sexual exploitation, it is imperative that forensic and genital examination is carried out by specially trained personnel. You must not interrupt the chain of evidence so always seek advice before proceeding. In the course of your examination you may find evidence of FGM and this should always be documented.

General examination of the pubic area and groin

The patient is best examined in the lithotomy position, exposed from umbilicus to knees. Start by inspecting the skin of the supra-pubic, pubic, inguinal, perineal and perianal areas. Palpate the inguinal area and note the size, shape, contour, firmness, mobility and tenderness of any swellings you find. In males inspect the skin of the scrotum and the dorsal and ventral surfaces of the penis and in females the labia majora and minora.

Note if pubic hair is shaved or waxed and the presence of any folliculitis. In a patient presenting with genital itch, examine the pubic hair closely for the ectoparasite *Phthirus pubis* (and its eggs) which causes 'crabs'.

Look at the skin creases for evidence of fungal and bacterial intertrigo. Tinea cruris gives rise to an erythematous rash with a well-defined border. In cutaneous candidiasis the border is poorly defined with satellite lesions surrounding it.

Tiny dark-red papules of angiokeratoma (Fig. 18.1), or round, firm, whitish nodules of sebaceous cysts may be seen on the scrotum or the vulva. Both are harmless and the patient can be reassured.

Multiple small yellow-white papules may be seen on the underside of the penis or the inner vulva. These are ectopic sebaceous glands (Fordyce's spots) (Fig. 18.2) that do not require treatment.

An inflamed, red and thickened (lichenified) scrotum or vulva with added excoriations is typical of lichen simplex and suggests an underlying chronic skin condition such as atopic eczema or a contact dermatitis.

Itchy pink or hyperpigmented nodules on the genitals are typical of scabies. The itch tends to be worse at night. Excluding the face and neck, other lesions can be found on the abdomen, the axilla, the elbows, wrists and hands where classical interdigital linear burrows are seen.

Lichen sclerosus (LS) is an inflammatory skin condition of unknown aetiology that can affect any part of the skin, but is most often symptomatic at the genitals. LS affects both sexes, although the distribution differs; in males it typically presents on the glans, meatus, frenulum and prepuce whilst in females on the vulval and perianal skin leading to a 'figure of eight' distribution (Fig. 18.3). Active LS causes erythema, which in turn leads to thinning, tightening and hypopigmentation of the skin (sclerosis). Telangiectasia (owing to friable bloods vessels), fissures and blisters can also be seen. The chronic inflammatory process (particularly if untreated) can lead to squamous cell carcinoma in a small proportion of cases.

You may find pigmented naevi and non-pigmented groin and anal skin tags which can be confused with genital warts (condylomata acuminata).

Genital warts are benign epithelial skin tumours predominately caused by HPV types 6 and 11. They appear on the genital skin as single or multiple broad-based or pedunculated growths with a cauliflower-like appearance. They are usually soft to touch but also karatinized and can arise anywhere on the anogenital skin, inside the urethral meatus, the vagina, the cervix and inside the anus (Fig. 18.4).

Genital molluscum are benign epithelial skin eruptions caused by the *Molluscum contagiosum* virus. They typically appear in the pubic area as pearly, pink or yellow dome-shaped papules with a central umbilicus and are smooth to touch.

Both warts and molluscum are sexually transmitted. Occasionally they can appear sore and inflamed, particularly if they have been manipulated.

Painful anogenital sores are most commonly caused by herpes simplex virus (HSV), but other causes of genital ulceration should be considered and guided by the sexual history. In primary herpes the characteristic shallow ulcers are preceded by a crop of blisters, although it is typical for the patient to present after they have broken (Fig. 18.5). They

Figure 18.1   Angiokeratoma.

Figure 18.2   Fordyce spots.

Figure 18.3   Lichen sclerosus.

Figure 18.4   Genital warts.

may experience intense dysuria owing to infection of the urethral mucosa and develop painful inguinal lymphadenopathy and a flu-like illness that correlates with seroconversion. Owing to nerve invasion that establishes viral latency, paraesthesia of the skin of the genitals, buttocks and lower limbs is not uncommon. Recurrences tend to be less severe and can present atypically as itchy spots or fissures so always take a detailed history of previous similar episodes.

A solitary painless genital ulcer should lead to suspicion of syphilis, particularly if the patient is in a high-risk group (e.g. MSM or a sex-worker). The primary syphilitic chancre is typically hard (indurated) with a clear serous fluid oozing from its base and regional lymphadenopathy that is painless and rubbery. The coronal sulcus of the penis is the most common site (Fig. 18.6).

Figure 18.5   Genital herpes.

Tropically acquired causes of genital ulceration include chancroid and donovanosis, but these infections are becoming exceedingly rare in the countries in which they were once endemic. Lymphogranuloma venereum is another cause of genital ulceration that has become more common in MSM in recent years; however, it is more likely to present with proctitis. Other causes of genial ulcer include trauma, fixed drug reactions, dermatitis and Behcet's disease.

A groin swelling is likely to be inguinal lymphadenopathy. Anal, penile and vulval carcinoma may metastasize to the inguinal lymph nodes giving rise to hard, irregular and fixed lymphadenopathy. Inguinal lymphadenopathy may also be part of a generalized disorder, such as lymphoma, secondary syphilis, infectious mononucleosis or HIV infection.

Male genital examination

Palpate the scrotal contents by anchoring each testis between the fingers and smoothing the fingertips over surface noting the size (they should be roughly equal) and any tenderness or masses. Next palpate the epididymis (a soft structure that runs alongside the testis) and the tubular structure of the vas deferens within the spermatic cord as it passes through the neck of the scrotum. Examine the patient standing to check for hernias.

A varicocele is a tortuous dilatation of the veins contained within the spermatic cord (known as the pampiniform plexus) and it feels like a 'bag of worms' in the scrotum. A hydrocele is a painless fluctuant scrotal swelling that can be demonstrated by transillumination. Small, firm lumps within the epididymis are harmless cysts. A sudden onset of severe pain in the scrotum is concerning for a testicular torsion or a strangulated inguinal hernia. Urgent ultrasonography and surgical review are recommended if in doubt. A painless, hard enlargement of a testis must be considered malignant and should also be investigated without delay.

If the patient presents with penile lump or curvature, on palpation you may find a hard, fibrotic mass within the shaft which is typical of Peyronie's disease. Occasionally (following rigorous sexual activity) a boggy tender swelling known as a lymphocele can form just proximal to the neck of the glans. The patient can be reassured that it will settle spontaneously.

Retract the prepuce (if present) to reveal the sub-prepuce, coronal sulcus, glans penis, external urethral meatus and frenulum. Inspect inside the meatus and swab any discharge present before carefully drawing the prepuce forwards.

Smegma is greyish-white cheesy material arising from Tyson's glands (which lie either side of the frenulum) and may accumulate under the prepuce if unwashed. Tiny regular papules arranged in rows around the coronal sulcus are coronal papillae (pearly penile papules), which may be mistaken for warts.

Phimosis is the inability fully to retract the prepuce, which may be a late complication of lichen sclerosus. Phimosis may predispose to recurrent episodes of infection of the glans (balanitis), the prepuce (posthitis) or both (balanoposthitis) which is often fungal in aetiology and also seen in poorly controlled diabetes. Always perform a urinalysis.

A paraphimosis is painful swelling of a trapped retracted prepuce and may need urological intervention.

Female genital examination

Carefully inspect the skin of the intralabial folds, the clitoral hood and clitoris. Part the labia to expose the vestibule and the opening of the vagina (introitus) and note the presence of any discharge.

Vulval papillae appear as small, smooth finger-like projections at the vestibule of the vagina; often they are confused with genital warts. A Bartholin's cyst or a tender abscess can be found at the inferior aspect of the labia either side of the vaginal opening. It may result from gonococcal or chlamydial infection, and purulent discharge may be observed from Bartholin's duct, which is between the upper two-thirds and lower one-third of the labia.

If visualization of the vagina and cervix is required, use your non-dominant hand to anchor the labia away from the vestibule and using your dominant hand place a lubricated speculum into the introitus. Gently insert it into the vagina and advance slowly. When fully inserted, open the speculum to reveal the cervix and fix it in place. Inspect the vaginal walls and the cervix. Samples of discharge can be taken from the lateral wall and posterior fornix of the vagina as well as the cervical opening (os).

Nabothian follicles appear as yellow cysts on the cervix, which may have prominent vessels on their surface but are normal. A cervical ectropion (ectopic columnar epithelium) may be visible surrounding the cervical os, which is also normal. Purulent discharge and friability of the cervical os can be a sign of mucopurulent cervicitis. A retained foreign body, such as a tampon, causes a very offensive odour; if not removed, may, rarely, lead to toxic shock syndrome.

A bimanual examination (BME) is indicated in cases of suspected PID or other pelvic pathology. Insert two fingers of the dominant hand into the vagina to palpate the cervix. Use the non-dominant hand to apply pressure on the lower abdomen enabling you to palpate the uterus and each adnexa

Figure 18.6 Primary syphilis.

between the fingers. Note the approximate size of the uterus and any abnormal masses. Pain elicited on palpation of the cervix is known as cervical excitation tenderness and this may co-exist with uterine and adnexal tenderness. All are positive findings suggestive of PID.

Proctoscopy

If the patient presents with symptoms suggestive of proctitis or has lumps and ulceration extending into the anal canal, then proctoscopy is indicated. The patient should be in the left lateral position with knees drawn up to chest. Place a lubricated proctoscope at the anal verge and apply gentle pressure onto the external anal sphincter, allowing it to open. Slowly advance the proctoscope into the anal canal and rectum. Remove the obturator to allow examination

Figure 18.7 Condylomata lata.

of the rectal mucosa. Proctitis appears as purulent discharge with friable mucosa. Ulceration may also be seen. Samples can be taken from the rectal wall before carefully removing the proctoscope.

Anal itch (pruritus ani) may be secondary to rectal discharge, anal warts, hemorrhoids, perianal dermatitis or poor anal hygiene. If the itch is worse at night, then threadworm infestation should be considered. Both primary syphilis and genital herpes can present with anal fissures. Flat warty lesions of condylomata lata can be confused with anal warts but, in fact, are the highly infectious lesions of secondary syphilis (Fig. 18.7).

General examination

A widespread maculopapular rash should raise suspicion for HIV seroconversion or secondary syphilis. Other signs of secondary syphilis include a palmoplantar rash, patchy alopecia of the scalp and erythematous lesions of the oral mucosa known as mucous patches. In cases of suspected secondary or late syphilis, then a dedicated cardiovascular and neurological examination may be indicated according to symptomatology.

Dermatological conditions (e.g. atopic eczema, seborrheic dermatitis, psoriasis and lichen planus) can all affect the genital skin and, in some cases, may be the only presentation of it. If you find evidence of these in the genitals make sure to examine the remaining skin, nails, scalp and oral cavity for other features to support your diagnosis.

Testing

A combination of nucleic acid amplification tests (NAAT), serology, microscopy and culture is used to screen for and diagnose STI. Point-of-care tests (POCT) (e.g. for HIV, *Trichomonas vaginalis* (TV) and syphilis) are particularly useful in outreach and resource poor settings.

Asymptomatic

The NAAT performed on urine and self-taken swabs from the oropharynx, vulvovagina and rectum are

Table 18.1 Site-specific screening using NG/CT NAAT according to gender and sexual behaviour			
	Urine	**Oropharynx + rectum**	**Vulvovaginal**
Cis MSM	All	All	
Trans men and women	All	Sex worker	If a vagina present
		According to sexual risk	
Cis women		Sex worker	All
		Age <25 years	
		According to sexual risk	
Cis men (heterosexual)	All		

validated to detect *Neisseria gonorrhoea* (NG) and *Chlamydia trachomatis* serovars D-K (CT) with a high sensitivity and specificity. See Table 18.1 for guidance on site-specific testing according to gender and sexual behaviour. It is important to note that all sexually active MSM should be tested at three sites, regardless of sexual roles and practices.

Alongside NG/CT NAAT, serological tests are the main screening method for diagnosing HIV and syphilis and should be offered to all those who attend sexual health services or request a sexual health screen.

Syphilis is caused by the spirochete bacterium *Treponema pallidum* (TP). Specific serological tests for treponemes are used as screening tools to diagnose syphilis. False-positive results can occur occasionally, so a positive result on one specific test (e.g. treponemal enzyme immunoassay (EIA)) is always repeated on another (e.g. *Treponema pallidum* particle agglutination (TPPA)). Non-specific tests (e.g. the anticardiolipin antibody also known as the Venereal Disease Research Laboratories (VDRL) and the rapid plasma reagin (RPR)) are used to quantify the degree of treponemal disease activity. The VDRL and RPR are expressed as a titre (e.g. 1:4, 1:8, etc.); following treatment a two-fold reduction in titre is considered an adequate response. Specific tests for syphilis will remain positive lifelong. Past infection with endemic treponematoses, such as yaws, bejel and pinta, may also result in positive specific serological tests for syphilis and it is custom to treat presumptively.

Additional serological tests to screen for HAV, HBV and HCV are offered to MSM, sex workers, people living with HIV (PLWH) and others according to endemic risk, lifestyle and sexual practices.

An understanding of testing window periods is useful. GC/CT NAAT can reliably exude infection 2 weeks after exposure. The combined fourth generation HIV antigen/antibody test will reliably exclude HIV 45 days following exposure. HIV POCT, as well as hepatitis B and C antibodies, may take up to 90 days.

Symptomatic

Urethral discharge should be investigated with Gram-stain microscopy and the patient should not have passed urine for at least 2 hours. A sample is taken from the urethra using a plastic loop or swab and smeared onto a microscope slide ready for staining.

A short history of continuous thick yellow urethral discharge following recent condomless sex is typical of gonococcal urethritis (GU). This diagnosis is strongly supported by the presence of polymorphonucleocytes (PML) with Gram-negative intracellular diplococci (GNID) on microscopy (Fig. 18.8) and ultimately confirmed with positive NAAT and culture for NG. Culture is also used for

antimicrobial sensitivity testing of NG diagnosed by NAAT. Symptomatic NG proctitis and cervicitis may also be diagnosed on microscopy, albeit with lower sensitivity.

Lower genital NG infections may be complicated by epididymo-orchitis, PID and disseminated infection involving the skin and joints. Autoinoculation to the eye can give rise to gonococcal conjunctivitis (an ophthalmic emergency).

A cloudy grey-white discharge would imply non-gonococcal urethritis (NGU); for a list of causes see Box 18.1. The diagnosis of NGU is confirmed by greater than 5 PML per high power field (×1000) on microscopy of urethral smear. Urine NG/CT and *mycoplasma genitalium* (MGen) NAAT are performed in the first instance, whereas persistent NGU may require additional NAAT for TV. NGU can be complicated by epididymo-orchitis, PID and sexually acquired reactive arthritis (SARA) which, in addition to urethritis, classically gives rise to bilateral kerato-conjunctivitis and oligoarthritis. Circinate balanitis is a cutaneous manifestation of SARA that appears on the glans penis as erythematous eroded

Figure 18.8   Gram-negative intracellular diplococci.

Box 18.1	Causes of non-gonococcal urethritis
Sexually transmitted infection (STI)	
Chlamydia trachomatis D-K serovars (~30%)	
Mycoplasma genitalium (~30%)	
Trichomonas vaginalis	
Ureaplasma urealyticum	
Herpes simplex virus	
Intrameatal warts	
Meatal chancre	
Non-STI	
Bacterial urinary tract infection	
Adenoviruses	
Candidiasis	
Urethral stricture	
Chemical irritation	
Foreign body	
Trauma	

lesions that coalesce with a slightly raised and polycyclic edge.

Epididymo-orchitis is a clinical diagnosis characterized by acute onset of pain in the scrotum with tenderness of the testes and epididymis on examination. In sexually active men under the age of 35 the most likely cause is STI. Gram stain of a urethral smear may be normal, show NGU or GU. In older men, a bacterial urinary tract infection is a more common cause. The diagnosis is supported by positive urine dip for leukocytes, blood and nitrites; a urine culture should be performed in addition to urine NG/CT NAAT.

Vaginal discharge should be investigated with two forms of microscopy. A sample taken from the vaginal wall using a cotton tip is smeared onto a microscope slide for Gram-staining. A second sample taken from the posterior fornix using a plastic loop is mixed into a drop of saline on a microscope slide, known as a wet preparation. Vaginal discharge may also be pH tested using litmus paper. STI is a common cause of vaginal discharge so perform vulvovaginal swab (VVS) NG/CT NAAT in all cases.

Bacterial vaginosis (BV), which is an imbalance of the normal vaginal microflora, presents as an offensive classically 'fishy' off-white discharge with no inflammatory symptoms. It may arise following a change in sexual partner or unprotected sex, but it is not considered to be an STI.

The diagnosis is confirmed by the absence of lactobacilli and the presence of mixed flora and 'clue cells' (Hay-Ison criteria) on Gram-stain microscopy of vaginal smear. 'Clue cells' are vaginal epithelial cells covered with *Gardnerella vaginalis*, which are Gram-variable but mainly Gram-negative coccobacilli. The vaginal pH is typically elevated more than 4.5.

A thick white, yellow or green 'cottage-cheese' like discharge associated with vulval irritation is suggestive of vulvovaginal candidiasis (VVC) which is not an STI. External or false dysuria may occur when urine makes contact with inflamed vulva, so be wary of confusing this presentation with a urinary tract infection, particularly because it can be triggered and indeed worsened by a course of broad-spectrum antibiotics. The diagnosis is confirmed by the presence of fungal spores and hyphae on Gram-stain microscopy of vaginal smear. In recurrent infections, culture of candida species may be useful in identifying intrinsic and acquired anti-fungal resistance.

Infection with TV may give rise to a fishy, frothy yellow-green discharge which can be intensely itchy and sore. The diagnosis is confirmed by the direct visualization of jerky motile trichomonads under light-field illumination (Fig. 18.9). The sensitivity of microscopy for detecting TV is variable, so consider performing VVS TV NAAT if there is vulval inflammation with an offensive discharge and no cause found on microscopy.

Abnormal vaginal bleeding, deep dyspareunia and LAP should be investigated as per vaginal discharge, but additional examination of the cervix and pelvic organs is required. With clinical features of mucopurulent cervicitis or PID on examination, then endocervical Gram-stain microscopy is indicated. Mucopurulent cervicitis has a similar infective aetiology to urethritis and is investigated accordingly. PID is an ascending infection of the pelvic organs and usually the result of bacterial STI; however, bacterial vaginosis and anaerobic infections are implicated. The diagnosis should be considered in any sexually active women with recent onset LAP and a positive BME in whom no other cause is found. The absence of endocervical or vaginal PMN on microscopy has good negative predictive value for diagnosing PID; however, their presence is non-specific. Right upper quadrant pain in association with PID is known as Fitzhugh-Curtis syndrome and is caused by perihepatic inflammation.

Infectious proctitis should be suspected in any patient with a history of receptive anal intercourse; typical symptoms and inflamed rectal mucosa are noted on proctoscopy. Microscopy of rectal smear should be performed and greater than 5 PML ×1000 is supportive of the diagnosis. Rectal NG/CT NAAT

Figure 18.9 *Trichomonas vaginalis.*

should be performed in all cases. MSM and other people based on risk assessment should have additional rectal swab NAAT for CT serovars 1–3 also known as lymphogranuloma venereum (LGV) and HSV 1 and 2, particularly if ulcers are seen. Rarely, LGV may progress to colitis or mimic inflammatory bowel disease in presentation.

HSV 1 and 2 NAAT should be performed on all cases of genital ulcers. Where a genital syphilitic chancre is suspected, either by history or appearance, then a sample of serious fluid should be removed from the ulcer base with a cover slip. The diagnosis is confirmed by direct visualization of the motile spirochete under dark-ground microscopy (DGM) (Fig. 18.10). Ulcer swabs for TP NAAT can be performed (where available) and may be useful in cases where DGM is negative or not possible (e.g. a chancre in the oral cavity). Contemporaneous syphilis serology should always be performed at the time of presentation and may be negative early in the disease (Table 18.2).

HIV infection

The spread of HIV infection and the emergence of the acquired immune deficiency syndrome (AIDS) in the early 1980s resulted in a dramatic fall in life expectancy across the world. Increased access to HIV testing and the development and uptake of combined antiretroviral therapy (ART) mean that people living with HIV (PLWH), if treated early, will have a normal life expectancy and cannot transmit the virus. Nevertheless, a significant proportion remains at risk of the infective and non-infective complications, especially if they are undiagnosed and develop late-stage infection, or once diagnosed are unable to access or adhere to ART.

Primary HIV infection may present with a seroconversion illness that is non-specific and can feature any of fever, headache, myalgia, malaise, diarrhea, lymphadenopathy, pharyngitis and a widespread erythematous, maculopapular rash. Night sweats, weight loss, meningism, neuropathy and oral

thrush may rarely occur in the context of the acute severe viraemia and associated CD4 T-lymphocyte (CD4) decline. HIV seroconversion can also be very mild or asymptomatic. Anyone presenting with rash and fever should be tested for HIV, particularly if having recently engaged in high- risk sexual activity or IVDU. The differential diagnosis would also include viral hepatitis, cytomegalovirus (CMV), Epstein-Barr virus (EBV), secondary syphilis and drug reactions. If HIV is diagnosed during the primary illness and it is acceptable to the patient, then rapid initiation of ART is appropriate and will have the benefit of reducing the viral reservoir and be associated with a significant decline in onward transmission.

Following seroconversion, the immune system attempts to control HIV and, in doing so, brings the level of HIV-RNA in the blood (known as the viral load) down to a set point. The CD4 count partially recovers and also stabilizes to a baseline level that is typically within the normal range. A period of clinical latency ensues and the CD4 count decline correlates with advancing immunosuppression (Fig. 18.11).

In the UK routine screening for HIV is recommended in the following circumstances:
1. MSM, female partners of MSM, people who inject drugs, sex workers, trans women, people from countries with a high seroprevalence (>1%) and their sexual contacts.
2. Anyone accessing health services for sexual health, addiction and substance misuse, antenatal care, termination of pregnancy and the management of hepatitis B and C, TB and lymphoma.
3. Anyone accessing health care settings in areas where the prevalence is high (2–5 per 1000) or extremely high HIV (>5 per 1000).
4. Anyone presenting with symptoms or signs of an indicator condition which be AIDS-defining or non-AIDS-defining but associated with an undiagnosed HIV prevalence of more than 1 per 1000. (Tables 18.3 and 18.4).
5. The sexual partners of those diagnosed with HIV.

When assessing all PLWH, gather information on current symptoms and past medical history, including any infections or cancers and treatment given. If HIV has been newly diagnosed, then a detailed social history is required to ascertain if sexual partners and/or children are also at risk which would necessitate further contact tracing and testing. If a patient is already known to have HIV, then gather information on the latest CD4 count and HIV viral load and record the current ART regimen and any prophylactic antimicrobials. It is prudent to find out the centre the patient attended for HIV care so that outstanding information can be obtained at the earliest convenience. An assessment of sexual wellbeing, relationships and the psychological impact

Figure 18.10   Treponema pallidum.

Table 18.2 Investigations and diagnoses in symptomatic patients

Syndrome	Features	Near patient test results	Presumptive diagnosis	Laboratory tests
Urethral discharge	Thick Yellow	Urethral Gram stain: GNID	Gonococcal urethritis	Urine NG/CT NAAT Urethral NG culture
	Cloudy grey-white	Urethral Gram stain: >5 PML	Non-gonococcal urethritis	Urine NG/CT, MGen, TV NAAT
Tender testis or epididymis	Age <35 years Urethral discharge	Urethral Gram stain: Normal	Epididymo-orchitis	Urine NG/CT, MGen NAAT
		Urethral Gram stain: >5 PML		
		Urethral Gram stain: GNID	Gonococcal Epididymo-orchitis	Urine NG/CT NAAT Urethral NG culture
	Age >35 years Urinary symptoms	Urinalysis: normal	UTI epididymo-orchitis	Urine NG/CT NAAT
		Urinalysis: leucocytes, blood, nitrites		Urine culture
Vaginal discharge	Thin Fishy odour pH: >4.5	Vaginal Gram stain: Clue cells, no lactobacilli	Bacterial vaginosis (BV)	VVS NG/CT NAAT
		Wet prep: negative		
	Frothy Yellow green Fishy odour Inflammation	Wet prep: Motile trichomonads Vaginal Gram stain: PML/normal	Trichomonas vaginalis (TV)	VVS NG/CT, TV NAAT
	Thick cheesy White Inflammation	Vaginal Gram stain: Spores and hyphae Wet prep: negative	Vulvovaginal candidiasis (VVC)	VVS NG/CT NAAT ±Yeast culture
Abnormal vaginal bleeding Pain ±positive BME	Purulent Inflamed friable cervix	Vaginal Gram stain: PML/clue cells, no lactobacilli/ normal Wet prep: negative	Mucopurulent cervicitis ±PID	Endocervical NG/CT, MGen NAAT
		Endocervical Gram stain: GNID	Gonococcal cervicitis ± PID	Endocervical NG/CT NAAT NG culture
Anorectal symptoms	Purulent Inflamed friable Rectum	Rectal Gram stain: >5 PML	Proctitis	Rectal NG/CT, LGV, HSV, MGen NAAT
		Rectal Gram stain: GNID	Gonococcal proctitis	Rectal GC/CT NAAT NG culture
Genital ulcers	Painful Multiple Shallow	N/A	Genital herpes	Ulcer HSV 1+2 NAAT
	Painless Solitary Indurated	Ulcer fluid dark ground: Motile spirochetes	Primary syphilis	Ulcer TP NAAT

BME, Bimanual examination; CT, chlamydia trachomatis; GNID, gram negative intracellular diplococci; HSV, herpes simplex virus; LGV, lymphogranuloma venereum; MGen, mycoplasma genitalium; NAAT, nucleic acid amplification test; NG, neisseria gonorrhea; PML, polymorphonucleocyte; TP, treponema pallidum TV, trichomonas vaginalis; VVS, vulvulo-vaginal swab.

of living with HIV is appropriate in all situations. Complete your assessment with a systematic review and examination looking for features of immunosuppression and indicator conditions.

Persistent lymphadenopathy may be the only positive finding in early asymptomatic infection and the CD4 count is expected to be above 500 cells/mm^3.

As the CD4 count falls below normal, mild symptoms and signs of immune activation and immunosuppression may appear. These include repeated upper respiratory tract infections (e.g. sinusitis, otitis media, tonsillitis and pharyngitis), oral ulcers, herpes zoster (shingles) and seborrheic dermatitis.

As the CD4 count falls below 350 cells/mm^3 and the HIV viral load rises, the patient's health will begin to deteriorate. Oral candidiasis presents with a painful mouth and examination reveals white plaques on the tongue and palate over inflamed and bleeding mucosa (Fig. 18.12). Oral hairy leucoplakia may also be seen on the lateral border

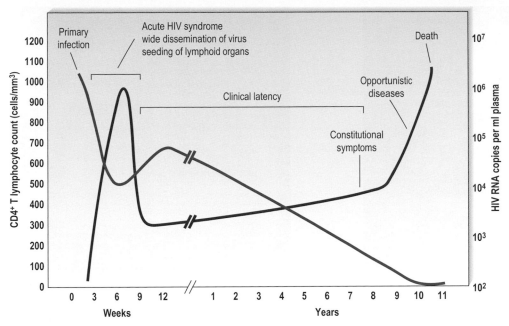

Figure 18.11 The natural history of HIV infection.

Table 18.3	AIDS-defining indicator conditions in people living with HIV
Category	**AIDS-defining condition**
Neoplasms	Cervical cancer, non-Hodgkin lymphoma, Kaposi's sarcoma
Bacterial infections	Mycobacterium tuberculosis, pulmonary or extrapulmonary
	Mycobacterium avium complex/Mycobacterium kansasii, Mycobacterium, other species or unidentified species, disseminated or extrapulmonary
	Pneumonia, recurrent (two or more episodes in 12 months) Salmonella septicaemia, recurrent
Viral infections	Cytomegalovirus retinitis
	Cytomegalovirus, other (except liver, spleen, glands)
	Herpes simplex, ulcer(s) >1 month/bronchitis/pneumonitis
	Progressive multifocal leukoencephalopathy
Parasitic infections	Cerebral toxoplasmosis
	Cryptosporidiosis diarrhoea >1 month
	Isosporiasis >1 month
	Atypical disseminated leishmaniasis
	Reactivation of American trypanosomiasis (meningoencephalitis or myocarditis)
Fungal infections	Pneumocystis carinii pneumonia
	Candidiasis, oesophageal, bronchial/tracheal/pulmonary
	Cryptococcosis, extrapulmonary
	Histoplasmosis, disseminated/extrapulmonary
	Coccidioidomycosis, disseminated/extrapulmonary
	Penicilliosis, disseminated

Source: BHIVA/BASHH/BIA Adult HIV Testing Guidelines 2020.

Table 18.4	Non-AIDS-defining HIV indicator conditions (associated with an undiagnosed HIV prevalence of >1 per 1000)
Category	**Condition**
Hematological	Unexplained leukocytopenia/thrombocytopenia lasting >4 weeks
Neoplasm	Malignant lymphoma, anal cancer/dysplasia, cervical dysplasia, primary lung cancer
Neurological	Peripheral neuropathy, mononeuritis, Guillain-Barré syndrome, subcortical dementia, multiple sclerosis-like disease
Dermatological	Seborrheic dermatitis/exanthema, severe or atypical psoriasis
Renal	Unexplained chronic renal impairment
Gastro-intestinal	Unexplained weight loss, unexplained chronic diarrhea
Infective	Community-acquired pneumonia, herpes zoster (shingles), hepatitis B or C (acute of chronic), hepatitis A, unexplained oral candidiasis, candidaemia, STI, mononucleosis-like illness, visceral leishmaniasis, invasive pneumococcal disease
Other	Unexplained lymphadenopathy, unexplained fever, oral hairy leukoplakia

Source: BHIVA/BASHH/BIA Adult HIV Testing Guidelines 2020.

Figure 18.12   Oral candidiasis.

Figure 18.14   Cerebral toxoplasmosis.

Figure 18.13   Kaposi sarcoma.

of the tongue. Bacterial pneumonia becomes more common, presenting with fever, a productive cough, dyspnoea and typical radiographic features. PLWH are more likely to acquire or reactivate *Mycobacterium tuberculosis* (TB). Pulmonary *Mycobacterium tuberculosis* is the most common presentation, although atypical presentations and multisystem involvement are also seen. The typical presentation of recurrent fever, weight loss, night sweats and lymphadenopathy is equally suggestive of lymphoma, so investigations should exclude both diagnoses. HIV has a cytotoxic effect on the gut, which may lead to HIV enteropathy, and it presents with chronic diarrhoea and weight loss. HIV also has a cytotoxic effect on the kidney, leading to HIV nephropathy and renal failure.

As the CD4 count falls below 200 cells/mm^3 many more of the classic AIDS-defining illnesses arise. General examination may reveal severe weight loss and cachexia and Kaposi sarcoma (KS) (Fig. 18.13). KS, which is caused by human herpesvirus 8 (HHV-8), presents with purple or brown macules on the skin and oral mucosa that are not typically pruritic or painful. An affected soft palate is a strong indicator of visceral involvement. *Pneumocystis jirovecii* (formerly *P. carinii*) pneumonia can present with progressive exertional dyspnoea and a dry cough, with or without fever. The patient often has an increased respiratory rate and will desaturate on exertion; however, respiratory examination findings can be subtle. Disseminated histoplasmosis may appear and is acquired abroad, so country of birth and lifetime travel history will be relevant.

Neurological complications of HIV are varied. Intracranial infections may present atypically, particularly in severe immunosuppression. Cross-sectional imaging of the central nervous system (CNS) and lumbar puncture (LP) for cerebrospinal fluid (CSF) analysis is recommended. Cryptococcal meningitis is caused by *Cryptococcus neoformans* and typically presents with headache and fever. LP often has raised opening pressure and a positive CSF India ink and cryptococcal antigen (CrAg) is diagnostic. CNS space-occupying lesions generally present with focal neurological signs or seizures. Cerebral toxoplasmosis abscesses arise from reactivation of chronic infection with *Toxoplasma gondii*. The classic appearance of multiple ring-enhancing lesions on MRI of the brain is usually sufficient to commence empirical therapy (Fig. 18.14). Differential diagnosis includes primary cerebral lymphoma, tuberculoma or bacterial abscess.

Peripheral neuropathy, HIV encephalopathy (HIVE) and HIV-associated dementia (HAND) are more common in older PLWH. They are also a result of HIV cytotoxicity. Neuropathy presents with symmetrical distal numbness and allodynia of the lower limbs. On examination strength is usually preserved and reflexes are depressed or absent and there is impaired sensation to pain and temperature. HIVE/HAND can result in poor concentration, depression, memory loss, personality changes and language impairment. Examination may reveal impaired saccadic eye movements, generalized hyperreflexia and tremor. MRI may show cerebral atrophy and diffuse white matter signal change or could be normal. Other causes of abnormal neurology and white matter change in advanced immunosuppression include progressive multifocal encephalopathy (PML) and CMV encephalitis.

Oral candidiasis may involve the oesophagus; it presents with painful and difficult swallowing. The differential diagnoses include HSV and CMV oesophagitis. CMV, *Cryptosporidium*, *Isospora*, *Cyclospora* and *Microsporidium* are important causes of diarrhoea in advanced immunosuppression.

Severely immunocompromised patients presenting with floaters, an increasing blind spot, visual blurring or sudden visual loss in one or both eyes may have sight-threatening retinitis caused by CMV, varicella zoster virus (VZV) or toxoplasmosis. Fundoscopy is obligatory. In CMV retinitis multiple granular white dots with haemorrhages are seen.

Disseminated *Mycobacterium avium* complex (DMAC) infection also occurs in severe immunosuppression; it often presents with non-specific features, including diarrhoea, weight loss, anorexia and hepatomegaly. Mycobacterial blood and/or bone marrow cultures are useful in aiding the diagnosis.

Endocrine and metabolic disorders | 19

Tahseen A. Chowdhury and William M. Drake

Introduction

The endocrine system is composed of the classic endocrine organs:

- Hypothalamus/pituitary
- Thyroid
- Parathyroid
- Adrenal
- Pancreatic islet cells
- Gonads

The mode of presentation of endocrine disorders does not fit neatly into a system-based model, the symptoms rarely being specific to a particular system. Frequently, endocrine disease is suggested by a constellation of non-specific symptoms.

The endocrine history

As in other systems, the history consists of presenting symptoms, the history of the development of the illness and the family history.

Presenting symptoms

A number of symptom complexes particularly suggests endocrine disease.

Thirst and polyuria

Excessive thirst (polydipsia) and increased urine output (polyuria) are important symptoms for which careful history taking is crucial for accurate diagnosis. The word 'excessive' appears in almost all dictionary definitions of polydipsia and polyuria, but no accepted number of episodes of fluid intake or excretion indicate a definite abnormality, largely because individual habitual fluid intake is so variable in health. If the symptoms form the basis of a patient's complaint, they require careful and sympathetic evaluation. Polyuria and polydipsia are common presenting symptoms of diabetes mellitus; these are discussed in detail below. These symptoms may also be caused by impairment of renal concentrating capacity as a result of a deficiency of antidiuretic hormone (ADH) or a failure of ADH action (cranial and nephrogenic diabetes insipidus, respectively). The latter may be inherited or may occur secondary to impairment of ADH action by hypercalcaemia or hypokalaemia. An important distinction must be made between frequency of urination and polyuria. Prostatic enlargement in men and childbirth-related pelvic damage in women are common causes of frequent urination, but in these situations the volumes of urine passed will usually be small and the symptoms will not be accompanied by thirst. Nocturia (the passage of urine during conventional sleeping hours) is common in men with prostatic enlargement, but is not accompanied by thirst; indeed, most men will make conscious efforts to restrict evening fluid intake in an attempt to reduce nocturia with its associated fatigue. In contrast, a patient with diabetes insipidus, characteristically, will take at least a glass, often a whole bottle, of water to bed in order to quench his nocturnal thirst. Probing the details of nocturnal symptoms is also useful in distinguishing the reported polydipsia and polyuria caused by increased fluid intake, which at its most extreme may be vastly excessive (primary, sometimes referred to as psychogenic, polydipsia). In general, nocturnal polyuria is not a feature of primary polydipsia, because the capacity of the pituitary to release ADH and of the kidney to respond to it are not disturbed. In contrast, it is often the nocturia and the associated urge to drink that most disturb patients with diabetes insipidus. However, this is not an absolute distinction and further investigation of urine concentrating capacity is sometimes required.

Weight loss

Loss of weight is a feature of decreased food intake or increased metabolic rate. Sometimes both factors may operate to reduce body weight, as in the cachexia of malignant disease. Thyroid overactivity (hyperthyroidism) is nearly always associated with a combination of unintentional or effortless weight loss and increased appetite, although occasionally the latter may be stimulated more than the former so that a paradoxical increase in weight occurs. Weight loss is rarely the sole presenting symptom of hyperthyroidism and other clinical features often predominate, particularly in younger patients (Box 19.1). In the elderly, however, hyperthyroidism may be occult or may simulate the gradual weight loss of malignant disease. Cardiac arrhythmias are a

Box 19.1	Clinical features of hyperthyroidism

- Tachycardia
- Atrial fibrillation/heart failure
- Eye signs
- Lid lag
- Lid retraction
- Exophthalmos (Graves' disease)
- Sweating
- Thyroid gland enlargement and bruit (Graves' disease)
- Fine distal tremor
- Thinning of hair
- Proximal weakness; cannot rise from squat
- Chorea

Box 19.2	Endocrine and metabolic diseases in which weight loss is a clinical feature

- Hyperthyroidism
- Type 1 diabetes mellitus
- Hypopituitarism
- Adrenocortical failure (Addison's disease)
- Anorexia nervosa

Box 19.3	Conditions in which increased body weight is a feature

- Simple obesity: energy intake/expenditure imbalance
- Primary hypothyroidism
- Cushing's syndrome
- Hypothalamic lesions
- Leptin deficiency

Box 19.4	Conditions in which metabolic myopathy is a feature

Painless

- Hyperthyroidism
- Cushing's syndrome, including iatrogenic steroid myopathy
- Acromegaly

Painful

- Vitamin D deficiency
- Osteomalacia
- Hypothyroidism

Box 19.5	Conditions in which temperature intolerance is a feature

- Intolerance to cold: hypothyroidism
- Intolerance to heat: hyperthyroidism

Box 19.6	Clinical features of hypothyroidism

- Weight gain
- Sallow complexion and dry skin
- Thinning of scalp and lateral eyebrow hair
- Cold intolerance
- Deepened, gruff voice
- Slow physical and mental activity
- Unsteadiness and slightly slurred speech
- Tingling in toes and fingers
- Aching muscles with cramp
- Mild proximal weakness
- Slow pulse and shortness of breath

Weight gain is therefore a common feature of primary hypothyroidism. However, obesity is rarely a consequence of specific endocrine dysfunction, an exception being the very rare phenomenon of leptin deficiency. In the majority of patients, 'simple obesity' is owing to a long-standing imbalance between energy intake and expenditure; it frequently begins in childhood and is often present in more than one family member. Glucocorticoid hormone excess (Cushing's syndrome) results in an increase in body fat predominantly involving abdominal, omental and interscapular fat (truncal obesity), with paradoxical thinning of the limbs owing to muscle atrophy.

Muscle weakness

Symptomatic muscular weakness not caused by neurological disease is a feature of several metabolic disorders, including thyrotoxicosis, Cushing's syndrome and vitamin D deficiency. In all these conditions, the metabolic myopathy (Box 19.4) causes symmetrical proximal weakness, mainly involving the shoulder and hip girdle musculature. There is usually associated muscle wasting. The major reported symptom is difficulty in climbing stairs, boarding a bus or rising from a sitting position. Most patients with hyperthyroidism have proximal weakness. This may be subclinical; it is best demonstrated by asking the patient to rise from the squatting position. The proximal myopathy of vitamin D deficiency is often painful, in contrast to other causes. The differential diagnosis of painful proximal muscular weakness includes polymyositis and polymyalgia rheumatica, as well as spinal root or plexus disease.

Cold intolerance

An abnormal sensation of cold, out of proportion to that experienced by other individuals, may indicate underlying hypothyroidism (Boxes 19.5 and 19.6).

frequent feature in the elderly. Anorexia nervosa, a psychogenic disorder characterized by a long history of low body weight in the absence of other features of ill health, must be considered, especially in young women. Any form of weight loss may be associated with oligo-amenorrhoea.

Other endocrine conditions in which weight loss is a major feature are listed in Box 19.2.

Weight gain or redistribution

An increase in body weight (Box 19.3) is a predictable result of a reduction in metabolic rate.

This symptom differs from the localized vasomotor symptoms in the hands found in Raynaud's phenomenon and is rather non-specific, especially in the elderly.

Heat intolerance

The increased metabolic rate of thyrotoxicosis may be associated with heat intolerance in which, at its most extreme, the patient is comfortable at an ambient temperature that others find unpleasantly cold. This is an important symptom, highly specific for thyroid overactivity, which may partly explain some of the seasonal variation in presentation of the condition.

Increased sweating

Hyperhidrosis (excessive sweating) may be a constitutional abnormality, characterized by onset in childhood or adolescence and sometimes by a family history. A recent increase in sweat secretion, on the other hand, may be an early indication of thyroid overactivity. Paroxysmal sweating is a common feature of anxiety. Increased catecholamine secretion from a phaeochromocytoma of the adrenal medulla is a rare cause of hyperhidrosis. Intermittent sweating after meals (gustatory hyperhidrosis) may occur in patients with autonomic dysfunction. Growth hormone excess (acromegaly) also increases sweating, perhaps because of hypertrophy of the sweat glands, and this feature can be used to assess the activity of the disease in the clinic. Increased sweating should be distinguished from flushing that occurs physiologically at the time of the natural menopause. Flushing may be a presenting feature of serotonin-secreting carcinoid tumours of the gut and usually indicates extensive disease with hepatic metastases.

Tremor

A fine rapid resting tremor is one of the cardinal clinical features of thyrotoxicosis. This must be distinguished from the coarser and more irregular tremor of anxiety, which is usually associated with a cool peripheral skin temperature, in contrast to the warm skin of the thyrotoxic patient. Tremor owing to neurological disease is greater in amplitude, slower in rate and may be present at rest, as in Parkinson's disease, or on movement, as in cerebellar tremor. It therefore rarely simulates thyrotoxic tremor. Essential tremor is not so rapid as thyrotoxic tremor; it is variable and is worse in certain postures. It often involves the head and neck.

Palpitations

Palpitations are a heightened, unpleasant awareness of the heartbeat. They may be a feature of thyrotoxicosis, but more likely are caused by anxiety. Awareness of the heartbeat while lying down is normal. Other causes of rapid heart rate include paroxysmal tachyarrhythmias. The sensation of intermittent forceful cardiac contraction, sometimes described by the patient as a missed beat, is often owing to a compensatory pause following an ectopic beat and is usually a normal phenomenon.

Postural unsteadiness

Dizziness, or a sensation of faintness on standing, should prompt measurement of lying and standing blood pressure. Postural hypotension, a fall of diastolic blood pressure on standing, occurs with reduced blood volume. In the absence of obvious bleeding or gastrointestinal fluid loss, adrenal insufficiency should be considered. Postural hypotension is frequently caused by autonomic neuropathy, especially in patients with long-standing diabetes mellitus. It is also a common complication of any drug therapy for essential hypertension. The drug history is particularly important in the elderly patient with dizziness.

Visual disturbance

Several endocrine conditions may cause visual symptoms. Blurred vision is common in uncontrolled hyperglycaemia. Decreased visual acuity may be caused by space-occupying lesions compressing the optic nerve. For example, severe dysthyroid eye disease and orbital or retro-orbital tumours may present in this way. Bitemporal hemianopia (bilateral loss of part or all of the temporal fields of vision), often asymmetrical or incongruous, is a major feature of suprasellar extension of pituitary adenomas compressing the optic chiasm, but may occur in other tumours in this location. Double vision (diplopia) on lateral or upward gaze often results from medial or lateral rectus muscle tethering in dysthyroid eye disease. Apparent magnification of vision (macropsia) can occur in hypoglycaemia.

Fasting symptoms

Tachycardia, sweating and tremor occurring intermittently, especially when fasting, are suggestive of hypoglycaemia. These symptoms resemble those associated with the increased sympathetic drive found in states of fear or with excess secretion of noradrenaline (norepinephrine), as in phaeochromocytoma. In severe persistent hypoglycaemia, these symptoms may progress to decreased consciousness. This is a serious emergency implying neuroglycopenia sufficient to impair brain function. Spontaneous or fasting hypoglycaemia may be caused by the following:

- Autonomous insulin production owing to an insulinoma
- Glucocorticoid deficiency, with or without thyroxine and growth hormone deficiency (e.g. primary adrenal failure or hypopituitarism)
- Inappropriate insulin or excessive sulfonylurea drug administration in a diabetic patient
- Rarer causes of hypoglycaemia, for example hepatic failure and rapidly growing malignant lesions, especially thoracic or retroperitoneal

mesothelial tumours secreting proinsulin-like growth factor II.

Cramps and 'pins and needles'

Intermittent cramps and 'pins and needles' (paraesthesiae), especially if bilateral, can be caused by a decreased level of circulating ionized calcium. This may occur in hypoparathyroidism or be associated with a fall in the ionized component of serum calcium because of an increased extracellular pH (alkalosis). The latter may occur with any alkalosis, but is particularly well recognized in hyperventilatory states (respiratory alkalosis) and hypokalaemia (metabolic alkalosis). Refractory cramping symptoms after correction of hypocalcaemia may be owing to an associated hypomagnesaemia. However, the differential diagnosis of paraesthesiae in the hands includes median nerve compression at the wrist (carpal tunnel syndrome), a syndrome usually accompanied by typical sensory and motor disturbance suggestive of a lesion in the median nerve (see Chapter 16). Paraesthesiae in the feet are a common symptom of diabetic peripheral sensory neuropathy.

Nausea

Nausea is a rare symptom of endocrine disease. It is an important presenting feature of adrenal insufficiency, in which typically it is maximal in the morning and may be associated with vomiting. Similar symptoms may occur with severe hypercalcaemia and may be the sole manifestation of this condition. These two conditions should be considered early in the differential diagnosis of a patient presenting with upper gastrointestinal symptoms in the absence of demonstrable structural disease. Occasionally, thyrotoxicosis may present with nausea and vomiting, although looseness of stools is the more common gastrointestinal manifestation of this condition.

Dysphagia

Difficulty in swallowing is an unusual manifestation of endocrine disease, but it may be the presenting feature of multinodular thyroid enlargement with retrosternal extension. Smaller goitres only rarely result in dysphagia. Severe hyperthyroidism with generalized weakness may be associated with a reversible myopathy of the pharyngeal musculature and consequent dysphagia.

Neck pain and swelling

Superficial discomfort in the neck may lead to the incidental finding of thyroid enlargement. Modest degrees of thyroid enlargement are very common, whereas pain arising from the thyroid is comparatively unusual. The most common cause of local discomfort and tenderness in the neck is inflammatory lymphadenopathy. Severe tenderness of the thyroid itself, especially when accompanied by fever and signs of thyrotoxicosis, suggests a diagnosis of viral subacute thyroiditis (de Quervain's thyroiditis). Occasionally, autoimmune thyroiditis may give rise to pain and tenderness, which mimics a viral thyroiditis but is less severe. The sudden onset of localized pain and swelling in the thyroid is indicative of bleeding into a pre-existing thyroid nodule and is a recognized complication of multinodular goitre. The symptoms are self-limiting. Painless enlargement of the thyroid gland (goitre) presents either with pressure effects, resulting in dysphagia progressing to tracheal compression and stridor, or cosmetic disturbance. The underlying cause of thyroid enlargement is often difficult to establish. The family history and subsequent investigation may point to autoimmune thyroiditis or dyshormonogenesis. A history of rapid enlargement of the gland, especially in an elderly patient, suggests an anaplastic thyroid carcinoma. Coexisting severe diarrhoea points towards a diagnosis of medullary carcinoma of the thyroid. In the differential diagnosis, goitrogenic drugs, for example lithium, should be considered, as should residence in an iodine-deficient area. Previous exposure to neck irradiation or to radioactive iodine in childhood may also be important.

Impotence

Reduced erectile potency may be a consequence of primary abnormalities, such as the following:
- Decreased blood supply to the penis (e.g. atherosclerosis)
- Neural dysfunction (e.g. autonomic neuropathy complicating diabetes)
- Testosterone deficiency (e.g. hypopituitarism and primary testicular failure)
- Hyperprolactinaemia
- Drug therapy (e.g. certain antihypertensives)
- Psychological factors
- A combination of several causes

It is often difficult to distinguish with certainty between impotence owing to organic factors and that which is psychological, although total erectile failure and the absence of nocturnal and morning erections suggest a physical cause. Impotence in a diabetic patient should not be assumed to be inevitably owing to autonomic neuropathy, and other causes should be considered. Most importantly, it should be recognized that male impotence is often complicated by a psychological disturbance, which may serve to exacerbate the problem.

Gynaecomastia

Gynaecomastia refers to a smooth, firm, mobile, often tender disc of breast tissue under the areola in the male. It should be distinguished from the soft, fatty enlargement often seen in obesity. Mild gynaecomastia (sometimes unilateral or asymmetrical) frequently occurs as a temporary phenomenon in normal puberty and may persist for several years or sometimes indefinitely (termed

Increased oestrogen/testosterone ratio

- Chronic liver disease
- Thyrotoxicosis
- Phenytoin therapy

Androgen receptor antagonists

- Spironolactone, digoxin

Inherited androgen receptor defects

- Testicular feminization syndrome

Testosterone deficiency or oestrogen excess

- Primary and secondary hypogonadism
- Tumour production of human chorionic gonadotrophin (hCG)
- Oestrogen production by Leydig cell tumour of testis

Congenital and hereditary

- X-linked spinal muscular atrophy (Kennedy syndrome)
- Klinefelter's syndrome (karyotype XXY)

persistent pubertal gynaecomastia). In adults, gynaecomastia may result from:
- Excess oestrogen stimulation
- Reduction in circulating androgen
- Antagonism of androgen action
- Androgen insensitivity (Box 19.7)

Therefore, clinical assessment of the patient with gynaecomastia should include an enquiry about any change in libido and an examination of thyroid status, the genitalia, the muscles and for stigmata of chronic liver disease.

Amenorrhoea

The term amenorrhoea describes absence of menstrual periods (menses). Perhaps the most common cause of failure of onset of menses (primary amenorrhoea) is physiological delay of puberty, a diagnosis that can be made only with certainty in retrospect. Important pathological causes include:
- Hypothalamic–pituitary dysfunction (e.g. owing to tumours)
- Ovarian failure (e.g. failure of normal ovarian marked development or cytotoxic chemotherapy)
- Thyroid dysfunction
- Defects in lower genital tract development

Important diagnostic pointers in the history include symptoms suggestive of thyroid disease, or any visual disability that might indicate compression of the optic chiasm by a hypothalamic or pituitary tumour. Secondary amenorrhoea (cessation of previously established menses) has similar causes. In addition, marked weight loss may lead to amenorrhoea, as in anorexia nervosa or inflammatory bowel disease. Amenorrhoea or oligomenorrhoea (infrequent scanty periods) may occur in women subject to excessively rigorous physical training programmes. Normal pregnancy is the most common cause of secondary amenorrhoea.

Galactorrhoea

Occasionally, physiological lactation may persist after breastfeeding has ceased. Inappropriate lactation is usually bilateral. There are a number of causes, which include the following:
- Prolactin-secreting tumours of the pituitary gland
- Idiopathic galactorrhoea, in which there is an apparent increased sensitivity to normal levels of serum prolactin
- Hyperprolactinaemia owing to hypothyroidism
- Hyperprolactinaemia owing to dopamine antagonist drugs (most commonly anti-emetic and anti-psychotic medications)
- Hyperprolactinaemia caused by lactotroph disinhibiting lesions of the hypothalamopituitary region

Inappropriate secretion of breast milk should therefore always prompt enquiry for symptoms referable to the thyroid and pituitary glands, and a thorough drug history should be taken. Even with very high prolactin levels, galactorrhoea is rare in men.

Excess hair growth

An increase in the growth of facial and body hair in adult females is a relatively common symptom that may be caused by increased circulating androgens. However, it is most commonly a normal, constitutional characteristic. Pathological causes of hirsutism include:
- Polycystic ovary syndrome
- Late presentation of congenital adrenal hyperplasia
- Androgen-secreting ovarian or adrenal tumours

The history is vital in the clinical assessment. If the symptoms commenced shortly after the menarche, then a tumour source of androgen is unlikely. A regular menstrual cycle is good evidence against severe androgen excess, but does not exclude polycystic ovary syndrome. Increased libido suggests substantially increased androgen secretion, which may be either ovarian or neoplastic in origin. The latter symptom requires sensitivity to elicit, particularly if a partner is present.

Bowel disturbance

Constipation and abdominal distension may be features of hypothyroidism, hypercalcaemia or panhypopituitarism. Diarrhoea may occur as part of autonomic neuropathy involving the gut in diabetes mellitus. Peptic ulceration may occur in Zollinger–Ellison syndrome, in which gastrin-secreting tumours of the gut result in increased gastric acid secretion. The combination of dyspepsia and marked diarrhoea (the latter owing to inactivation of pancreatic enzymes by excessive acid production) is highly suggestive of Zollinger–Ellison syndrome.

Skin changes

Pallor often occurs in primary testicular failure and in panhypopituitarism. Excessive pigmentation occurs in adrenocorticotrophic hormone (ACTH)-dependent Cushing's syndrome, and increased sebum production causing greasy skin and acne on the face and shoulders may occur in all causes of glucocorticoid excess. In carcinoid tumours of the gut or lung, increased humoral secretion results in a violaceous cyanosis-like skin discolouration. A variegate, patchy rash is a feature of porphyria, an inherited abnormality of haem metabolism. In primary hypoadrenalism, there is increased pigmentation of the conjunctival membrane beneath the eyelids and of the inside of the mouth, the axillae and the palmar skin creases. In hypothyroidism, the skin appears dry, pale, sallow or even slightly yellow; scalp hair is coarse and lateral eyebrow hair is thinned. In hyperthyroidism, the skin is dry and hot, but often not flushed. In hypocalcaemia, the nails are friable. In uraemia, the skin is pale or yellow and slightly pigmented, and in terminal uraemia, a 'uraemic frost' may appear on the skin.

Vitiligo, a patchy depigmentation of the skin, is common in association with many autoimmune disorders, particularly autoimmune hypothyroidism and vitamin B$_{12}$ deficiency.

Family history

The family background in endocrine or metabolic disease may be particularly useful in the evaluation of several of the more common disorders. It is also particularly important in the assessment of less common inherited disorders of metabolism.

Thyroid disease

Autoimmune hypothyroidism and hyperthyroidism frequently show familial aggregation. Dyshormonogenetic goitre is also often inherited. A family history of organ-specific autoimmune disease (e.g. pernicious anaemia, vitiligo, Addison's disease) may also point to an autoimmune aetiology of thyroid disease.

Renal calculi

Primary hyperparathyroidism, an important cause of renal stones, may be familial, occurring either as an isolated disorder or as a part of the syndrome of multiple endocrine neoplasia (type I).

The examination

General assessment

Begin the general assessment by observing the general appearance of the patient. Start by assessing the state of nutrition and by measuring weight and height. Calculate the body mass index (BMI). The distribution of fat should be noted. Deposition of fat in the intra-abdominal, thyrocervical and interscapular regions with relative sparing of the

Figure 19.1 Typical facial appearance of Cushing's syndrome. Note the increased fat deposition and the plethoric appearance. The patient presented with a 2-year history of secondary infertility, easy bruising and central adiposity.

limbs (truncal obesity) is characteristic of Cushing's syndrome and is accompanied by a typical plethoric appearance (Fig. 19.1) because of a combination of increased subcutaneous fat and thinning of the skin.

Patients with growth hormone hypersecretion resulting from somatotroph pituitary adenomas also demonstrate a classic facial appearance, with increased fullness and coarsening of soft tissues, including the lips and tongue which, in patients with long-standing disease, may be accompanied by overgrowth of the zygoma, orbital ridges and mandible (prognathism) (Fig. 19.2). Acromegaly in young people occurring before epiphyseal fusion causes abnormally tall stature (gigantism). Increased adiposity in a child who is growing poorly suggests the possibility of growth hormone deficiency, hypothyroidism, craniopharyngioma or, rarely, Cushing's syndrome. Simple obesity is associated with normal or increased linear growth velocity.

The skeletal proportions should be noted: a long-limbed appearance may indicate delayed epiphyseal fusion owing to hypogonadism (eunuchoidism) or the connective tissue abnormality Marfan syndrome. A eunuchoid body habitus is confirmed by demonstrating that the leg length (top of symphysis pubis to ground) exceeds the sitting height or that the span exceeds the total height. Shortening of the limbs occurs with a variety of skeletal dysplasias.

The cytogenetic disorder Turner syndrome (karyotype 45XO), which is characterized by gonadal dysgenesis and the variable presence of

Figure 19.2   The facial **(A)** and hand **(B)** appearance of acromegaly. There is overgrowth of the facial skeleton, coarsening of features and an increase in soft tissues, most obvious in the hands. The patient had a 4-year history of excessive sweating, increased shoe size, frontal headache and 'pins and needles in fingers'.

other visceral abnormalities, has a typical phenotypic appearance, including short stature, failure of secondary sexual development, decreased or absent secondary sexual hair, an increase in the normal angulation between the humerus and the lower arm, a low posterior hairline and an exaggerated fold of skin between the neck and shoulder. It is most important that accurate wall-mounted stadiometers be used in the assessment of normal growth and its possible disorders.

Figure 19.3   The hands in pseudohypoparathyroidism. Note the characteristic shortening of the fourth and fifth metacarpals.

Figure 19.4   Circumoral pigmentation in a patient with hypersecretion of ACTH.

The hands should be carefully examined for evidence of finger clubbing which, among other things, may be a rare manifestation of thyrotoxic Graves' disease (called thyroid acropachy). Palmar erythema may also be found in thyrotoxicosis of any cause as well as in patients with chronic liver disease or rheumatoid arthritis, and in pregnancy.

A unique selective shortening of the fourth and fifth metacarpals may be found as the major somatic manifestation of a group of recessively inherited disorders of parathormone action (pseudohypoparathyroidism; Fig. 19.3).

The skin

Pigmentation, especially buccal, circumoral or palmar, may indicate the increased secretion of ACTH that occurs with adrenal failure (Addison's disease; Fig. 19.4); patches of depigmentation, or vitiligo (Fig. 19.5), may also be found in Addison's disease or other organ-specific autoimmune disorders. Violaceous striae, arising as a result of stretching of thin skin with exposure of the dermal capillary circulation, suggest the possibility of glucocorticoid excess

Figure 19.5 Extensive areas of depigmentation (vitiligo) in a patient with organ-specific autoimmune disease.

Figure 19.7 The facial appearance of hypothyroidism. The patient demonstrates periorbital puffiness and coarsening of scalp hair. (Source: Figure 14.18 in Jarvis C: Physical examination & health assessment, ed 4, Philadelphia, 2004, Saunders, p 295.)

The thyroid

The anatomical landmarks relevant to inspection and palpation of the thyroid are shown in Fig. 19.8. Immediately inferior to the thyroid cartilage (with its superior notch) is the cricoid cartilage, with the thyroid isthmus lying just below in the midline. The right and left lobes of the thyroid curve posterolaterally around the trachea and oesophagus and are partially covered by the sternomastoid muscles. The attachment of the thyroid to the pretracheal fascia dictates that it moves superiorly on swallowing; absence of this movement raises the possibility of an infiltrative thyroid carcinoma. Remember that the right lobe is slightly larger than the left; hence, diffuse thyroid enlargement, as in Graves' disease, is often apparently asymmetrical. There are several methods for examining the thyroid, but a suggested routine is as follows.

Figure 19.6 Violaceous striae typical of Cushing's syndrome.

(Fig. 19.6), and abnormal dryness of the skin and coarseness of the hair are found in hypothyroidism (Fig. 19.7). Localized thickening of the dermis owing to mucopolysaccharide and inflammatory cell deposition, particularly on the anterior aspects of the legs when it is known as pretibial myxoedema, is one of the classic, although relatively rare, extrathyroidal manifestations of Graves' disease.

In females, dermatological examination should also include attention to any abnormality of hair distribution, either excess hair growth in an androgen-dependent distribution (hirsutism) or hair loss in a male pattern, both of which may indicate increased circulating androgen and should prompt examination for evidence of virilization (see below).

With the patient's neck slightly extended, inspect the area below the cricoid cartilage. Ask him to take a sip of water, extend the neck again and swallow. Watch for the superior movement of the gland, carefully noting its contour and any asymmetry.

Thyroid palpation is best carried out from behind, with the patient's neck slightly extended, but not so much that the neck musculature is tightened. This may feel awkward initially, but with time and practice it will become more comfortable. Have a glass of water available throughout the examination so the patient may take repeated sips and swallow, as necessary. Position both hands to encircle the neck (see Fig. 19.8A) with the fingers slightly flexed, such that the tips of the index fingers lie just below the cricoid in order to palpate the isthmus. Now rotate the fingers down and slightly laterally in order to feel the lateral lobes, including the inferior border (see Fig. 19.8B). The anterior surface of each lobe should be no larger than the terminal phalanx of the patient's thumb.

The following points should be addressed:

- Is the thyroid diffusely enlarged, as in thyroid-stimulating hormone (TSH)-mediated or autoimmune enlargement (see Fig. 19.8D)? If

so, is it soft (e.g. dyshormogenesis, diffuse goitre of puberty) or firm/hard (e.g. autoimmune thyroiditis). In general, the firmer the texture of an enlarged thyroid, the more likely is the pathology to be autoimmune.

- Are there two or more identifiable nodules (see Fig. 19.8E, Fig. 19.9)? If so, is the patient thyrotoxic and does the gland extend downward behind the sternum? (If the gland is partially or completely retrosternal, the inferior border may not be palpable or palpable only on swallowing.) Most multinodular goitres are benign, but a history

(A) Feeling the isthmus

(B) Feeling the lateral lobes

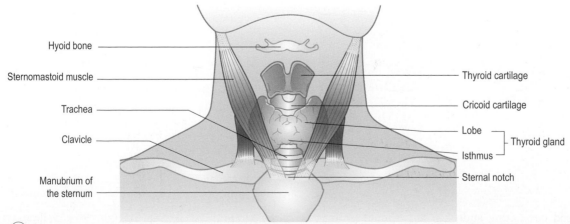

Hyoid bone

Sternomastoid muscle

Trachea

Clavicle

Manubrium of the sternum

Thyroid cartilage

Cricoid cartilage

Lobe ⎤
　　　⎬ Thyroid gland
Isthmus ⎦

Sternal notch

(C)

Figure 19.8 Examination of the thyroid. **(A)** Feeling the isthmus; **(B)** feeling the lateral lobes; **(C)** anatomical landmarks; **(D)** diffuse enlargement; **(E)** multinodular goitre; **(F)** single nodule.

Figure 19.9 A large multinodular goitre. Note the asymmetrical growth of the nodules.

of neck irradiation, enlarged cervical lymph nodes or progressive enlargement of one of the nodules raises the suspicion of malignancy.

- Is the palpable abnormality a single focal nodule (see Fig. 19.8F), suggesting a cyst, adenoma or carcinoma? Rapid growth, hard texture, lack of movement on swallowing (see above), enlarged regional lymphadenopathy, male gender and a history of neck irradiation all increase the probability of malignancy.
- Is the goitre firm and asymmetrical?
- Are there features of local pressure effects or local infiltration (e.g. dysphonia from recurrent laryngeal involvement)?
- Are there weight loss and debility? These suggest anaplastic carcinoma or lymphoma.

- Is there a bruit, indicating increased blood supply? This is frequently found in untreated Graves' disease, but should not be confused with a transmitted bruit from the carotid.

The cardiovascular system

Particular attention should be paid to any postural drop in blood pressure. This may indicate a depleted extracellular fluid volume, for example in patients with adrenal insufficiency, or autonomic dysfunction, the most common cause of which is diabetes mellitus. Additional indicators of the latter include failure of reflex bradycardia during the Valsalva manoeuvre and loss of beat-to-beat variation in cardiac cycle length, as determined by electrocardiography. A hyperdynamic circulation, sinus tachycardia or atrial fibrillation may be found in thyrotoxicosis; this may progress to cardiac decompensation and cardiac failure.

The breasts and genitalia

A detailed description of growth and pubertal development is beyond the scope of this chapter. In brief, however, in the average adolescent female, pubertal development usually commences between the ages of 10 and 11 and takes 3 to 4 years to complete. A growth spurt starts about 1 year before breast development, peak height velocity is reached on average 1 year later and menarche follows in an average of 1 year. In males, pubertal development usually commences between the ages of 11 and 12, takes approximately 3 years to complete and has a characteristic sequence of adrenarche (onset of adrenal androgen secretion with the appearance of secondary sexual hair), testicular development, beginning of pubic hair, beginning of growth spurt and peak height velocity.

The breasts should be examined for mass lesions and, if suggested by the history, for galactorrhoea. In the adolescent female, physiological breast enlargement provides a precise index of pubertal status and signals the onset of the pubertal growth spurt (Tanner stage 3 breast development). Onset of menses (menarche) is a relatively late pubertal event at which point pubertal breast development is virtually complete. In males, any tendency to gynaecomastia should be noted (Fig. 19.10). This may range from minor degrees of subareolar glandular enlargement to substantial breast prominence; breast enlargement associated with generalized adiposity should not be confused with true gynaecomastia.

Genital examination in the male should document testicular volume. This is particularly important in the assessment of pubertal development, for which volume should be measured by comparison with calibrated ovoids (Prader orchidometer; Fig. 19.11). Prepubertal testicular volume is less than 4 ml; increased volume implies pubertal gonadotrophin stimulation. Onset of the pubertal growth spurt in boys is associated with a testicular volume of 10 ml and normal adult testicular volume is in the range of 15 to 25 ml. In the assessment of normal puberty, it is important to establish that growth velocity and gonadal changes (testicular volume or breast stage) are concordant, because a discordance of puberty proceeding ahead of growth implies an abnormal source of sex steroid (e.g. androgen-secreting tumours

Figure 19.11 Prader orchidometer. **(A)** Testicular volume (in ml) may be estimated by comparison with calibrated ellipsoids. **(B)** Gently grip the testis in one hand and compare its volume (including the scrotal skin, but excluding the epididymis) with that of the ellipsoids. The patient shown has a reduced testicular volume of 8 ml, caused by Klinefelter's syndrome; the normal secondary sexual hair is owing to the provision of exogenous testosterone.

Figure 19.10 Gynaecomastia. There is enlargement of both breasts in this man.

Figure 19.12 Corneal calcification (band keratopathy) in a patient with long-standing hyperparathyroidism.

Figure 19.13 Lid retraction and proptosis in a patient with thyrotoxic Graves' disease. In this patient, there had been a 6-month history of effortless weight loss, tremulousness, shortness of breath on exertion and palpitations.

or congenital adrenal hyperplasia). Testicular atrophy in the adult male indicates hypogonadism, owing to primary testicular failure, hypothalamopituitary dysfunction or chronic liver disease. Tumours of Leydig cells are usually palpable and should be sought in any patient with gynaecomastia.

Examination of the external genitalia in the female is important when androgen hypersecretion is suspected. Enlargement of the clitoris is a feature of excess androgen secretion.

Ambiguity of the external genitalia is indicative of foetal androgen excess in the karyotypic female and of testosterone or dihydrotestosterone deficiency or resistance in the male; these conditions are rare and require specialized investigation.

The eyes

The hypercalcaemic patient should be carefully examined for corneal calcification, evident as a narrow band on the medial or lateral border of the cornea (Fig. 19.12); this usually indicates long-standing hypercalcaemia and a diagnosis of primary hyperparathyroidism.

In patients with thyroid disease, the presence of exophthalmos (proptosis) should be noted. This may be unilateral or bilateral and may be associated with apparent ophthalmoplegia owing to tethering of the extraocular muscles, particularly the medial and inferior rectus muscles, such that diplopia occurs on upward or lateral gaze (dysthyroid eye disease; Fig. 19.13). These ocular signs are especially important in the diagnosis of autoimmune thyroid disease (Graves' disease). Remember that unilateral proptosis may also occur with an orbital tumour. Lid retraction, evident as a wide-eyed staring expression, and lid lag, in which depression of the upper lid lags behind the eye in a downward gaze, are caused by increased activity of the sympathetic innervation of levator palprebae superioris and are not specific to Graves' disease. Any degree of corneal exposure

owing to the failure of complete lid apposition should be documented.

Visual acuity should be measured, both with and without a pinhole, to correct for any refractive error. Reduced acuity may be a feature of optic nerve compression in severe dysthyroid eye disease or of asymmetrical pressure on the optic chiasm owing to hypothalamopituitary space-occupying lesions. In the latter, assessment of the visual fields may reveal a bitemporal hemianopia; this is frequently incomplete and incongruous, reflecting the asymmetrical growth of the tumour. A detailed description of the visual pathways and examination of the visual fields is given in Chapter 16. In the context of suspected pituitary/peripituitary disease, use of a red object (e.g. a hat pin) is preferable to finger movements because this provides a more sensitive marker of early visual pathway compression. Examination of the optic discs with the ophthalmoscope may show papilloedema, indicating recent onset of optic nerve compression, or pallor, indicating neural atrophy resulting from long-standing pressure. In the context of a pituitary mass lesion, pallor of the optic discs suggests that full visual recovery is improbable.

The nervous system

In thyrotoxicosis, examination of the nervous system reveals a rapid fine tremor. Proximal weakness, with or without wasting of the shoulder and hip girdle musculature (proximal myopathy), is a typical feature of thyrotoxicosis, glucocorticoid excess and vitamin D deficiency. Osteomalacic myopathy is often associated with myalgia.

Hypocalcaemia is associated with increased neural excitability, which may be demonstrated by gentle percussion over the proximal part of the facial nerve (as it exits from the parotid gland). The test is positive if this manoeuvre evokes involuntary facial muscular twitching (Chvostek's sign).

Tendon reflexes will be abnormally brisk in patients who are thyrotoxic and may show a slow relaxation phase in hypothyroidism. Both hypothyroidism and acromegaly may give rise to nerve entrapment syndromes, particularly of the median nerve at the wrist (carpal tunnel syndrome).

Investigation

The investigation of endocrine and metabolic disorders usually involves (a) the measurement of electrolytes, minerals, metabolites or hormones in plasma and (b) isotopic, ultrasonographic, radiological or magnetic resonance (MR) imaging of specific endocrine glands. In investigating endocrine disease, one is usually interested in whether a specific gland is overactive or underactive. An important principle of endocrine testing is that if underactivity of a gland is suspected then blood samples taken at a time of day when the hormone level, in health, is maximum are most informative; a good example of this is the measurement of an early morning cortisol to assess adequacy of the hypothalmo-pituitary-adrenal axis given the circadian rhythm of cortisol secretion. Conversely, if overactivity of a gland is suspected, sampling at a time of day when the relevant hormone levels should be minimal provides useful diagnostic information; this explains the common practice of measuring cortisol in blood or saliva at midnight in patients with suspected Cushing's syndrome. For many patients the relevant clinical questions may be answered by basal hormone measurements; for example, serum free thyroxine and TSH in thyrotoxicosis and hypothyroidism. In many instances, however, the lack of a clear distinction between basal hyposecretion, normal secretion and hypersecretion necessitates the use of stimulation and suppression tests. If underperformance of an endocrine gland is suspected and basal testing has not provided sufficient clarity, then a stimulation test may be necessary. If hormonal overproduction is suspected, a suppression test may be needed.

Endocrine stimulation tests

Endocrine stimulation tests are designed to demonstrate how much hormone a gland can secrete in response to a near-maximal stimulus. Examples include the following:

- Insulin tolerance testing, in which carefully controlled insulin-induced hypoglycaemia stimulates hypothalamopituitary secretion measured by serum growth hormone, cortisol and prolactin
- Tetracosactrin testing, in which an injection of a synthetic ACTH analogue is used to assess adrenocortical reserve
- Oral glucose tolerance test, which is an indirect test of insulin secretion and action as determined by the rise and subsequent fall in the plasma glucose level following an oral glucose load

Endocrine suppression tests

Endocrine suppression tests indicate whether a physiological feedback mechanism is intact or if secretion of the hormone in question has become at least partly autonomous. For example, the suppression of plasma cortisol by the synthetic glucocorticoid dexamethasone is incomplete in Cushing's syndrome, and suppression of serum growth hormone by an oral glucose load fails to occur in acromegaly. These tests are needed because of the huge variation in serum levels of cortisol and growth hormone in health, making isolated, random measurements of both almost valueless in diagnosis.

Endocrine imaging

Plain X-ray imaging is of limited value in the investigation of endocrine disorders. However, lateral and anteroposterior views of the pituitary fossa can be useful in demonstrating abnormal calcification in the fossa or gross expansion and erosion of the fossa owing to large intrasellar or suprasellar tumours. Plain abdominal radiology may show renal calcification (nephrocalcinosis; Fig. 19.14) in patients with long-standing hypercalcaemia or renal tubular acidosis.

Figure 19.14 Widespread renal calcification typical of nephrocalcinosis in a patient with long-standing hyperparathyroidism.

Figure 19.15 Axial CT scan of the abdomen in a patient with a right adrenal medullary phaeochromocytoma. Note the extensive tumour mass, with areas of hypodensity indicating episodes of partial tumour infarction.

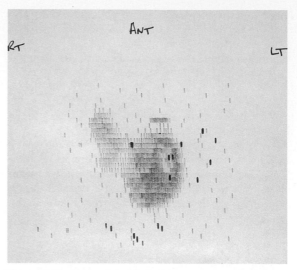

Figure 19.17 Technetium-labelled isotope scan of the thyroid in a patient with a focal thyroid nodule. Note the focal area of uptake corresponding to the palpable lesion, with surrounding inactivity indicating autonomous function within the nodule.

Figure 19.16 Magnetic resonance imaging (sagittal view) of the pituitary, demonstrating a large pituitary adenoma with suprasellar extension.

Computed tomography (CT) imaging is useful in assessing the pituitary, adrenal glands (Fig. 19.15) and thorax. However, MR imaging of the pituitary (Fig. 19.16) offers definite advantages over CT in terms of improved precision in detecting small intrasellar tumours and better definition of the lateral border of the pituitary and the cavernous sinus.

Isotopic imaging is particularly useful for demonstrating autonomous function within endocrine tumours. This technique is applicable to the thyroid gland (radiolabelled pertechnetate; Fig. 19.17), the adrenal medulla (radiolabelled metaiodobenzylguanidine) and parathyroids (combined radiolabelled sesta-methoxy-isobutyl-isonitrile (MIBI) and pertechnetate differential scanning).

Diabetes mellitus

Diabetes is a Greek word meaning 'a passer through; a siphon', and mellitus derives from the Greek word for 'sweet'. The Greeks named it thus because of the excessive amounts of urine produced by sufferers that attracted insects because of its glucose content. The ancient Chinese tested for diabetes by observing whether ants were attracted to a person's urine.

Diabetes mellitus is the most common metabolic disorder encountered in clinical practice. It is strongly linked to obesity. Diabetes mellitus is characterized by abnormal carbohydrate and lipid homoeostasis, leading to elevation in plasma glucose, or hyperglycaemia, and abnormality of serum lipids, or dyslipidaemia. Glucose homoeostasis is modulated mainly by the release of insulin from the islet cells (β cells) of the pancreas. Diabetes develops as a result of a variable combination of absolute insulin deficiency caused by pancreatic islet cell dysfunction and tissue insulin resistance owing to reduced cellular responsiveness to insulin.

The World Health Organization (WHO) has developed a classification of diabetes mellitus based on its pathogenesis (Box 19.8). Type 1 is characterized by absolute insulin deficiency owing to autoimmune-mediated pancreatic islet cell destruction. In contrast, type 2 diabetes is associated with a variable degree of tissue insulin resistance, leading—at least in the early stages—to high plasma insulin levels, then subsequently to relative insulin deficiency as pancreatic islet cell function fails to overcome this resistance. The diagnostic criteria for disorders of glucose metabolism are shown in Box 19.9. Note that glycosuria itself (glucose in the urine) is not a reliable diagnostic test for diabetes mellitus.

Box 19.8 The World Health Organization classification of diabetes mellitus

Type	Common subtypes/pathogenesis	Treatment
Type 1	Destruction of pancreatic islet cells leading to insulin deficiency	Insulin
Type 2	Ranges from predominantly insulin resistance with relative insulin deficiency (often associated with obesity) to predominantly insulin deficiency	Diet/oral hypoglycaemic agents/insulin
Other types		
Genetic defects of β-cell function	Diabetes associated with glucokinase, hepatic nuclear factor (HNF) 1α, HNF1β, HNF4α, Neurod1 and insulin promotor factor mutations (all previously grouped under maturity-onset diabetes of the young (MODY)) Mitochondrial diabetes	Tablets or insulin, depending on genetic defect
Genetic defects of insulin action	Insulin-resistance syndromes (type A insulin resistance, leprechaunism, Rabson-Mendenhall syndrome lipoatrophic diabetes)	Insulin-sensitizing agents and insulin
Diseases of the exocrine pancreas	Fibrocalculous pancreatic diabetes, pancreatitis, trauma/pancreatectomy, neoplasia, cystic fibrosis, haemochromatosis, others	Frequently insulin required
Endocrinopathies	Cushing's syndrome, acromegaly, phaeochromocytoma, glucagonoma, hyperthyroidism, somatostatinoma, others	Treatment of underlying cause
Drug- or chemical-induced	Glucocorticoids, α-adrenergic agonists, β-adrenergic agonists, thiazides, interferon-α therapy	Avoid
Uncommon forms of immune-mediated diabetes	Insulin autoimmune syndrome (antibodies to insulin), anti-insulin receptor antibodies, 'stiff man' syndrome	Variable
Other genetic syndromes associated with diabetes	Down's syndrome, Friedreich's ataxia, Huntington's chorea, Klinefelter's syndrome, Lawrence-Moon-Biedl syndrome, myotonic dystrophy, porphyria, Prader-Willi syndrome, Turner's syndrome, Wolfram's syndrome	Variable
Gestational diabetes		Diet/insulin
Hybrid forms of diabetes	Slowly evolving immune-mediated diabetes of adults Ketosis prone type 2	

Box 19.9 World Health Organization criteria for diagnosis of diabetes mellitus

	Fasting plasma glucose (mmol/l)		2-hour plasma glucose (mmol/l)	Random plasma glucose (mmol/l)	Glycated haemoglobin (mmol/mol (%))
Diabetes mellitus	≥7.0	or	≥11.1	≥11.1	>48 [6.5] (if asymptomatic should be repeated)
Impaired glucose tolerance (IGT)	<7.0	and	Between 7.8 and 11.0	–	42–47 [6.1–6.4] – pre-diabetes
Impaired fasting glucose (IFG)	Between 6.1 and 6.9	and	<7.8	–	

Presenting symptoms of diabetes

Many people with type 2 diabetes may be asymptomatic at diagnosis, for example by routine screening of blood or urine, when there may be only mildly increased levels of hyperglycaemia. Once diagnosed, however, many patients do admit to some long-standing, often mild symptoms. Acute metabolic decompensation, leading to marked hyperglycaemia, occurs infrequently.

In contrast, type 1 diabetes is often abrupt in onset, and characterized by severe hyperglycaemia with acute life-threatening decompensation (diabetic ketoacidosis).

The cardinal symptoms of diabetes mellitus are unintentional (effortless) weight loss, polyuria and polydipsia, and their presence should always result in an immediate test for blood glucose and urine for ketones.

Polyuria, polydipsia and nocturia

Acute hyperglycaemia causes polyuria and polydipsia. These presenting symptoms of diabetes mellitus are also termed 'osmotic symptoms'. Raised plasma glucose leads to increased renal tubular delivery of glucose, which then exceeds the resorptive capacity of the renal tubule, leading to glycosuria. Therefore, despite hyperglycaemia, people with an increased renal threshold for glucose may have no osmotic symptoms. Conversely, people with a low renal threshold for glucose may have glycosuria despite being normoglycaemic. For this reason, glycosuria is an unreliable feature in the diagnosis of diabetes mellitus. Nocturia is also common in patients presenting with osmotic symptoms of diabetes, and enquiry regarding the frequency of passing urine at night can be helpful in evaluating symptoms.

Weight loss and lethargy

Loss of more than 5% of total body weight should be considered clinically important in a person not deliberately attempting to lose weight. Weight loss is a common presenting symptom in people with type 1 diabetes and occasionally in type 2 diabetes with marked hyperglycaemia. Loss of weight in diabetes is predominantly caused by renal glucose loss as a result of lack of insulin to enable cellular uptake of glucose. The weight loss usually occurs despite a normal appetite and dietary intake. This is in contrast to the weight loss of malignant disease, which is usually associated with reduced appetite and oral intake.

Lethargy and fatigue are also common presenting symptoms of diabetes mellitus, particularly type 2, where the symptoms may have been present for some time.

Skin problems

Dermatological manifestations of diabetes are common at diagnosis, especially in patients with poor glycaemic control. Skin infections, such as staphylococcal infection leading to boils, carbuncles or abscesses, which are often recurrent, may occur. Severe infection itself can lead to hyperglycaemia, and a new diagnosis of diabetes should be reconsidered once the acute infection has cleared.

Oral and genital candidiasis can also be presenting features of diabetes mellitus. The presence of the characteristic white plaques on the tongue and oropharynx in a previously healthy person not on antibiotic therapy should alert the physician to the possibility of diabetes mellitus, although other conditions leading to immune paresis, such as HIV infection or haematological malignancy, can also lead to candidiasis. Genital candidiasis in women leads to a thick white discharge and vaginal soreness. Similarly, in men it can lead to a severe balanitis (inflammation of the glans penis). Always check the blood glucose in people with recurrent candidiasis.

Visual disturbance

Hyperglycaemia can lead to blurred vision, owing to osmotic changes within the aqueous humour of the lens of the eye. This can also occur when chronic hyperglycaemia is treated, causing further osmotic shifts in the lens. The symptom usually settles once normoglycaemia is achieved.

Other important aspects of a diabetic history

Family history

A history of diabetes in first-degree relatives is a potent risk factor for diabetes. Type 2 diabetes appears to have a stronger genetic component than type 1, with around a third of patients having a positive family history compared with around 10% of type 1 diabetic patients.

A family history of premature cardiovascular disease is also important. Patients with diabetes are at risk of cardiovascular disease, and this risk is increased when there is a family history of vascular disease in fathers or brothers aged less than 55 years, or mothers or sisters aged less than 65.

Diet and lifestyle history

The cornerstone of management of diabetes is lifestyle; accordingly, periodic reassessment is important. Regularity of meals, the quality and quantity of foods eaten and the frequency of snacks should be known. Enquire about the following:
- Regularity of meals: three meals a day is ideal.
- Content of fatty/greasy foods: particularly discourage saturated (animal) fats, as this type of fat is linked to heart disease.
- Content of fruit and vegetables: at least five portions a day are recommended.
- Content of sugar and sugary foods: avoid carbonated drinks, cakes, sweets and biscuits.
- Content of salt: a high salt intake can lead to hypertension.
- Alcohol intake: a maximum of two units of alcohol per day is recommended.

The smoking history is of paramount importance; smoking with diabetes is strongly linked to cardiovascular disease. Occupational history may be important, because if insulin therapy is required, this may have an impact on legal requirements for driving. Assess physical activity to ascertain whether increased activity may improve glycaemia and weight. At least 30 minutes of moderate exercise per day, for example brisk walking, is recommended.

Assessment of other cardiovascular risk factors

Cardiovascular risk is greatly increased in people with diabetes, and additional cardiovascular risk factors multiply the risk. Thus, any history of hypertension, hyperlipidaemia or previous vascular disease (cerebro-, cardio- or peripheral vascular) should be noted. Take a full medication history, including the use of antiplatelet, antihypertensive and lipid-lowering drugs.

Home glucose testing

In a patient previously diagnosed with diabetes, assess his self-monitoring of glucose. This will enable a reasonable judgement of glycaemic control. Self-monitoring can be done by home capillary blood testing or by urine testing for glycosuria.

Insulin injections

In patients taking insulin, it is important to ascertain whether the patient self-injects, the delivery device used (disposable pen, cartridge pen or syringe/vial), the sites chosen and whether they experience any problems.

Symptoms of complications of diabetes

Chronic complications of diabetes mellitus can be subdivided usefully into large blood vessels (macrovascular), small blood vessels (microvascular) and others (Box 19.10)

Symptoms of macrovascular disease

The features of ischaemic heart disease are described elsewhere (see Chapter 13). People with diabetes have fewer, less severe symptomatic chest pains, possibly owing to autonomic neuropathy leading to reduced deep pain sensation—so-called 'silent ischaemia'. Thus, the only symptom of ischaemic heart disease in a diabetic patient may be breathlessness.

Peripheral vascular disease presents with claudication. In addition, in patients with diabetes, a combination of peripheral neuropathy and peripheral vascular disease can lead to foot ulceration, particularly at sites of pressure (Fig. 19.18).

Cerebrovascular disease in diabetic patients can present with any stroke syndrome (see Chapter 16). Transient ischaemic attacks are common.

Symptoms of microvascular disease

Diabetic retinopathy is frequently asymptomatic until it causes significant visual loss, which may be acute in onset (e.g. because of a sudden retinal haemorrhage) or insidious (e.g. because of cataract or maculopathy). Diabetic nephropathy is similarly asymptomatic until renal dysfunction becomes so severe that uraemia ensues (see Chapter 17). Uraemic symptoms include fatigue, breathlessness and tachypnoea, pleuritic chest pain owing to pericarditis and pruritus. Heavy proteinuria may lead to the development of a nephrotic syndrome.

In contrast, diabetic neuropathy can manifest in a number of ways. Chronic peripheral sensory

Box 19.10	Chronic complications of diabetes	
Macrovascular	Coronary artery disease Peripheral vascular disease Cerebrovascular disease	
Microvascular	Retinopathy	Non-proliferative (mild, moderate and severe) Proliferative Maculopathy
	Neuropathy	Peripheral sensory neuropathy Autonomic neuropathy Mononeuropathy Proximal motor neuropathy
	Nephropathy	
Other	Dermatological	Diabetic dermopathy Necrobiosis lipoidica diabeticorum Bullosis diabeticorum Granuloma annulare Acanthosis nigricans
	Rheumatological	Diabetic cheiroarthropathy Flexor tendinopathy Adhesive capsulitis Diabetic osteoarthropathy Charcot neuroarthropathy Diffuse idiopathic skeletal hyperostosis
	Hepatic	Non-alcoholic steatohepatitis

Figure 19.18   Diabetic neuropathic ulcer in a patient with Charcot neuroarthropathy.

Figure 19.19 Diabetic amyotrophy. Note the marked wasting of the thigh muscles (Source: Charles D. Forbes and William F. Jackson. Color Atlas and Text of Clinical Medicine. 3 ed. Mosby Ltd. 2003.)

neuropathy is the most common form, affecting around 5% of patients with diabetes. This can present with symptoms varying from numbness, a feeling of 'walking on cotton wool' and paraesthesiae (pins and needles) to burning, sharp and shooting pains. The latter is a feature of selective involvement of small pain fibres. Typically, the symptoms start distally and spread up in a stocking distribution and are characteristically worse at night, frequently leading to insomnia.

Proximal motor neuropathy (diabetic amyotrophy or femoral neuropathy) is uncommon, but is seen predominantly in middle-aged men with type 2 diabetes. The condition is characterized by severe, deep pain and paraesthesiae in the upper anterior thigh, followed by weakness and wasting of the quadriceps muscle (Fig. 19.19). The condition is often unilateral, generally short-lived (around 3 months) and usually resolves spontaneously. Associated weight loss and cachexia are common.

Mononeuropathies, particularly affecting the median nerve of the hand (carpal tunnel syndrome; see Chapter 16), are common in patients with diabetes. This frequently presents with paraesthesiae and numbness in the median nerve distribution of the hand (lateral two-and-half digits) and is again worse at night. Similar symptoms may occur in the foot (tarsal tunnel syndrome). Cranial mononeuropathies

are rare, but palsies of cranial nerves III, VI and VII are seen in patients with diabetes, leading to blurred or double vision owing to ophthalmoplegia or a lower motor neuron facial palsy (see Chapter 16). The pupillomotor fibres are usually spared in diabetic third-nerve palsy.

Diabetes can cause autonomic neuropathy, the symptoms of which can be very troublesome. They include impotence, gustatory sweating (severe facial sweating on tasting food), urinary retention or incontinence, dizziness or syncope owing to postural hypotension, constipation or diarrhoea (so-called diabetic diarrhoea) and recurrent nausea and vomiting owing to diabetic gastroparesis.

Hypoglycaemia

Treatment of diabetes is aimed at reducing symptoms and also the risk of diabetic complications. In attempting to reduce hyperglycaemia using oral hypoglycaemic tablets or insulin therapy, the patient with diabetes is at risk of hypoglycaemia.

Physiological responses to hypoglycaemia start at a plasma glucose of around 3.8 mmol/l, with the release of counter-regulatory hormones such as glucagon or adrenaline (epinephrine). Symptoms of hypoglycaemia normally occur at around this level because of sympathetic overactivation. Such symptoms include sweating, palpitations, hunger, agitation or blurred vision, and most patients recognize them as hypoglycaemia and are able to treat themselves rapidly. A further drop in plasma glucose leads to neuroglycopenic symptoms, in which cerebral glucose is low, leading to impaired intellectual activity or diminished psychomotor skills. Further drops in glucose levels can lead to severe agitation, confusion, coma and epileptiform seizures. The symptoms of hypoglycaemia can be distressing and have a significant adverse impact on quality of life. Loss of awareness of hypoglycaemia is sometimes a problem in diabetic patients with autonomic neuropathy; in insulin-treated diabetes this can lead to unexpected hypoglycaemia. Patients at risk should be warned against driving motor vehicles and taught the early symptoms of hypoglycaemia in order to raise their awareness of this potentially serious complication of therapy.

Examination of the diabetic patient

General assessment

Patients with diabetes can present with acute metabolic decompensation, leading to diabetic ketoacidosis (DKA), hyperosmolar hyperglycaemic syndrome (HHS) or, in treated patients, hypoglycaemia. Thus, it is mandatory for all patients

Box 19.11   The diabetic annual review

History

- Patient concerns
- Events: life and medical
- Glucose diary (urine or blood)
- Current treatment
- Hypoglycaemia
- Driving
- Pregnancy/contraception in women
- Impotence
- Symptoms of coronary artery disease or peripheral vascular disease
- Smoking habit

Examination

- Weight/body mass index
- Blood pressure: erect and supine
- Injection sites
- Urinalysis
- Eye examination
- Foot examination

Tests

- Renal function, liver function
- Glycated haemoglobin (HbA$_{1c}$)
- Lipids
- Urine for albumin excretion

Figure 19.20   Necrobiosis lipoidica diabeticorum.

Figure 19.21   Granuloma annulare. (Courtesy of Dr David Peterson.)

presenting with coma or reduced conscious level to have their blood glucose checked immediately.

Characteristically, the cardinal symptoms of severe polyuria, polydipsia and weight loss will have been present for some time prior to coma; such symptoms should never be ignored in a diabetic person. Patients with acute hyperglycaemic crises are frequently severely dehydrated, with hypotension (including postural hypotension), tachycardia, dry mucous membranes and reduced skin turgor. Other signs of DKA include rapid deep sighing respiration (Kussmaul breathing—a respiratory compensation for metabolic acidosis) and ketones on the breath (a sweet odour reminiscent of nail polish remover). Diabetic ketoacidosis can occasionally present with symptoms of an acute abdomen.

In the non-acute setting, it is desirable for all patients with diabetes to undergo a full medical assessment once a year—the so-called diabetic annual review (Box 19.11).

Skin, nails and hands

Dermatological manifestations of diabetes are common. Fungal nail infections, particularly of the feet, are common, as are dermatophyte infections of the skin of the feet (tinea pedis). Staphylococcal skin infections leading to pustules, abscesses or carbuncles can also be seen. Other skin lesions seen in diabetes include necrobiosis lipoidica diabeticorum (Fig. 19.20). This is a rare complication of diabetes, predominantly seen in young women aged 15 to 40 years. This presents as a painless red macule, usually over the anterior shin, which then heals with scarring to form a yellowish/brown lesion. The condition can be unsightly, and little effective treatment is available. Vitiligo is seen in a small number of patients with type 1 diabetes, reflecting its autoimmune nature.

Diabetic dermopathy is characterized by brown macules on the lower legs that heal to form atrophic, shiny white scars. A further skin lesion seen in patients with diabetes is granuloma annulare, pale, shiny rings and nodules usually seen on the arms or hands (Fig. 19.21). Bullosis diabeticorum is a rare manifestation, characterized by tense blistering, mainly on the feet. Acanthosis nigricans

Figure 19.22 Acanthosis nigricans.

Figure 19.23 Lipohypertrophy. (Courtesy of Dr David Peterson.)

Figure 19.24 Lipoatrophy. (Courtesy of Dr David Peterson.)

Figure 19.25 The prayer sign in diabetic cheiroarthropathy.

Figure 19.26 Tinel's sign in carpal tunnel syndrome: tapping on the median nerve at the wrist induces pain in the median nerve distribution.

injected near fat cells; Fig. 19.23) or lipoatrophy (an allergic response to non-human insulins—now rarely seen) (Fig. 19.24). Continuous glucose monitoring and continuous subcutaneous insulin infusion (insulin pump) devices are increasingly common in people with type 1 diabetes and has transformed the quality of life and susceptibility to dangerous hypoglycaemia in many. The sampling and delivery needles remain in the subcutaneous space for several days at a time and careful inspection of these sites is particularly important.

Diabetic cheiroarthropathy ('stiff hand syndrome' or 'limited joint mobility') is seen in some patients with long-standing diabetes. It is characterized by skin thickening and sclerosis of the tendon sheaths, leading to reduced joint mobility and the characteristic prayer sign (Fig. 19.25). Examination of the hands for signs of carpal tunnel syndrome (see Chapter 16) is important if the patient has suggestive symptoms. Thus, the presence of Tinel's sign

is characterized by a dark velvety appearance in the axillae or neck of people with insulin resistance (Fig. 19.22) and frequently accompanies type 2 diabetes, but may occur in people with insulin resistance in the absence of diabetes.

Diabetic patients treated with insulin should have their injection sites examined for signs of lipohypertrophy (a physiological response to insulin

Figure 19.27 Phalen's sign in carpal tunnel syndrome: hyperflexion of the wrist leads to pain in the median nerve distribution.

Figure 19.29 Diabetic cataract.

Figure 19.28 Corneal arcus and xanthelasmata in a patient with diabetic dyslipidaemia.

Box 19.12	Characteristic features of diabetic retinopathy

Non-proliferative retinopathy

- Microaneurysms
- Dot haemorrhages
- Hard exudates (lipid deposits) not involving the macula

Mild

- <5 microaneurysms
- Haemorrhages and/or exudates

Moderate

- Extensive (>5) blot haemorrhages and/or microaneurysms and/or cotton wool spots (retinal ischaemia)
- Venous beading
- Looping or reduplication
- Intraretinal microvascular anomaly (IRMA)

Severe

- Intraretinal deep blocked haemorrhages in four quadrants
- Venous beading in two quadrants
- Severe IRMA in one quadrant

Proliferative retinopathy

- New vessels on disc (NVD) or elsewhere (NVE)

Maculopathy

- Any retinopathy 1 disc diameter around the macula
- Focal or exudative maculopathy
- Diffuse
- Ischaemic

(Fig. 19.26) and Phalen's sign (Fig. 19.27) should be sought. Thenar eminence wasting may also be seen.

Eyes

Examination of the eyes is mandatory in patients with diabetes. External examination may indicate signs of dyslipidaemia (corneal arcus and xanthelasmata; Fig. 19.28). A reduced pupillary response to light may indicate autonomic neuropathy. Visual acuity should be assessed yearly with a Snellen chart, and unexplained loss of acuity should be investigated. Fundoscopy should be undertaken with pharmacological dilatation of the pupils in order to obtain an adequate view. Loss of the red reflex on fundoscopy may indicate cataract formation, and the lens should be assessed for opacities (Fig. 19.29). The vitreous and retina should be examined carefully, starting from the optic disc and radiating into each quadrant of the eye. The macula is examined last, because this can be quite uncomfortable for the patient. The use of green light may aid the detection of microaneurysms. Ideally, all patients with diabetes should have annual fundal photography. A classification of diabetic retinopathy is shown in Box 19.12 (Figs 19.30–19.34).

Cardiovascular system

Examination of the heart and vasculature is important in patients with diabetes. Palpation of peripheral pulses, especially of the feet, is extremely important,

Figure 19.30 Background retinopathy (dot haemorrhages and microaneurysms) in the inferior nasal region. (Courtesy of Dr Paul Dodson.)

Figure 19.31 Preproliferative changes with multiple dot and blot haemorrhages and cotton wool spots. (Courtesy of Dr Paul Dodson.)

Figure 19.32 Retinal haemorrhage owing to new vessel formation in severe proliferative retinopathy. (Courtesy of Dr Paul Dodson.)

Figure 19.33 New vessel formation and laser photocoagulation burns in severe proliferative retinopathy. (Courtesy of Dr Paul Dodson.)

Figure 19.34 Exudative diabetic maculopathy. (Courtesy of Dr Paul Dodson.)

in patients with diabetes) or postural hypotension (drop in systolic BP >20 mmHg on standing). A resting tachycardia, loss of sinus arrhythmia (reflex bradycardia on expiration) and loss of reflex bradycardia during a Valsalva manoeuvre can indicate autonomic neuropathy, although these are best assessed by electrocardiography (ECG).

Feet

The feet of patients with diabetes should be examined at least once a year. Signs of deformity; callus (a sign of excessive pressure at this site); fungal infection, especially between the toes; nail care and ulceration should be carefully assessed. Peripheral pulses and nail-fold refill should be assessed for signs of peripheral vascular disease. Nerve function should be assessed by testing vibration sense at the great toe, medial malleolus and knee, and testing fine touch on the toes, metatarsal heads, heels and dorsum of the feet with a 10-g monofilament (Semmes Weinstein monofilament) (Fig. 19.35). Loss of ankle jerks

as is auscultation of the carotid and femoral arteries to detect bruits. Blood pressure should be measured frequently in patients with diabetes to detect hypertension (classed at >140/80 mmHg

Figure 19.35 Testing for neuropathy using a Semmes Weinstein monofilament giving standard 10 g of fine touch.

is also a sign of early diabetic peripheral sensory neuropathy.

A complication of diabetic peripheral neuropathy is the neuropathic joint—Charcot neuroarthropathy (see Fig. 19.18). This usually affects the ankle and presents with a painless, swollen, hot red joint, sometimes with a history of minor local trauma. The natural history is of progressive deformity until the process settles, usually over a few months. Untreated, the joint develops severe deformity, which then puts the foot at high risk of ulceration, infection and amputation. Treatment is with immobilization in a plaster-cast boot and intravenous bisphosphonates.

Diabetic patients with signs of peripheral vascular disease or peripheral neuropathy, even if asymptomatic, should be classified as at high risk for ulceration and be given careful education on foot care by a podiatrist.

Investigation

Diagnosis of diabetes is based on a fasting plasma glucose, oral glucose tolerance test (OGTT) or glycated haemoglobin (HbA_{1c}) using the WHO criteria (see Box 19.9). Although clinically it is relatively simple to distinguish between type 1 and type 2 diabetes, occasionally the diagnosis is not clear, especially in younger-onset type 2 diabetes without a family history. In these circumstances, the use of immunological tests, such as anti-islet cell (ICA), anti-glutamic acid decarboxylase (GAD), anti-zinc transporter 8 (ZnT8) or anti-islet antigen-2 (IA2) antibody, may be helpful. Positivity of either is a good indicator of autoimmune islet cell destruction (and hence probable type 1 diabetes), insulin deficiency and a subsequent requirement for insulin therapy. Measurement of C-peptide may also be helpful; this is the connecting peptide that joins the A and B chains of insulin in the proinsulin molecule. Insulin and C-peptide are secreted in equimolar amounts, but a combination of its longer half-life and the fact that the liver metabolizes large amounts of portal vein insulin, but not C-peptide, dictates that it is a good measure of endogenous insulin secretory capacity. Close to the diagnosis of type 1 diabetes when there may be some, but reduced, insulin secretion, levels of C-peptide can overlap with those seen in type 2 diabetes. However, 3 to 5 years after the diagnosis, if there is still diagnostic uncertainty between type 1, type 2 or monogenic diabetes, measurement of C-peptide may be extremely helpful because low-undetectable levels confirm the absolute need for insulin replacement therapy.

In acute hyperglycaemic decompensation of diabetes, urgent investigations are required, including a laboratory glucose estimation, assessment of renal function (urea and electrolytes), urinalysis testing for ketones and glucose and arterial blood gas assessment to determine pH and bicarbonate level. A search for precipitating causes should be undertaken, including a chest radiograph, ECG, white cell count and, in younger women, a pregnancy test.

To reduce the risk of chronic complications, it is important to ensure a full biochemical assessment is undertaken yearly as part of an annual diabetic review. Renal and liver function should be checked, along with assessment of urine albumin excretion. Glycaemic control can be assessed using the HbA_{1c}, which is well correlated to prevailing glycaemic control over the preceding 10 to 12 weeks. Glycaemic targets are individualized according to the patient's age, comorbid conditions, risk of hypoglycaemia and the patient's own preferences. An HbA_{1c} less than 53 mmol/mol (7.0%) is generally deemed to show acceptable glycaemic control. Lipid profile (cholesterol, triglycerides, low-density lipoprotein (LDL) cholesterol and high-density lipoprotein (HDL) cholesterol) should be checked yearly.

Communication, phraseology and mental health

Diabetes is a lifelong condition, with relentless self-care requirements, from which there are no holidays. Maintaining euglycaemia whilst avoiding hypoglycaemia is extremely difficult, particularly in type 1 diabetes, and oscillations in blood glucose can be very dispiriting. Although the long-term outcome studies in diabetes relate almost exclusively to prevailing levels of HbA_{1c}, this can sometimes translate into this value forming the sole focus of the clinical interaction, with the unintended consequence that the person with diabetes feels 'adversely judged' if the result is unfavourable. Be careful when presenting cases to colleagues and avoid phrases such as 'poorly controlled diabetic' or 'frequent flyer' if someone has repeated admissions to hospital. People live with diabetes; they are not 'diabetics'. Always remember that most people with diabetes are likely to have more experience and understanding of the condition than you.

Depression, eating disorders and anxiety are more common in people with diabetes than in the background population. The interaction between insulin replacement therapy and body weight has potential consequences for mental health and self-esteem. Insulin is an anabolic hormone and its deliberate omission or restriction by people with type 1 diabetes can sometimes be used as a strategy for weight control. Many experienced diabetes physicians make use of the diabetes distress scale: a clinical instrument for opening a conversation with a person with diabetes that uses a 17-item scale to capture four critical dimensions of distress: emotional burden, regimen distress, interpersonal distress and physician distress. Others take a less structured approach and simply start the consultation with an open-ended question such as: 'Before we get on to the glucose measurements, how is life in general?' Even if the person with diabetes is coping well and has no mental health issues, he will appreciate that you understand living with diabetes is hard work.

Lipid disorders

The two circulating lipids, cholesterol and triglyceride, are transported within lipoproteins in the circulation. The apolipoproteins over the surface of these molecules enable their recognition by cells in organs such as the liver. Lipid disorders, which are common, contribute significantly to the burden of cardiovascular disease. Primary lipid disorders are usually inherited, whereas secondary disorders are acquired as a result of other medical disorders, such as thyroid disease, diabetes, liver disease, nephrotic syndrome or alcohol excess.

History

Lipid disorders rarely cause significant symptoms, unless the patient presents with an acute feature, such as acute pancreatitis or myocardial infarction. Thus, any previous history of vascular disease or acute abdominal pain should be sought. Acute pancreatitis, a rare complication of severe hypertriglyceridaemia, presents with acute, severe, generalized abdominal pain. Although alcohol and cholelithiasis are the two most common causes of acute pancreatitis, hypertriglyceridaemia is a well-recognized and easily overlooked cause of the condition; any patient presenting with acute pancreatitis should have his serum lipids checked.

In the assessment of patients with lipid disorders, it is important to enquire about symptoms of ischaemic heart disease (chest pain history, admissions for ischaemic heart disease and any cardiological/cardiothoracic interventions), peripheral vascular disease (intermittent claudication) and

Figure 19.36   Tendon xanthoma of the hands. (Courtesy of Dr David Peterson.)

cerebrovascular disease (transient ischaemic attacks, amaurosis fugax and strokes). Other cardiovascular risk factors should also be assessed. The smoking history is very important and a family history of premature vascular disease (under the age of 55 years) should be carefully sought. In familial hypercholesterolaemia, half of men and a fifth of women die before the age of 60 from coronary artery disease. Possible symptoms of secondary causes should also be assessed. Thus, symptoms of hypothyroidism (above), diabetes (above), renal failure or nephrotic syndrome (see Chapter 17) and liver disease (see Chapter 14) should be sought. Alcohol intake and dietary history should also be assessed.

Examination

The diagnostic hallmark of familial hyper-cholesterolaemia is tendon xanthomata. These are localized infiltrates of lipid-containing macrophages that resemble atherosclerotic plaques; they develop from the third decade onwards. The most common sites are the Achilles tendon and the extensor tendons of the hands, particularly over the knuckles (Fig. 19.36). Other sites include the tibial tuberosities, at the site of insertion of the patellar tendon (subperiosteal xanthomata) or at the triceps tendon at the elbow.

As the cholesterol deposition is deep within the tendon and the swelling is fibrous, tendon xanthomata are felt as hard nodules along the length of the tendon. They occasionally become inflamed, and a tenosynovitis develops. On the extensor surface of the hands, they may overlie the knuckle and be very hard and quite easy to miss.

Xanthelasmata are deposits of lipid in the skin of the eyelids, more commonly the upper rather than the lower (see Fig. 19.28). Although a dramatic sign, they are not present in the majority of patients with familial hypercholesterolaemia. More common is a corneal arcus, seen as a rim of lipid deposit around the iris (see Fig. 19.28). This can be seen at any age, although it is more common in older people;

Figure 19.37   Eruptive xanthomata in severe hypertriglyceridaemia. (Courtesy of Dr David Peterson.)

Figure 19.38   Lipaemia retinalis. (Courtesy of Dr Paul Dodson.)

only in the minority is this sign associated with hypercholesterolaemia.

The characteristic sign of hypertriglyceridaemia is eruptive xanthomata (Fig. 19.37). These are yellow nodules or papules that usually appear on the extensor surface of the elbows, knees, buttocks and back. Striate palmar xanthomas are yellowish discolouration of the skin creases, usually seen best in the hands; they are caused by hypertriglyceridaemia. In severe forms of hypertriglyceridaemia, hepatosplenomegaly may be seen. Fundoscopy in severe hypertriglyceridaemia may show lipaemia retinalis, characterized by optic pallor and the retinal vessels appearing white (Fig. 19.38).

A careful cardiovascular examination should be performed in all patients with significant hyperlipidaemia, including a search for carotid or femoral bruits and signs of peripheral vascular disease. Patients with homozygous familial hypercholesterolaemia may have signs of aortic stenosis.

Investigation

All patients with lipid disorders should undergo a fasting lipid profile, composed of total cholesterol, LDL cholesterol, HDL cholesterol and triglycerides. In severe hypertriglyceridaemia, the serum may become turbid and take on the appearance of milk. Investigations to exclude secondary causes should include thyroid, liver and renal function and fasting glucose. Resting or exercise ECG may be checked to look for signs of ischaemic heart disease. Genotyping to determine the type of familial lipid abnormality may be required, especially for familial hypercholesterolaemia, although usually this is available only in specialist centres.

Acute pancreatitis can be diagnosed using serum amylase or lipase, which is frequently very elevated in the condition. In severe hypertriglyceridaemia, however, falsely low serum amylase can lead to diagnostic confusion, because triglycerides interfere with the amylase/lipase assay. Severe hypertriglyceridaemia can lead to a pseudohyponatraemia, and care should be exercised when interpreting serum sodium levels in the condition.

Skin, nails and hair | 20

Rino Cerio

Introduction

The skin is the largest organ in the human body. Forming a major interface between man and his environment, it covers an area of approximately 2 m and weighs about 4 kg. The structure of human skin is complex (Figs 20.1 and 20.2), consisting of four distinct layers and tissue components with many important functions (Box 20.1). Reactions may occur in any of the components of human skin and their clinical manifestations reflect, among other factors, the skin level in which they occur, and sometimes they act as a 'window' of systemic changes elsewhere in the body, e.g. medical conditions discussed later in the chapter, such as those associated with pruritus (see Box 20.9), systemic causes of erythema nodosum (see Box 20.10) or paraneoplastic skin conditions (Box 20.2).

The accurate diagnosis of most skin lesions requires an adequate history, careful examination of the patient and, occasionally, laboratory investigation, but dermatology is predominantly a visual specialty.

History

Detailed information should be sought concerning the present skin condition. This should include the site of onset, mode of spread and duration of the disorder. Any personal history or family history of skin disease, including skin cancer and atopy (an allergic skin reaction becoming apparent more or less immediately on contact), is important. Previous medical conditions should be noted and a full drug history obtained, including the use of over-the-counter and other preparations. The social and occupational history and, in some circumstances, details of recent travel, environmental exposure, especially sunshine and artificial ultraviolet light, and sexual activity are often important (Box 20.3).

Examination

The whole skin, including hair, nails and assessable mucosae, should be fully inspected (preferably in natural light), but the patient's modesty should be protected. Sometimes a magnifying lens or dermatoscope is useful.

Colour and pigmentation

Before inspecting any rash or lesion, note the colour of the skin. Normal skin colour varies, depending on lifestyle and light exposure as well as constitutional and ethnic factors.

Pallor can have many causes. It may be:

- Temporary, owing to shock, haemorrhage or intense emotion
- Persistent, owing to anaemia or peripheral vasoconstriction

Vasoconstriction is seen in patients with severe atopy—an inherited susceptibility to asthma, eczema and hay fever. Pallor is a feature of anaemia, but not all pale persons are anaemic; conjunctival and mucosal colour is a better indication of anaemia than skin colour. A pale skin resulting from diminished pigment occurs with hypopituitarism and hypogonadism.

Normal skin contains varying amounts of brown melanin pigment. Brown pigmentation owing to deposited haemosiderin is always pathological. Albinism is an inherited generalized absence of pigment in the skin; a localized form is known as piebaldism. Patches of white and darkly pigmented skin (vitiligo) (Fig. 20.3) are owing to a local and complete absence of melanocytes. Several autoimmune endocrine disorders are associated with vitiligo.

Abnormal redness of the skin (erythema) is seen after overheating, extreme exertion and sunburn and in febrile, exanthematous and inflammatory skin diseases. Flushing is a striking redness, usually of the face and neck, which may be transient or persistent. Local redness may be caused by telangiectasia, especially on the face. Cyanosis is a blue or purple-blue tint caused by the presence of excessive reduced haemoglobin, either locally, as in impaired peripheral circulation, or generally, when oxygenation of the blood is defective. The skin colour in methaemoglobinaemia is more leaden than in ordinary cyanosis; it is caused by drugs, such as dapsone, and certain poisons.

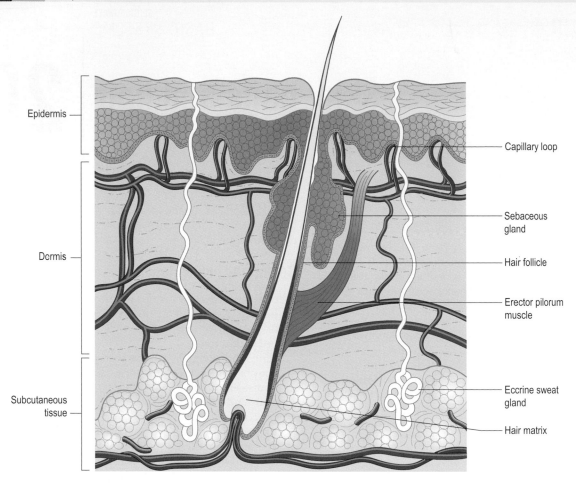

Figure 20.1 The anatomy of the full thickness of the skin in section.

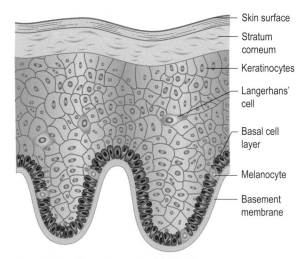

Figure 20.2 The anatomy of the epidermis.

Jaundice varies from the subicteric lemon-yellow tints seen in pernicious anaemia and haemolytic jaundice to various shades of yellow, orange or dark olive-green in obstructive jaundice. Jaundice, which stains the conjunctivae, must be distinguished from the rare orange-yellow of carotenaemia, which does

---

| Box 20.1 | Functions of the human skin |

- Protection: physical, chemical, infection—immune and innate
- Physiological: homoeostasis of electrolytes, water and protein
- Thermoregulation
- Sensation: specialized nerve endings—pain, touch and temperature
- Lubrication and waterproofing: sebum
- Immunological reactions: Langerhans' cells, lymphocytes, macrophages
- Wound healing
- Ultraviolet-induced vitamin D synthesis
- Body odour: apocrine glands
- Psychosocial: cosmetic

---

not. Slight degrees of jaundice cannot be seen in artificial light.

Increased pigmentation may be racial, owing to sunburn or connected with various diseases. In Addison's disease, a brown or dark-brown pigmentation affects exposed parts and parts not normally pigmented, such as the axillae and the

Box 20.2	Paraneoplastic skin disorders
Dermatosis	**Associated tumour**
Dermatomyositis	Lung, gastrointestinal (GI) tract, genitourinary tract
Acanthosis nigricans	GI tract, lung, liver
Paget's disease of the nipple/extra-mammary Paget's disease of the perineum	Adenocarcinoma
Erythroderma	Haematological
Tylosis-thickening of palms and soles	Oesophageal carcinoma
Ichthyosis	Lymphoma
Erythema gyratum repens	Lung, breast
Necrolytic migratory erythema	Glucagonoma

Figure 20.3   Vitiligo, a disorder of cutaneous pigmentation that is often autoimmune in origin and associated with other autoimmune disorders.

Box 20.3	Approach to dermatological patient history

- Time course of skin eruption
- Distribution of lesions including initially
- Symptoms: pruritus
- Family history: atopy and psoriasis
- Drug/allergy history
- Past medical history
- Contacts: family and partners
- Provoking factors: sunlight and foods
- Previous and current treatments

Figure 20.4   Flat-topped papules of lichen planus.

palmar creases; the lips and mouth may exhibit dark bluish-black areas. Note, however, that mucosal pigmentation is a normal finding in a substantial proportion of black patients.

More or less generalized pigmentation may also be seen in the following:

- Haemochromatosis, in which the skin has a peculiar greyish-bronze colour with a metallic sheen, owing to excessive melanin and iron pigment
- Chronic arsenic poisoning, in which the skin is finely dappled affecting covered more than exposed parts
- Argyria, in which the deposition of silver in the skin produces a diffuse slate-grey hue
- The cachexia of advanced malignant disease

In pregnancy, there may be pigmentation of the nipples and areolae, of the linea alba and sometimes a mask-like pigmentation of the face (chloasma). Chloasma may also be induced by oral contraceptives containing oestrogen. A similar condition, melasma, may be seen in Asian and Afro-Caribbean males.

Localized pigmentation may be seen in pellagra and in scars of various kinds, particularly those owing to X-irradiation therapy. Venous hypertension in the legs is often associated with chronic purpura, leading to haemosiderin pigmentation. The mixture of punctate and fresh purpura and haemosiderin may produce a golden hue on the lower calves and shins. Pigmentation may also occur with chronic infestation by body lice. Erythema ab igne, a reticular pattern of pigmentation, can be seen in patients who use local heat to relieve chronic pain or on the shins of people who habitually sit too near a fire. Livedo reticularis, a web-like pattern of reddish-blue discolouration mostly involving the legs, occurs in autoimmune vasculitis, especially in systemic lupus erythematosus (SLE) and antiphospholipid syndrome, when it is associated with cerebral infarction. The violet-coloured lesions of lichen planus are slightly raised, flat-topped papules (Fig. 20.4). Psoriasis usually presents as a symmetrical plaque on extensor surfaces (Fig. 20.5). Keloid consists of raised and inflamed, overgrown tender scar tissue (Fig. 20.6). Dermatomyositis often produces swelling and heliotrope-coloured erythema of the eyelids without scaling of the skin.

Figure 20.5 Salmon-pink plaque of psoriasis on elbow covered in characteristic silver scale.

Figure 20.6 Multiple keloid scarring of the back caused by acne vulgaris. There is a genetic predisposition to the formation of keloid in scar tissue.

Box 20.4	Primary skin lesions: a glossary of dermatological terms
Macule	Non-palpable area of altered colour
Papule	Palpable elevated small area of skin (<0.5 cm)
Plaque	Palpable flat-topped discoid lesion (>2 cm)
Nodule	Solid palpable lesion within the skin (>0.5 cm)
Papilloma	Pedunculated lesion projecting from the skin
Vesicle	Small fluid-filled blister (<0.5 cm)
Bulla	Large fluid-filled blister (>0.5 cm)
Pustule	Blister containing pus
Wheal	Elevated lesion, often white with red margin owing to dermal oedema
Telangiectasia	Dilatation of superficial blood vessel
Petechiae	Pinhead-sized macules of blood
Purpura	Larger petechiae that do not blanch on pressure
Ecchymosis	Large extravasation of blood in skin (bruise)
Haematoma	Swelling owing to gross bleeding
Poikiloderma	Atrophy, reticulate hyperpigmentation and telangiectasia
Erythema	Redness of the skin
Burrow	Linear or curved elevations of the superficial skin owing to infestation by female scabies mite
Comedo	Dark horny keratin and sebaceous plugs within pilosebaceous openings

Skin lesions and eruptions

Skin eruptions and lesions should be examined with special reference to their morphology, distribution and arrangement. The terminology of skin lesions is summarized in Boxes 20.4 and 20.5. Colour, size, consistency, configuration, margination and surface characteristics should be noted.

Morphology of skin lesions

Inspection and palpation

Assessment of morphology requires visual and tactile examination. Do not be afraid to feel the lesions. You will rarely be exposed to any infection risk, with the exception of herpes simplex, herpes zoster, syphilis, hepatitis B and human immunodeficiency virus (HIV) disease. If these infections are suspected, it is wise to wear disposable plastic gloves when examining open or bleeding cutaneous lesions. Begin with palpation of the skin. Pass the hand gently over

it, pinching it up between the forefinger and thumb, and note the following points:

- Is it smooth or rough, thin or thick?
- Is it dry or moist?
- Is there any visible sweating, either general or local?

The elasticity of the skin should be investigated. If a fold of healthy skin is pinched up, it immediately flattens itself out again when released. Sometimes, however, it only does so very slowly, remaining creased for a considerable time. This is found frequently in healthy old people, but may be an important sign of dehydration, for example after severe vomiting and diarrhoea, or in uncontrolled diabetes mellitus.

Subcutaneous oedema

When oedema is present, firm pressure on the skin with a finger produces a shallow pit that persists for some time. In some cases, especially when the oedema is very long standing, pitting is not found. The best place to look for slight degrees of oedema in cardiac disease is behind the malleoli at the ankles in patients who are ambulant and over the sacrum in

Box 20.5	Secondary skin lesions that evolve from primary lesions
Scale	Loose excess normal and abnormal horny layer
Crust	Dried exudate
Excoriation	A scratch
Lichenification	Thickening of the epidermis with exaggerated skin margin
Fissure	Slit in the skin
Erosion	Partial loss of epidermis which heals without scarring
Ulcer	At least the full thickness of the epidermis is lost. Healing occurs with scarring
Sinus	A cavity or channel that allows the escape of fluid or pus
Scar	Healing by replacement with fibrous tissue
Keloid scar	Excessive scar formation (see Fig. 20.6)
Atrophy	Thinning of the skin owing to shrinkage of epidermis, dermis or subcutaneous fat
Stria	Atrophic pink or white linear lesion owing to changes in connective tissue

Figure 20.7   Hansen's disease. A depigmented area of anaesthetic and slightly pink skin is seen on the exposed cheek. In this lepromatous lesion, acid-fast bacilli were found in scrapings.

those who are confined to bed. The finger pressure should be maintained for 20–30 seconds or slight degrees of oedema will be overlooked. Pitting is minimal or absent in oedema owing to lymphatic obstruction, where the skin is usually thickened and tough.

Subcutaneous emphysema

Air trapped under the skin gives rise to a characteristic crackling sensation on palpation. It starts in, and is usually confined to, the neighbourhood of the air passages. On rare occasions, it may result from the clostridial infection of soft tissues after injury (gas gangrene).

Distribution of skin lesions

Consider the distribution of an eruption by looking at the whole skin surface:

- Is it symmetrical or asymmetrical? Symmetry often implies an internal causation, whereas asymmetry may imply external factors.
- Is the eruption centrifugal (radiating from the centre) or centripetal (radiating to the centre)? Certain common diseases, such as chickenpox and pityriasis rosea, are characteristically centripetal, whereas erythema multiforme and erythema nodosum are centrifugal. Smallpox, now eradicated, was also centrifugal.
- A disease may exhibit a flexor or an extensor bias in its distribution: atopic eczema in childhood is characteristically flexor, whereas psoriasis in adults tends to be extensor.

- Are only exposed areas affected, implicating sunlight or some other external causative factor?
- If sunlight is suspected, are areas normally in shadow involved?
- Are the genitalia involved?
- Localized distributions may point immediately to an external contact as the cause, for example contact dermatitis from nickel earrings, lipstick dermatitis, etc.

Swelling of the eyelids is an important sign. Without redness and scaling, bilateral periorbital oedema may indicate acute nephritis, nephrosis or trichinosis. If there is irritation, contact dermatitis is the probable diagnosis. Dermatomyositis often produces swelling and heliotrope-coloured erythema of the eyelids without scaling of the skin. In Hansen's disease (leprosy), the skin lesions may be depigmented or reddened, with a slightly raised edge; they are also anaesthetic to pinprick testing (Fig. 20.7) and mainly located in skin that is normally cooler than core body temperature.

Configuration of skin lesions

Once the morphology of individual lesions and their distribution has been established, it is useful to describe their configuration on the skin (Box 20.6).

The hair

Hair colour and texture are racial characteristics that are genetically determined. The yellow-brown Mongol race has black straight hair, negroid people have black curly hair and Caucasians have fair, brown, red or black hair. Secondary sexual hair begins to appear at puberty and has characteristic male and female patterns. Androgenic male pattern baldness is genetically determined, but requires adequate levels of circulating androgens for its expression. It occurs in women only in old age.

Growth of hair

Unlike other epithelial mitotic activity that is continuous throughout life, the growth of hair is cyclic (Fig. 20.8), the hair follicle going through alternating phases of growth (anagen) and rest (telogen). Anagen in the scalp lasts 3–5 years; telogen is much shorter, about 3 months. Catagen is the conversion stage from active to resting and it usually lasts a few days. The duration of the anagen phase determines the length to which hair in different body areas can grow. On the scalp, there are on average about 100 000 hairs. The normal scalp may shed as many as 100 hairs every day as a normal consequence of growth cycling. These proportions can be estimated by looking at plucked hairs (trichogram); the 'root' of a telogen hair is non-pigmented and visible as a white, club-like swelling. Normally 85% of scalp hairs are in anagen and 15% in telogen.

Box 20.6	Configuration of individual lesions

- Nummular/discoid
- Round or coin-like
- Annular
- Ring-like
- Circinate
- Circular
- Arcuate
- Curved
- Gyrate/serpiginous
- Wave-like
- Linear
- In a line
- Grouped
- Clustered
- Reticulate
- Net-like

Alopecia

Hair loss (alopecia) has many causes. It is convenient to subdivide alopecia into localized and diffuse types. In addition, the clinician should determine whether the alopecia results in scarring and hence, permanent hair loss (Box 20.7).

Any inflammatory or destructive disease of the scalp skin may destroy hair follicles in its wake. Thus, burns, heavy X-ray irradiation or herpes zoster infection in the first division of the trigeminal nerve may cause scarring and alopecia. Alopecia in the presence of normal scalp skin may be patchy and localized, as in traction alopecia in nervous children, ringworm infections (tinea capitis) or autoimmune alopecia areata. Secondary syphilis is a rare cause of a patchy alopecia with a 'moth-eaten' appearance.

Scalp hair loss at the temples and crown, with the growth of male-type body hair, is characteristic of women with virilizing disorders. Metabolic causes of diffuse hair loss in women include hypothyroidism and severe iron deficiency anaemia. Antimitotic drugs may affect the growing hair follicles, producing a diffuse loss of anagen hairs, which are pigmented throughout their length. Dramatic metabolic upsets, such as childbirth, starvation and severe toxic illnesses, may precipitate follicles into the resting phase, producing an effluvium of telogen hairs 3 months later, when anagen begins again. This is called telogen alopecia. In the autoimmune disorder alopecia totalis (Fig. 20.9), there is complete loss of hair. Self-inflicted traction alopecia (Fig. 20.10) may indicate psychological problems.

The nails

The nails should be examined carefully. The structure of the nail and nail bed is shown in Figs 20.11 and 20.12. The nail consists of a strong,

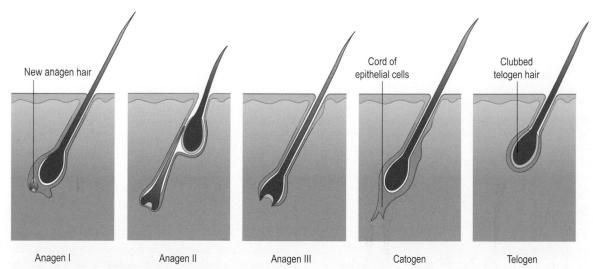

New anagen hair

Cord of epithelial cells

Clubbed telogen hair

Anagen I   Anagen II   Anagen III   Catogen   Telogen

Figure 20.8 Hair follicle growth stages.

Box 20.7	Causes of alopecia

Non-scarring

- Alopecia areata
- Trichotillomania (self-induced hair pulling)
- Traction alopecia
- Scalp ringworm (human)
- Metabolic iron deficiency, hypothyroidism
- Drugs (e.g. heparin, retinoids, chemotherapy)
- Sarcoidosis

Scarring

- Burns, trauma
- Aplasia cutis
- Discoid lupus erythematosus, lichen plakophilins
- Dissecting folliculitis
- Pseudopelade
- Kerion (see Fig. 20.30)
- X-irradiation
- Necrobiosis

Figure 20.10 Traction alopecia in a psychologically troubled patient.

Figure 20.9 Alopecia totalis.

Figure 20.11 Structure of the nail (lateral view).

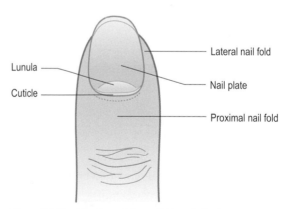

Figure 20.12 Structure of the nail (dorsal view).

relatively inflexible keratinous nail plate over the dorsal surface of the end of each digit, protecting the fingertip.

Nail matrix abnormalities

Thimble pitting of the nails is characteristic of psoriasis (Fig. 20.13), but eczema and alopecia areata may also produce pitting. A severe illness may temporarily arrest nail growth; when growth starts again, transverse ridges develop. These are called Beau's lines and can be used to date the time of onset of an illness. Inflammation of the cuticle or nail fold (chronic paronychia) may produce similar changes. The changes described above arise from disturbance of the nail matrix.

Nail and nail-bed abnormalities

Disturbance of the nail bed may produce thick nails (pachyonychia) or separation of the nail from the bed (onycholysis). This occurs in psoriasis, but may be idiopathic. Long-term tetracyclines may induce separation when the fingers are exposed to strong sunlight (photo-onycholysis). The nail may be destroyed in severe lichen planus (Fig. 20.14) or epidermolysis bullosa (a genetic abnormality in which the skin blisters in response to minor trauma). Nails

Figure 20.13   Psoriasis of the nail beds.

Figure 20.14   Lichen planus, showing longitudinal ridging of the nails and overgrowth of the cuticle on the nail plate (pterygium).

Figure 20.15   Typical heliotrope-coloured erythema seen in dermatomyositis (periungual and Gottron's papules over the knuckles).

Figure 20.16   Yellow nail syndrome in bronchiectasis.

are missing in the inherited nail-patella syndrome. Splinter haemorrhages under the nails may result from trauma, psoriasis, rheumatoid arthritis or other 'collagen vascular' diseases, bacterial endocarditis and trichinosis.

The nails in systemic disease

In long-lasting iron-deficiency states, the fingernails and toenails become soft, thin, brittle and spoon-shaped. They lose their normal transverse convex curvature, becoming flattened or concave (koilonychia). The 'half and half nail', with a white proximal and red or brown distal half, is seen in some patients with chronic renal failure. Whitening of the nail plates may be related to hypoalbuminaemia, as in cirrhosis of the liver (leukonychia). Some drugs, notably antimalarials, antibiotics and phenothiazines, may discolour the nail. Nail-fold telangiectasia or erythema is a useful physical sign in dermatomyositis (Fig. 20.15), systemic sclerosis and systemic lupus erythematosus. In dermatomyositis, the cuticle becomes ragged. In systemic sclerosis, loss of finger pads may lead to curvature of the nail plates. An impaired peripheral circulation, as in Raynaud's phenomenon, can lead to thinning and longitudinal ridging of the nail plate, sometimes with partial onycholysis. In bronchiectasis, the nails may take on a curved, yellow appearance (Fig. 20.16).

Clubbing

Clubbing is probably caused by hypervascularity and the opening of anastomotic channels in the nail bed. Rarely, clubbing may be congenital. The distal end of the digit becomes expanded, with the nail curved excessively in both longitudinal and transverse planes. Viewed from the side, the angle at the nail plate is lost and may exceed 180°. In normal nails, when both thumbnails are placed in apposition, there is a lozenge-shaped gap whereas, in clubbing, there is a reduction in this gap (Schamroth's window test; Fig. 20.17). In hypertrophic pulmonary osteoarthropathy, there is clubbing of the fingers and thickening of the periosteum of the radius, ulna, tibia and fibula, which can be tender. (The causes of clubbing are listed in Box 20.8.)

Cutaneous manifestations of internal disease

Genodermatoses (lesions of inherited origin)

White macules shaped like small ash leaves and present at birth may be the first sign of tuberous

Normal nail

Clubbed nail

Figure 20.17   Schamroth's window test.

Box 20.8	Causes of clubbing of the fingers

Cardiopulmonary disorders

- Severe chronic cyanosis
- Cyanotic congenital heart disease
- Chronic fibrosing alveolitis
- Chronic suppuration in the lungs:
  —Bonchiectasis
  —Empyema
  —Lung abscess
- Carcinoma of the bronchus
- Bacterial endocarditis

Chronic abdominal disorders

- Crohn's disease
- Ulcerative colitis
- Cirrhosis of the liver

sclerosis. Sometimes they are difficult to see by natural light, but show up under ultraviolet light (Wood's light). They should be looked for in infants with seizures. Pigmentation of the lips is a feature of the genetically determined Peutz-Jeghers syndrome, in which multiple polyps of the stomach or colon appear that may later undergo malignant transformation. Café au lait type macules, sometimes multiple, are a common sign of neurofibromatosis (NF). Another valuable sign in von Recklinghausen's neurofibromatosis is bilateral freckling of the axillary skin. The characteristic soft neurofibromata may

Figure 20.18   Discoid lupus erythematosus, showing atrophic scars.

be solitary or a few or hundreds may be scattered over the body. Ichthyosis (scaly fish skin) is usually present from childhood and is genetic. If ichthyosis is acquired in adult life, a search should be made for malignancy or other underlying disease.

Non-organ-specific autoimmune disorders

Several of the so-called collagen vascular diseases show characteristic cutaneous eruptions. Systemic lupus erythematosus, seen in women between puberty and the menopause, may show a symmetrical 'butterfly' erythema of the nose and cheeks. In discoid lupus, the cutaneous lesion is localized (Fig. 20.18). In polyarteritis nodosa, reticular livedo of the limbs with purpura, vasculitic papules and ulceration occurs. In scleroderma (systemic sclerosis), acrosclerosis of the fingertips with scarring, ulceration and calcinosis follows a Raynaud's phenomenon of increasing severity. Dermatomyositis often presents with a heliotrope-coloured discolouration and oedema of the eyelids and with fixed erythema over the dorsa of the knuckles and fingers (see Fig. 20.15) and over the bony points of the shoulders, elbows and legs. There is usually weakness of the proximal limb muscles. Dermatomyositis in the middle-aged is associated with internal malignancy in about 10% of cases.

Skin pigmentation

Acanthosis nigricans is a brownish velvety thickening of the axillae, groins and sides of the neck. Sometimes there is thickening of the palms and soles, and warty excrescences may develop on the skin, eyelids and oral mucosa. In the middle-aged, acanthosis nigricans is strongly associated with internal malignancy, but benign minor forms are seen in obese young women, especially in Arab people, and in children with endocrinopathies characterized by insulin resistance. Patchy depigmented macules which are hypoanaesthetic and associated with enlargement of the peripheral nerves are a feature of certain types of leprosy (Hansen's disease).

Generalized, severe persistent pruritus in the absence of obvious skin disease may be caused by systemic disease (Box 20.9). However, in older people with dry skin, it is common and of no systemic significance. Diabetes mellitus has a number of skin manifestations; of these, pruritus vulvae, pruritus ani, balanoposthitis and angular stomatitis are caused by *Candida* overgrowth. Boils, follicular pustules or ecthyma are staphylococcal in origin. Impetigo and erysipelas, both streptococcal infections, are uncommon (Fig. 20.19). Eruptive xanthomata are a rare feature of uncontrolled diabetes mellitus. Necrobiosis lipoidica diabeticorum (Fig. 20.20) produces reddish-brown plaques, usually on the shins, with central atrophy of the skin. It has to be distinguished from peritibial myxoedema (which is hypertrophic, not atrophic), the dermatoliposclerosis of chronic venous disease in the legs and the epidermal hypertrophy of chronic lymphatic obstruction.

Neuropathic ('perforating') ulcers, which are found on pressure points of the heel, ball of the foot or toes, are characteristically painless. Arteriopathic ulceration resulting from large vessel disease is seen on the foot and on the calves in small vessel disease.

Box 20.9	Causes of pruritus in systemic disease

- Iron deficiency anaemia
- Diabetes mellitus
- Thyrotoxicosis or hypothyroidism
- Chronic renal failure
- Chronic hepatic failure
- Biliary obstruction, including primary biliary cholangitis
- Lymphoma and other internal malignancies
- Drugs (e.g. cocaine, morphine)
- HIV infection
- Polycythemia vera
- Parasites (e.g. onchocerciasis)
- Psychogenic

Spider naevi consist of a central arteriole feeding a cluster of surrounding vessels. Many young people have up to seven naevi on the face, shoulders or arms. In others, pregnancy, the administration of oestrogens (as in oral contraceptives) and liver disease may cause multiple lesions. Pregnancy and liver disease may also produce a blotchy erythema of the thenar and hypothenar eminences ('liver palms'). Leuconychia are seen in liver disease.

Erythema nodosum is a condition in which tender, painful, red nodules appear, typically on the shins. They fade slowly over several weeks, leaving bruising, but never ulcerate. Sarcoidosis, inflammatory bowel disease and drug sensitivity are the most common causes, but other systemic disorders should be considered (Box 20.10).

Xanthomata are yellow or orange papules or nodules in the skin caused by dermal aggregations of lipid-loaded cells. Different patterns of hyperlipoproteinaemia may induce varying patterns of xanthomatosis. Thus, the type Ia (hypercholesterolaemia) pattern typically causes tuberous xanthomata on the extensor aspects of the knees and elbows and on the buttocks, sometimes associated with tendon xanthomata. Widespread eruptive xanthomata are more characteristic of hypertriglyceridaemia. White deposits of lipid (arcus senilis) in the cornea may have a similar explanation, but may be a normal feature in those over 60. Flat lipid deposits around the eyes (xanthelasma) may be caused by hyperlipidaemia, but they are also seen in the middle-aged and elderly without any general metabolic upset.

Carotenaemia produces an orange-yellow colour to the skin, especially of the palms and soles. It occurs in those who eat great quantities of carrots and other vegetables, in hypothyroidism, in diabetic patients and also in those taking β-carotene for the treatment of porphyria.

Figure 20.19 **(A)** Impetigo. **(B)** Erysipelas.

Figure 20.20 Necrobiosis lipoidica diabeticorum.

Box 20.10	Causes of erythema nodosum

- Sarcoidosis
- Drugs (e.g. sulphonamides)
- Streptococcal infection
- Tuberculosis
- Inflammatory bowel disease
- Behçet's disease
- Other infections (e.g. leprosy, systemic mycoses, toxoplasmosis, lymphogranuloma venereum)

Haemorrhage in the skin

Aggregations of extravasated red blood cells in the skin cause purpura (Fig. 20.21). Purpura may punctate from capillary haemorrhage or may form larger macules, depending on the extent of haemorrhage and the size of vessels involved. Palpable purpura should raise suspicion of leucocytoclastic vasculitis. The Hess test for capillary fragility involves deliberately inducing punctate purpura on the forearm by inflating a cuff above the elbow at 100 mmHg for 3 minutes. Sensitivity to drugs such as aspirin may cause widespread 'capillaritis'.

The term ecchymosis implies a bruise, usually with cutaneous and subcutaneous haemorrhage causing a palpable lump. A frank fluctuant collection of blood is a haematoma. Unlike erythema and telangiectasia, purpura cannot be blanched by pressure. It must not be confused with senile haemangioma (cherry angioma or Campbell de Morgan spot), which is common in later life on the trunk and has no pathological significance. Haemorrhage into the thick epidermis of the palm or sole caused by trauma (e.g. 'jogger's heel') may induce brown or almost black macules that take weeks to disappear, inviting confusion with melanoma.

The skin in sexually transmitted diseases

The skin is involved in various sexually transmitted diseases. The primary chancre of syphilis may occur

Figure 20.21 Purpura in Henoch-Schönlein disease.

on the genitalia of either sex, at or near the anus, on the lip or, rarely, elsewhere. The rash of secondary syphilis is brownish-red and maculopapular; it is one of the few rashes involving the palms and soles. It does not itch. Other manifestations of the secondary stage are condylomata lata around the anogenital area and snail-track ulceration and 'mucous patches' in the mouth. There may be low-grade fever, lymphadenopathy and splenomegaly.

Septicaemia is a rare complication of gonorrhoea that occurs particularly in pregnant women presenting with pustular skin lesions. Recurrent type II herpes simplex is common on the penis; it occurs less often on the buttocks, where relapses may be heralded by a radiating neuralgia. Genital viral warts are common in both sexes. They are particularly important in females because evidence indicates that certain viral subtypes are responsible for chronic cervical dysplasia with malignant potential.

HIV-related syndromes have many cutaneous manifestations, including disseminated Kaposi's sarcoma, candidiasis, molluscum contagiosum, seborrhoeic dermatitis, folliculitis and oral hairy leukoplakia (Fig. 20.22).

Viral infection of the skin

Several of the most common viral infections and illnesses of childhood are characterized by fever and a distinctive rash (exanthem), including measles, varicella and rubella. In measles, upper respiratory symptoms are quickly followed by a characteristic maculopapular and erythematous rash. In rubella (German measles), the rash is more transient, with small papules, and associated

Figure 20.22   Hairy leukoplakic.

Figure 20.24   Herpes zoster vesicles on the ear lobe involving the C2 dermatome.

Figure 20.23   Herpes simplex (type I).

with occipital lymphadenopathy and only slight malaise. The exanthem of varicella (chickenpox) is papulovesicular and centripetal, and there may be lesions in the mouth. In herpes zoster and herpes simplex infections (Fig. 20.23), there is a non-follicular papulovesicular rash in which the vesicles are planted in an inflamed base. The rash is painful. In herpes zoster, the rash follows a segmental distribution, corresponding with skin of a dermatome. The vesicular lesion becomes encrusted (Fig. 20.24) and later, secondary infection may occur.

Other less common viral infections associated with a rash include erythema infectiosum, caused by a parvovirus, in which the exanthem on the face gives a 'slapped-cheek' appearance, and roseola infantum, a disease of toddlers which mimics rubella.

Drug eruptions

In the last 40 years, eruptions caused by drugs have become common. Most such rashes are caused by an allergic hypersensitivity. Drug rashes can mimic almost every pattern of skin disease. Thus, urticaria may be caused by penicillin or opiates; a measles-like (morbilliform) rash may be induced by ampicillin, especially when given to patients with infectious mononucleosis; eczema-like rashes are seen with methyldopa and phenylbutazone therapy; and gold and chloroquine rashes mimic lichen planus.

A palpable rash looking like Henoch-Schönlein purpura indicates leucocytoclastic vasculitis. Generalized exfoliative dermatitis may be induced by sulfonylureas, indomethacin and allopurinol. Increasing use of biologics in clinical medicine has identified unusual skin eruptions.

Drugs that may sensitize the skin to sunlight (phototoxic reaction) include tetracyclines, sulfonamides and nalidixic acid. Acne-like rashes may follow high-dose prednisolone therapy and are common with phenytoin therapy. Certain cytotoxic drugs and sodium valproate cause hair loss. Both erythema nodosum and erythema multiforme may be induced by sulfonamides, including co-trimoxazole. Laboratory tests are of little value in the diagnosis of drug eruptions. A carefully taken history and knowledge of the common patterns of drug reactions usually allow accurate diagnosis (Box 20.11).

Tumours in the skin

Exposure to the sun may, after many years, result in the development of many common skin tumours, for example squamous or basal cell carcinoma or melanoma. These tumours are especially common in fair-skinned people. Basal cell carcinoma arises especially on the face, near the nose or on the forehead (Fig. 20.25). The lesion may be ulcerated with a firm, rounded edge, or papular. Melanomas

Box 20.11 | Common drug eruptions

Morphological type	Drug
Maculopapular	Penicillin/amoxicillin
Urticaria	Penicillin, non-steroidal drugs
Vasculitis	Hydralazine
Fixed drug eruption	Tetracyclines, phenolphthalein
Pigmentation	Amiodarone, minocycline
Photosensitivity	Thiazides, sulfonamides
Lupus erythematosus	Isoniazid, penicillamine
Erythema nodosum	Oral contraceptive pill, sulfonamides
Erythema multiforme	Barbiturates
Acneform	Steroids
Pustular	Carbamazepine
Lichenoid	Thiazides, antimalarials, allopurinol
Psoriasiform	Beta-blockers, lithium, antimalarials
Toxic epidermal necrolysis/ Stevens-Johnson syndrome/ erythema multiforme	Carbamazepine, non-steroidal drugs, co-trimoxazole
Pemphigus	Angiotensin converting enzyme (ACE) inhibitors
Linear IgA disease	Vancomycin
Erythroderma	Sulfonylureas, ACE inhibitors, allopurinol

Figure 20.26 Malignant melanoma on a male chest. The nodule is invasive.

Figure 20.27 A pigmented basal cell papilloma (seborrhoeic keratosis) on the face. This is a benign lesion.

Figure 20.25 Basal cell carcinoma.

may develop on the torso in men and legs in females. They may be pigmented or amelanotic and may in about a third of cases develop rapidly in a pre-existing benign mole (Fig. 20.26). Staging by assessing draining regional sentinel lymph nodes is becoming increasingly routine in cutaneous oncology. Seborrhoeic keratoses are familial, resulting in a raised warty pigmented lesions found in the sun-exposed elderly, especially on the dorsa of hands as 'liver spots' (Fig. 20.27). A symptomatic pigmented skin lesion having an asymmetric, ragged border, three or more colours and diameter of more than 7

mm, particularly if it is increasing in size or bleeding and found on sun-damaged freckled skin, should be regarded as suspicious of malignant melanoma.

Special techniques in examination of the skin

The skin is uniquely available to the examining physician. There are a number of diagnostic procedures and blood tests (Box 20.12).

Tzanck preparation

Tzanck preparation, an often forgotten old but valuable technique, is useful for emergency diagnosis of vesicular infections or blistering eruptions, such as pemphigus. The intact blister is opened and the base gently scraped. The material obtained is smeared onto the microscope slide, allowed to air dry and then stained. Viral lesions will show typical multinucleated giant cells, and pemphigus will show acantholytic cells.

Microscopic examination—dermatoscopy (direct assessment of skin lesions)

Dermatoscopic and/or microscopic examination is useful in the diagnosis of scabies, pediculosis (lice) and fungal infection (tinea and candidiasis). The established routine use of the dermatoscope has become essential in the assessment of pigmented skin lesions and aids in diagnosis of skin malignancy, especially malignant melanoma.

Scabies

Scabies is caused by the mite *Acarus (Sarcoptes) scabei*. The female is larger than the male and burrows in the epidermis, depositing eggs. These burrows should be looked for between the fingers, on the hands or wrists and on the sides of the feet. They can be recognized with the naked eye as short dark lines terminating in a shining spot of skin. The eggs lie in the dark line, the mite in the shining spot. It may be picked out by means of a flat surgical needle and placed on a microscope slide for more detailed examination.

Pediculosis

Three forms of pediculosis or louse infestation occur: *Pediculus capitis* on the head, *Pediculus corporis* on the trunk and *Pediculus pubis* on the pubic and axillary hairs. The eggs or nits of *P. pubis* and *P. capitis* adhere to the hairs. From their position on the hairs, one can judge roughly the duration of the condition: they are fixed at first near the root of the hair and are carried up as the hair grows, so the higher the nits are, the longer the pediculi have been present. *P. corporis* should be looked for in the seams of the clothes, especially where the clothes come into contact with the skin, for example over the shoulders. The bites of the parasite produce haemorrhagic spots, each with a dark centre and a paler areola. Marks of scratching should be looked for on parts accessible to the patient's nails. *P. pubis* is venereally acquired and causes intense pubic itching. The nits are laid on the pubic hair and the lice themselves are easily visible. *P. corporis* is seen only in the grossly deprived, living in rough conditions of war or social upheaval. In contrast, *P. capitis* is common in school children,

however clean they and their families may be, and is endemic in many schools.

Fungal infections

Fungus may grow in the skin, nails or hair and can cause disease (ringworm or tinea), for example athlete's foot (tinea pedis).

The most common sites of fungal infection are the skin between the toes (tinea pedis) and the soles of the feet and the groin (tinea cruris). The lesions may be scaly or vesicular, tending to spread in a ring form with central healing (Fig. 20.28); macerated, dead, white, offensive-smelling epithelium is found in the intertriginous areas, such as the toe clefts.

Nail discolouration, deformity, hypertrophy and abnormal brittleness may result from fungus infection (tinea unguium).

Ringworm of the scalp (tinea capitis) is most common in children. It presents as round or oval areas of baldness covered with short, lustreless broken-off hair stumps. These hair stumps may fluoresce bright green under Wood's light. Some fungi do not fluoresce with Wood's light, however, and these can be detected only by microscopy and culture (Figs 20.29 and 20.30).

Microscopic examination for fungus infection

Scales from the active edge of a lesion are scraped off lightly with a scalpel or the roofs of vesicles are snipped off with scissors. The material is placed in a drop of 10% to 20% aqueous potassium hydroxide solution on a microscope slide, covered with a coverslip and left for 30 minutes to clear. It is then examined under the light microscope with the 8-mm or 4-mm objective using low illumination. The mycelia are recognized as branching, refractile threads that boldly transgress the outlines of the squamous cells. Nails are examined in much the same way, but it is necessary to break up the snippings

Box 20.12	Dermatology blood investigations
Blood test	**Clinical example**
Full blood count (FBC)	Pruritus
Ferritin and iron studies	Hail and nail
Biochemistry renal and liver function	Pruritus
Streptococcal serology	Cellulitis
Autoantibodies	Autoimmune disorders
Hepatitis screen	Lichen planus
HSV 1 and 2 serology	Erythema multiforme
Syphilis serology	Secondary syphilis
HIV	Persistent infections
HLA typing	Dermatitis herpetiformis
DNA analysis	Epidermolysis bullosa

Figure 20.28 Tinea rubrum (ringworm infection).

Figure 20.29 Lactophenol blue preparation showing macronidia of Microsporum species, isolated from skin scrapings from a patient with ringworm.

Figure 20.31 Disposable punch skin biopsy, especially useful where minimal scarring is desirable.

Figure 20.32 A 4-mm punch diagnostic biopsy.

Figure 20.30 Kerion owing to localized deep dermatophyte infection in the scalp.

and shavings into small fragments. These are either heated in potassium hydroxide or are left to clear in it overnight before being examined.

A scalp lesion is cleaned with 70% alcohol or with 1% cetrimide; infected stumps and scales are removed by scraping with a scalpel. The hairs are cleaned in potassium hydroxide in the same way as skin scales. Examination under the microscope reveals spores on the outside of the hair roots and mycelia inside the hair substance. The species of fungus responsible may be established by culture on Sabouraud's glucose-agar.

Wood's light

A Wood's light lamp emits long-wave ultraviolet light at a peak of 360 nm. Wood's light examination is performed in a darkened room and is useful to identify the fluorescence of fungi and corynebacterial infection (erythrasma), elevated porphyrins in urine or in the localization of pigmentary abnormalities.

Contact allergy patch testing

Contact allergy patch testing is an important and valuable tool for the diagnosis of suspected allergic dermatitis owing to contact (contact dermatitis). The formulation of the allergens is critical, and various standard contact allergen test batteries have been developed in different countries and clinics to include the most common culprits. Patch testing is simple, but the results are not always easy to interpret. Allergens are placed in shallow aluminium 1-cm^2 wells and applied in strips to the patient's back for 48 hours for initial reading and a second reading at 96 hours. This ensures that any delayed-type hypersensitivity (e.g. Coomb's type IV reaction to an allergen) can be identified.

Skin biopsy

Biopsy of the skin is used not only to excise benign and malignant tumours but also to identify the nature of reactive and/or inflammatory lesions. Punch biopsy (Figs 20.31 and 20.32) is popular because of its convenience and its minimal scarring. The biopsy can be studied by conventional histology, often supplemented by immunofluorescence and sometimes immunohistochemistry or molecular biology, to identify specific proteins or genetic abnormalities. Skin biopsy of fresh tissue can be sent for the microbiology of unusual infections and is increasingly used in diagnosis and in assessing the progress of skin diseases.

Eyes | 21

Andrew Coombes

Introduction

Although proportionally a greater contribution towards the diagnosis of ophthalmic disorders is made by the examination compared with the history, it is important to obtain a detailed account of the presenting complaint and associated visual symptoms from the patient with an ocular problem.

History

Disturbance of vision, the most important ocular symptom, may be sudden or gradual, unilateral or bilateral, and lead to loss of central vision or partial field loss. Simultaneous, bilateral visual symptoms are usually owing to disease in optic pathways at or posterior to the optic chiasm. Sudden visual disturbance should be assessed urgently. Visual hallucinations may be formed or unformed. Some visual symptoms have particular significance (Table 21.1). For example, haloes around lights occur in acute angle-closure glaucoma caused by corneal oedema. 'Floaters' and flashes (photopsia) are indicative of vitreous or retinal disorders, respectively. The latter may also cause objects to appear smaller (micropsia), larger (macropsia) or distorted (metamorphopsia). Disorders of ocular movement may cause double vision (diplopia) or visual blurring. Are the visual symptoms binocular or monocular? Are they related to eye movements?

Other common presentations include a red eye, abnormal lid position, protrusion of the globe and pupillary or eyelid abnormality. Ocular pain is often associated with a red eye (Table 21.2). Ocular pain owing to a foreign body may be described as 'a gritty sensation' in the eye, often worsened by blinking. It may be associated with sensitivity to light (photophobia) but this, particularly in conjunction with ocular aching, usually indicates serious corneal or intraocular disease. Severe ocular pain with vomiting may indicate acute glaucoma. Migraine often presents with bilateral visual symptoms and headache. Raised intracranial pressure and giant cell arteritis should also be considered when headache is associated with visual symptoms. Pain may be referred to the eye because of neighbouring disease, for example

sinusitis. Excessive tear production (lacrimation) associated with discomfort may indicate ocular surface disease. There may be abnormal secretions from the eye, such as mucus or pus. With insufficient tears, the eye typically feels dry, whereas a painless overflow of tears (epiphora) typically indicates blockage of the lacrimal drainage system.

Note any previous ophthalmic history, such as a squint in childhood, and any pre-existing poor vision or previous ocular injury or surgery. Note what type of glasses or contact lenses are worn: extended-wear soft contact lenses are associated with an increased risk of corneal infection. The family history may reveal glaucoma, decreased visual acuity, colour blindness, squint or neurological disease associated with visual loss. In addition to the ocular history, the medical, drug and social histories are important.

Examination

Eye examination is part of the cranial nerve examination. It includes ocular movements (cranial nerves III, IV and VI), corneal sensation (ophthalmic division of the trigeminal nerve) and eye closure (VII). Assess the optic (II) nerve by testing visual acuity, colour vision, the visual fields and the pupillary light reaction. Inspect the optic nerve head (the optic disc and cup) with the ophthalmoscope. Detailed examination of the anterior segment of the eye requires use of the slit lamp which, with additional equipment, can also be used to test the intraocular pressure (IOP) and examine the retina.

Visual acuity

Visual acuity is most reliably tested at 6 m (20 ft) using a standard chart such as the Snellen (Fig. 21.1A) or Log MAR chart (Fig. 21.1B). Tests of acuity in near vision are portable, but limited by age-related loss of accommodation (presbyopia), which necessitates refractive correction in older patients. These use test types of varying sizes, based on the point system of the printers (Fig. 21.2), and the smallest type that can be read comfortably at a distance of 33 cm is recorded (normally N4.5 or N5 type).

Table 21.1 Sudden visual disturbance

Diagnosis			History: visual symptoms
Vascular	Ocular	Amaurosis fugax	Transient (minutes), unilateral
		Retinal artery/vein occlusion	Permanent, unilateral, often associated with systemic vascular disease (e.g. ischaemic heart disease, hypertension, diabetes)
		Non-arteritic ischaemic optic neuropathy (NAION)	Permanent, unilateral, often associated with systemic vascular disease (e.g. ischaemic heart disease, hypertension, diabetes)
		Arteritic ischaemic optic neuropathy (AAION)	Permanent, unilateral, typically associated with symptoms of giant cell arteritis (e.g. temporal headache/tenderness, jaw claudication, features of polymyalgia rheumatica)
		Papilloedema/optic disc swelling	Transient (seconds), bilateral visual obscurations, often precipitated by coughing or bending
	Cortical	Transient ischaemic attack (TIA)	Transient (minutes), bilateral, associated with systemic vascular disease (e.g. ischaemic heart disease, hypertension, diabetes, etc.)
		Migraine	Transient, bilateral, typically followed by nausea and headache
		Cerebrovascular accident (CVA)	Permanent homonymous field defect, may be preceded by TIA symptoms; note central acuity usually preserved except in bilateral occipital lobe infarction
Non-vascular	Vitreous	Posterior vitreous detachment (PVD)	Transient (weeks), unilateral, floaters, occasional photopsia, central vision normal
		Vitreous haemorrhage	Transient (weeks), unilateral, multiple floaters, central vision typically reduced
	Retina	Wet age-related macular degeneration (AMD)	Progressive, unilateral central visual distortion (metamorphopsia) This condition is also known as exudative or neovascular AMD
		Retinal detachment	Progressive, unilateral field loss, central vision reduced if macula involved, often associated with symptoms of PVD
	Optic nerve	Optic neuritis	Transient (months), unilateral, may be associated with features of multiple sclerosis
		Acute compression	Progressive, unilateral, bilateral if chiasm involved (e.g. pituitary apoplexy (infarction of a pituitary tumour))
Pseudo		Suddenly noticed	Unilateral gradual visual loss from (e.g. dry AMD or cataract)
		Functional	Bilateral or unilateral; diagnosis of exclusion

Snellen distance vision

On the Snellen chart, each line of letters is designated by a number that corresponds to the distance at which those letters can be read by someone with 'normal' distance vision. For example, the largest letter, at the top of the chart—designated 60—would be read at 60 m by a person with 'normal' vision.

Technique

The patient sits or stands 6 m (20 ft) from the chart. Where space is limited, a mirror may be used 3 m from both patient and chart, with the patient facing away from the chart and reading the letters in the mirror, giving a total of 6 m. However, increasingly, electronic computer screens are being used and the letter size can be adjusted to allow test distance to be varied between 3 and 6 m. Distance glasses should be worn if necessary and each eye tested separately. The patient should read line by line from the top of the chart. If a patient cannot see the largest letter,

designated 60, then the test distance should be reduced. If at 1 m the 60 letter cannot be seen, assess the following:

- Counting fingers held up at about 1 m (CFs)
- Hand movements (HMs)
- Perception of light (PL)

When testing low vision, ensure that the eye not being tested is completely covered. If a patient cannot read 6/6 or better in either eye, check the vision again using a pinhole occluder (Fig. 21.3). This test distinguishes patients with poor vision owing to refractive error from those who have ocular or neurological conditions. In a myopic (short-sighted) eye, the rays of light are focused in front of the retina. In hypermetropia (long-sightedness), light is focused behind the eye, because the eye is abnormally short. In astigmatism, the cornea is not uniformly curved and light is not focused evenly on the retina. When using a pinhole, only the central rays of light pass through to the retina and refractive errors are significantly reduced.

Table 21.2 Red eye

Diagnosis	History	Examination
Subconjunctival haemorrhage	Typically asymptomatic, spontaneous May be associated with trauma	Unilateral (except some trauma), contiguous red area
Viral conjunctivitis	FB sensation, watering, no visual loss or photophobia Recent contact with person with red eye or URTI?	Bilateral, prominent inflamed conjunctival vessels and follicles, enlarged tender preauricular lymph node
Bacterial conjunctivitis	FB sensation, discharge, no visual loss or photophobia	Bilateral, prominent inflamed conjunctival vessels, mucopus
Allergic conjunctivitis	Itch, watering, no visual loss or photophobia, history of atopy	Bilateral, prominent inflamed conjunctival vessels and follicles
Iritis (anterior uveitis)	Reduced vision, aching sensation, photophobia PMH or systemic enquiry may elicit underlying disease	Unilateral, prominent pericorneal vessels, small pupil, aqueous cells and flare (protein) (at slit lamp), hypopyon
Acute angle-closure glaucoma	Severe pain, haloes/rainbows around lights, reduced vision, hypermetropic, elderly	Unilateral, pericorneal prominent vessels, semidilated (oval) pupil, corneal oedema, shallow anterior chamber (slit lamp)
Episcleritis	Mild discomfort, tenderness, no visual loss or photophobia, young adult, otherwise fit and well	Unilateral, typically sectorial prominent inflamed subconjunctival vessels (may also be nodular or diffuse)
Scleritis	Significant aching pain, tender, photophobia, occasionally reduced vision, systemic enquiry may elicit underlying disease	Unilateral, typically sectorial prominent inflamed deep scleral vessels (may also be nodular or diffuse)
Bacterial keratitis	FB sensation, watering/discharge, visual loss, photophobia Pre-existing ocular surface disease, recent trauma or contact lens wear?	Unilateral, opacity in cornea (slit lamp) stains with fluorescein
Herpetic viral keratitis	FB sensation, watering/discharge, visual loss, photophobia Cold sores or ophthalmic shingles?	Unilateral, branching linear dendrite(s) on cornea (slit lamp) stains with fluorescein

FB, foreign body; PMH, past medical history; URTI, upper respiratory tract infection.

Recording visual acuity

The top figure, the numerator, records the distance of the subject from the test chart—usually 6 m. The bottom figure records the line read by the patient. The normal person can read the line designated 6 at 6 m (i.e. 6/6 (20/20) vision).

Record a mistake of one letter in a line as '−1' and a single letter read from the next smaller line as '+1'. Thus, if all except one of the letters on the line designated 6 are read correctly, the visual acuity is recorded 6/6 −1. If only one letter on that line is read correctly, the visual acuity is recorded 6/9 +1. Like all ophthalmic findings except visual fields, right eye visual acuity is traditionally written on the left side of the page (as the patient's eye appears to you) and vice versa. Whether the patient was using glasses, pinhole (ph) or was unaided (ua) is recorded in the middle (Fig. 21.4).

Log MAR charts

Increasingly, Snellen acuity tests are being replaced by use of a Log MAR chart, which superficially appears similar to a Snellen chart but addresses its problems, namely different number of letters per line, irregular spacing between letters/lines and unequal graduation from one line to the other. On a Log MAR chart each letter has a score value of 0.02 log units with 5 letters per line (each line therefore scores 0.1 log units). 6/6 is equivalent to Log MAR score 0.00 and 6/60 is 1.00. Each letter read contributes to the score; for example, 6/6−1 would be recorded as 0.02. The digital output is also helpful for research and audit purposes.

Colour vision

Tests of colour vision are important because colour perception, especially for red, is affected in optic nerve disease before changes in visual acuity can be detected. Show the patient a red target one eye at a time (any bright red target can be used) and ask if there is a difference between the eyes. In the affected eye, red appears 'washed out' (desaturated). Acquired defects of colour vision may also occur in macular disease. The Ishihara test (Fig. 21.5) was devised to test for congenital colour anomalies (colour blindness), but is often used to assess acquired visual disorders. Most inherited colour blindness occurs in males (sex-linked recessive inheritance). It ranges from total colour blindness (monochromatopsia) to subtle confusion between colours, typically between red and green. About 8% of men and 0.5% of women

Figure 21.1 **(A)** Snellen chart for testing distance vision. **(B)** Log MAR chart for testing distance vision.

in the UK have congenital colour perception defects. Blue/yellow deficiencies and total colour blindness are uncommon.

Visual field testing

Visual field testing is described in Chapter 16. Field defects may affect one or both eyes. Symmetrical bilateral (homonymous) field defects are characteristic of lesions posterior to the optic chiasm, and asymmetrical field defects are usually caused by lesions anterior to the chiasm (i.e. in the optic nerves or retinae). Characteristic field defects (scotoma) occur in glaucoma, when damage to nerve fibres occurs at the optic disc, typically at the inferior or superior aspect of the optic cup. Fundoscopy shows an increase in vertical length of the optic cup (see later in the chapter for details about how to examine the fundi) and field loss is arc-shaped (arcuate scotoma). If both the inferior and superior fields are involved, a ring-shaped scotoma develops. Untreated glaucoma results in loss of the peripheral field so that only a small central island of vision remains (tunnel vision). Computerized perimetry is useful in identifying early visual field loss. The Humphrey field test analyser (Carl Zeiss), for example, provides statistical information indicating the reliability of the test in comparison with a group of age-matched controls (Fig. 21.6).

Pupils

Examination of the pupils in neurology is discussed in Chapter 16. In ophthalmic practice, there are three key aspects to pupil examination: size, shape and reactions.

Pupil size: anisocoria

In 12% of normal individuals, the pupils are slightly unequal, particularly in bright light (anisocoria), but in these subjects they react normally. Abnormal pupils dilate and constrict abnormally, and the degree of anisocoria varies with the ambient illumination. However, it is often difficult to decide which pupil is abnormal. In the absence of local eye disease, a small pupil may be owing to paralysis of the dilator pupillae muscle (sympathetic innervated), part of Horner's syndrome (Fig. 21.7), in which anisocoria is more pronounced in low ambient light. An enlarged pupil suggests a parasympathetic lesion, which may be preganglionic in oculomotor lesions or postganglionic as in the tonic pupil of Adie's syndrome. Adie's tonic pupil tends to be dilated in bright light and is very slow to react. A feature of both parasympathetic and sympathetic lesions is denervation hypersensitivity caused by upregulation of receptors at the neuromuscular junction (adrenergic in sympathetic and cholinergic in parasympathetic). This is the basis of pharmacological pupil testing. In both pre- and postganglionic parasympathetic blockade, the pupil is supersensitive to weak cholinergic drops (e.g. pilocarpine 0.1%). In sympathetic block, dilute adrenergic agonists, such as phenylephrine 1%, are unreliable, so the uptake blocker, cocaine 4%, is used. This dilates normal pupils but has no effect in pre- or postganglionic lesions. Hydroxyamfetamine 1% causes noradrenaline (norepinephrine) release from normal or intact postganglionic neurons and allows pre- and postganglionic lesions to be distinguished (the synapse is located in the superior

Figure 21.2 Near vision chart based on the point system of the printer.

READING TEST TYPES

as approved by

THE FACULTY OF OPHTHALMOLOGISTS,

LONDON, ENGLAND

N. 5

He moved forward a few steps: the house was so dark behind him, the world so dim and uncertain in front of him, that for a moment his heart failed him. He might have to search the whole garden for the dog. Then he heard a sniff, felt something wet against his leg — he had almost stepped upon the animal. He bent down and stroked its wet coat. The dog stood quite still, then moved forward towards the house, sniffed at the steps, at last walked calmly through the open door as though the house belonged to him. Jeremy followed, closed the door behind them; then there they were in the little dark passage with the boy's heart beating like a drum, his teeth chattering, and a terrible temptation to sneeze hovering around him. Let him reach the nursery and establish the animal there and all might be well, but let them be discovered, cold and shivering, in the passage, and out the dog would be flung. He knew so exactly what would happen.

(From "Jeremy" by Hugh Walpole).

wire sons vain error unwise cream remove

N. 6

The camp stood where, until quite lately, has been pasture and ploughland; the farm house still stood in a fold of the hill and had served us for battalion offices; ivy still supported part of what had once been the walls of a fruit garden; half an acre of mutilated old trees behind the wash-houses survived of an orchard. The place had been marked for destruction before the army came to it. Had there been another year of peace, there would have been no farmhouse, no wall, no apple trees. Already half a mile of concrete road lay between bare clay banks, and on either side a chequer of open ditches showed where the municipal contractors had designed a system of drainage. Another year of peace would have made the place part of the neighbouring suburb. Now the huts where we had wintered waited their turn for destruction.

(From "Brideshead Revisited" by Evelyn Waugh)

nervous manner immune over unanimous wear

N. 8

And another image came to me, of an arctic hut and a trapper alone with his furs and oil lamp and log fire; the remains of supper on the table, a few books, skis in the corner; everything dry and neat and warm inside and outside the last blizzard of winter raging and the snow piling up against the door. Quite silently a great weight forming against the timber; the bolt straining in its socket; minute by minute in the darkness outside the white heap sealing the door, until quite soon when the wind dropped and the sun came out on the ice slopes and the thaw set in a block would move, slide and tumble high above, gather way, gather weight, till the whole hillside seemed to be falling, and the little lighted place would crash open and splinter and disappear, rolling with the avalanche into the ravine.

(From "Brideshead Revisited" by Evelyn Waugh)

immense snow came near arrow use.

cervical ganglion). In complex pupil abnormalities, for example bilateral Horner's syndrome, infrared pupil imaging can be valuable. Causes of anisocoria are highlighted in Box 21.1. In congenital Horner's syndrome, the affected iris is depigmented and appears blue.

Pupil reactions: afferent and central defects

The swinging light test is used to detect a relative afferent pupillary defect (RAPD) resulting from retinal or optic nerve disease. The test loses sensitivity in symmetrical bilateral optic nerve disease, but this is rare; in most bilateral cases the defect will be detected on the more abnormal side. RAPD is often associated with reduced vision, but if central vision is retained, the acuity will be normal, although severe peripheral field damage may cause RAPD. In neurosyphilis, the pupils are small and irregular and show the Argyll Robertson phenomenon (normal pupil constriction to a near target but reduced reaction to light) owing to a midbrain defect. In Parinaud's syndrome, the pupils are typically large and poorly reactive to light, with abnormal vertical gaze, convergence retraction nystagmus and lid retraction on attempted upgaze (Collier's sign). The causes of light-near dissociation are given in Box 21.2.

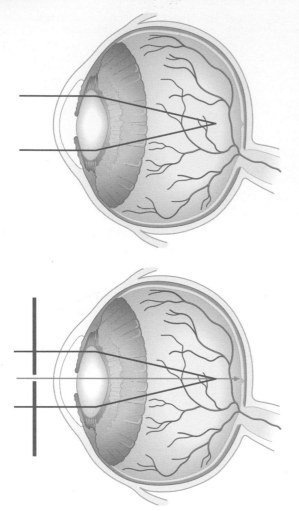

Figure 21.3 Testing vision with a pinhole. Top: light is not focused on the retina owing to refractive error (in this case in front of the retina, as in myopia, or short-sightedness). Bottom: the use of a pinhole selects rays of light not needing to be focused, giving a better indication of a patient's true best corrected visual acuity despite refractive error.

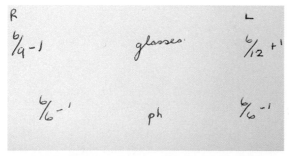

Figure 21.4 Recording visual acuity: the numerator is the test distance. ph, pinhole.

Pupil shape

Slit-lamp examination is the best technique to assess intrinsic ocular disease that may affect the shape and position of the pupil (Box 21.3).

Direct ophthalmoscopy

The direct ophthalmoscope is an indispensable clinical instrument that allows direct visualization of the retina, which is part of the central nervous system (CNS), and its circulation. It consists of a bright, focused light source that illuminates the retina to allow the observer to see the image, magnified about 15 times.

Preparation

1. Decide the objective of the examination.
2. Consider dilating the pupils with 1% cyclopentolate (Mydrilate) (0.5% in children under 6 months) or 1% tropicamide (Mydriacyl). This blurs the vision for at least 2 hours, so patients should be forewarned and instructed not to drive. Some patients have a predisposition to closed-angle glaucoma (Box 21.4) and dilation may precipitate an attack. At-risk individuals must be warned to return if symptoms of acute angle closure occur.
3. Briefly explain the examination so that the patient can cooperate fully. Ask the patient to fixate on a distant target: the patient should continue to look in this direction even if the examiner's head obscures the target.
4. Dim the room lights.
5. Set the ophthalmoscope lens wheel to zero dioptres (D), unless correcting for your own short- or long-sightedness.
6. Ensure that the ophthalmoscope light is bright. Unless the pupil is small, select a large light spot size (Box 21.5, Fig. 21.8).

Examining the fundi

Look carefully at the optic disc/cup, the retinal vessels and the retina and macula (Fig. 21.9).

Optic disc

The optic disc marks the point where the retinal axons exit the back of the eye to form the optic nerve. It corresponds to the physiological blind spot. The normal disc is round or slightly oval. With astigmatism, the disc may appear more oval than normal. There are four key questions to consider when viewing the optic disc:

1. Is the colour normal? The normal disc is yellow-pink and its temporal side is paler. An abnormally pale disc is a sign of optic atrophy (Fig. 21.10). In addition, in optic atrophy there is a reduction in the number of capillaries crossing the edge of the disc, from the normal 10 to 7 or fewer (Kestenbaum's sign). The causes of optic atrophy are listed in Box 21.6. In primary optic atrophy owing to optic nerve lesions, the disc is flat and white, with clear-cut edges. Secondary optic atrophy follows swelling of the optic disc owing to papilloedema: the disc is greyish-white, with indistinct edges.

Figure 21.5   Ishihara colour vision test.

Figure 21.6   Automated static perimetry: the Humphrey field test analyser.

Figure 21.7   Horner's syndrome. On the affected side there is ptosis, which may be very slight, and a small pupil (miosis) that reacts to both light and accommodation. (Reproduced with permission from Mir, 2003 Atlas of Clinical Diagnosis, ed 2. Saunders, Edinburgh.)

Box 21.1	Causes of anisocoria

- Idiopathic (12% population)
- Parasympathetic:
    - Third nerve palsy (external ophthalmoplegia)
    - Tonic pupil (internal ophthalmoplegia, e.g. Holmes-Adie)
- Sympathetic:
  Horner's syndrome
- Argyll Robertson
- Pharmacological
- Ocular:
    - Iris inflammation (e.g. iritis)
    - Iris ischaemia
    - Trauma
    - Iatrogenic

Box 21.2	Light-near dissociation

- Argyll Robertson pupil
- Holmes-Adie pupil
- Parinaud's syndrome
- Aberrant third nerve regeneration
- Myotonic dystrophy
- Diabetes mellitus

Box 21.3	Causes of abnormal pupil shape

- Congenital: Rieger's anomaly (anterior segment cleavage anomalies)
- Trauma
- Iatrogenic (sphincterotomies, iridectomy, cataract surgery)
- Inflammatory (posterior synechiae in iritis)
- Tumour (ectropion uveae in ciliary body malignancies)
- Ischaemic: herpes zoster, angle-closure glaucoma
- Idiopathic: iridocorneal endotheliopathy (ICE) syndrome (which also features multiple pupils (polycoria) and misplaced pupils (correctopia))

Figure 21.8 Examining the right eye with the direct ophthalmoscope.

Figure 21.9 Normal fundus anatomy. OC, optic cup; OD, optic disc. Retinal vascular arcades: F, fovea; IN, inferonasal; IT, inferotemporal; M, macula; SN, superonasal; ST, superotemporal.

2. Are the margins distinct? The disc margin should be sharply defined. In optic disc swelling, this clear edge is obscured (Fig. 21.11) and venous pulsations are abolished. However, venous pulsations may be difficult to see in some normal subjects. Some important causes of disc swelling are listed in Box 21.7. In papilloedema, caused by raised intracranial pressure, the disc is abnormally red and its margins are blurred, especially at the upper and lower margins, and particularly in the upper nasal quadrant. The physiological cup becomes obliterated and the retinal veins are slightly distended. As the condition progresses, the disc becomes more definitely swollen (Fig. 21.12). In order to measure the degree of swelling, start with a high plus lens in the ophthalmoscope and reduce the

Figure 21.10 Primary optic atrophy. The disc is pale and whiter than normal, and its edges are unusually sharply demarcated from the retina. The retinal vessels are slightly attenuated.

Box 21.6	Causes of optic atrophy

- Congenital:
  - Dominant and recessive
- Optic neuritis
- Chronic papilloedema
- Toxic:
  - Tobacco, lead, alcohol
- Optic nerve compression:
  - Thyroid
  - Tumour
- Post-traumatic (direct optic nerve or indirect vascular damage)

Box 21.7	Causes of the appearance of optic disc swelling

- Raised intracranial pressure (papilloedema)
- Infiltration:
  - Lymphoma
  - Sarcoid
- Vascular:
  - Hypertension (grade 4)
  - Central retinal vein occlusion
  - Anterior ischaemic optic neuropathy
- Pseudopapilloedema:
  - Congenital small discs
  - High hypermetropia
- Optic disc drusen

Figure 21.11 Papilloedema: optic disc swelling caused by raised intracranial pressure.

Figure 21.12 Severe papilloedema with retinal haemorrhages.

power until the centre of the disc is just in focus. The retina, a short distance from the disc, is then brought into focus by further reduction of the lens power. This further reduction indicates the degree of swelling of the disc (3D is equivalent to 1 mm of swelling). If papilloedema develops rapidly, there will be marked engorgement of the retinal veins with haemorrhages and exudates on and around the disc, but with papilloedema of slow onset there may be little or no vascular change, even though the disc may become very swollen. The retinal vessels will, however, bend sharply as they dip down from the swollen disc to the surrounding retina. The oedema may extend to the adjacent retina, producing greyish-white striations near the disc (Paton's lines), and a macular fan of hard exudates temporal to the fovea may develop in some cases.

3. Is the central cup enlarged? The cup is a physiological central depression formed at the optic disc as nerve fibres leave the retina to form the optic nerve. It marks the point where the retinal vessels enter and leave the eye. It is paler than the surrounding rim of the disc. The optic cup-to-disc ratio is estimated by comparing their ratios vertically. In chronic open-angle glaucoma, the ratio is increased (>0.3)—optic disc cupping. When the cup is deep, in advanced glaucoma,

Figure 21.13 Glaucomatous disc cupping. The cup is oval in the vertical plane and appears pale. The retinal vessels are displaced nasally.

retinal vessels disappear as they climb from the floor to the rim, and reappear as they bend sharply over the edge of the rim (bayonetting); in less advanced cases, the cup appears as a vertical oval extending to the edge of the disc (Fig. 21.13). In myopic individuals, the disc and cup appear large, and mimic glaucoma. Myopes often have a partial ring of pigmentation or white sclera surrounding the disc, which is

Figure 21.14   Myelinated nerve fibres: the white area obscures the disc; this is a normal variant.

Figure 21.15   Retinal arteriolar emboli. Cholesterol emboli in the retinal arteries of a patient with atheromatous disease of the internal carotid artery in the neck.

easily mistaken for the edge of the cup. In severe myopia, degenerative chorioretinal changes may occur in the fundus, which can involve the macula and impair central vision.

4. Are there any other abnormal features? In proliferative diabetic retinopathy, new blood vessels (neovascularization) develop at the optic disc. Myelinated nerve fibres have a dramatic white appearance, but they are a unilateral, harmless and non-progressive congenital anomaly (Fig. 21.14). They have a characteristic feathered edge that may obscure the retinal vessels.

Blood vessels

Four pairs of arterioles and venules form the main retinal vascular arcades that emerge from the optic disc: superotemporal (above the macula), infero-temporal (below the macula), superonasal and inferonasal. Study each in turn. Arterioles are thin, bright red in colour and with a longitudinal streak of light reflection. In branch arteriolar occlusion, a bright yellow (cholesterol) embolus may occa-sionally be seen (Fig. 21.15). In diabetes or venous occlusion, the venules are larger, darker and often dilated or tortuous. Look carefully at arteriolar/venous crossings: compression and localized dila-tation of venules (arteriovenous (AV) nipping) with arteriolar narrowing (attenuation) is a sign of hypertension (Box 21.8, Fig. 21.16). Spontane-ous arteriolar pulsation is an abnormal finding that may occur if the intraocular pressure (IOP) is very high or the central retinal artery pressure very low. Spontaneous venous pulsation is frequently seen in normal eyes, but is reduced in papilloedema.

Retina and macula

As each main vascular arcade is followed and exam-ined, the adjacent and peripheral retina can be systematically assessed. The macula is the central retinal area bounded by temporal vascular arcades. It measures approximately five disc diameters across.

Box 21.8	Appearance and classification of hypertensive retinopathy

- Grade 1: arteriolar narrowing (attenuation) and vein concealment
- Grade 2: profound arteriolar attenuation and venous deflections at crossings (arterior venous (AV) nipping)
- Grade 3: severe attenuation 'arteriolar copper wiring', haemorrhages, cotton wool spots and hard exudates
- Grade 4: all of the above, plus very severe attenuation 'arteriolar silver wiring' and optic disc swelling

Figure 21.16   Hypertensive retinopathy. The arteries are irregular in calibre and show 'silver wiring'. Arteriovenous nipping is present. Characteristic 'flame-shaped' haemorrhages and 'cotton wool' spots (*arrow*) can be seen.

Box 21.9	Common retinal abnormalities

White

- Cotton wool spots: white, fluffy, indistinct areas indicative of retinal ischaemia. This is the accumulation of axonal proteins in the nerve fibre layer. Causes include severe hypertension, diabetes and retinal vein occlusion.
- Chorioretinal atrophy: well-defined, 'punched-out' lesions (the white is the sclera). May occur in conjunction with retinal pigment hypertrophy. Associated with previous retinal inflammation or injury (including retinal laser).

Yellow

- Hard exudates: bright yellow with well-demarcated edges consisting of lipid deposits that have leaked out of abnormal blood vessels. Most commonly associated with microaneurysms in diabetes (Fig. 21.17).
- Drusen: small multifocal round yellow features, usually located in the central macula. Generally smaller and less bright yellow than hard exudates. Typically bilateral and relatively symmetrical. Common in elderly people associated with 'dry' age-related macular degeneration.

Red

- Microaneurysms: the dots that typify diabetic retinopathy. They may leak to cause exudates or bleed to cause blot haemorrhages (Fig. 21.17).
- Blot haemorrhages: rounded localized intraretinal blood, typically caused by diabetic retinopathy, but other causes include severe hypertension and retinal vein occlusion.
- Deep large haemorrhages: associated with retinal ischaemia when numerous.
- Flame haemorrhages: have a characteristic feathery shape as the blood is in the nerve fibre layer; may be present in retinal vein occlusion (Fig. 21.18). Not typically associated with ischaemia.

Black

- Retinal pigment hypertrophy: well-defined black lesions, often in conjunction with chorioretinal atrophy. May occur with previous retinal inflammation or injury (including retinal laser therapy).

Figure 21.17 Diabetic retinopathy. Microaneurysms (tiny red dots), blot haemorrhages, hard exudates and areas of new vessel formation (*arrow*) are characteristic of this condition. In many patients, hypertensive retinopathy is also present.

Figure 21.18 Branch retinal vein occlusion. There are flame-shaped retinal haemorrhages, but the disc is normal.

The fovea at its centre is one disc diameter in size. The fovea, with its high density of cone photoreceptors, is responsible for fine discriminatory vision. To find the fovea, locate the optic disc and move the ophthalmoscope beam temporally (move yourself towards the nose). Alternatively, ask the patient to look directly into the light. However, if the pupil is not dilated, it tends to constrict at this point, and the patient may recoil because of dazzle (you can dim the light beam to make it more comfortable). In young patients, the retina is very reflective and there is often a small yellow dot in the middle of the fovea (macula lutea or fovea centralis). Box 21.9 and Figs 21.17 and 21.18 identify common retinal abnormalities by their colour and appearance.

Slit lamp and intraocular pressure

The slit lamp (Fig. 21.19) provides a stereoscopic, magnified view of the eye and is the key examination tool for ophthalmologists. Many accident and emergency departments have a slit lamp, and it can be invaluable for assessing suspected foreign bodies and corneal abrasions. Some direct ophthalmoscopes are equipped with a slit-lamp beam, which can be useful. Alternatively, the anterior orbital structures and globe can be examined with a bright torch and basic magnification, and the same principles of systematic examination apply. The slit lamp is composed of a table-mounted binocular microscope column with an adjustable illumination source that produces a narrow, slit beam of light.

Figure 21.19 Slit lamp.

The patient is seated with forehead and chin supported. The slit beam illumination and microscope have a common axis of rotation and coincident focal lengths, allowing the angle of illumination to be varied along with its width, length and intensity. Projected onto the globe, the slit beam illuminates an optical cross-section of the eye's transparent structures, and this can be viewed with magnification varying from 10× to 40× power. An attachment allows the IOP to be measured (tonometry). The drainage angle can be seen with a special contact lens (gonioscopy) and, with the aid of a hand-held lens or a contact lens, the retina can also be viewed.

The following structures can be examined:

- Lid margins, meibomian gland orifices and lashes. Inflammation of the lid margins (blepharitis) is one of the most common ophthalmic conditions. It is related to chalazia, blocked meibomian glands and infected lash follicles (styes). The puncta, on the medial aspect of the lids, drain tears into the canalicular tear drainage pathway. Misdirected lashes (trichiasis) causing foreign body sensations occur with chronic lid disease.
- Conjunctival surfaces (tarsal, forniceal and bulbar). This mucous membrane lines the eyeball (bulbar conjunctiva) and the inner surface of the eyelids (tarsal conjunctiva). The conjunctiva may be pale in anaemia, yellow in jaundice or red (injected) in conjunctivitis and other inflammatory eye disorders. Directing the patient's gaze up, down, left and right ensures that all the bulbar conjunctiva is viewed. To examine the inferior tarsal conjunctiva of the lower lid, the lower lid should be gently everted and the patient asked to look upwards. To examine the superior tarsal

Figure 21.20 Everting the upper eyelid to expose the tarsal conjunctiva.

Figure 21.21 Fluorescein used to stain the cornea and tear film.

conjunctiva—for example if a foreign body is suspected—ask the patient to look downwards (Fig. 21.20). Grasp the lashes between the forefinger and thumb, gently pull down on them and rotate the eyelid upwards over either the other thumb or a cotton bud.

- Cornea and tear film. The transparent cornea can be viewed in cross-section. The addition of a drop of 2% fluorescein reveals defects or foreign bodies in the corneal epithelium and the tear film can be assessed (Fig. 21.21). The tear meniscus on the lower eyelid should be symmetrical and less than 1 mm thick, and the tear break-up time should be more than 10 seconds. Fluorescein also aids the identification of aqueous leakage in a penetrating corneal injury (Seidel's test). Arcus senilis is a common crescentic opacity near the periphery of the cornea. It usually starts at the lower part of the cornea, extending to form a complete circle. It is common in old people, but may occur in the young (arcus juvenilis) in association with type IV hyperlipoproteinaemia. Corneal sensation should be tested.

■ Anterior chamber (filled with aqueous). In iritis, a cause of red eye, there is inflammation in the aqueous, with flare (protein) and cells (typically leukocytes). In severe iritis, the inflammatory exudate settles inferiorly to create a white fluid level in the anterior chamber (hypopyon). Hyphaema has a similar but red appearance caused by bleeding into the anterior chamber, usually owing to trauma.

■ Iris. Note any difference in the colour of the two eyes (heterochromia), abnormality in the shape or size of the pupils or signs of iritis. In iritis, the pupil may be constricted (miosis) or irregular owing to the formation of adhesions (posterior synechiae) between the edge of the pupil and the anterior surface of the lens. Blunt trauma can cause a dilated (mydriasis) unreactive pupil with radial ruptures in the iris. An irregular or teardrop-shaped pupil and a history of a high-velocity foreign body is highly suspicious of a penetrating eye injury where the iris has plugged the leaking wound. Other abnormalities of the pupils are described in Chapter 16.

■ Lens. Cataracts are usually caused by ageing (central nuclear sclerosis), but also occur in diabetes mellitus, after injury and in certain hereditary diseases, for example myotonic dystrophy. Posterior subcapsular cataract is a common side effect of corticosteroid therapy. Blunt eye injury may cause partial dislocation of the lens (subluxation) or complete dislocation into the vitreous cavity.

■ Anterior vitreous. This is best examined when the pupil is dilated. Opacities may be observed, most easily using a green light. Cells in the vitreous may be associated with ocular inflammation (vitritis), trauma (vitreous haemorrhage) or retinal holes/ detachment (retinal pigment).

Measuring intraocular pressure: applanation tonometry

Intraocular pressures between 10 and 21 mmHg are considered normal. An increased IOP is a characteristic feature of glaucoma. A diminished IOP occurs in diabetic coma and in severe dehydration from any cause. The IOP may be assessed by palpating the eyeball, although only gross variations from normal can be appreciated. More accurate is applanation tonometry, in which the force required to flatten (applanate) an area of a sphere (the cornea) is proportional to the pressure within the sphere (Fig. 21.22). Topical anaesthetic and fluorescein are

Figure 21.22   Goldman tonometry.

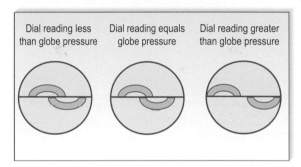

Figure 21.23   Diagrammatic representation of tonometry.

applied to the cornea and a bright cobalt blue filter is used to illuminate the sterile tonometer head. Contact between the tonometer head and the cornea creates a thin green circular outline of fluorescein, and a prism in the head splits this into two semicircles. The tonometer force is adjusted manually until the semicircles just overlap and then it is read in millimetres of mercury (mmHg; Fig. 21.23).

Eyelid, lacrimal and orbital assessment

Eyelids

People of Asian origin have a long, narrow palpebral aperture with an upward and outward obliquity and a characteristic fold of skin along the upper lid. The highest point of the aperture is typically at the junction of its middle and inner thirds. In Down's syndrome, the palpebral fissure is also oblique. However, it is also short and wide, with its highest point at the centre of the lid.

Normally no sclera is visible above the limbus (the corneoscleral junction). The most common cause of scleral show is eyelid retraction (Fig. 21.24) owing to

Figure 21.24 Thyroid eye disease with upper eyelid retraction and mild exophthalmos (bilateral proptosis).

Figure 21.25 Lower eyelid entropion causing infective keratitis and corneal opacification.

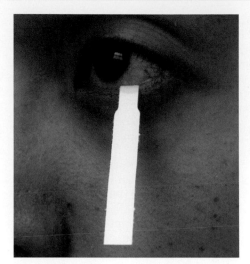

Figure 21.26 Schirmer's test for dry eyes.

dysthyroid eye disease, accompanied by other signs, such as lid lag, in which movement of the upper lid seems to lag behind that of the eyeball when the patient looks downwards. In Parkinsonism, there may be reduced blink frequency. Look for reduced eyelid closure (lagophthalmos) and levator muscle function. Ptosis (drooping of the upper lid) may be congenital or acquired (check old photographs). In age-related ptosis, owing to levator disinsertion, levator function is retained and there is a high upper eyelid skin crease. In ptosis owing to myogenic or neurogenic lesions, there is reduced levator function (see Chapter 16). In entropion, there is inversion of the lid margin with associated malpositioning of the lashes, which may rub on the cornea (Fig. 21.25); and, in ectropion, eversion of the eyelid is often associated with watering. The lower lid is susceptible to skin tumours, particularly basal cell and squamous cell carcinomas (see Fig. 20.25). Xanthelasmas are fatty deposits that develop in the upper and lower eyelids in patients with long-standing hypercholesterolaemia.

Lacrimal gland

Examine the lacrimal gland by pulling up the outer part of the upper lid while the patient looks downwards and inwards. Acute inflammation (dacryoadenitis)

causes a tender swollen gland, with oedema of the upper lid and localized conjunctival injection. Chronic dacryoadenitis, a painless enlargement of the lacrimal gland which is frequently bilateral, occurs in sarcoidosis and lymphoproliferative disorders. Tumours of the lacrimal gland produce a hard swelling of the gland associated with displacement of the globe. Involvement of the lacrimal gland by any disease process may cause a dry eye.

Assess the position and size of the puncta (see above). Painless watering is a feature of obstruction of the tear drainage pathway, but exclude reflex tearing and overflow from, for example, a dry eye. Schirmer's test uses a standardized strip of filter paper to detect dry eyes by assessing the extent of wetting at 5 minutes (Fig. 21.26). Overt nasolacrimal duct blockage can be excluded if the patient reports fluid at the back of the throat on probing and syringing with normal saline (Fig. 21.27).

Orbit

The most common cause of forward displacement of the eyeball—proptosis when unilateral, or exophthalmos when bilateral—is thyroid eye disease (TED) (see Fig. 19.13). This can cause corneal exposure and ulceration. Optic nerve damage may occur despite minimal proptosis. Axial proptosis, in the primary direction of the eye in forward gaze, is typical of TED and of tumours in the extraocular muscle cone behind the eye (intraconal mass lesions) (Fig. 21.28). Non-axial proptosis occurs in association with space-occupying orbital lesions outside the muscle cone: for example, lacrimal gland tumours; these displace the globe forward and inferomedially. Apparent ('pseudo') proptosis causes diagnostic confusion: for example, in ipsilateral eyelid retraction or myopia (where the eye is longer than normal) or when there is contralateral ptosis or enophthalmos.

Figure 21.27 Syringe and probing to assess nasolacrimal duct function.

Figure 21.28 Axial CT orbits in TED. Left-sided thyroid eye disease (TED) with exophthalmos and marked hypertrophy (inflammation) of the medial and lateral rectus muscles on that side. These muscles in the other eye are also slightly enlarged. The optic nerve can clearly be seen between the enlarged muscles on the left side.

Proptosis and enophthalmos can be measured with the Hertel exophthalmometer (Fig. 21.29). A difference of more than 2 mm between sides is abnormal. A proptosis that increases while the patient performs a Valsalva manoeuvre is suggestive of a venous abnormality. Pulsatile proptosis with an orbital bruit is a feature of carotid cavernous fistula.

Blunt trauma to the orbit may cause a blowout fracture of the thin orbital floor. Orbital contents may prolapse through the fracture, restricting the movement of the inferior rectus muscle and limiting upgaze. A full orbital examination should include palpation, eye movement examination, optic nerve assessment and testing of the trigeminal nerve for altered sensation.

Figure 21.29 Hertel exophthalmometry to quantify proptosis or exophthalmos.

Examination of the eye in children

The advice given in Chapter 6 on the examination of children in general is also important when examining children's eyes. Children may object strongly to lights and instruments, particularly when they are wielded by white-coated strangers. Allow the child to get used to the surroundings while taking a history from the parent, but do not ignore the child. Constantly observe the child, noting visual behaviour, the position and movements of the eyes and the general appearance of each eye.

Visual maturation continues after birth and without a focused retinal image, the visual pathways fail to develop properly, a condition known as amblyopia. Untreated, sight loss from amblyopia becomes irreversible. It is therefore important to assess visual acuity in preverbal and young children. Babies should rapidly fix a large object—for example the examiner's face—and follow it. After 6 months, 'continuous' and 'steady' fixation that is 'maintained' ('CSM') during a blink should be demonstrable. If an infant strongly objects to your covering an eye for even a short time, consider whether the non-covered eye may not be seeing well. A more sophisticated assessment can be made using 'preferential looking'. Cards are presented to the child with a grating drawn at one end and none at the other. The child will prefer to look at the image rather than nothing. Successively smaller spatial gratings are shown until the child does not see them. The grating seen can be converted to an approximate Snellen acuity (the vision of a 1-year-old equates to approximately 6/12), although testing each eye independently in this age group is difficult. From the age of 2 years, a more accurate estimate of acuity can be made using the Kay picture-matching test (Fig. 21.30), and from 3 years the Sheridan-Gardiner letter-matching test. In these tests, the child, or the child's parent, holds a card with a number of pictures or numbers on it. The examiner holds up an image and asks the child to match this target to one on the card; the targets vary in size.

Next, the position and movements of the eyes should be assessed. The least disturbing method is to observe the corneal light reflex: a light held at about 1 m should produce a reflection in the centre of each pupil. If the reflection in one eye is at a different location from that in the other, there may be a squint (although a wide intercanthal distance may give this appearance). If a squint is suspected, a cover

Figure 21.30 Kay picture-matching test to assess the visual acuity of children 2 years of age and older.

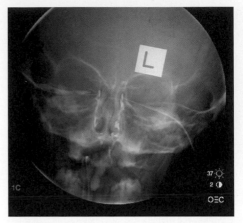

Figure 21.31 Dacryocystogram showing restricted flow of radiopaque dye in the right nasolacrimal duct.

and alternate cover test should be performed. Assess the ocular movements and the pupillary responses to light and accommodation. Examine the media and fundi with the ophthalmoscope through the dilated pupil. Because of limited cooperation, refraction testing may be limited to the retinoscopy assessment. In general, only children with refractive errors so severe that there is a risk of amblyopia require treatment.

Imaging

Plain X-rays

Plain X-rays have a limited role in the detection of foreign bodies, but have been largely superseded by computed tomography (CT) or magnetic resonance imaging (MRI). Ultrasound is used to assess the globe. A dacryocystogram uses a radiopaque dye introduced into the lacrimal drainage system to identify sites of lacrimal duct obstruction (Fig. 21.31). It is particularly useful in the watering eye, when carcinoma is suspected, when repeat surgery is planned or when trauma has occurred.

Computed tomography and magnetic resonance imaging

Computed tomography and MRI are used extensively in the diagnosis of orbital disease. CT is often considered superior because it defines the bony orbit, but the X-ray dose to the eye and lens is not inconsiderable. CT is the investigation of choice in blunt orbital trauma and blowout fractures (see above), where fine-cut coronal spiral images are desirable (Fig. 21.32).

A- and B-mode ultrasound

The A-mode scan is a one-dimensional time-amplitude study commonly used to assess axial length, which is an essential measurement for lens implant calculation prior to cataract surgery. The B-mode scan gives a two-dimensional cross-sectional view of the eye for the diagnosis of both intraocular and orbital tumours,

Figure 21.32 Coronal CT orbits in blowout fracture. The right bony orbital floor is fractured and the orbital contents prolapsed.

retinal detachments and intraocular disorders when the fundal view is impaired (e.g. with vitreous haemorrhage; Fig. 21.33).

Retinal photography and fundus fluorescein angiography

Retinal photography alone is useful to document posterior segment abnormalities and allow monitoring, for example, of a choroidal naevus. In conjunction with the intravenous injection of sodium fluorescein photography it gives a detailed assessment of the retinal and choroidal vasculature (Figs 21.34 and 21.35). A blue filtered light excites fluorescence (530 nm) as the dye circulates. Fundus fluorescein angiography is useful in investigating diabetic retinopathy, age-related macular degeneration and retinal ischaemia. Minor side effects, including transient nausea and yellow discolouration of the skin and urine, are common. Severe anaphylaxis is, fortunately, very rare.

Retinal and optic disc tomography

Optical coherence tomography and optic disc tomography

Becoming increasingly widely used clinically, optical coherence tomography (OCT) is based on interferometry, typically using near infrared light, to obtain high-resolution (2–20 μm) cross-sectional images of the retina (Fig. 21.36) and optic disc. Optical coherence tomography angiography (OCTA) is a newer development that compares motion contrast imaging with high-resolution volumetric blood flow information to generate non-invasive retinal angiography images without injection of fluorescein. OCT has also been developed to generate images of the anterior segment (ACOCT), for example showing the angle structures in high resolution. In addition to OCT, a variety of techniques have been developed to image and assess the shape of the optic disc that are particularly useful in the management of glaucoma. These include scanning laser polarimetry (SLP) and the scanning laser ophthalmoscope (SLO) that assesses nerve fibre thickness indirectly.

Figure 21.33 B-mode ultrasound scan showing lens opacity and vitreous opacities, but no retinal detachment following penetrating trauma. C, cornea; L, lens; ON, optic nerve; V, vitreous.

Special examination techniques

Refraction and refractive assessment

A refraction test will ascertain the optical power of an eye, with a view to prescribing glasses or contact lenses. An objective refraction is performed using neutralizing lenses in conjunction with a retinoscope. In adults and cooperative children, this is then refined subjectively by placing neutralizing

Figure 21.34 Fluorescein retinal angiogram of fundus in papilloedema. Note the late-phase leakage of the dye.

Figure 21.35 Fluorescein retinal angiogram of fundus in pseudopapilloedema.

Figure 21.36 Ocular coherence tomography image of a normal macula. C, choroid; RPE, retinal pigment epithelium; PR, photoreceptor layer; ICN, inter-connecting neurone layer; NFL, nerve fibre layer; FD, foveal depression.

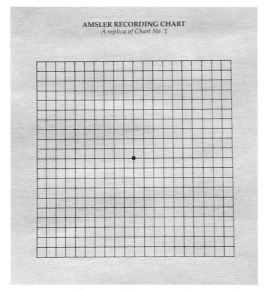

Figure 21.37 Amsler grid for testing macular function.

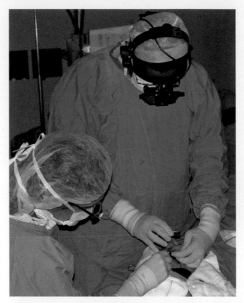

Figure 21.38 Indirect ophthalmoscopy, here used intraoperatively. Note the head light and hand-held 20 D lens.

Indirect ophthalmoscopy

Binocular indirect ophthalmoscopy, using a light source supported on the examiner's head and a hand-held lens in front of the patient's eye, allows a much greater area of the fundus to be visualized (Fig. 21.38). The retinal periphery is more readily seen.

Electrophysiological tests

Visual evoked potentials (VEP), recorded from the occipital cortex using scalp electrodes while the patient views an alternating black-and-white chequerboard stimulus, have a role in the diagnosis of disease of the visual pathway. The principal waveform recorded from the scalp is a positive deflection occurring about 100 ms after the stimulus (the P100 wave). This is attenuated in amplitude and increased in latency in disease of the optic nerve, for example optic neuritis or optic nerve compression. Electroretinograms (ERG) measure the electrical potential across the eye, recorded with a corneal electrode, with a reference electrode placed on the forehead. Flash, flicker or pattern stimuli are used to generate electrical responses from retinal activation. This is useful in assessing hereditary or acquired retinal degeneration.

lenses in front of the eye and simultaneously assessing visual acuity. Increasingly, the retinoscope is being replaced by an automated technique (the autorefractor).

Amsler grid

The Amsler grid is a sensitive test of macular function. It is composed of a series of vertical and horizontal lines with a central spot for fixation (Fig. 21.37). The patient is asked to look at this spot and describe any distortions or missing areas in the grid.

Ear, nose and throat | 22

Michael J. Wareing and Elinor Warner

Introduction

This chapter describes the assessment of potential diseases of the ear, nose and throat. The formal title of the specialty is otorhinolaryngology, also known as ear, nose and throat (ENT). The specialty has many interactions with oral and maxillofacial specialties, although extensive details of the latter are too specialized for an undergraduate textbook.

A close functional and anatomical relationship exists between the ear, the nose and the throat. Disease in one area may have manifestations in another area. Symptoms in one area may likewise refer to another area, so an accurate assessment requires a thorough history and examination of the entire area to elucidate a cause. Ear, nose and throat is a highly clinical subject because much is visible, especially with modern examination techniques, and so a lot of imaging and other investigations are often unnecessary.

The ear

Anatomy

The ear (Fig. 22.1) consists of the external, middle and inner ears. The external ear consists of the pinna and external auditory canal (meatus). The cartilaginous pinna is covered with perichondrium and skin, forming the helix and antihelix. The meatus has an outer cartilaginous and an inner bony component. The skin overlying the external auditory meatus contains hair cells and modified sebaceous glands, which produce wax (cerumen). Desquamated skin debris, mixed with cerumen, migrates outward from the drum and deep canal and makes the external ear a self-cleaning system.

The opaque or semitranslucent eardrum (tympanic membrane) separates the middle and external ears (Fig. 22.2). The pars tensa, the lower part of the drum, is formed from an outer layer of skin, a middle layer of fibrous tissue and an inner layer of middle ear mucosa. It is attached to the annulus, a fibrous ring that stabilizes the drum to the surrounding bone. The pars flaccida, the upper part of the drum, may retract if there is prolonged negative middle ear pressure secondary to Eustachian tube dysfunction. The malleus, incus and stapes are three small connecting bones (ossicles) (Fig. 22.3) that transmit sound across the middle ear from the drum to the cochlea. The handle of the malleus lies within the fibrous layer of the pars tensa.

Within the middle ear, the head of the malleus articulates with the incus in the attic, the upper portion of the middle ear space. The long process of the incus articulates with the stapes. This articulation (the incudostapedial joint) is liable to disruption from trauma or chronic infection owing to a tenuous blood supply, which may be compromised when these situations occur. The stapes footplate sits in the oval window, and transmits and amplifies sound to the fluid-filled inner ear. The inner ear has two portions. The cochlea (Fig. 22.4), the spiral organ of hearing, is a transducer that converts sound energy into digital nerve impulses that are transmitted by the eighth cranial nerve (cochlear) to the brainstem and thence to the auditory cortex. The organ of Corti (Fig. 22.5) within the cochlea contains hair cells that detect frequency-specific sound energy; low-frequency sounds are detected in the apical region and high-frequency sounds are detected in the basal region. The inner ear is also concerned with balance. The semicircular canals and the vestibule contain receptors that detect angular and linear motion in the three cardinal x, y and z planes. The inner ears are only one component of the balance system; visual input and proprioception from joints and muscles are also important.

The facial (seventh cranial) nerve (Fig. 22.6) is important in otological practice. It runs from the brainstem through the cerebellopontine angle to the internal auditory meatus (IAM) with the cochlear and vestibular (eighth) nerves. The facial nerve passes through the temporal bone and leaves the skull through the stylomastoid foramen near the mastoid process. It may be damaged in cases of suppurative middle ear disease or trauma. The chorda tympani leaves the descending portion of the facial nerve in the temporal bone to provide taste fibre innervation to the anterior two-thirds of the tongue. The facial

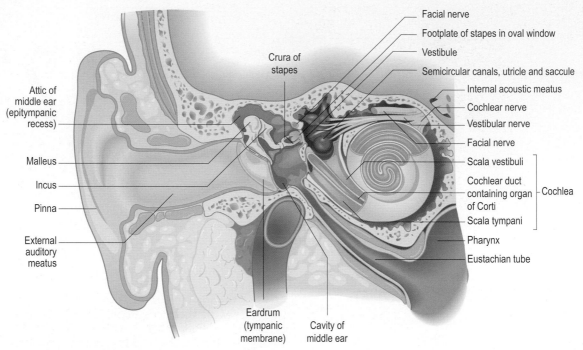

Figure 22.1 Anatomy of the ear.

Figure 22.2 A normal left tympanic membrane.

nerve supplies the facial muscles through upper and lower divisions that arise as it passes through the parotid gland.

Symptoms of ear disease

The five main symptoms of ear disease are:
- Otalgia: earache or pain
- Otorrhoea: discharge
- Hearing loss
- Tinnitus: a perception of sound in the absence of an appropriate auditory stimulus
- Vertigo: an illusion of movement

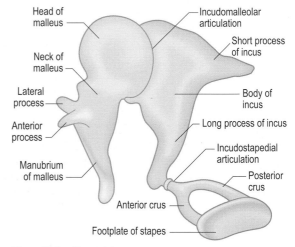

Figure 22.3 The ossicles.

Otalgia

Pain from disease of the external ear, tympanic membrane and middle ear reaches the brain by branches of the fifth, ninth and tenth cranial nerves, together with nerves from C2 and C3 roots. Because branches of these nerves also supply the larynx and pharynx, as well as the temporomandibular joint and teeth, diseases of these structures may give rise to referred pain in the ear. Therefore, if otoscopic examination is normal, examination of these other sites should be considered. In half of patients with otalgia, the pain is referred.

The main causes of otalgia are listed in Box 22.1. Of the otological causes, acute infection of the cartilage caused by the pinna (perichondritis) can be

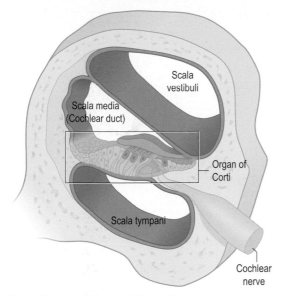

Figure 22.4   Section through the cochlea.

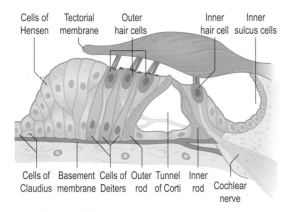

Figure 22.5   The organ of Corti.

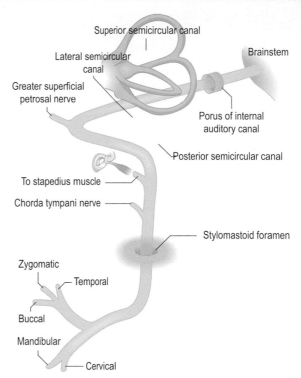

Figure 22.6   The course of the peripheral facial nerve.

Box 22.1	Causes of otalgia

Otological

- Acute otitis media, mastoiditis
- Acute otitis externa
- Barotrauma
- Furunculosis
- Perichondritis
- Herpes zoster (Ramsay Hunt syndrome—shingles of the facial nerve)
- Myringitis bullosa—viral myringitis
- Necrotizing external otitis (malignant otitis externa)
- Neoplasia

Non-otological

- Tonsillitis or quinsy
- Dental disease
- Temporomandibular joint pathology
- Cervical spine disease
- Carcinoma in the upper air and food passages

very painful. Malignant otitis externa (also known as necrotizing otitis externa) is not neoplastic. It is due to infection (usually *Pseudomonas*) and can spread to the skull base, especially in diabetic or immunocompromised patients, and its incidence is increasing exponentially in the UK.

Otorrhoea

Pus draining from the ear varies in character depending on its origin (Table 22.1). A profuse mucoid discharge with pulsation suggests a tympanic membrane perforation. The length of history is important. Persistent discharge suggests chronic otitis media with perforation (Table 22.2). Cholesteatoma usually begins with tympanic membrane retraction and blockage of migrating desquamated skin from the drum and external meatus. The retraction deepens and infection leads to destruction of middle ear structures, sometimes causing damage to the facial nerve or inner ear. The infection may spread outside the temporal bone, even causing meningitis or intracranial abscess. Bleeding from a chronically discharging ear is usually caused by infection, but may rarely indicate malignant change. Cranial trauma followed by bleeding and leakage of cerebrospinal fluid (CSF) indicates fracture of the base of the skull.

Hearing loss

Deafness may be gradual or sudden, bilateral or unilateral. There may be an obvious precipitating cause, such as trauma or noise exposure. There are two characteristics of hearing loss: to use the analogy of a radio, a decrease in volume or a change in the tuning corresponding to impaired speech

Table 22.1 Characteristics of otorrhoea in relation to site and aetiology

Diagnosis	Purulent	Mucopurulent	Mucoid	Serous	Watery
Acute otitis externa (OE)	✓✓	✓		✓	
Chronic OE	✓✓	✓		✓✓	
Acute otitis media (AOM)	✓	✓✓	✓		
Chronic OM	✓	✓✓	✓✓		
Cerebrospinal fluid leak				✓	✓✓

Table 22.2 Classification of chronic otitis media (COM)

COM classification (synonym)	Otoscopic abnormalities
Healed COM (healed perforation with or without tympanosclerosis)	Thinning and/or local or generalized opacification of the pars tensa without perforation or retraction
Inactive mucosal COM (dry perforation)	Permanent perforation of the pars tensa, but the middle ear mucosa is not inflamed
Active mucosal COM (discharging perforation)	Permanent defect of the pars tensa with an inflamed middle ear mucosa that produces mucopus which may discharge
Inactive squamous epithelial COM (retraction)	Retraction of the pars flaccida or pars tensa (usually posterosuperior) which has the potential to become active with retained debris
Active squamous epithelial COM (cholesteatoma)	Retraction of the pars flaccida or tensa that has retained squamous epithelial debris and is associated with inflammation and the production of pus, often from the adjacent mucosa

Box 22.2 Causes of deafness

Conductive

- Occluding wax in the external meatus
- Middle ear effusion: otitis media with effusion
- Acute otitis media
- Chronic otitis media: perforation, ossicular erosion, cholesteatoma
- Otosclerosis
- Trauma to the drum or ossicular chain
- Otitis externa
- Congenital atresia of the external meatus or congenital ossicular fixation
- Carcinoma of the middle ear

Sensorineural

- Age-associated hearing loss: presbycusis
- Noise-induced hearing loss
- Genetic: syndromal or non-syndromal
- Ménière's disease
- Infective: meningitis, measles, mumps, syphilis
- Sudden sensorineural hearing loss: idiopathic
- Perinatal: hypoxia, jaundice
- Prenatal: rubella
- Trauma: head injury, surgery
- Ototoxicity: aminoglycosides, diuretics, cytotoxics
- Neoplastic: vestibular schwannoma, other cerebellopontine angle lesions

discrimination so that words are not clear even with a hearing aid. Hearing loss may be conductive, sensorineural or mixed, with both conductive and sensorineural components (Box 22.2). Conductive deafness is caused by disease in the external ear canal, tympanic membrane or middle ear. Characteristically, the patient retains normal speech discrimination. Sensory deafness implies pathology in the cochlea, and neural deafness implies pathology in the cochlear nerve or the central connections of hearing. In practice this distinction is difficult to make and rarely useful, and the term sensorineural deafness is used instead. Sensorineural deafness causes impairment of speech discrimination with recruitment; the latter is an abnormal perception of the increase of intensity of sound with increasing signal volume that results from damage to the hair cells in the cochlea. This leads to a decreased functional dynamic range, so that a small increase in sound intensity is uncomfortable (which is why a

deaf grandparent might not be able to hear you one minute, but as you raise your voice, then ask you not to shout). The patient may also notice an apparent difference in the pitch or frequency of a tone between the two ears (diplacusis).

Most hearing loss is gradually progressive and related to ageing. There are also occupational causes of deafness, owing to loud sound exposure through work or social noise exposure and a predisposition to an early onset of hearing loss is often inherited. Many drugs are ototoxic, and there are associations between hereditary hearing loss and neurological and renal disorders. Occasionally, sensorineural hearing loss occurs suddenly. A cause is only rarely identifiable.

Tinnitus

Tinnitus is a ringing, rushing or hissing sound in the absence of an appropriate auditory stimulus. It can be caused by almost any pathology in the auditory pathways. It is strongly associated with hearing loss, although it occasionally occurs with normal hearing. It is common, affecting up to 18% of the population of industrialized countries. In a small proportion (0.5%), daily life is affected. Correction of coexisting depressive illness may be of value. Management of tinnitus includes the use of hearing aids, masking devices and stress management techniques. It usually improves with time, but in most cases there is no specific treatment.

Vertigo

Vertigo is an illusion of movement such that the patient either feels the world moving or has a sensation of moving in the world. Patients frequently have difficulty describing the symptom. Higher centre dysfunction, as in anxiety states or drug effects, may also cause dizziness. There are therefore many causes for symptomatic 'dizziness' (Box 22.3). A feeling of the room spinning associated with nausea or vomiting suggests an acute labyrinthine cause, especially if there are changes in hearing or tinnitus. Fortunately, most acute vestibular events are self-limiting, because even if one vestibular system is abnormal, the central connections can 'reset' the system over a period of a few days. The elderly are less able to compensate. In all age groups, vertigo may cause residual vague imbalance, particularly in association with movement or after alcohol ingestion. It is important to test for positional changes; the most common cause of vestibular vertigo is benign paroxysmal positional vertigo (BPPV), secondary to loose debris floating in the posterior semicircular canal.

Clinical examination of the ear and hearing

Pinna and postauricular area

First, inspect the pinna and the surrounding skin. Congenital abnormalities may be associated with accessory skin tags, abnormal cartilaginous fragments in the skin surrounding the ear or small pits and sinuses. Look also for any lymphadenopathy (associated with otitis externa or scalp cellulitis) and for surgical scars. A hot, tender postaural swelling, pushing the pinna forward, suggests mastoid infection or mastoid abscess (Fig. 22.7). Incomplete development of the ear (microtia) occurs with narrowing (atresia) of the external meatus, but the auricle can also be displaced from its normal position (melotia) or pathologically enlarged (macrotia). These abnormalities may be associated with cysts or infection in a preauricular sinus.

External ear canal

Inspect the external auditory canal using a hand-held otoscope (Fig. 22.8). To bring the cartilaginous meatus into line with the bony canal, retract the pinna backwards and upwards. Always use the largest speculum that will comfortably fit the ear canal.

Box 22.3	Causes of vertigo

Of sudden onset
- Acute viral labyrinthitis
- Vestibular neuritis
- Migraine

With focal features
- Brainstem ischaemia (transient ischaemic attack)
- Multiple sclerosis
- Migraine
- Temporal lobe epilepsy

With deafness and tinnitus
- Ménière's disease
- Vestibular schwannoma
- Migraine

With positional change
- Benign paroxysmal positional vertigo (BPPV)
- Cervical vertigo

After trauma
- BPPV
- Perilymph fistula

With motion
- Motion sickness

Drug-induced
- Vestibulotoxic drugs (e.g. aminoglycosides, salicylate, quinine, furosemide, platinum-based chemotherapy)

With aural discharge
- Middle ear disease

With systemic disorders
- Postural hypotension
- Syncope
- Cardiac dysrhythmia
- Carotid sinus hypersensitivity
- Anxiety and panic attacks
- Hyperventilation syndrome

Hold the otoscope like a pen between thumb and index finger, with the ulnar border of your hand resting gently against the side of the patient's head. In this way, any movement of the patient's head during the examination causes synchronous movement of the speculum, limiting any risk of accidental injury to the ear canal. With a young child, sit him on his parent's lap with the head and shoulder held (Fig. 22.9).

Wax may be removed with a Jobson Horne probe or wax hook or by syringing with water. Never syringe if there is a history of previous perforation or discharge. It is important to use water at 37°C lest vertigo be induced by caloric stimulation of the labyrinth. Keratin debris, pus or mucopus in the meatus can be removed and can be sent for microbiology. Foreign bodies in the ear canal are sometimes found in children; they may be difficult to remove without a general anaesthetic.

Figure 22.7 Acute mastoiditis (**A**) before and (**B**) after incision.

Figure 22.8 Examining the ear in an adult.

The tympanic membrane

The hand-held otoscope is satisfactory for most examinations, but the outpatient microscope offers the best view. Be familiar with the variability in appearance of the normal drum. The most common abnormality is tympanosclerosis (Fig. 22.10), which consists of white chalky patches in the drum caused by hyaline degeneration of the fibrous layer due to previous infection.

Prolonged negative middle ear pressure may cause the drum to become thinned and atelectatic (Fig. 22.11), either diffusely or with a retraction pocket. Eustachian tube dysfunction and/or acute otitis media may cause a middle ear effusion (Fig. 22.12). Fluid behind the drum is often obvious, but when the drum is opaque, increased vascularity and retraction are useful clues.

Perforations of the pars tensa are either central or marginal (Fig. 22.13). Marginal perforations extend to the annulus and may be associated with cholesteatoma (Fig. 22.14), whereas with central perforations a rim of membrane is retained between the defect and the annulus. Both are described by their position in relation to the handle of the malleus (anterior, posterior or inferior) and by their size (Fig. 22.15). The fistula test is indicated if the patient is dizzy with middle ear pathology. Press on the tragus to occlude the meatus and then apply more pressure. If the labyrinth is open, this pressure change will be applied to the inner ear. The patient will be dizzy and nystagmus may be induced. Typical computerized tomography (CT) scan findings of a positive fistula test are shown in Figure 22.27.

The facial nerve

Test the facial movements. Unilateral weakness is much easier to identify than bilateral weakness. A peripheral facial palsy can be graded using the House-Brackmann scale (Table 22.3). Function of the greater superficial petrosal nerve can be tested with Schirmer's test: absorbent paper strips are applied to the inferior margin of the eye to detect tear formation (see Chapter 21). Chorda tympani function can be tested by the sense of taste and by electrogustometry, although this is rarely used in practice.

Clinical assessment of hearing

Conversational hearing will indicate any possible deafness. The television may be too loud or varying amounts of background noise make conversation unexpectedly difficult. Establish which is the patient's better-hearing ear. Test using words or numbers. Stand to the side of the ear to be tested and mask the non-test ear by gently rubbing the tragus. The test starts with a whispered voice at 60

Figure 22.9 Examining the ear in a child.

Figure 22.10 A right tympanic membrane showing marked posterior tympanosclerosis and a small anterior perforation.

Figure 22.12 A left tympanic membrane with a middle ear effusion.

Figure 22.11 A left tympanic membrane showing atelectasis and posterior retraction on to the long process of the incus.

Figure 22.13 A left tympanic membrane with an anterior central perforation.

Figure 22.14 A left tympanic membrane with cholesteatoma in the posterosuperior quadrant.

Figure 22.15 A left tympanic membrane with a subtotal perforation. The chorda tympani and long process of the incus can clearly be seen, as can the round window niche.

Table 22.3	The House-Brackmann facial nerve grading scale
Grade	**Function**
I	▪ Normal
II	▪ Normal at rest
	▪ Slight weakness on close inspection
	▪ Complete eye closure with minimal effort
	▪ Slight asymmetry of mouth with movement
	▪ Good to moderate forehead movement
	▪ Normal at rest
	▪ Obvious asymmetry on movement
	▪ Synkinesis ± hemifacial spasm
	▪ Complete eye closure with effort
	▪ Slight to moderate forehead movement
	▪ Slight weakness of mouth with maximal effort
III	▪ Normal at rest
	▪ Asymmetry on movement is disfiguring
	▪ Incomplete eye closure
	▪ No perceptible forehead movement
	▪ Asymmetrical mouth motion with maximal effort
IV	▪ Asymmetric at rest
	▪ Barely noticeable movement
	▪ No forehead movement
	▪ Incomplete eye closure
	▪ Slight mouth movement with effort
	▪ No facial function perceptible

cm (approximate intensity 15 dB) and proceeds with a whispered voice at 15 cm (35 dB). If there is no response, try a conversational voice at 60 cm (50 dB); this is then repeated, if necessary, at 15 cm (55–60 dB) from the test ear. With experience, a surprisingly accurate assessment can be made. It is valuable in correlating the history and results of more formal audiometry.

The Rinne test (Fig. 22.16) compares hearing by air and bone conduction using a 512- or 256-Hz tuning fork. Strike the tuning fork and hold it near the external ear canal with the prongs vibrating towards the meatus (air conduction) and then against the mastoid process (bone conduction). Ask the patient which sound was louder. In subjects with normal hearing and those with sensorineural loss, air conduction is better than bone conduction (Rinne positive). In conductive deafness, bone conduction is louder (Rinne negative), although patients with a small conductive loss (up to 30 dB) may remain Rinne positive; it is only when the difference between air and bone conduction exceeds 40 dB that the Rinne test is consistently negative. Moreover, patients with a profound unilateral sensorineural hearing loss will report a Rinne-negative response if the contralateral ear has normal or reasonable hearing. This is because, although the vibrating tuning fork held adjacent to the test ear will only be heard in that ear, the same tuning fork placed on the mastoid process will also be heard in the non-test ear. For these reasons, masking (by rubbing) the non-test ear should always validate a negative response. If there is doubt, a Barany box should be used to mask the contralateral ear.

In the Weber test, the base of the vibrating tuning fork is placed firmly on the vertex or forehead in the midline. With eyes shut, ask the patient whether the sound is heard in the midline or whether it is lateralized. With normal response or with hearing symmetrically reduced, the sound is heard in the midline. However, when one ear is normal, the noise will be louder on the side opposite to an ear with pure sensorineural loss and on the same side as an ear with purely conductive hearing loss. The Weber test is simple and quick, but there is a high test-retest

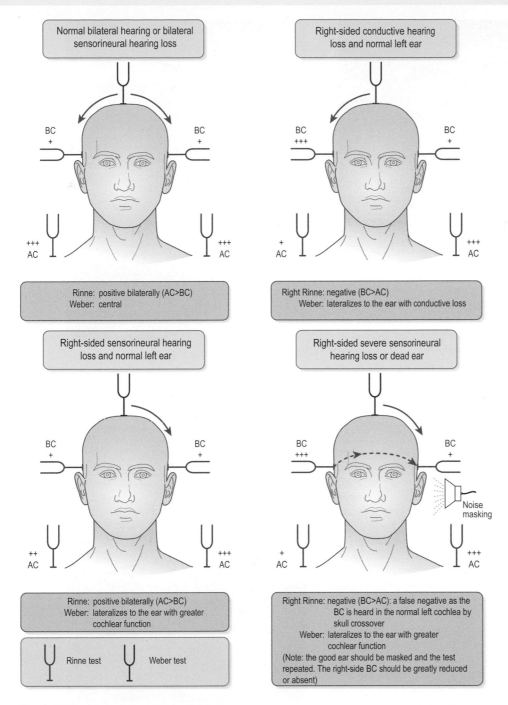

Normal bilateral hearing or bilateral sensorineural hearing loss

BC +

BC +

+++ AC

+++ AC

Rinne: positive bilaterally (AC>BC)
Weber: central

Right-sided conductive hearing loss and normal left ear

BC +++

BC +

+ AC

+++ AC

Right Rinne: negative (BC>AC)
Weber: lateralizes to the ear with conductive loss

Right-sided sensorineural hearing loss and normal left ear

BC +

BC +

++ AC

+++ AC

Rinne: positive bilaterally (AC>BC)
Weber: lateralizes to the ear with greater cochlear function

Rinne test   Weber test

Right-sided severe sensorineural hearing loss or dead ear

BC +++

BC +

Noise masking

+ AC

+++ AC

Right Rinne: negative (BC>AC): a false negative as the BC is heard in the normal left cochlea by skull crossover
Weber: lateralizes to the ear with greater cochlear function
(Note: the good ear should be masked and the test repeated. The right-side BC should be greatly reduced or absent)

Figure 22.16 Interpretation of tuning fork tests.

variability. Because all clinical tests of hearing have limited reliability, accurate formal audiometry in the ENT clinic is essential.

Clinical assessment of balance

The unsteady patient requires a full neuro-otological examination. It is also necessary to examine the cardiovascular system (see Chapter 13). The aim is to localize the site of any potential lesion and possibly confirm a diagnosis, although sometimes all that is possible is to differentiate between central (brainstem) and peripheral (labyrinthine) lesions.

- Examine the cranial nerves (see Chapter 16), particularly testing the eyes and for nystagmus.
- Nystagmus (see Chapters 16 and 21). The characteristic saw-toothed nystagmus of vestibular disease has a slow (labyrinthine) and a fast (central) component and is enhanced by movement of the eyes in the direction of the fast phase. Eye movements can also be assessed using Frenzel's glasses (Fig. 22.17). These are illuminated and

Figure 22.17 Frenzel's glasses.

have 20-dioptre lenses that abolish visual fixation for the patient, thereby possibly unmasking nystagmus. Horizontal nystagmus can be peripheral or central; pure vertical upbeat or downbeat nystagmus usually indicates a central process.

■ Pursuit (slow) movements, which depend on the fovea and the occipital cortex of the brain, are seen when the patient tracks an object moved slowly horizontally and vertically across the visual field about 35 cm away. If these are jerky rather than smooth this can indicate a central lesion.

■ Saccadic movements are driven by the frontal lobes and the pontine gaze centres are seen when the patient alternates the gaze rapidly between two objects held approximately 30° apart. Disorders of saccadic accuracy indicate a central lesion.

■ All these eye movement disorders can be identified by videonystagmography (Fig. 22.18) in which a test battery is run using video cameras to monitor the eyes and measure and record eye movements to identify signs of vestibular (peripheral) or neurological (central) disorders.

■ Romberg's test. The patient stands with the feet together, initially with the eyes open and then closed. Patients with disorders of the spinal posterior columns (impaired position sense) will sway or fall with closed eyes, but will stand normally if eyes are open. Patients with uncompensated unilateral labyrinthine dysfunction are unstable, tending to fall to the side of the lesion. Patients with central dysfunction sway to both sides, whether the eyes are open or shut. Patients with persistent postural perceptual dizziness (PPPD), a cause of chronic dizziness, will feel excessively unsteady on Romberg's testing despite not exhibiting particularly pronounced sway. Computerized dynamic posturography tests postural stability and an ability to maintain an upright posture under different test conditions using information from the muscles/joints, eyes and ears. This can be used in a rehabilitative setting

Figure 22.18 Videonystagmography.

Figure 22.19 Computerized dynamic posturography.

as well as to aid diagnosis of balance dysfunction (Fig. 22.19).

■ Unterberger's stepping test has the patient standing with arms outstretched and eyes closed and taking steps on the spot. Unilateral vestibular hypofunction leads to rotation to the affected side.

■ Gait assessment. The patient walks heel to toe with eyes first open and then closed. The patient with a cerebellar lesion is unable to do either (ataxic gait). The patient with a peripheral

Figure 22.20   The Dix–Hallpike test position.

Figure 22.21   (**A**) Pure tone audiometry. (**B**) Bone conduction testing with masking being performed.

vestibular lesion will struggle, particularly with the eyes closed.

- The Dix–Hallpike test assesses the effect of positional change. The patient sits on an examination couch. First test neck movements, to make sure they are free and painless. The head is then turned 45° to the side of test. The patient is laid back rapidly with his head extended over the end of the bed (Fig. 22.20). The classic response in BPPV involves a variable latent period when nothing happens. Then a torsional nystagmus beating occurs to the lower ear, with a variable feeling of vertigo. This lasts perhaps 5–30 seconds. With repetition, the response becomes less or absent. The condition is caused by debris in the posterior semicircular canal. It is frequently self-limiting, but if it persists it may be cured by the Epley particle repositioning manoeuvre. Other positive results are possible. Persistent immediate positional nystagmus without vertigo implies central pathology.

Special investigations of hearing

Pure tone audiometry

A single-frequency tone is presented at standardized levels into each ear in turn. This is done in noise-free surroundings, usually in a soundproofed booth (Fig. 22.21). Air conduction is tested first through headphones. A level well above threshold, as predicted by free field testing, is chosen and the patient responds when he hears the sound. The intensity is then reduced in 10-dB steps until the patient cannot hear it. It is then increased in 5-dB steps to establish the quietest sound that can be heard—the threshold. The better ear is tested first at 1, 2, 4 and 8 kHz, then at 250 and 500 Hz (Fig. 22.22). In conductive loss, the difference is called the air–bone gap. This may be correctable by surgery to the middle ear and tympanic membrane.

Speech audiometry

A pure tone audiogram does not test discrimination (i.e. whether speech is intelligible). A speech

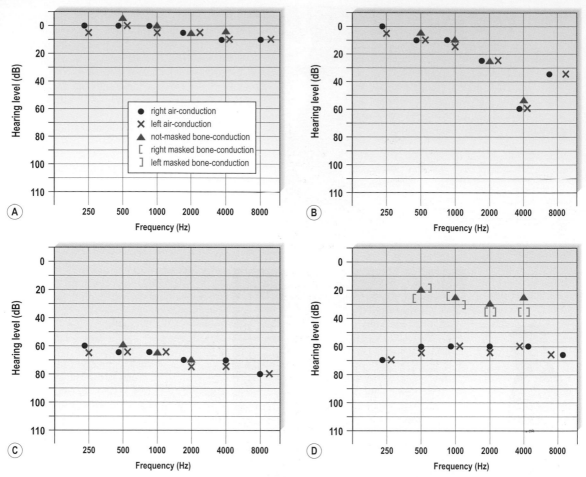

Figure 22.22 Pure tone audiograms. (**A**) Normal; (**B**) noise-induced hearing loss; (**C**) presbycusis; (**D**) bilateral conductive hearing loss.

audiogram measures the patient's ability to recognize words from phonetically balanced lists delivered at different sound levels to the test ear from a tape recording. The percentage of words correctly repeated by the subject is noted at each level. With normal hearing, all words are heard (100% optimal speech discrimination (ODS)) at a sound intensity of 40 dB. Patients with sensorineural deafness are often unable to achieve 100% ODS and, in particular, patients with neural/retrocochlear loss have poor ODS (Fig. 22.23).

Tympanometry

An earpiece is inserted into the external meatus, through which pass three channels. The first delivers a continuous tone into the ear canal during the test (probe tone); the second has a microphone to record the sound intensity level within the ear canal; the third channel connects to a manometer so that the pressure within the canal can be altered (Fig. 22.24A).

The external meatus is a rigid tube with a compliant end (the drum). Normally the middle ear and ear canal pressures are equal, and most of the sound introduced into the meatus is transmitted into the ear; only a minimum of sound energy is reflected

back and measured by the microphone. Changing the pressure difference between the external and the middle ear causes the tympanic membrane to become less compliant. This increases the sound energy reflected back to the probe. These changes are plotted graphically on a tympanogram (Fig. 22.24B). The test also measures the volume of the canal: a large volume indicates a tympanic perforation.

Impedance (the reciprocal of compliance) is increased when the tympanic membrane is thickened or the middle ear has fluid and is decreased when the drum is hypermobile or atrophic. Tympanometry is an objective test. It has particular value in children in the assessment of glue ear.

Otoacoustic emissions

When a click or tone-burst is played into the ear, a very small noise is emitted in return, probably arising from the outer hair cells. These emissions are particularly prominent in neonates, but become increasingly difficult to elicit with age. Testing does not require cooperation. When there is hearing loss there is no response. The technique is valuable in the screening of neonates and forms the backbone of the Universal Neonatal Hearing Screen programme.

SPEECH MATERIAL

FREE FIELD / EARPHONE

SCORING: PHONEME / WORD / SENTENCE

SPEECH LEVEL	RIGHT %	LEFT %
30	50	
40	80	
50	93	
60	97	
70	100	17
80		30
90		53
100		67

COMMENTS:

100% at 70 dB in the right ear

67% at 100 dB in the left ear

(maximum level of the audiometer reached with appropriate masking)

Figure 22.23   A speech audiogram.

Evoked-response audiometry

A click presented to the ear causes a nerve impulse to be sent to the auditory cortex via the brainstem. If a large number (>2000) of responses are averaged, then evoked responses in brainstem and cortex can be seen and amplitudes and latencies measured. The auditory brainstem response is not affected by sedation and the main indication is in the establishment of hearing thresholds, especially in infants. Cortical-evoked responses are less widely used. They require an awake and alert patient.

Special tests of balance

Caloric testing is the most commonly performed routine test of the vestibular end-organ. The patient lies on a couch with the head up 30° in order to bring the lateral semicircular canals into the vertical plane. With the patient fixing on a point in central gaze, each external ear canal is irrigated with water at 30°C, and then at 44°C for 30–40 seconds, with suitable intervals. Cold water induces nystagmus away from the irrigated ear and the opposite for warm water (COWS: *c*old *o*pposite, *w*arm *s*ame). The modern testing technique involves using hot and cold air rather than water, to avoid causing ear infections or perforations. The induced nystagmus is recorded and analysed using videonystagmography, which uses infrared video systems for a more detailed observation, recording and analysis of these eye movements, whilst preventing optical fixation (Fig. 22.25) (see also Frenzel's glasses above). Peripheral lesions tend to cause a diminished response on one side (a canal paresis). A directional preponderance may be caused by central disorders, especially in the brainstem. An alternative to caloric testing is the video head impulse test (vHIT), an objective test of the vestibulo-occular reflex (VOR) and indicative of peripheral vestibular dysfunction if abnormal (Fig. 22.26).

Radiological examination

Computed tomography scanning is the investigation of choice, but it is not a substitute for clinical assessment of chronic ear disease. It is not specifically diagnostic of cholesteatoma (Fig. 22.27), but is useful

GSI TIMESTAR MIDDLE EAR ANALYZER
PROBE S/N: 13153900

TYMP SCREENING   TEST 1

Ytm 226 Hz   R

m1

EARCANAL VOLUME: 0.9

	daPa	ml
TYMP 1:	20	0.5
GRADIENT:	65	daPa
REFLEX:	I 1000 Hz	NT

TYMP SCREENING   TEST 2

Ytm 226 Hz   L

m1

EARCANAL VOLUME: 1.0

	daPa	ml
TYMP 1:	25	1.0
GRADIENT:	60	daPa
REFLEX:	I 1000 Hz	NT

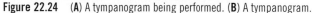

Figure 22.24 (**A**) A tympanogram being performed. (**B**) A tympanogram.

in cranial trauma (Fig. 22.28) and in the evaluation of temporal bone neoplasia. Magnetic resonance imaging (MRI) is more useful in identifying soft tissue abnormalities in the cerebellopontine angle, especially vestibular schwannoma (Fig. 22.29).

These tumours present with asymmetric sensorineural hearing loss. MRI also helps assess tumour spread outside the temporal bone. CT angiography helps in assessment of pulsatile tinnitus and vascular lesions. Formal angiography is useful for embolization of vascular tumours.

The nose and paranasal sinuses

Anatomy

The nose (Box 22.4) is formed by the two nasal bones which articulate with the nasal process of the maxilla on each side. The lateral cartilages provide support for the nostrils, especially in inspiration (Fig. 22.30). The nasal cavity is divided by the nasal septum, formed of cartilage anteriorly and bone posteriorly (Fig. 22.31). The lateral wall of the nose is formed by the three nasal turbinate bones: inferior, middle and superior (Fig. 22.32). Under each turbinate is a corresponding meatus. The nose constantly produces mucus—a pint a day—which is constantly propelled backwards by the cilia to the posterior choanae, whence it is swallowed, usually unnoticed.

The paranasal sinuses are air-filled spaces in the bones of the facial skeleton (see Figs 22.32 and 22.33). They comprise the paired maxillary, frontal and ethmoid sinuses and the unpaired but bisected sphenoid sinus, and form the structure of the adult face. The ethmoidal cells or labyrinth comprises a number of small bony cells. The sinuses open into the nose via small drainage channels (ostia). Their

Caloric

| UW: 32% Right Weaker ◆ | DP: 32% LB Stronger ◆ | Total:85 d/s ✓ |

Figure 22.25 (**A**) A caloric test being performed. (**B**) A computerized caloric test result.

mucus is swept by cilia through the ostia to be mixed with mucus secreted by the nose. The middle meatus is the common pathway for drainage from the maxillary, the anterior ethmoid and the frontal sinuses. The anterior ethmoids are important because disease in these areas will compromise maxillary and frontal sinus drainage. Blockage of the ostia owing to inflammation in the nose, with retention of mucus and secondary infection, is the presumed mechanism for sinus infection (rhinosinusitis). The upper teeth are closely related to the floor of the maxillary sinus; infection here may lead to sinus problems.

The olfactory neuroepithelium of the nose is located in the roof of the nasal cavity. Neurons run through the cribriform plate to the olfactory bulb lying on the floor of the anterior cranial fossa. The postnasal space contains the adenoids, which are lymphoid tissue, part of Waldeyer's ring, which includes the palatine tonsils. These are largest in childhood and regress from the age of about 8 years onwards, although rarely they may persist into adult life. The inferior opening of the Eustachian tube is on the lateral wall of the postnasal space.

Symptoms of nasal disease

The important symptoms of nasal and sinus disease are:
- Nasal blockage
- Rhinorrhoea: nasal discharge
- Epistaxis: nasal bleeding
- Sneezing and itching
- Disturbances of smell
- Facial pain

Figure 22.26 A vHIT test being performed.

Figure 22.28 Computerized tomography (CT) scan of a right ear showing a fracture across the rmiddle ear. There is disruption and widening of the incudo-malleolar joint.

Figure 22.27 Computerized tomography (CT) scan of right ear showing a lateral semicircular canal fistula in a patient with cholesteatoma.

General features

Orbital and facial pain, proptosis, diplopia, periorbital swelling and conjunctival chemosis may develop if infection or neoplasia spread outside the sinuses. Pathology in the postnasal space may lead to otological symptoms secondary to Eustachian tube involvement.

Nasal blockage

Unilateral or bilateral blockage of the nose is common. Maximum resistance to airflow occurs at the front of the nose near the inferior turbinate. In the nasal cycle (2–6 hours long), one side is congested and one side decongested at any one time. The most common cause of bilateral or alternating nasal blockage is allergic rhinitis. A constant blockage suggests a structural abnormality (deviated nasal septum, nasal polyposis, adenoidal hypertrophy (children)).

Rhinorrhoea

Nasal discharge may be mucoid, purulent or watery. It may contain blood. A purulent discharge suggests infection, either in the nose or in the sinus. In a child, unilateral discharge may be caused by a foreign body retained in the nose. Mucoid discharge is more suggestive of allergic rhinitis. Watery discharge is indicative of vasomotor rhinitis. CSF leak is a rare but important cause; the discharge is clear, watery and salty in taste. Epistaxis (a nose bleed) varies in severity from a minor intermittent problem to a life-threatening major haemorrhage that may require cautery. It tends to occur in children and the elderly. The arterial supply of the nose is from branches of the sphenopalatine artery (external carotid), and from the anterior and posterior ethmoidal arteries (internal carotid). These vessels anastomose in the anterior nasal septum, the site of most epistaxis. Epistaxis is associated with hypertension, trauma (including nose-picking), rhinitis and bleeding disorders.

Itching and sneezing

Sneezing is a protective expulsive reflex that helps clear the nasal airway of irritants. Paroxysmal sneezing, associated with rhinorrhoea, nasal obstruction and palatal and conjunctival itching, occurs with allergic rhinitis.

Figure 22.29   Magnetic resonance imaging (MRI) scan (**A**) T2 weighted (**B**) T1 weighted demonstrating a small left-sided intracanalicular vestibular schwannoma confined to the internal auditory meatus.

Box 22.4	Functions of the nose

- Respiration
- Filtration
- Heating
- Humidification
- Smell

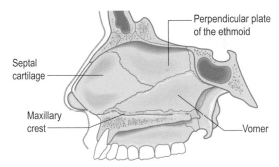

Figure 22.31   The nasal septum.

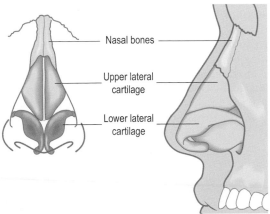

Figure 22.30   The external nose.

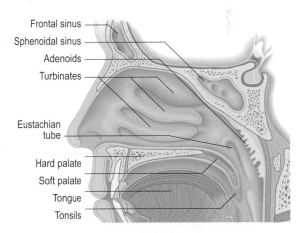

Figure 22.32   The lateral wall of the nose.

Disturbances of smell

Loss of smell (anosmia) or impaired sense of smell is most often caused by nasal obstruction, for example with nasal polyposis or allergic rhinitis. It also follows damage to nerve fibres passing through the cribriform plate after craniofacial trauma. Rarely, viral infection may cause permanent anosmia. Cacosmia is an unpleasant smell, sometimes unnoticed by the patient, caused by chronic anaerobic sepsis in the nose.

Facial pain

Pain in the face is very common, but pain limited to the nose is rare. Pain centred over a sinus may indicate infection or, rarely, a malignancy. There are many causes of facial pain. Some, such as cluster headache (causing transient nasal blockage and rhinorrhoea) and trigeminal neuralgia, are functional disorders, with well-defined features (see Chapter 16). Structural disorders, such as infection or tumour involving facial structures, may also present with facial pain.

Investigation should usually include imaging by CT and MRI.

Other symptoms

Always enquire about any history of allergy. Most people are aware of hay fever, but house dust mite allergy is also common and can be easily tested for with skin prick testing.

Examination of the nose and face

Inspect the nose and face from the front, side and back in a good light. Note the colour of the skin and any asymmetry of facial contours. Observe for scars and pigmentary changes. With age, the tip of the nose tends to droop. Deformities of the nasal bone

and cartilage, such as saddle deformity, often follow a nasal fracture or other destructive disorders of the bony or cartilaginous septum. Palpate the nose and facial skeleton, especially the orbital margins, noting tenderness and any swelling, expansion or depression of bone. Facial swelling is unusual in maxillary sinusitis, but occurs with dental root infections and in carcinoma of the maxillary antrum. Inspect and palpate the palate and alveoli from inside the mouth using a gloved finger.

Examine the nasal vestibule and intranasal contents by gently pushing the tip of the nose upwards with a finger, preferably using reflected illumination from a head mirror. The nasal vestibule is lined with skin and contains vibrissae (thicker hairs); these become prominent in older men. Inspect the anterior nasal cavity with Thudicum's nasal speculum or an otoscope (Fig. 22.34). The nasal septum is rarely completely straight, but should not be so bent that it is not possible to see the anterior end of the inferior turbinate. The majority of nasal resistance to airflow occurs in the front of the nose. Look for any area of granulation on the nasal septum and for any perforation (Fig. 22.35). Perforations may be secondary to cocaine snorting, digital trauma (nose-picking), surgical trauma, granulomatous conditions or inhalation of industrial dusts, notably nickel and chrome.

Nasal polyps are usually easily identifiable by their pale colour (Fig. 22.36) and their softness and lack of sensitivity to probing. In a child, an apparent polyp may be seen arising from the roof of the nose; this should not be probed because it may be the intra-nasal presentation of a meningocele. In children and adults, airflow through a patent nostril causes misting on a cold metal tongue depressor or mirror held at the nose. In a neonate, nasal patency is best estimated by observing any movement of a wisp of cotton wool held in front of each nostril after blocking each in turn with the thumb. Nasal endoscopy (Fig. 22.37), after applying a topical decongestant

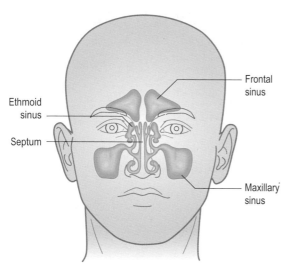

Figure 22.33 Cross-section through the sinuses (semischematic).

Frontal sinus

Ethmoid sinus

Septum

Maxillary sinus

Figure 22.34 Examining the nose.

Figure 22.35 A septal perforation.

Figure 22.37 Rigid nasal endoscopy.

Figure 22.36 A large polyp in the right nasal cavity.

Figure 22.38 Endoscopic view of the Eustachian tube orifice and the postnasal space.

such as xylometazoline with topical lidocaine anaesthesia, allows inspection of the middle meatus for oedema, draining pus or polyps. The postnasal space and the opening of the Eustachian tube (Fig. 22.38) can be seen, with the fossa of Rosenmuller, the site of origin of postnasal space carcinomas, lying directly above and behind. In children and young adults, look for adenoidal swelling.

Special tests

Allergy testing

If allergic symptoms are severe, there is merit in confirming extrinsic allergy by skin-prick testing (see Chapter 20). An important component of treating allergy is allergen avoidance, and the certainty of responsible allergens may encourage compliance. The common inhalant allergens (Box 22.5), together with any agents that have been suspected from the history, should be tested and compared with positive and negative controls (histamine and saline). Unfortunately, however, a negative response does not definitely exclude atopy. The radioallergosorbent test (RAST), which measures specific IgE in blood,

Box 22.5	Common inhalant allergens

- House dust and house dust mite
- Grass pollen
- Tree pollen
- Weed pollen
- Animal dander: cat, dog, rabbit
- Feathers
- Moulds

may be considered for certain food allergens, although generally this type of testing is less specific than skin prick testing. Nasal provocation tests are time consuming, because only one allergen can be tested at a time.

Nasal patency

Objective assessment of nasal patency is difficult. Rhinomanometry, which measures nasal airflow and

Figure 22.39 Coronal computerized tomography (CT) scan of the nose showing an opaque left maxillary antrum and evidence of periapical lucency indicating dental infection around the adjacent molar tooth.

resistance, and acoustic rhinometry, which measures nasal volume and

cross-sectional area, remain specialized research tools.

Mucociliary clearance

Mucociliary clearance is a test of impaired ciliary function used, for example, in Kartagener's syndrome of impaired ciliary motility. A strong, sweet taste, such as saccharin placed on the anterior end of the inferior turbinate, should be tasted in the mouth about 20 minutes later.

Radiological examination

Plain X-rays are unreliable in the management of sinus disease. Previously, lateral X-rays were commonly used in estimating the degree of adenoidal hypertrophy in young children. More commonly now, clinicians would use a paediatric nasoendoscope, which is mostly well tolerated, avoids radiation exposure and allows direct visualization of the postnasal space even in young children. Endoscopic nasal examination and CT scanning are the investigations of choice for sinus disease (Fig. 22.39). CT is useful in the management of chronic infection, trauma and neoplasia. However, there is a radiation dosage to the eyes, and the investigation should be used only when the diagnosis is uncertain or to provide accurate anatomical information before surgery. MRI is less useful in sinus disease because of difficulties in interpretation. MRI is highly sensitive to changes in the mucosal lining of the sinuses. However, it tends to over diagnose and interpretation requires caution. It does have value in assessing the spread of sinus neoplasia.

The throat

Anatomy

The throat includes the oral cavity, the pharynx (oropharynx, nasopharynx and hypopharynx),

the larynx and the major salivary glands. The oral cavity extends from the lips to the anterior faucial pillars. The oral cavity proper is bounded by the teeth laterally, the tongue and floor of the mouth inferiorly and the hard and soft palate superiorly. The pharynx extends from the base of the skull to the cricopharyngeal sphincter (Fig. 22.40). The oropharynx is bounded above by the soft palate and below by the upper surface of the epiglottis. Its anterior margin is defined laterally by the anterior faucial pillar, containing the palatoglossus muscle, and by the posterior third of the tongue. The posterior pharyngeal wall is its posterior boundary. The palatine tonsils are situated laterally between the anterior and posterior pillars of the fauces. The base of the tongue contains the lingual tonsils. This lymphoid tissue, together with the adenoids and the tubal tonsil (lymphoid tissue around the Eustachian tube opening), makes up Waldeyer's ring, an important line of immunological defence. The hypopharynx consists of the posterior pharyngeal wall, the piriform fossae and the postcricoid area. The piriform fossae, which comprise the lateral walls of the pharynx adjacent to the larynx, are the routes by which food is passed into the upper oesophagus. The larynx is a rigid structure consisting of cartilages, the most prominent of which are the paired thyroid cartilages, which articulate with the cricoid cartilage below. The epiglottis is attached to the inner surface of the thyroid cartilage and aids the separation of air and food passages during swallowing. The larynx consists of three compartments (Fig. 22.41): glottis, supraglottis and subglottis. The glottis is formed by the vocal folds. The glottis has poor lymphatic drainage, which may help to delay the spread of malignancy from this area. The epiglottis extends from the false cords below to the hyoid bone above. It has a rich lymphatic drainage, and therefore malignancy in this area is more frequently associated with metastatic disease. The subglottis, which is the narrowest part of the upper respiratory tract, extends from the glottis to the lower border of the cricoid.

Torus tubarius

Pharyngeal tonsil

Pharyngeal recess

Nasal cavity

A

Torus levatorius (fold overlying levator veli palatini)

Fold overlying palatopharyngeal sphincter

B

Salpingopharyngeal fold

Palatine tonsil

Tongue

Lingual tonsils

Palatopharyngeal arch (overlies palatopharyngeus muscle)

C

Laryngeal inlet

Vallecula

Oesophagus

A Nasopharynx

Trachea

B Oropharynx

C Laryngopharynx

Figure 22.40   Midline sagittal section demonstrating the pharynx.

The prime function of the larynx is to separate breathing and swallowing, thereby protecting the airway. Voice production is a secondary function that has arisen with evolution. Phonation occurs with movement of the vocal folds into the midline (Fig. 22.42). Changes in voice volume are caused by alterations in the subglottic pressure, whereas alterations in pitch are owing to modification of the length and tension of the vocal folds. The quality of this basic laryngeal sound is modulated by resonance in the pharynx, air sinuses, mouth and nose.

The pharynx is innervated from the pharyngeal plexus (cranial nerves IX, X and XI). Interruption of this nerve supply by lesions at the jugular foramen leads to swallowing problems and severe morbidity. All the muscles of the larynx, except the cricothyroid, are supplied by the recurrent laryngeal branch of the vagus (cranial nerve X). In the chest, this nerve loops around the arch of the aorta on the left and the subclavian artery on the right, before running up to enter the larynx. The long course of

the left recurrent laryngeal nerve means it is more frequently affected by disease. The cricothyroid muscle, which is supplied by the external branch of the superior laryngeal nerve (cranial nerve X), controls vocal pitch.

There are three paired major salivary glands (Fig. 22.43). The parotid gland lies anterior to the ear. Its duct opens opposite the second upper molar tooth. The submandibular gland lies far posterior in the floor of the mouth and may be palpated in the neck, under the mandible. Its duct opens anteriorly in the floor of the mouth adjacent to the frenulum of the tongue. The smaller sublingual gland lies anteriorly in the floor of the mouth and its duct joins the submandibular duct.

The lymph nodes of the head and neck (Fig. 22.44) provide a barrier to the spread of disease, whether inflammatory or neoplastic. Enlargement implies either primary disease within the nodes or that they have become involved secondary to pathology in the areas they drain. Occasionally they may become involved by pathology below the clavicle.

Symptoms of throat disease

Patients with throat disorders present with:

- Pain
- Ulceration
- Stridor, or stertorous (noisy) breathing
- Dysphonia (hoarseness)
- Dysphagia (difficulty in swallowing)
- A mass in the neck

Occasionally lesions in the upper airway may present with overspill of food and fluids into the upper trachea or nose or with weight loss. Malignant mouth, throat and airway disease is very strongly associated with smoking, with alcohol intake an important synergistic factor.

Oral ulceration and pain

An ulcer is the most common oral lesion. Traumatic ulcers heal quickly although, if caused by ill-fitting dentures or broken teeth, they will rapidly recur, if not fail to heal. Aphthous ulcers are small, painful superficial ulcers of the tongue, buccal mucosa and

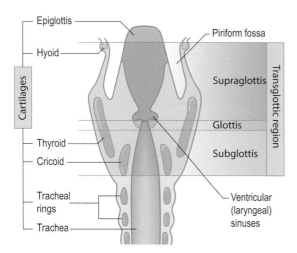

Figure 22.41 The divisions of the larynx.

palate, of uncertain cause, which are painful but generally heal quickly. There is a high incidence of recurrence. Oral carcinoma may present as an ulcer and is frequently painless. Sometimes there will be other symptoms, such as bleeding, loose teeth or halitosis, but suspicious non-resolving lesions need to be biopsied.

Thrush (fungal infection with *Candida albicans*) is a frequent cause of white patches or pain. Rare causes of ulceration include Crohn's disease and Behçet's syndrome. The sensation of 'burning mouth' has a number of causes outlined in Box 22.6.

Sore throat

A sore throat is one of the most frequently reported symptoms. Viral pharyngitis is the most common cause. Tonsillar inflammation is also common. Acute follicular tonsillitis begins with local redness, developing into a punctate or confluent yellow exudate on the tonsils, often caused by group A *Streptococcus* infection. In glandular fever (Epstein–Barr virus infection), the tonsils are covered with a white membrane with palatal petechiae. A grey membrane is the classic feature of the now-rare infection with *Corynebacterium diphtheriae*. A throat swab for culture and sensitivity is a useful test. Find out the frequency and severity of attacks of tonsillitis, as estimated by the amount of time lost from school or work, and any antibiotic treatment; such considerations help to decide whether tonsillectomy is merited. Generally in children, at least five attacks a year for 2 years is the minimum indication for tonsillectomy.

An abscess adjacent to the tonsil (quinsy) is very painful, causing dysphagia and trismus (spasm in the jaw). Surgical drainage is usually required. Squamous cell carcinoma of the tonsil is also often painful. It presents as an exophytic mass or ulcer. In the early stages, diagnosis is difficult. Ulceration in the oropharynx also occurs in glandular fever, rubella and streptococcal tonsillitis.

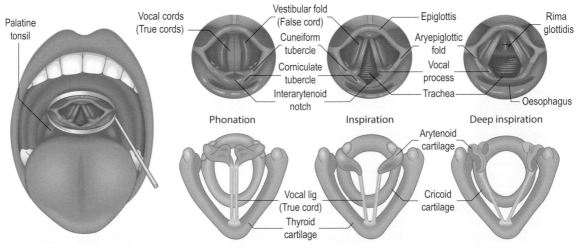

Figure 22.42 The mechanism of phonation.

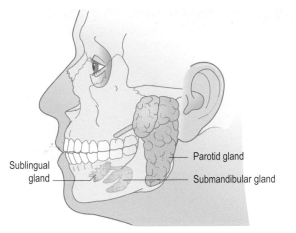

Figure 22.43 The major salivary glands.

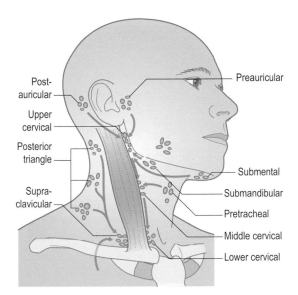

Figure 22.44 The cervical lymph node groupings.

Box 22.6	Causes of a burning sensation in the mouth

Deficiency states
- Iron deficiency
- Vitamin B12 deficiency
- Folate deficiency

Infection
- Candidiasis

Diabetes mellitus

Erythema migrans (lyme disease)

Psychogenic
- Anxiety
- Depression
- Cancer phobia

Box 22.7	Causes of stridor

Neonatal
- Congenital tumours and cysts
- Laryngomalacia
- Subglottic stenosis

Children
- Supraglottitis (epiglottitis)
- Laryngotracheobronchitis
- Acute laryngitis
- Foreign body
- Retropharyngeal abscess
- Papillomatosis

Adults
- Acute laryngitis
- Laryngeal trauma
- Laryngeal carcinoma
- Supraglottitis (epiglottitis)

Stridor and stertor

Stridor is noisy breathing associated with upper airway obstruction at the laryngeal level (Box 22.7). Stertor is noisy breathing at the oropharyngeal level and is nearly always caused by adenotonsillar hypertrophy. Epiglottitis is particularly important in infants and small children up to the age of 7 years. It is associated with infection by *Haemophilus influenzae* type B, and may present with rapidly progressive airway obstruction and dyspnoea, fever, pharyngeal pain and drooling. Vaccination has reduced its incidence. Immediate antibiotic therapy may need to be supplemented by intubation or even tracheostomy. In adults, laryngeal carcinoma may cause stridor owing to direct blockage of the airway, to fixation of the vocal fold or with recurrent laryngeal nerve involvement. Croup, acute laryngotracheobronchitis in young children, causes less severe airway obstruction. The thick tenacious secretions are relieved by air humidification and nebulized adrenaline and steroids are used until symptoms settle. Rarely, children may require intubation.

Dysphonia

Dysphonia or hoarseness covers a range of symptoms, from subtle changes noticed by professional voice users to aphonia, when there is no voice. It may be caused by structural problems affecting the vocal fold or by neurological disease (Box 22.8). Hoarseness followed by increasing airway obstruction is the typical presentation of a laryngeal neoplasm (Fig. 22.45).

Damage to the recurrent laryngeal nerve anywhere along its course usually leads to hoarseness, although compensation from the unaffected side will limit symptoms. A lesion of the vagus above the exit of the superior laryngeal nerve produces a more breathy voice, as there is also loss of cricothyroid function. Acute vocal abuse and acute inflammation cause dysphonia, which is usually self-limiting. Long-term vocal abuse may lead to a number of changes of the

Box 22.8	Causes of dysphonia

Inflammatory

- Acute and chronic laryngitis
- Smoke inhalation

Neoplasia

- Carcinoma
- Laryngeal papillomatosis

Recurrent laryngeal nerve

- Post thyroidectomy
- Carcinoma of lung/breast

Neurological

- Myasthenia gravis
- Spasmodic dysphonia

Systemic

- Hypothyroidism
- Rheumatoid arthritis

Habitual dysphonias

- Reinke's oedema
- Singer's nodules
- Vocal cord polyps
- Vocal process granuloma

Gastro-oesophageal/laryngopharyngeal reflux

Psychogenic

- Musculoskeletal
- Spasmodic
- Conversion disorders
- Mutational falsetto (pubophonia, habitual use of a high-pitched voice after puberty)

Figure 22.45 Laryngeal carcinoma at the anterior commissure with hyperkeratosis of the right vocal cord.

Figure 22.46 A traumatic right vocal cord polyp.

vocal folds: singer's nodules, polyps (Fig. 22.46) or Reinke's oedema. These will often respond to speech therapy, although surgery may be necessary. It is also worth considering whether gastro-oesophageal (laryngo-pharyngeal) reflux may be implicated. Malignancy should be considered in any patient with dysphonia of more than 4 weeks' duration.

Dysphagia

Any lesion that interrupts the normal sequence of coordinated muscular activity necessary for swallowing may cause dysphagia (Box 22.9). Dysphagia results from structural disease of the pharyngo-oesophagus or from neurological disorders. Persistent dysphagia, especially if associated with regurgitation of undigested food, weight loss, dysphonia, otalgia or a mass in the neck, requires urgent investigation. Pooling of saliva in the piriform fossa seen at laryngoscopy implies obstruction in the cervical oesophagus or in the postcricoid area (see Chapter 14 for discussion of dysphagia below the cricopharyngeus).

Lump in the neck

The causes of salivary gland swelling are outlined in Box 22.10.

Box 22.9	Causes of dysphagia

- Neuromuscular: motor neuron disease, multiple sclerosis, myasthenia gravis
- Intrinsic lesions: oesophageal stricture, oesophageal web, achalasia, pharyngeal pouch, pharyngeal and oesophageal neoplasia
- Extrinsic lesions: thyroid enlargement, primary or secondary neoplasia, aortic aneurysm
- Systemic: scleroderma
- Psychosomatic: globus pharyngeus

Box 22.10	Salivary gland enlargement

- Bacterial infection: acute usually unilateral painful swelling (sialadenitis)
- Viral infection: mumps; painful bilateral swelling and rash
- Obstruction by stone: calculus; variable swelling and pain
- Salivary tumour: gradual increase in size, may be painless

The neck has a rich lymphatic system of nodes and channels that drain the head and neck (see Fig. 22.44). The deep cervical lymph nodes run in the carotid sheath. The most prominent of these is the jugulodigastric node, which can be palpated just posterior to the angle of the mandible and anterior to the anterior edge of sternomastoid. This is the most commonly enlarged node in upper respiratory tract infections, especially following tonsillitis. The most common mass in the neck is a lymph node following infection, especially in children.

Tuberculosis and atypical mycobacterial infection should always be considered with persistent cervical lymphadenopathy. The diagnosis of a neck lump is partly suggested by the age of the patient (Box 22.11). Features that suggest malignancy are progressive enlargement, hardness, lack of tenderness, fixation to deep structures and size (a node more than 1 cm in diameter is more likely to be malignant). Ultrasound is a valuable investigation, particularly combined with fine needle aspiration cytology.

Examination of the mouth and throat

With practice it is possible to inspect all of the oral cavity, the pharynx and the larynx. Use a headlight or a head mirror to ensure adequate illumination and keep both hands free to manipulate the instruments. First check the lips, teeth and gums, the floor of the mouth and the openings of the submandibular and parotid ducts. Observe the corners of the mouth for cracks or fissures (angular stomatitis or cheilitis). In children, this is usually owing to bacterial infection, but poor dentition in the elderly leads to cracks and candidiasis (thrush). This may also be seen in severe iron-deficiency anaemia and in vitamin B2 (riboflavin) deficiency. Grouped vesicles on the lips on a red base with crusted lesions are seen in herpes simplex labialis. This viral infection is acute and the lack of induration and ulceration serves to distinguish it from malignancy. If salivary gland pathology is suspected, bimanual palpation, with one gloved finger in the mouth and synchronous palpation of the gland, may help to define the pathology. Palpation is also valuable for examining the cheeks, tongue and even the tonsils, on occasion. Tongue mobility (cranial nerve XII) should be assessed by protrusion and side-to-side movement. Look for wasting or fasciculation. Depress the tongue to inspect the tonsillar pillars, the palatine tonsils, soft palate and uvula. The tonsils and soft palate should be nearly symmetrical. Check the gag reflex (cranial nerve IX). The more distant portions of the pharynx can be inspected only with a laryngeal mirror or fibreoptic laryngoscope. The flexible fibreoptic nasal endoscope (Fig. 22.47) allows a good view in almost every case; currently, it is much more commonly used than indirect laryngosopy because it provides a superior view and allows recording and photodocumentation of the examination for clinical review.

Box 22.11	Causes of neck lumps by age (these groupings are not exclusive)

Less than 20 years
- Inflammatory/infective lymph nodes
- Thyroglossal and branchial cysts, midline dermoid, cystic hygroma
- Lymphoma

20–40 years
- Salivary gland pathology: calculus, infection, tumour
- Thyroid pathology: goitre, inflammatory thyroiditis, tumour
- Chronic infection: HIV, tuberculosis, actinomycosis
- Lymphoma

Over 40 years
- Secondary malignancy
- Primary malignancy: lymphoma
- Thyroid pathology: goitre, tumour

Figure 22.47 Flexible fibreoptic nasoendoscopy.

Videolaryngostroboscopy (Fig. 22.48) is a specialized endoscopic examination, useful for detailed visualization of the vocal folds. In this technique, stroboscopic light is used through the endoscope to visualize the mucosal wave of the vocal fold and heighten diagnostic capabilities and pick up submucosal lesions, such as vocal cord cysts.

Examination of the neck

Examination of the neck is part of the routine assessment of any patient with suspected or proven disease in the throat. The neck is exposed and inspected from the front and side before the

Figure 22.48 (**A**) Videolaryngostroboscopy and (**B**) the image.

Figure 22.49 Examination of the neck.

examiner stands behind the patient (Fig. 22.49) and follows a well-rehearsed routine so that no area is missed. Start by palpating the nodes in the posterior auricular region and then progressively feel for the nodes on the anterior border of the trapezius muscle

Figure 22.50 Thyroglossal cyst.

down to the supraclavicular fossa. The latter area is palpated forwards from behind. The examining fingers then pass up the jugular vein, where the most important groups of nodes in the head and neck are situated, towards the ear. The jugular, parotid and preauricular areas are then examined, followed by submandibular and submental nodes. Finally, the nodes associated with the anterior jugular chain are examined. This brings the fingers to the thyroid gland (details of thyroid examination are in Chapter 19). Midline lumps should also be assessed with the patient protruding the tongue. Movement suggests attachment to the base of the tongue and implies the presence of a thyroglossal cyst (Fig. 22.50). The larynx should be mobile from side to side and, if the thyroid cartilage is held between thumb and first finger and gently moved against the cervical spine, it should grate. This laryngeal crepitus is a normal phenomenon. It may be reduced or abolished by hypopharyngeal pathology or a mass in the prevertebral space displacing the larynx away from the cervical spine. Finally, auscultate the carotid arteries and the thyroid gland.

Tissue sampling

Fine-needle aspiration cytology is useful in virtually all neck lumps. If correctly performed, this will diagnose the vast majority of metastatic squamous carcinomas. It is less accurate in distinguishing lymphoma from reactive changes. If doubt remains, then core or excision biopsy should be performed. Accessible lesions in the oral cavity and oropharynx may be biopsied in the clinic with either topical anaesthesia or a local anaesthetic injection (usually with lidocaine).

Radiological examination

A soft-tissue lateral neck X-ray is not a sensitive investigation, even for detecting foreign bodies but is used first line if suspecting an ingested foreign body alongside a flexible fibreoptic nasoendoscope examination. A barium swallow, a dynamic investigation, can locate obstruction in the oesophagus or demonstrate uncoordinated swallowing. It can be combined with video recording (videofluoroscopy).

Figure 22.51   Magnetic resonance imaging (MRI) scan of the neck demonstrating a large metastatic lymph node.

It is less helpful in evaluating the hypopharynx, where endoscopy under a general anaesthetic is the preferred investigation. Endoscopy is also helpful in taking biopsies in suspected malignancy. Ultrasound is useful for the evaluation of neck masses and the thyroid gland. Doppler ultrasound assesses the cervical vasculature. CT scanning helps to stage neoplastic disease, particularly of lesions of the larynx and below, and may demonstrate metastatic spread that has eluded palpation. MRI evaluation is most useful for suspected tumours above the larynx (e.g. the oropharynx and tongue base) and can detect extracapsular spread of metastatic lymph nodes, a poor prognostic sign (Fig. 22.51).

Acknowledgements

Ashok Adams, Consultant Neuroradiologist, for helping with the radiological images, and Rachael Mcfarlane, Senior Audiologist, for helping with the vestibular testing and audiological testing images.

SARS-CoV-2 and the COVID-19 pandemic

Teresa Cutino-Moguel

Severe acute respiratory syndrome coronavirus-2 (SARS-CoV-2) is a novel coronavirus that belongs to the same family of viruses as the Severe Acute Respiratory Syndrome Coronavirus (SARS-CoV) and the Middle East respiratory syndrome coronavirus (MERS-CoV). It was first identified in Wuhan, China and subsequently spread worldwide, leading the World Health Organization to declare a pandemic on the 30th January 2020.

SARS-CoV-2 and other human coronaviruses

Human coronaviruses (hCoV) were identified in 1965 as causing around 30% of the cases of common cold and flu-like illnesses in humans. The CoVs belong to the order *Nidovirales*, subfamily *Orthocoronavirida*, family *Coronoviridae*. They owe their name to the club-shaped glycoproteins on their surface or 'spikes' that give them a crown-like appearance (*corona* in Latin).

CoVs are classified into four genera according to their genomic organization: α-CoV, β-CoV, γ-CoV and δ- CoV. The α-CoVs and β-CoVs infect various mammals (such as bats, cattle and domestic animals) including humans. All hCoV are zoonotic (able to jump from animals to humans) and most originate in bats that are considered their natural reservoir, including SARS-CoV-2. Zoonotic transmission then can occur using domesticated animals or other animals that are in closer contact with humans, such as the palm civets for SARS-CoV or camels for MERS-CoV. The emergence of novel variants of CoV was predictable owing to their genetic variability and frequent recombination between strains.

Seven strains of hCoV have been identified. Four are responsible for causing mild respiratory infection: NL63, 229E, OC43 and HKU1. A further three highly pathogenic strains have also been identified as causes of acute respiratory distress syndrome with high fatality rate: SARS-CoV, MERS-CoV and SARS-CoV-2. In 2002, SARS-CoV caused an outbreak that spread to 27 countries, infecting approximately 8000 people with 774 deaths. In 2012, an outbreak of MERS-CoV started in the Arabic peninsula where it remains endemic; so far, it has involved around 2500 individuals with 30% mortality. SARS-CoV and MERS-CoV are both beta coronaviruses.

The first reports of an atypical pneumonia originated in November 2019 in Wuhan province, in China. The viral agent responsible was identified shortly thereafter as a new beta coronavirus and was initially called 2019 novel coronavirus (2019-nCoV). The virus was renamed SARS-CoV-2 in February 2020. The genome of SARS-CoV-2 was fully sequenced in January 2020 and it was found to be 96.2% identical to the bat CoV RaTG13 and 79.5% identical to SARS-CoV indicating that both SARS-CoV and SARS-CoV-2 originated from a common ancestor.

Genomic organization and structure of SARS-CoV-2

SARS-CoV-2 is an enveloped, single-stranded, positive sense RNA virus with a genome of 29 Kb in size. Its genome contains a 5' leader untranslated region (UTR) followed by a replicase (R), spike (S), envelope (E), matrix (M), nucleocapsid (N) genes and a 3' UTR with a poly (A)tail. It also contains 6 to 12 open reading frames (ORFs) between the conserved genes (S,E,M and N), 9 transcription regulatory elements and 9 subgenomic RNAs. The first ORF is ORF1a/b and it constitutes two-thirds of the genome at the 5'end. It codes two long polypeptides that can produce 16 non-structural proteins after processing by proteases encoded by the virus. At the 3' end are ORFs 10 and 11 encoding the 4 structural proteins SEMN (Fig. A1).

The viral particle has a pleomorphic structure; on its surface are located the spikes that are peplomers formed by projections of glycoproteins with an important role in the immunogenicity and pathogenesis of the virus. The M protein lies between the viral nucleocapsid and the envelope. The E protein is a transmembrane protein that, along with S and M, constitutes the viral envelope. Proteins E and M have important roles in the viral replication. The N protein is associated with genomic RNA forming the nucleoprotein (Fig. A2).

Figure A1 Genomic organization of SARS-CoV-2. (Adapted from Mishra SK, Tripathi T. 2021. One year update on the COVID-19 pandemic: Where are we now? Acta Tropica 214: 105778. https://doi.org/10.1016/j.actatropica.2020.105778.)

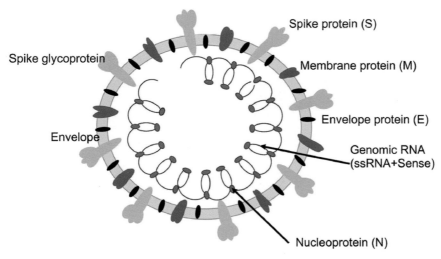

Figure A2 Structure of SARS-CoV-2 viral particle. (Adapted from Mishra SK, Tripathi T. 2021. One year update on the COVID-19 pandemic: Where are we now? Acta Tropica 214: 105778.Med2020. https://doi.org/10.1016/j.actatropica.2020.105778.)

Emergence of variants of SARS-CoV-2

A large number of mutations in the original Wuhan strain of SARS-CoV-2 have emerged owing to the huge number of infections that have occurred in a small period of time. Most changes are expected to have no or minimal consequence for virus biology, but tracking these changes allows a better understanding of the virus evolution and its impact on treatment or vaccine effectiveness. Data sharing and dissemination are crucial for the surveillance of any organism, particularly in the setting of a pandemic. To this end, global initiative on sharing avian influenza data (GISAID), a public and private initiative that was established in 2008 as a result of the H1N1 influenza pandemic, provided a free platform on which information on SARS-CoV-2 sequences could be uploaded and shared. This allowed the analysis of data from all over the world. Making use of this sequenced data, CoV-GLUE analysed the mutations that resulted in amino acid replacements in viral proteins or changes in sequence lengths as a result of insertions or deletions (indels). CoV-GLUE is thus an amino acid database.

In March 2020, a new strain of SARS-CoV-2 emerged with a mutation in position 614 of the viral S protein that resulted in the substitution of an aspartic acid (single-letter code: D) with glycine (single-letter code: G). This mutation (D614G) was associated with a selective advantage that resulted in this variant taking over the original strain and becoming the dominant strain circulating all over the world. This variant was not associated with higher mortality or disease severity, but appeared to be more transmissible, which probably explained its fixation in the global population. Towards the end of 2020, more variants started to be identified all over the world. The identification of these variants was of particular concern because it coincided with the approval of COVID-19 vaccines, the efficacy of which could be threatened by the new variants or lineages of SARS-CoV-2. Lineage B.1.1.7 is a variant of SARS-CoV-2 that was identified originally in November 2020 in the southeast of the UK and was termed the 'Kent variant'. It was calculated to be 40–80% more transmissible than the wild-type SARS-CoV-2 or D614G. It rapidly spread first in the UK and then all over the world and this is thought

Table A1 WHO nomenclature of SARS-CoV-2 variants as per June 2021

WHO label	Variant type	Country of first detection	Date of designation	Earliest documented samples	GISAID clade/ variant	Pango lineage
Alpha	VOC	United Kingdom	18 December 2020	September 2020	GRY (formerly GR/501Y.V1)	B.1.1.7
Beta	VOC	South Africa	18 December 2020	May 2020	GH/501Y.V2	B.1.351
Gamma	VOC	Brazil	11 January 2021	November 2020	GR/501Y.V3	P1
Delta	VOC	India	4 April 2021 (VOI); 11 May 2021 (VOC)	October 2020	G/452R.V3	B.1.617.2

to be at least partly owing to some of the mutations that this variant presents in its spike protein, such as E484K and N501Y.

One of the mutations, N501Y, was also identified in further variants of concern (VOC), such as one identified originally in South Africa (Lineage B.1.351) and another one identified in Brazil (Lineage B). More recently, another VOC has been identified in India (B612.7) that appears to be replacing the previous B.1.1.7 in the UK. The nomenclature of the different variants has been changed by the WHO and they are all now denominated with Greek letters rather than numbers or the place where they were first identified (Table A1). An updated list of variants can be found in updated list of names that can be found at https://www.who.int/activities/tracking-SARS-CoV-2-variants.

SARS-CoV-2 pathogenesis

The spike protein (S) of SARS-CoV-2 has a receptor-binding domain (RBD) that binds the angiotensin-converting enzyme 2 (ACE2) receptor in tissue and triggers a conformational change that produces membrane fusion between the virus and host cell. The S protein has two subunits (S1 and S2). S1 contains the RBD in its C-terminal domain that determines cellular tropism. S2 mediates the fusion of the viral envelope and the cellular membrane. The binding affinity of RBD with ACE2 determines its transmissibility; it has been observed that the affinity of the S protein of SARS-CoV-2 is higher than, for example, SARS-CoV or MERS-CoV.

Diagnosis

Clinical specimens

The diagnosis of COVID-19 can be made with a variety of tests, including molecular and serological tests, and it can be performed in different clinical samples. The choice of clinical specimens will depend on the clinical symptoms, stage of the disease and the environment in which the test is performed. During an active infection, samples from the upper and lower respiratory tracts (i.e. nasopharyngeal swabs and aspirates, or throat swabs) and saliva are currently the main samples used to make a diagnosis. Saliva has been shown to work as a less-invasive sample for SARS-CoV-2 RNA detection during active infection. Faecal samples have also been reported to remain positive for viral RNA in some individuals, beyond the period of detection of SARS-CoV-2 RNA in respiratory samples. Hence, in some patients, it may be possible to make a retrospective diagnosis where the window for detection in a respiratory or salivary sample has been missed, although the utility of this remains to be established. In some studies, the detection of viral RNA in faecal or anal swabs was associated with more severe or critical illness.

The main consideration when choosing either clinical specimens or methodology to test for the presence of SARS-CoV is sensitivity and specificity. The sensitivity of a test describes its ability to correctly identify patients with a disease. Specificity denotes the ability of the test to correctly identify people without the disease.

Nasal swabs have higher viral loads than oropharyngeal swabs, so a combination of these sites gives a higher yield. Lower respiratory specimens have higher viral loads compared with upper respiratory specimens in patients in later stages of COVID-19. Examples of the former are sputum, bronchoalveolar lavage or endotracheal secretions. However, some can carry the risk of generating aerosols when collected.

SARS-CoV-2 can rarely be detected in blood samples. When this is positive, it can be a marker of severe disease. Nevertheless, viraemia is not common, so plasma is not considered a useful specimen to diagnose COVID-19.

Laboratory tests

Nucleic acid amplifications tests (NAAT)

NAAT are the best tests to diagnose most viral infections, including detection of SARS-CoV-2. Real time polymerase chain reaction (RT-PCR) can detect SARS-CoV-2 RNA in many different clinical specimens with high sensitivity and specificity. This method begins with the isolation and purification of the viral nucleic acids and the conversion of the single-stranded RNA genome into complementary DNA (cDNA). This is what is called reverse transcription; traditionally transcription in a cell occurs from DNA to RNA. After this, a subsequent series of temperature cycles follow. These enable denaturation, then annealing (binding) of the primers to their complementary sequence in the viral cDNA, polymerization (replication) of the regions amplified by the primers, all of which results in the exponential production of multiple copies of such regions. These copies work as templates for further cycles of annealing and polymerization that use the deoxynucleotides (dNTs) and *Taq* polymerase provided to the reaction and with each cycle of amplification a fluorescent signal is produced. This signal is detected in real time by the instrument where the reaction is taking place. This fluorescence reaches a certain threshold and when this is crossed, the platform registers the number of cycles that this took, producing a cycle threshold (CT) that is used as a semi-quantitative measure of the amount of viral nucleic acids in the sample. The targets in the viral genome detected by RT-PCR vary in the different commercial assays and often include at least two, such as the nucleocapsid (N gene), envelope (E gene) and regions in the first open reading frame (orf1a and orf1b) or RNA-dependent RNA polymerase (RdRp) gene. These targets are generally chosen as they are more conserved than the spike gene. Mutations in PCR targets can affect the performance of the assays and, in some cases, these mutations are enough to render the assay unable to detect the target entirely, such as the S-gene dropout observed with the emergence of the alpha variant (B.1.1.7 lineage) in the UK. Variants can be efficiently detected by viral whole genome sequencing. However, this is not available widely so is not useful for screening or initial diagnosis.

Other NAAT include the loop-isothermal amplification (LAMP)-based detection of SARS-CoV-2 RNA that has also been implemented as a rapid test for the detection of the virus in saliva samples.

The difference between these two technologies is a higher turnaround time (time from sample collection to result) for RT-PCR, but a lower sensitivity of LAMP. This means that RT-PCR will be able to detect most positive cases, whereas LAMP will miss some cases owing to its lower sensitivity (RT PCR cited to be around 95% vs 80% for LAMP). RT-PCR requires a laboratory setting and has to be performed by highly skilled laboratory staff, whereas LAMP can be performed in a simpler environment.

Antibody tests or serological tests

Antibodies against SARS-CoV-2 are produced during the first week after infection with neutralizing antibodies detected in around 50% of infected individuals by day 7 and in all infected individuals by day 14. IgM production peaks around week 2 post infection and then falls. IgG production goes on for longer and is detectable for at least 3 months after the infection. The neutralization ability of these antibodies appears to protect against subsequent reinfections or against severe disease, but it will take time to develop a better understanding and establish the clinical meaning of a positive anti-SARS-CoV-2 antibody with certainty. Serological tests to detect these antibodies are immunoassays that can be N protein or S protein-based, depending on the specificity of the IgG (± IgM) that they detect. They are not useful in the diagnosis of acute infection, but can help establish previous exposure to the virus or vaccination so their utility is mainly epidemiological.

Antigen tests

Antigen tests were developed as rapid diagnostic tests to identify acute infection. They can detect the presence of SARS-CoV-2 proteins or antigens in respiratory samples or the saliva of infected individuals. These antigens bind to antibodies fixed on a paper strip enclosed in a plastic device producing a visible band in 15–30 minutes. Although their reported sensitivity is around 80%, their ease of use, availability and low price make them good alternatives for self-testing in a variety of settings in hospital and the community.

Clinical presentation

Symptoms and signs of COVID-19 vary widely amongst individuals, ranging from completely asymptomatic infection to severe respiratory infection and multi-organ failure. During the different pandemic waves, up to two-thirds of infected individuals remained symptom-free, whereas the other third had mild flu-like symptoms. Symptoms observed include fever, cough, fatigue, sore throat, headache and, interestingly, anosmia and dysgeusia (altered sense of taste). Gastrointestinal symptoms, which are also commonly reported, can include diarrhoea, nausea and vomiting. The latter are observed particularly in children. Of the symptomatic population, around 10% can present with dyspnoea and severe pneumonia. Critical illness can develop in about 5% of total cases and these patients develop respiratory failure without perception of dyspnoea, also called 'silent hypoxaemia'. However, most of the patients with severe disease have underlying medical issues, such as diabetes, cardiovascular disease, obesity and hypertension. Mortality is higher amongst the elderly, frail population.

The typical course of the severe disease is 6 days of flu-like symptoms followed by dyspnoea at around 6–7 days with hospitalization around day 8 and intubation around day 12 after the onset of symptoms. It is important to consider that

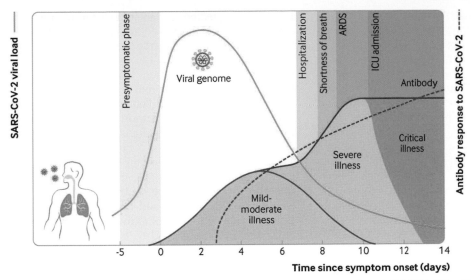

Figure A3   Natural course of COVID-19 disease. (Adapted from Cevik M, Kuppalli K et al. BMJ 2020; 371:m3862. https://doi.org/10.1136/bmj.m3862.)

patients are infectious 2–3 days before the onset of symptoms and that they remain infectious for about 6 days after. This also translates into the window of positivity of upper respiratory samples during which the virus can be detected to confirm a clinical diagnosis. Figure A3 shows the typical evolution of the disease as well as the type of test that is useful at the different stages.

Laboratory abnormalities

Amongst hospitalized patients with COVID-19, the most common abnormalities found in basic laboratory tests are leucopaenia or leucocytosis, lymphopaenia, thrombocytopaenia and elevated alanine aminotransferase and aspartate aminotransferase. An increased lactate dehydrogenase has also been reported. Clinical severity and oxygen saturation are associated with reduced procalcitonin and increased C-reactive protein. A correlation between these inflammatory markers and mortality has also been observed. Increased troponin, D-dimer and ferritin levels are indicators of higher mortality.

Radiological features

Chest computed tomography (CT) abnormalities may be evident even before RT-PCR positivity in patients with and without symptoms. Chest CT abnormalities may precede symptom onset in 44% of the patients with COVID-19. However, conventional chest X-ray has a sensitivity of only 60% to detect initial COVID-19-related pulmonary disease that can include bilateral consolidation in the lower zone and peripherally with hazy opacities.

More than 90% of patients with respiratory symptoms have distinctive chest CT imaging appearances consisting of bilateral pulmonary parenchymal ground-glass opacification. However, it is not recommended to do a chest CT routinely in COVID-19 patients; rather, this is reserved for hospitalized patients.

COVID-19 in children

The most common symptoms in children with acute infection with SARS-CoV-2 are fever and cough. Children can also present sore throat, rhinorrhoea, myalgia, headache and fatigue. Gastrointestinal symptoms, such as diarrhoea, nausea and vomiting, are also relatively common in paediatric patients.

A small proportion of children can present with severe COVID-19 requiring hospitalization. This is generally because of respiratory compromise and multisystem inflammatory syndrome in children (MIS-C). Although hospitalization amongst children with SARS-CoV-2 infection is much lower compared with infected adults, of those hospitalized children one in three requires intensive care. This is similar to adults. Children between 12 and 17 years of age account for around 40% of paediatric admissions and those with severe COVID-19 often have underlying conditions like obesity, asthma, immunosuppression or sickle cell disease. Nevertheless, mortality rate in paediatric patients is low. MIS-C clinical presentation includes persistent fever; gastrointestinal symptoms, such as abdominal pain, vomiting and diarrhoea; and mucocutaneous changes, including a rash or conjunctivitis. Some children also present with neurological symptoms, including headache or meningitis. Patients with MIS-C have some features of Kawasaki disease. In particular, fever and mucocutaneous changes may be evident, but MIS-C is considered a distinct clinical entity with cardiac dysfunction and gastrointestinal symptoms. MIS-C typically progresses within days to multi-organ dysfunction. It is important to keep in mind that the presenting signs and symptoms of MIS-C are similar to other common infections in children, such as sepsis, appendicitis or meningitis, so a wide differential should always be excluded because some other diagnoses are time sensitive and timely management can be life-saving.

Management of COVID-19

To date, the cornerstone of management is supportive care. Adjunctive treatments have a major role, mainly corticosteroids and anticytokines (i.e. tocilizumab).

During the first months of the COVID-19 pandemic, many medicines were re-purposed, despite the lack of evidence on their effectiveness, on the basis of *in vitro* antiviral activity. These included antivirals, such as remdesivir, favipiravir, lopinavir-ritonavir, ribavirin, interferon and hydroxychloroquine. The potential benefit of using a re-purposed drug rather than a new medicine is that safety data are already established and it is just the efficacy of the drug that needs to be evaluated in a particular, new, clinical setting. In the early days of the COVID-19 pandemic, re-purposing existing drugs was an attractive strategy, given the speed at which SARS-CoV-2 cases and deaths were progressing internationally. However, some of the re-purposed drugs showed a lack of effectiveness, but have been used widely. An example of this is hydroxychloroquine that, according to some estimates, has been given to almost one-third of COVID-19 patients globally.

The importance of rapidly acquiring data on the effectiveness of different treatment strategies was apparent from the beginning of the pandemic, so efforts to centralize clinical data were put in place as part of clinical trials that assessed different treatments. The Randomised Evaluation of COVid-19 thERapY (RECOVERY) trial in the UK evaluated different drugs used for the treatment of hospitalized patients. Two trials will assess the effectiveness of testing self-administered medications for individuals who are not sick enough to require hospitalization: Accelerating COVID-19 Therapeutic Interventions and Vaccines (ACTIV-6) in the USA and Platform Randomised Trial of Treatments in the Community for Epidemic and Pandemic Illnesses (PRINCIPLE) in the UK. Results from PRINCIPLE already indicate that inhaled budesonide can reduce recovery time in patients with COVID-19 managed in primary care.

Amongst antiviral preparations, remdesivir was the most promising against SARS-CoV-2. It is an adenosine nucleotide analogue that acts as an inhibitor of the viral polymerase (RdRp). Remdesivir initially was developed to treat Ebola virus, but it was shown to have broad-spectrum antiviral activity in tissue culture and animal models demonstrating activity against filoviruses, paramyxoviruses and coronaviruses, including SARS-CoV and MERS-CoV. Although it was approved to treat COVID-19 in the USA and Europe, randomized, controlled trials found no effect on mortality and only a modest effect on length of hospitalization. It is expensive and not widely available, so it is no longer used to treat patients with COVID-19. The US Food Drug Administration initially gave emergency authorization for the use of hydroxychloroquine, on the basis of its *in vitro* antiviral activity against SARS-CoV-2. Hydroxychloroquine is a generic antimalarial commonly used to treat amoebic liver abscess and rheumatic disease. Nevertheless, this was later found not to translate into clinical effectiveness in patients and its use was suspended. In the UK, the RECOVERY trial started on the 19th of March 2020 and to date is the world's largest randomized trial, including 177 sites and recruiting up to 39,780 participants at the time of writing. It is an international clinical trial that aims to identify treatments for people hospitalized with COVID-19. Findings of this trial have significantly improved and changed the management and prognosis for hospitalized patients with COVID-19. In its initial stages, results from this trial showed no benefit in clinical outcome of patients treated with the protease inhibitors, lopinavir/ritonavir, that are commonly used as antiretrovirals for HIV-1 positive patients. Evidence from the RECOVERY trial also concluded that there was no beneficial effect on hospitalization or other outcomes from hydroxychloroquine in hospitalized patients with COVID-19. This study demonstrated that tocilizumab reduced mortality, but aspirin did not improve survival of hospitalized patient with COVID-19. Amongst its most important findings, RECOVERY results showed that the drug dexamethasone reduces death by up to one-third in hospitalized patients with severe COVID-19. This finding was particularly striking as dexamethasone is a low-cost steroid widely available in resource-rich and poor settings. Tocilizumab, an intravenous anti-inflammatory used to treat rheumatoid arthritis, was also shown to reduce the risk of death in hospitalized patients with severe COVID-19 as well as to reduce the need for mechanical ventilator and to shorten the duration of hospitalization.

The Solidarity Therapeutics Trial, coordinated by the WHO, also confirmed that remdesivir, hydroxychloroquine, lopinavir/ritonavir and interferon had little or no effect on mortality at 28 days or clinical course of COVID-19 amongst hospitalized patients. The Solidarity trial is also an international collaboration including more than 30 countries looking at the effect of different treatment regimens on the initiation of ventilation, duration of hospitalization and mortality in hospitalized patients. At the time of writing, it includes 11,266 adults who have been randomized to receive remdesivir, and other drugs, and is considering anti-SARS COV-2 monoclonal antibodies for evaluation. It has confirmed the findings of RECOVERY and other major trials.

Finally, as well as pharmacological and supportive treatment, it is crucial to ensure patient isolation in hospital and in the community to avoid transmission to others, including healthcare providers. Quarantine measures are necessary to isolate infected individuals, including those with asymptomatic infection. Given the nature of the disease, individuals are infectious around 2–3 days before they develop symptoms, so it is also important to isolate those who have been in contact with a confirmed case to interrupt the chain of transmission.

COVID-19 vaccines

At the time of writing, there were 287 candidate vaccines in total, 102 in some clinical phase trial and 185 in pre-clinical phase according to the WHO Vaccine tracker (https://www.who.int/publications/m/item/draft-landscape-of-covid-19-candidate-vaccines). Multiple vaccine platforms have been explored, with most vaccines in clinical phase being a protein subunit (32%), 16% based in a viral vector, 10% and 16% being DNA or RNA based, respectively, and only 2% being live attenuated vaccines. The first approved vaccines were the mRNA vaccines from Pfizer-BioNTEch and Moderna, together with the adenoviral vector vaccine from Oxford-Astra Zeneca. They were initially approved for people 18 years and older.

Some developed countries had access to these vaccines from December 2020, but distribution across the world was not equitable. A WHO initiative called COVAX was created with the aim to ensure access to COVID-19 vaccines for all. Morbidity and mortality were reduced drastically with the administration of these vaccines, with efficacy reported from around 95% for the mRNA vaccines to around 80% for the adenoviral vector ones.

Despite the great success of COVID-19 vaccines, vaccine hesitancy continues to be an obstacle for their uptake. The amazing speed at which they were created has generated doubts in the public regarding their safety. This is generally owing to the perceived swiftness in the development of the clinical phases, particularly when compared with the traditional process to which most drugs and vaccines are subjected. However, the research that underpins their production spans decades and is often the lifetime work and dedication of multiple research groups. What was different in the production of these vaccines was the worldwide emergency that the pandemic created which focused the energy of governments and pharmaceutical companies on vaccine development. What has taken years for other medicines and vaccines took months for COVID-19 vaccines.

Technology and social media facilitated the recruitment of thousands of participants to clinical trials very quickly. This, along with the efficient analysis of the data and prompt evaluation done by regulatory agencies, produced one of the most successful achievements in modern medicine and may have turned the tide of the COVID-19 pandemic.

Index